# Algorithms in
# CRITICAL CARE MEDICINE

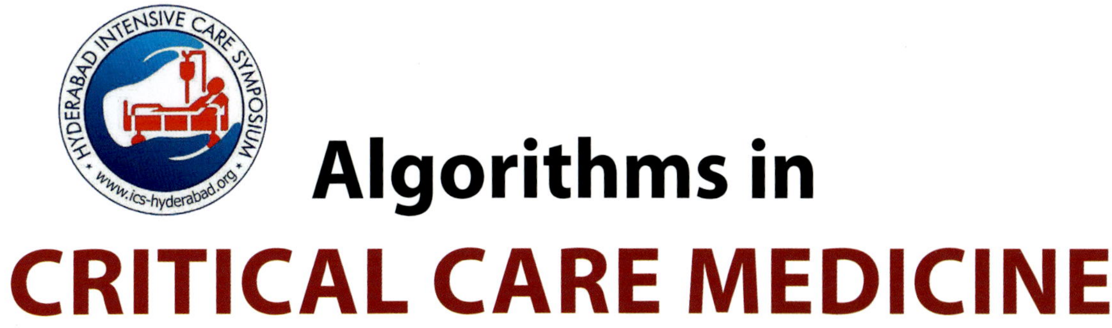


# Algorithms in CRITICAL CARE MEDICINE

***Editors***

**Srinivas Samavedam**
MD DNB FRCP FNB EDIC FICCM DMLE MBA
Chief Intensivist
Department of Critical Care
Ramdev Rao Hospital
Hyderabad, Telangana, India
Associate Editor, IJCCM

**Ganshyam M Jagathkar**
MBBS MD FNB FICCM MBA
Director
Department of Critical Care
Medicover Hospitals
Hyderabad, Telangana, India

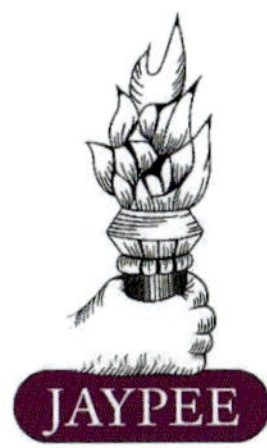


**JAYPEE BROTHERS MEDICAL PUBLISHERS**
*The Health Sciences Publisher*
**New Delhi | London**

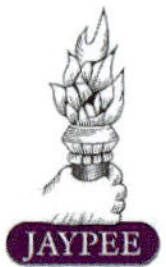

**Jaypee Brothers Medical Publishers (P) Ltd**

**Headquarters**

Jaypee Brothers Medical Publishers (P) Ltd
EMCA House, 23/23-B
Ansari Road, Daryaganj
New Delhi 110 002, India
Landline: +91-11-23272143, +91-11-23272703
+91-11-23282021, +91-11-23245672
Email: jaypee@jaypeebrothers.com

**Corporate Office**

Jaypee Brothers Medical Publishers (P) Ltd
4838/24, Ansari Road, Daryaganj
New Delhi 110 002, India
Phone: +91-11-43574357
Fax: +91-11-43574314
Email: jaypee@jaypeebrothers.com

**Overseas Office**

JP Medical Ltd.
83, Victoria Street, London
SW1H 0HW (UK)
Phone: +44 20 3170 8910
Fax: +44 (0)20 3008 6180
Email: info@jpmedpub.com

Website: www.jaypeebrothers.com
Website: www.jaypeedigital.com



**Inquiries for bulk sales may be solicited at:** jaypee@jaypeebrothers.com

***Algorithms in Critical Care Medicine***

*First Edition:* **2025**

ISBN: 978-93-6616-199-0

*Prinred at: Samrat Offset Pvt. Ltd.*

# Contributors

**A Karthick Ramalingam** MD
Critical Care Registrar
Critical Care Unit
Apollo Speciality Hospital
Chennai, Tamil Nadu, India

**Ajithkumar BR** MD MPH EDIC
Senior Consultant and Head
Department of Critical Care Medicine
Prashanth Hospital
Chennai, Tamil Nadu, India

**Aklesh Tandekar**
MBBS MD IDCCM EDIC FICCM FIMSA FCPS
Head
Department Critical Care
Wockhardt Hospitals
Mumbai, Maharashtra, India

**Alpesh Parmar** MD
Chest Physician
Consultant
Apple Hospital
Surat, Gujarat, India

**Ankit Sharma** MBBS MD
Professor
Department of Anesthesia and Critical Care
Govind Ballabh Pant Institute of Postgraduate Medical Education and Research
New Delhi, India

**Anuradha Pandey** MBBS DA DNB IDCCM
Anesthesiologist
Paras Hospital
Gurugram, Haryana, India

**Anusha Lakhinena** MD
Senior Resident
Department of Pulmonary Medicine
All India Institute of Medical Sciences
Guntur, Andhra Pradesh, India

**Ashwini Ajay Yadav**
MBBS MD DNB IDCCM
Junior Consultant and Intensivist
Department of Critical Care
Jupiter Hospital
Thane, Maharashtra, India

**Avadh Vithlani**
MBBS MD DM (Pulmonary and Critical Care Medicine)
Associate Consultant
Department of Pulmonary and Critical Care Physician
Zydus Hospitals
Ahmedabad, Gujarat, India

**Basjinder Kaur**
DA DNB IDCCM IFCCM CCIDC EDIC-1 FNCC
Senior Consultant
Department of Critical Care
SPS Hospitals
Ludhiana, Punjab, India

**Biji Thomas Philip**
MBBS MD PDCC SCE EDIC
Senior Consultant
Department of Critical Care Medicine
Rajagiri Hospital
Kochi, Kerala, India

**Binila Chacko**
MD (Gen Med) DNB FCICM (Australia) DM (Critical Care) FICCM
Professor and Head
Department of Critical Care
Christian Medical College
Vellore, Tamil Nadu, India

**Deeksha Singh Tomar**
DA IDCCM IFCCM EDIC
Senior Consultant
Department of Critical Care
Narayana Superspeciality Hospital
Gurugram, Haryana, India

**Devi Prasad Mohapatra** MD PDCC DM
Assistant Professor
Department of Neuroanesthesia and Neurocritical Care
Institute of Medical Sciences and SUM Hospital
Bhubaneswar, Odisha, India

**Dharmajivan Samantaray**
MBBS DNB (Anesthesia) IDCCM FICCC FTEE FIECMO FIECHO FIAMS CCEPC
Associate Clinical Director
Cardiac Anesthesiologist
Department of Critical Care Medicine
CARE Hospitals
Bhubaneswar, Odisha, India

**Dileep N**
MBBS MD DrNB (Critical Care Medicine)
Registrar
Department of Critical Care Medicine
Sir Ganga Ram Hospital
New Delhi, India

**Divya Dinakar**
MBBS MD (Anesthesiology) DrNB (Critical Care Medicine)
Assistant Professor
Department of Critical Care Medicine
St John's Medical College Hospital
Bengaluru, Karnataka, India

**Divya Rajasekaran** MBBS MD IDCCM
Clinical Associate
Department of Critical Care
Jupiter Hospital
Thane, Maharashtra, India

**Dnyanesh Kashikar**
MD IDCCM Fellowship in Regional Anesthesia
Senior Clinical Assistant
Department of Critical Care Medicine and Intensive Care Medicine
Sir HN Reliance Foundation Hospital and Research Centre
Mumbai, Maharashtra, India

**Dona Saha** MD PDCC DM
Consultant
Department of Anesthesiology
University Hospitals
Leicester, UK

**Gunchan Paul**
MD IDCCM FNCC
Professor
Department of Neurocritical Care and Obstetric Critical Care
Dayanand Medical College
and Hospital
Ludhiana, Punjab, India

**Hemalatha RV**
MD (Anesthesiology) DM (Critical Care Medicine)
Assistant Professor
Department of Critical Care Medicine
Sri Ramachandra Institute of Higher Education and Research
Chennai, Tamil Nadu, India

**Jacob George Pulinilkunnathil**
MBBS MD DM IDCCM IFCCM DrNB (Critical Care) EDIC
Senior Consultant and Head
Department of Critical Care Medicine
Caritas Hospital
Kottayam, Kerala, India

**Jaicob Varghese**
MBBS MD DM EDIC
Senior Consultant and Head
Department of Critical Care Medicine
Rajagiri Hospital
Kochi, Kerala, India

**Jasmine Nathani**
DNB (Medicine)
Clinical Associate
Department of Critical Care
Jupiter Hospital
Thane, Maharashtra, India

**Jitendra G Kotadiya**
MBBS DTCD DNB
Consultant and Interventional Pulmonologist
Zydus Hospital
Ahmedabad, Gujarat, India

**Jyotirmaya Prakash Pati** MD
Academic Senior Resident
Department of Critical Care
Atal Bihari Vajpayee Institute of Medical Sciences and
Dr Ram Manohar Lohia Hospital
New Delhi, India

**Kabilan Nallathambi**
MBBS MD IDCCM
Junior Consultant
Department of Critical Care Medicine
Apollo Proton Cancer Centre
Chennai, Tamil Nadu, India

**Kalavathy Swarna**
DNB (Anesthesiology) IDCCM
Senior Consultant
Department of Critical Care Medicine
SIMS Hospitals
Chennai, Tamil Nadu, India

**Kandaswamy N**
MD DNB (Anesthesiology) DM (Critical Care Medicine) EDIC
Assistant Professor
Department of Anesthesiology
and Critical Care
Jawaharlal Institute of Postgraduate Medical Education and Research
Puducherry, India

**Kanwalpreet Sodhi**
DA DNB IDCCM EDIC FICCM
Director and Head
Department of Critical Care
Deep Hospital
Ludhiana, Punjab, India

**Ketan Kargirwar**
MD FNB EDIC IDCCM PGDHHM
Senior Consultant
Department of Critical Care Medicine and Intensive Care Medicine
Sir HN Reliance Foundation Hospital
and Research Centre
Mumbai, Maharashtra, India

**Krishna Murari Dhaker**
MBBS CTCCM IDCCM
Attending Consultant
Department of Critical Care
Paras Hospital
Gurugram, Haryana, India

**Lakshmi Kanth Charan S**
MD IDCCM EDIC EDAIC
Consultant Intensivist
Department of Critical Care Medicine
Royal Care Super Speciality Hospitals
Coimbatore, Tamil Nadu, India

**Lalita Gouri Mitra**
MBBS DA MD DNB MNAMS FICCM
Professor and Head
Department of Anesthesia, Critical Care and Pain
Homi Bhabha Cancer Hospital
and Research Centre
Tata Memorial Hospital
New Chandigarh, India

**Leena Patil**
IDCCM DNB (Anesthesia)
Department of Critical Care
Dr KD Patil Multispeciality Hospital
Jalgaon, Maharashtra, India

**Lovely Thomas**
DNB (Gen Med) DM (Critical Care)
Associate Professor
Department of Critical Care
Christian Medical College
Vellore, Tamil Nadu, India

**M Srivatsa Nagachandan**
MBBS EDIC CTCCM MRCP
Registrar
Department of Critical Care Medicine
Apollo Adlux Hospital
Ernakulam, Kerala, India

**Mahender Prasad** MD FIACTA
Consultant
Department of Critical Care Medicine
Prashanth Hospital
Chennai, Tamil Nadu, India

**Manoj Job**
MD (Gen Med) DNB DM (Critical Care) MBA
Senior Registrar
Department of Critical Care
Christian Medical College
and Hospital
Vellore, Tamil Nadu, India

**Manoj K Singh**
DTCD MD DNB FCCP (Chest) FNB EDIC FICCM (Critical Care)
Senior Pulmonologist and
Critical Care Specialist
Zydus Hospital
Ahmedabad, Gujarat, India

**Manoj Y Singh**
MD (Med) FNB EDIC PGDip (Periop) FCICM AFRACMA
ICU Director and Senior ICU Specialist
Department of Intensive Care Unit
Canberra Hospital
Garran ACT, Canberra, Australia

**Mathew Antony**
MBBS MD (Anesthesiology) IDCCM
Registrar
Department of Critical Care Medicine
Caritas Hospital
Kottayam, Kerala, India

**Meenakshy Vijayakumar**
MBBS MD (Anesthesiology) IDCCM FNB (Critical Care Medicine)
Consultant (Surgical ICU, Trauma and Liver Transplant ICU)
Department of Critical Care Medicine
Rajagiri Hospital
Kochi, Kerala, India

**Melwin George**
MBBS MD DrNB EDIC
Consultant and Head
Department Critical Care Medicine
Lisie Hospital
Ernakulam, Kerala, India

**Minesh V Patel** MD IDCCM DAA
Consultant, Intensivist and
Pulmonologist
Department of Pulmonary and
Critical Care
Marengo CIMS Hospital
Ahmedabad, Gujarat, India

**Mohit Kharbanda**
MD (Medicine) IDCCM FNB (Critical Care) FICCM
Senior Director
Department of Critical Care
Desun Hospital
Kolkata, West Bengal, India

**Natesh Prabu R**
MBBS MD DNB (Anesthesiology) DM (Critical Care Medicine) ACME
Associate Professor
Department of Critical Care Medicine
St John's Medical College Hospital
Bengaluru, Karnataka, India

**Naveen Chandra Chinni** MD DM FNB
Critical Care Consultant
Department of Critical Care Medicine
Medicover Hospitals
Visakhapatnam, Andhra Pradesh, India

**Neeru Sahni** MD MAMS
Additional Professor
Department of Anesthesia and
Intensive Care
Postgraduate Institute of Medical
Education and Research
Chandigarh, India

**Neeta Bose**
MD (Anesthesiology) MBA (Healthcare & Hosp Management)
Professor
Department of Anesthesiology
GMERS Medical College and Hospital
Vadodara, Gujarat, India
BLS ACLS Instructor, BCLS CCLS
Instructor, ATLS Instructor

**Nilanjan Umesh**
MBBS DNB (Respiratory Medicine) FNB (Critical Care Medicine)
Consultant
Department of Critical Care Medicine
Rajagiri Hospital
Kochi, Kerala, India

**Niraj Tyagi** MBBS EDICM
Consultant
Department of Critical Care Medicine
Sir Ganga Ram Hospital
New Delhi, India

**Nishanth Baliga**
MBBS MD (Anesthesiology) DM EDIC FCCU
Assistant Professor
Department of Critical Care Medicine
Father Muller Medical College
Mangaluru, Karnataka, India

**Nitin Jain** MBBS MD EDIC
Director and Head
Department of Critical Care
Medicine
Fortis Memorial Research Institute
Gurugram, Haryana, India

**Nitin Saluja**
MBBS MD IDCCM FNB (Critical Care Medicine)
Senior Consultant
Department of Critical Care
Asian Institute of Medical Sciences
Faridabad, Haryana, India

**Nivedita J Bodra** MD
Assistant Professor
Department of Anesthesiology
Critical Care and Pain Medicine
All India Institute of Medical Sciences
Rajkot, Gujarat, India

**Parth Patel**
MBBS MD (Gold Medallist) FNB Critical Care Medicine (Bombay) Certified in Infectious Disease Control (Royal College, UK) Certified Antimicrobial Steward (Stanford, USA)
Consultant Intensivist and
Critical Care Medicine Specialist
Department of Critical Care Medicine
Sterling Hospitals, Ahmedabad
Civil Hospital, BJ Medical College
Ahmedabad, Gujarat, India
CCLS, BCLS, COLS, CPR Instructor, IRCF

**Pradip Dabhi**
DNB (Pulmonary Medicine) MD (Pulmonary Medicine) MBBS
Consultant Interventional
Pulmonologist and Lung Transplant
Physician
Department of Pulmonology and
Critical Care
KD Hospital
Ahmedabad, Gujarat, India

**Pragyan Kumar Routray**
MD (Medicine) IDCCM PGDGM
Head and Consultant
Department of Critical Care
CARE Hospitals
Bhubaneswar, Odisha, India

**Pratheema Ramachandran**
DNB IDCCM IFCCM EDIC FSNCC (Hon)
Senior Consultant and Coordinator
Department of Critical Care Medicine
Apollo Speciality Hospitals
Chennai, Tamil Nadu, India

**Priyanka KJ**
MBBS MD (Anesthesiology) DM (Critical Care Medicine) IDCCM
Assistant Professor
Department of Critical Care Medicine
St John's Medical College Hospital
Bengaluru, Karnataka, India

**Priyankar Datta**
DM (Critical Care Medicine)
Assistant Professor
Department of Anesthesia and Critical Care
All India Institute of Medical Sciences
New Delhi, India

**Pujith Chandaluri** MD
Senior Resident
Department of Respiratory Medicine
All India Institute of Medical Sciences
Guntur, Andhra Pradesh, India

**Raghvendra Kumar Giri**
MBBS MD FNB
Consultant
Department of Critical Care Medicine
Metro Cancer Institute
Faridabad, Haryana, India

**Rahul Baby Joseph**
MBBS MD (Anesthesiology) DrNB (Critical Care) IFCCM EDIC (European Diploma in Intensive Care)
Consultant
Department of Critical Care Medicine
Caritas Hospital
Kottayam, Kerala, India

**Rajan Bhupesh Pandya**
MBBS MD IDCCM
Clinical Associate
Department of Critical Care
Jupiter Hospital
Thane, Maharashtra, India

**Rajathadri Hosur Ravikumar**
MD (Anesthesiology) DM (Critical Care Medicine)
Assistant Professor
Department of Critical Care Medicine
Ramaiah Medical College
Ramaiah University of Applied Sciences
Bengaluru, Karnataka, India

**Ravindra Ghawat**
MBBS MD FNB IDCCM EDIC FSNCC
Director and Head
Department Critical Care
Jupiter Hospital
Thane, Maharashtra, India

**Ravirajsinh Gohil** MBBS MD IDCCM
Director and Head
Department of Critical Care
Aadicura Superspeciality Hospital
Vadodara, Gujarat, India

**Raymond Dominic Savio**
MD DM EDIC FICCM
Lead Consultant
Department of Critical Care Services
Apollo Proton Cancer Centre
Chennai, Tamil Nadu, India

**Reshu Gupta Khanikar**
MBBS DA IDCCM
Senior Consultant
Department of Critical Care Medicine
Health City Hospital
Guwahati, Assam, India

**Revathi Aiyer**
MD DNB (Med) IFCCM EDIC FICCM
Director and Head
Department of Critical Care
Sterling Hospitals
Vadodara, Gujarat, India

**Rishikant Birla** MD PDCC (Critical Care)
Consultant
Department of Critical Care Medicine
Paras Hospital
Gurugram, Haryana, India

**Robert James Premkumar**
MD DrNB (Critical Care) EDIC
Consultant
Department of Critical Care Medicine
Prashanth Hospital
Chennai, Tamil Nadu, India

**S Maniraj** MBBS MD DrNB
Senior Resident
Department of Critical Care Medicine
Sir Ganga Ram Hospital
New Delhi, India

**Sachin Gupta**
MD IDCCM IFCCM EDIC FCCM FICCM
Director
Department of Critical Care
Narayana Superspeciality Hospital
Gurugram, Haryana, India

**Sandeep Shyamsundar**
MD (Anesthesiology) DTCD DrNB (CCM)
Consultant
Department of Critical Care
Apollo Speciality Hospital
Chennai, Tamil Nadu, India

**Sandhya S** MBBS DTCD MD DrNB EDIC
Consultant
Department of Critical Care Medicine
Medical Trust Hospital
Ernakulam, Kerala, India

**Saswati Sinha** MD (Medicine) IDCCM EDIC
Senior Consultant
Department of Critical Care
Manipal Hospitals
Kolkata, West Bengal, India

**Shailesh Hiraman Chouksey**
MBBS MD DrNB EDIC
Consultant
Department of Critical Care
Criticare Hospital and Research Institute
Nagpur, Maharashtra, India

**Shrikanth Srinivasan**
MBBS MD DNB FNB EDIC FICCM
Chairman
Manipal Institute of Critical Care Medicine
Manipal Hospitals
New Delhi, India

**Sivakumar MN**
DA DNB IDCCM EDIC FICCM
Head
Department of Critical Care Medicine
Royal Care Superspeciality Hospitals
Coimbatore, Tamil Nadu, India

**Sri Lakshmi Tiruveedhula** MD DTCD
Senior Resident
Department of Pulmonology
All India Institute of Medical Sciences
Guntur, Andhra Pradesh, India

**Srinivasan Muthusamy** MBBS MD
Senior Resident
Department of Critical Care Medicine
Sir Ganga Ram Hospital
New Delhi, India

**Subhra Sen** MBBS DA IDCCM IFCCM
Junior Consultant and Intensivist
Department of Critical Care
Jupiter Hospital
Thane, Maharashtra, India

**Sultana Teslima Begum**
MBBS DA IDCCM
Consultant ICU
Nemcare Hospital
Guwahati, Assam, India

**Suma R Ahmad** MD EDAIC
Associate Professor
Department of Anesthesia and Critical Care
All India Institute of Medical Sciences
Bhubaneswar, Odisha, India

**Sunil Karanth**
MD (Int Med) FNB (Critical Care Med) EDIC FCICM (Aus/NZ)
Chairman
Department of Critical Care Medicine
Manipal Health Enterprises (P) Ltd
Consultant and Head
Department of Critical Care Medicine
Manipal Hospital
Bengaluru, Karnataka, India

**Sunil Kumar Karhana** MBBS IDCCM
Hospital Administration and Operations
Paras Hospitals
Faridabad, Haryana, India

**Suresh Kumar Sundaramurthy**
MBBS MD DNB EDAIC IDCCM IFCCM
Consultant
Department of Critical Care Medicine
Apollo Hospital
Chennai, Tamil Nadu, India

**Suvadeep Sen** MBBS MD FNB EDIC
Consultant Intensivist
Department of Critical Care
Apollo Hospital
Navi Mumbai, Maharashtra, India

**Swagata Tripathy**
MD DNB IDCCM IFCCM EDIC FSNCC (Hon)
Professor and In-charge ICU
Department of Anesthesia and Critical Care
All India Institute of Medical Sciences
Bhubaneswar, Odisha, India

**Swapnabharati Moharana** MD
Assistant Professor
Department of Anesthesia and Critical Care
All India Institute of Medical Sciences
Bhubaneswar, Odisha, India

**Thomas Isaiah Sudarsan**
MD (Internal Medicine) DM (Critical Care Medicine) IDCCM Fellowship in Critical Care
Assistant Professor
Department of Critical Care Medicine
Christian Medical College Hospital
Vellore, Tamil Nadu, India

**Tushar Patel**
MBBS MD DNB DrNB DM (Critical Care Medicine)
Head
Department of Critical Care Medicine
Shukan Multi-speciality Hospital and Trauma Center
Vadodara, Gujarat, India

**V Dedeepiya Devaprasad**
MD DNB EDIC (UK) IDCCM FICCM
Lead Critical Care Consultant
Critical Care Unit
Apollo Speciality Hospital
Chennai, Tamil Nadu, India

**Vadhan Prasanna S**
MBBS MD DNB DM EDIC PGDMLE
Consultant
Department of Critical Care Medicine
Kauvery Hospital
Salem, Tamil Nadu, India

**Vaishali Solao** MD FNB
Director
Department of Critical Care
Fortis Hospital
Mumbai, Maharashtra, India

**Vaishnavi R**
MBBS MD IDCCM DM (Critical Care)
Consultant
Department of Critical Care Medicine
Caritas Hospital
Kottayam, Kerala, India

**Vikram Damaraju**
MD (Internal Medicine) DM (Pulmonary and Critical Care Medicine) (PGIMER Chandigarh)
Assistant Professor
Department of Pulmonary Medicine
All India Institute of Medical Sciences
Guntur, Andhra Pradesh, India

**Vikrant Shamrao Pawar**
MBBS DA DNB IDCCM IFCCM EDIC FECMO
Consultant
Department of Critical Care Medicine
Sir HN Reliance Foundation Hospital and Research Centre
Mumbai, Maharashtra, India

**Vinay K**
MD (Int Med) DNB (Int Med) DrNB (Critical Care Medicine) EDIC
Consultant
Department of Critical Care Medicine
Manipal Hospital
Bengaluru, Karnataka, India

**Vipul P Parekh** MD FCCM
Consultant Intensivist and Head
Intensive Care Unit
Shree Bajrangdas Bapa Arogyadham Hospital
Bhavnagar, Gujarat, India

**Vishal Khandelwal** MD FNB
Consultant
Department of Critical Care
Sarvodaya Hospital
Faridabad, Haryana, India

**Vitrag H Shah** MBBS MD FNB EDIC
Physician and Intensivist
Vitrag Hospital
Surat, Gujarat, India

# Preface

Emergency clinical medicine and intensive care are areas where complex conditions present with overlapping clinical manifestations. Symptoms of several life-threatening conditions are often similar while the therapeutic options are diametrically opposite. Understanding the variability is crucial for quick initiation of appropriate therapy at the right time.

The vastness of medicine makes the recollection of all syndromes very difficult. In crucial situations, an algorithmic approach often helps to shortlist the differential diagnosis and prioritize the investigations and treatment.

An algorithmic approach to medical emergencies is well known and documented. The literature available so far deals with such algorithms as standalone documents. However, quite often, the endpoints of one algorithm end in clinical conditions which themselves need another algorithmic approach. It is therefore necessary for all algorithms to end seamlessly and lead to destination algorithms.

This initiative by the Hyderabad Intensive Care Symposium (HICS) team seeks to plug in a gap that exists in providing seamless algorithms. This collection of algorithms starts with a syndromic approach and leads to disease-specific algorithms. These algorithms have been curated and edited by Senior Practitioners of intensive care who, with their years of teaching and work experience, have molded clinical science into a practical framework. This collection of algorithms will be of immense help in emergency rooms, high-dependency units, and intensive care units as well as any location or facility where patients with acute presentations are cared for.

We hope that this publication will be well received and recommended.

**Srinivas Samavedam**
**Ganshyam M Jagathkar**

# Acknowledgments

This initiative by the HICS team is driven by the support and encouragement we get from students, trainees, and young intensivists. The stimulus to start this project comes from the numerous queries which the team gets in emergency situations. We are indebted to all those who trust us in tough decision-making situations.

The author pool for this publication is a list of the most erudite and accomplished teachers in the field. Generations of students have emerged from their tutelage and continue to do so. The fact that they took time out from their professional and academic commitments underlines their interest in enhancing patient safety and in advocating standard approaches to complex problems. We acknowledge their dedication and commitment wholeheartedly.

The team at M/s Jaypee Brothers Medical Publishers (P) Ltd, New Delhi, India, has been excellent as always in their communication and documentation. Their timely inputs and suggestions have made this publication more attractive to the readers.

Our greatest resource in formulating these algorithms has been the thousands of patients who taught us to be open minded and ever vigilant in dealing with acute medicine. The greatest acknowledgment is reserved for them.

# Contents

## SECTION 1
## SYNDROMIC APPROACH

***Section Editors:*** *Reshu Gupta Khanikar, Manoj Y Singh*

***Associate Editor:*** *Sultana Teslima Begum*



## SECTION 2
## SYSTEMWISE APPROACH

### PART 1: RESPIRATORY

***Editors:*** *Vikram Damaraju, Manoj K Singh*

***Associate Editors:*** *Alpesh Parmar, Anusha Lakhinena, Avadh Vithlani, Jitendra G Kotadiya, Minesh V Patel, Neeta Bose, Parth Patel, Pradip Dabhi, Pujith Chandaluri, Ravirajsinh Gohil, Revathi Aiyer, Sri Lakshmi Tiruveedhula, Tushar Patel, Vipul P Parekh, Vitrag H Shah*

## PART 2: CARDIOVASCULAR/HEMODYNAMICS

*Editors: Natesh Prabu R, Jacob George Pulinilkunnathil*

*Associate Editors: M Srivatsa Nagachandan, Vaishnavi R, Rahul Baby Joseph, Mathew Antony, Nishanth Baliga, Sandhya S, Kandaswamy N, Divya Dinakar, Priyanka KJ, Hemalatha RV, Vadhan Prasanna S, Thomas Isaiah Sudarsan*

## PART 3: CNS

*Editors: Swagata Tripathy, Pratheema Ramachandran*

*Associate Editors: Lakshmi Kanth Charan S, Sivakumar MN, Ajithkumar BR, Robert James Premkumar, Mahender Prasad, Kalavathy Swarna, Suresh Kumar Sundaramurthy, Kabilan Nallathambi, Dona Saha, Swapnabharati Moharana, Suma R Ahmad, Jyotirmaya Prakash Pati, Devi Prasad Mohapatra, Nivedita J Bodra*



## PART 4: GASTROENTEROLOGY/HEPATOLOGY

*Editors: Shrikanth Srinivasan, Lalita Gouri Mitra*

*Associate Editors: Krishna Murari Dhaker, Anuradha Pandey, Nitin Saluja, Priyankar Datta, Sunil Kumar Karhana, Nitin Jain, Vishal Khandelwal, Rishikant Birla, Raghvendra Kumar Giri, Ankit Sharma, Rajathadri Hosur Ravikumar*

## PART 5: RENAL

*Editor:* *Kanwalpreet Sodhi*
*Associate Editor:* *Neeru Sahni*



## PART 6: TRAUMA

*Editors:* *Sunil Karanth, Niraj Tyagi*
*Associate Editors:* *Vinay K, S Maniraj, Srinivasan Muthusamy, Dileep N*

## PART 7: METABOLIC ISSUES

*Editors:* *Aklesh Tandekar, Ravindra Ghawat*

*Associate Editors:* *Suvadeep Sen, Rajan Bhupesh Pandya, Ashwini Ajay Yadav, Divya Rajasekaran, Jasmine Nathani, Shailesh Hiraman Chouksey, Subhra Sen*



## PART 8: ENDOCRINE

*Editor:* *Jaicob Varghese*

*Associate Editors:* *Biji Thomas Philip, Melwin George, Nilanjan Umesh, Meenakshy Vijayakumar*



## PART 9: BLOOD GAS ANALYSIS

*Editors:* *Pragyan Kumar Routray, Dharmajivan Samantaray*

## PART 10: TOXICOLOGY

***Editor:*** ***Binila Chacko***

***Associate Editors:*** ***Lovely Thomas, Manoj Job***



## PART 11: SKIN AND SOFT TISSUE

***Editor:*** ***V Dedeepiya Devaprasad***

***Associate Editors:*** ***Sandeep Shyamsundar, A Karthick Ramalingam***



## PART 12: HEMATOLOGY

***Editor:*** ***Raymond Dominic Savio***

***Associate Editors:*** ***Suresh Kumar Sundaramurthy, Naveen Chandra Chinni***

## PART 13: INFECTIONS

*Editors: Saswati Sinha, Vaishali Solao*
*Associate Editor: Mohit Kharbanda*



## PART 14: AIRWAY

*Editors: Vikrant Shamrao Pawar, Ketan Kargirwar*
*Associate Editor: Dnyanesh Kashikar*



## PART 15: OBSTETRICS

*Editors: Gunchan Paul, Leena Patil*
*Associate Editor: Basjinder Kaur*

## PART 16: CHECKLISTS

***Editors:*** *Sachin Gupta, Deeksha Singh Tomar*

SECTION 1

# Syndromic Approach

***Section Editors:*** Reshu Gupta Khanikar, Manoj Y Singh
***Associate Editor:*** Sultana Teslima Begum

CHAPTER 1

# Hypoxia

## DEFINITION

It is the condition where tissue receives inadequate oxygen, this leads to anaerobic metabolism and subsequent lactic acidosis.

## ETIOLOGIES

- Hypoxemia (hypoxic hypoxia)
- Anemic hypoxia
- Ischemic/stagnant hypoxia
- Histotoxic hypoxia

### Hypoxemia (Hypoxic Hypoxia)

This refers to the state of low oxygen concentration in arterial blood. It depends on five key factors:

1. *Altitude:* As one moves to higher altitudes, the barometric pressure drops, resulting in the amount of low $O_2$ content in inspired air. Thus, at higher altitude the $O_2$ in the inspired air will not be able to adequately supply the metabolic needs of the tissues.
2. *Ventilation:* It refers to the supply of gases to the alveoli and directly related to $CO_2$ clearance. Hypoventilation leads to $CO_2$ build up, decrease clearance and subsequent decreased concentration of alveolar $O_2$.
3. *Oxygen diffusion:* This is the ability of $O_2$ to cross the alveoli and surround the capillary membranes effectively. Transport may be impaired because of a primary tissue disease process such as pulmonary fibrosis.
4. *Ventilation/Perfusion (V/Q) matching:* There is a balance between oxygenation of alveoli and blood flow through the capillaries. Mismatch between these two factors will occur when the blood flows through the alveoli with inadequate ventilation or when the blood does not reach those alveoli that have adequate ventilation, e.g., pulmonary embolism, in which perfusion is obstructed or in a case of status asthmaticus in which airway collapse causes air trapping further leading to ventilatory obstruction. It is important to note that ventilation and perfusion matching is heterogenous throughout different areas of the lung in normal state.
5. *Blood shunting:* Shunting of the blood refers to the bypassing of the process of oxygenation, i.e., blood enters the systemic circulation before receiving adequate oxygenation, e.g., congenital intracardiac septal defects;[1] mucous plugging of one mainstem bronchus.

### Anemic Hypoxia

Hypoxia may occur if there is critically low blood $O_2$ carrying capacity for e.g. -Acute changes in Hb level (acute blood loss), anemia and hypovolemic shock may result in decreased transport of $O_2$ to the tissues.[2] Hypoxia may also result from the changes in the Hb functionality; e.g., acute carbon monoxide poisoning, where there is plenty of Hb molecules which simply are not able to bind $O_2$.

### Ischemic/Stagnant Hypoxia

Hypoxia may result from a critical decrease in the flow of oxygenated blood to peripheral tissues. Systemic conditions such as cardiogenic shock may lead to decreased oxygenation of the blood during pulmonary gas exchange, as well as inadequate global delivery of blood to central and peripheral organs. Localized conditions may impede cellular diffusion of $O_2$ (such as with severe tissue edema) or focally impede blood flow of oxygenated blood (such as with arterial damage or obstruction).

### Histotoxic Hypoxia

Hypoxia may result from low tissue utilization of $O_2$. This may occur with direct cellular poison (cyanide, colchicine overdose) or abnormally high tissue oxygen demand (malignancy).

| | *Anemic hypoxia* | *Ischemic/stagnant hypoxia* | *Histotoxic hypoxia* |
|---|---|---|---|
| *Cause* | Hypoxia may occur if there is critically low blood $O_2$ carrying capacity | Hypoxia may result from a critical decrease in the flow of oxygenated blood to peripheral tissues | Hypoxia may result from low tissue utilization of $O_2$ |
| *Examples* | • Acute blood loss anemia<br>• Hypovolemic shock<br>• Acute carbon monoxide poisoning | • Cardiogenic shock<br>• Severe tissue edema<br>• Arterial damage or obstruction | • Cyanide, colchicine overdose<br>• Malignancy |

## WHEN SHOULD HYPOXIA BE SUSPECTED?

- There is no single lab value to directly measure hypoxia.
- It should be suspected in any patient with anxiety, confusion and restlessness which may be early signs of hypoxia and may precede changes in vital signs.[3]
- Low $SpO_2$ is the hallmark of hypoxemia and may be suspected in any pt with $SpO_2 < 90\%$ or $<88\%$ in pt with chronic lung disease.
- Lactic acidosis may develop from anaerobic metabolism from tissue hypoxia which can be detected from blood gas.[4]

### Approach to Patient of Hypoxia

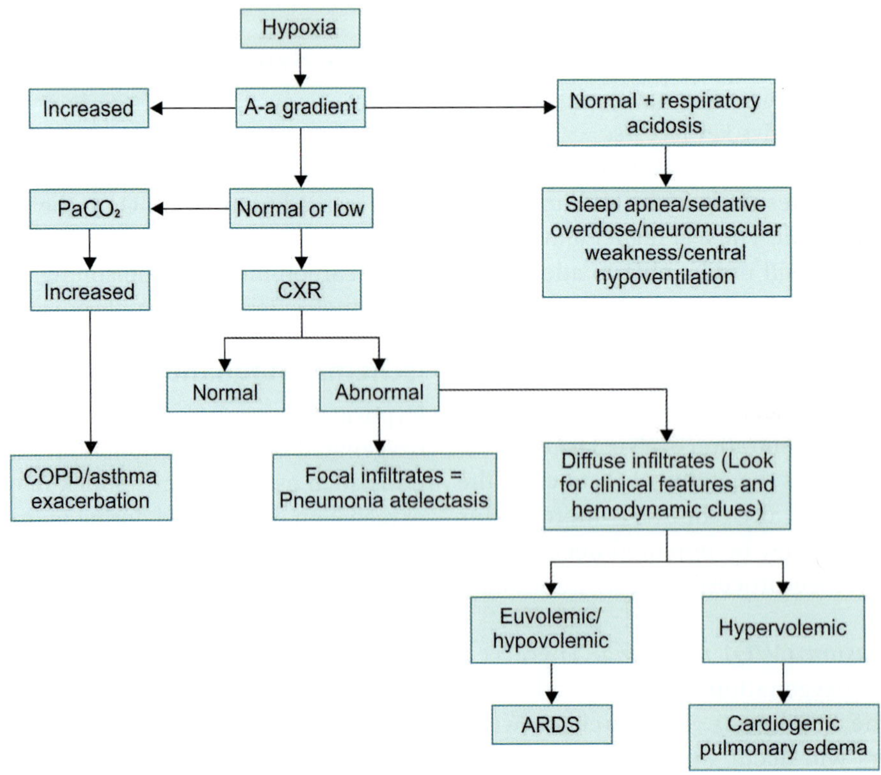

## GENERAL MANAGEMENT

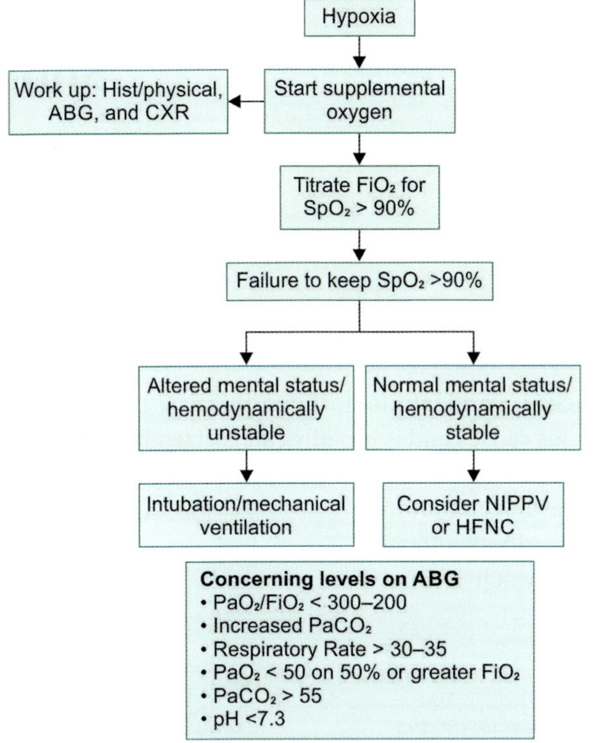


### Approach to Hypoxia

- Stabilize the patient—airway, breathing, and circulation
- History and physical examination
- *$SpO_2$:* <95% is abnormal.
- *ABG analysis:* Arterial oxygen pressure < 80 mm Hg is abnormal.
  $PaCO_2$-elevated level is seen in hypoventilation
  A-a gradient—alveolar oxygen pressure can be derived using alveolar gas equation

(alveolar oxygen pressure = ($FiO_2 \times \{760 - 47\}) - PaCO_2/.8$)

  Normal values indicate low $O_2$ content in the alveoli and abnormal values indicate diffusion or perfusion defect.
  $PaO_2/FiO_2$ ratio: Normal ratio—300–500 mm Hg. It is primarily used to gauge the severity of ARDS.
- *Imaging:* Chest X-ray and HRCT—to identify the underlying cause of hypoxia, e.g., pneumonia, pulmonary edema, or hyperinflated lungs in COPD.

## MANAGEMENT

- *Maintaining airway patency:*[5]
  - Maneuvers to prevent upper airway occlusion, e.g., head tilt, jaw thrust, and chin lift
  - Effective suctioning
  - Endotracheal tube or tracheostomy tube placement
  - CPAP or BIPAP for obesity hypoventilation syndrome
  - Lower airway patency is maintained through bronchodilators, aggressive chest physiotherapy
- *Increasing the $O_2$ content of inspired air:*
  - Supplemental $O_2$ is given when $SaO_2$ is <90% and $PaO_2$ is <60 mm Hg.[6]
  - *Low flow devices:* Nasal canula, simple face mask, partial rebreather mask, and nonrebreather mask[7]
  - *High-flow devices:* Venturi mask and high-flow nasal canula
  - *Positive pressure ventilation:* NIV (CPAP and BIPAP) and invasive ventilation
- *Improving $O_2$ diffusion through the alveolar interstitial tissues:* Find the root cause and treat accordingly, e.g., diuretics for pulmonary edema, steroids for ILD.
- *Extracorporeal membrane oxygenation (ECMO):* ECMO is a critical intervention for managing severe hypoxia when other treatments fail. Its application requires a specialized team and careful monitoring due to the complexity and potential risks associated with its use. Benefits of ECMO:
  - *Oxygenation:* ECMO provides high levels of oxygenation to the blood, bypassing the lungs if they are unable to function.
  - *Carbon dioxide removal:* It can effectively remove carbon dioxide from the blood, reducing the work of breathing and respiratory muscle fatigue.
  - *Lung rest:* By taking over the work of oxygenation, ECMO allows the lungs to rest and recover from injury or infection.

## REFERENCES


1. Mirwais S, Mirwais M, Altaf A, Collins J. Patent foramen ovale with platypnoea-Orthodeoxia syndrome. Cureus. 2020;12(10):e10958.
2. Gutierrez G, Reines HD, Wulf-Gutierrez ME. Clinical review of hemmorragic shock Crit Care. 2004;8(5):373-81.
3. Jardines T, Burton GG. Clinical Manifestation and Assessment of respiratory diseases, 6th edition. St Loius; MO: Elsevier Mosby; 2011.
4. Shanon TM, Celli B. Oxygen therapy. Emergency Med. 1991:23(21):63-70.
5. Grensemann J, Simon M, Kluge S. Airway management in intensive care and Emergency med; What is new? Med Klin Intensivemed Notfmed. 2019;114(4):334-41.
6. Wittebole X, Duprez F, Montiel V. Administration of supplemental Oxygen. Nengl J Med. 2021;385(17):e61.
7. Duprez F, Mashayekhi S, Cuvelier G, Legrand A Reychler G. A New Formula for predicting the fraction of delivered Oxygen during low flow oxygen therapy. Resp Care. 2018; 63(12):1528-34.

CHAPTER 2

# Shock

## DEFINITION

Shock is defined as a state of cellular and tissue hypoxia due to either reduced oxygen delivery, increased oxygen consumption, inadequate oxygen utilization, or a combination of these processes.[1]

"Undifferentiated shock" refers to the situation where shock is recognized but the cause is unclear.[2]

### Classification[1]

Shock is a critical medical condition. It can result from various causes and is broadly categorized into four types:

1. Hypovolemic shock
2. Cardiogenic shock
3. Distributive shock
4. Obstructive shock

| *Types of shock* | *Clinical presentation* | *Hemodynamics* | *Examples* |
|---|---|---|---|
| 1. Hypovolemic shock | Hypotension, Tachycardia, weak thready pulse, cool, pale moist skin, urine output (U/O) decreased | • Decreased Cardiac Output (CO)<br>• Increased Systemic Vascular Resistance (SVR) | Severe bleeding (hemorrhagic shock), dehydration, or burns |
| 2. Cardiogenic shock | Hypotension, Tachycardia, weak thready pulse, cool, pale moist skin, U/O <30 mL/h, crackles, tachypnea | • Decreased CO<br>• Increased SVR | Severe myocardial infarction, heart failure, or other cardiac conditions |
| 3. Distributive shock | | | |
| Neurogenic shock | Hypotension, bradycardia, warm dry skin | • Decreased CO<br>• Venous and arterial vasodilatation<br>• Loss of sympathetic tone | |
| Anaphylactic shock | Hypotension, Tachycardia, cough, dyspnea, pruritus, urticaria, restlessness, decreased LOC | • Decreased CO<br>• Decreased SVR | |
| Septic shock | Hypotension, tachycardia, full bounding pulse, tachypnea, pink warm flushed skin, decreased U/O, fever | • Decreased CO<br>• Decreased SVR | |
| 4. Obstructive shock | • Unusual<br>• Hypotension<br>• Tachycardia<br>• Altered consciousness<br>• Decreased U/O<br>• Cool, clammy skin<br>• Subcutaneous emphysema (air under your skin)<br>• Chest or abdominal pain | • Decreased cardiac output<br>• Increased SVR | Pulmonary embolism, cardiac tamponade, or tension pneumothorax |

## Shock Algorithm

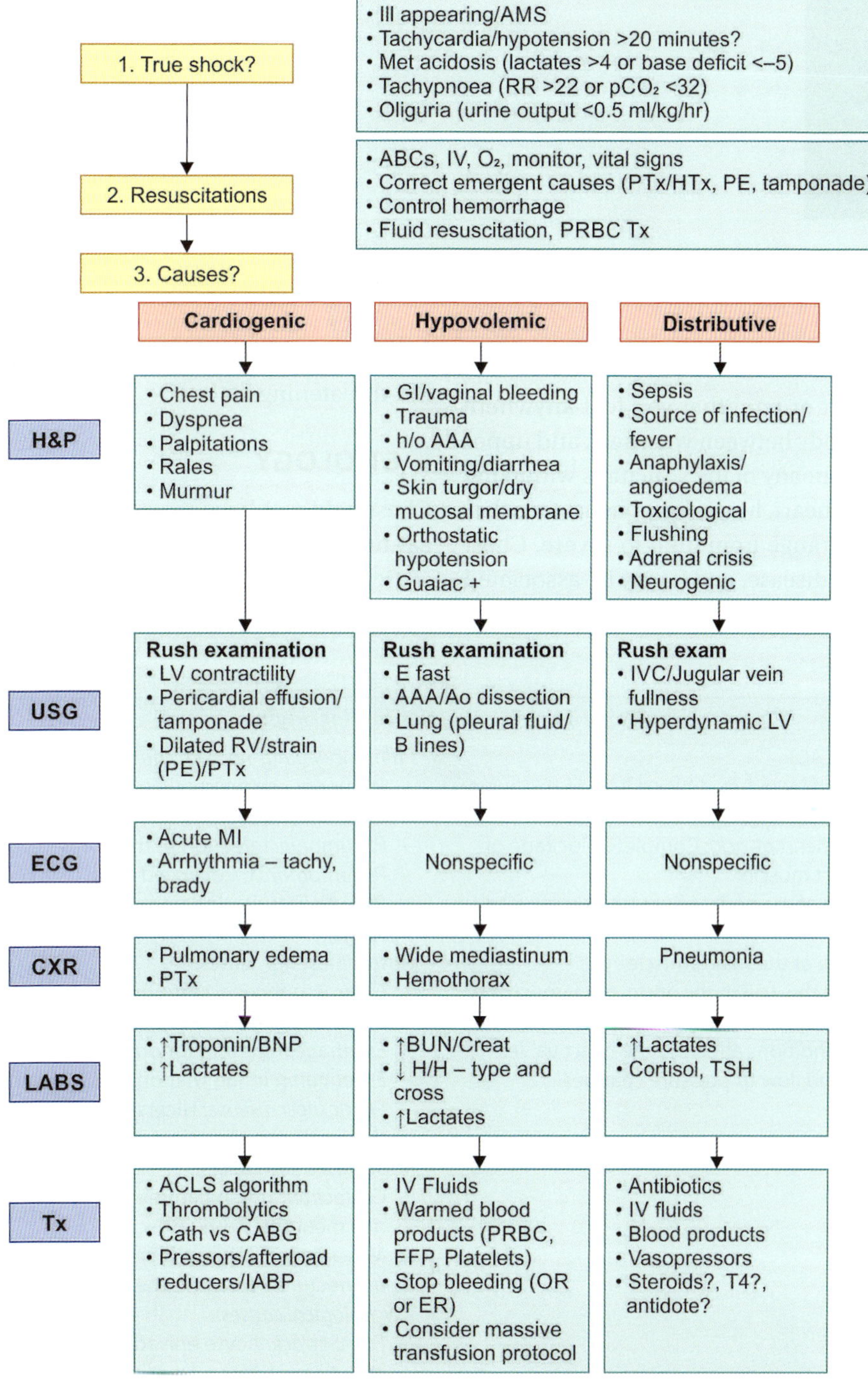


(AAA: abdominal aorta aneurysm; HTx: hypertension; PE: pulmonary embolism; PTx: pneumothorax)

## REFERENCES

1. Haseer Koya H, Paul M. Shock. In: StatPearls. Treasure Island (FL): StatPearls Publishing; 2024.
2. Manual of Medicine. (2021). Approach to Undifferentiated Circulatory Shock: Emergency and Acute Medicine. [online] Available from: https://manualofmedicine.com/topics/emergency-acute-medicine/approach-to-undifferentiated-shock/ [Last accessed February, 2025].

CHAPTER 3

# Chest Pain

## DEFINITION

Chest pain is discomfort or pain that you feel anywhere along the front of your body between your neck and upper abdomen. It can arise from any of the structures within the chest cavity, such as the heart, lungs, esophagus, muscles, ribs, or nerves, and can range from mild to severe. Chest pain is a *symptom*, not a disease, and it may be associated with various underlying conditions, some of which can be life-threatening.[1]

## ETIOLOGY

Chest pain can have many causes, broadly classified into cardiac (heart-related) and noncardiac origins.

| *Cardiac origin* | *Noncardiac origin* |
|---|---|
| • *Coronary artery disease (CAD):*<br>– *Angina pectoris:* Caused by reduced blood flow to the heart muscle (ischemia)<br>– *Myocardial infarction (heart attack):* Complete blockage of blood flow to the heart muscle<br>• *Pericarditis:* Inflammation of the pericardium (the sac around the heart)<br>• *Myocarditis:* Inflammation of the heart muscle<br>• *Aortic dissection:* A tear in the wall of the aorta, the large artery carrying blood from the heart<br>• *Valvular heart disease:* Conditions affecting the heart valves, leading to abnormal blood flow or pressure changes | • *Pulmonary (lung-related) causes*:<br>– *Pulmonary embolism (PE):* Blockage of an artery in the lungs by a blood clot<br>– *Pneumonia:* Infection of the lungs<br>– *Pneumothorax:* Collapsed lung<br>– *Pleuritis/Pleurisy:* Inflammation of the pleura (lining of the lungs)<br>• *Gastrointestinal causes:*<br>– *Gastroesophageal reflux disease (GERD):* Acid reflux causing esophageal irritation<br>– *Esophageal spasm:* Abnormal contraction of the esophagus<br>– *Esophagitis:* Inflammation of the esophagus<br>– *Peptic ulcer disease:* Ulcers in the stomach or upper part of the small intestine<br>• *Musculoskeletal causes:*<br>– *Costochondritis:* Inflammation of the cartilage where the ribs meet the sternum<br>– *Muscle strain:* Injury to the muscles of the chest wall<br>– *Rib fractures:* Breaks in the ribs due to trauma or injury<br>• *Psychological causes:*<br>– *Panic attack:* Acute episodes of intense fear and anxiety that may mimic heart-related chest pain<br>– *Anxiety or stress:* Can lead to chest tightness and pain without an underlying physical cause<br>• *Other causes:*<br>– *Herpes zoster (shingles):* A viral infection causing nerve pain in the chest area<br>– *Thoracic outlet syndrome:* Compression of nerves or blood vessels in the upper chest |

## CLASSIFICATION OF CHEST PAIN[2]

| | |
|---|---|
| **Based on location** | • *Central chest pain:* Pain in the middle of the chest (commonly cardiac-related)<br>• *Left-sided chest pain:* Pain on the left side of the chest (often cardiac in origin, but could be musculoskeletal or pulmonary)<br>• *Right-sided chest pain:* Pain on the right side (more commonly associated with lung or gastrointestinal issues) |
| **Based on nature of pain** | • *Sharp or stabbing:* Often seen in pleuritic conditions (e.g., pleuritis, pneumothorax)<br>• *Dull or aching:* Can indicate musculoskeletal pain, esophageal disorders, or even heart-related pain (e.g., angina)<br>• *Burning:* Frequently associated with GERD or heartburn<br>• *Tightness or pressure:* Typically associated with angina or myocardial infarction |
| **Based on duration** | • *Acute:* Sudden onset of pain (e.g., heart attack, pulmonary embolism)<br>• *Chronic:* Persistent or recurring pain (e.g., chronic stable angina, GERD) |
| **Based on severity** | • *Mild:* Often related to less serious conditions like muscle strain<br>• *Moderate to severe:* Can be a sign of life-threatening conditions such as myocardial infarction or aortic dissection |
| **Based on triggers** | • *Exertional chest pain:* Pain that occurs or worsens with physical activity (commonly associated with heart conditions like angina)<br>• *Positional chest pain:* Pain that changes with position, often seen in musculoskeletal causes or pericarditis<br>• *Postprandial (after eating):* Seen in GERD or peptic ulcer disease |

## DIAGNOSTIC WORKUP

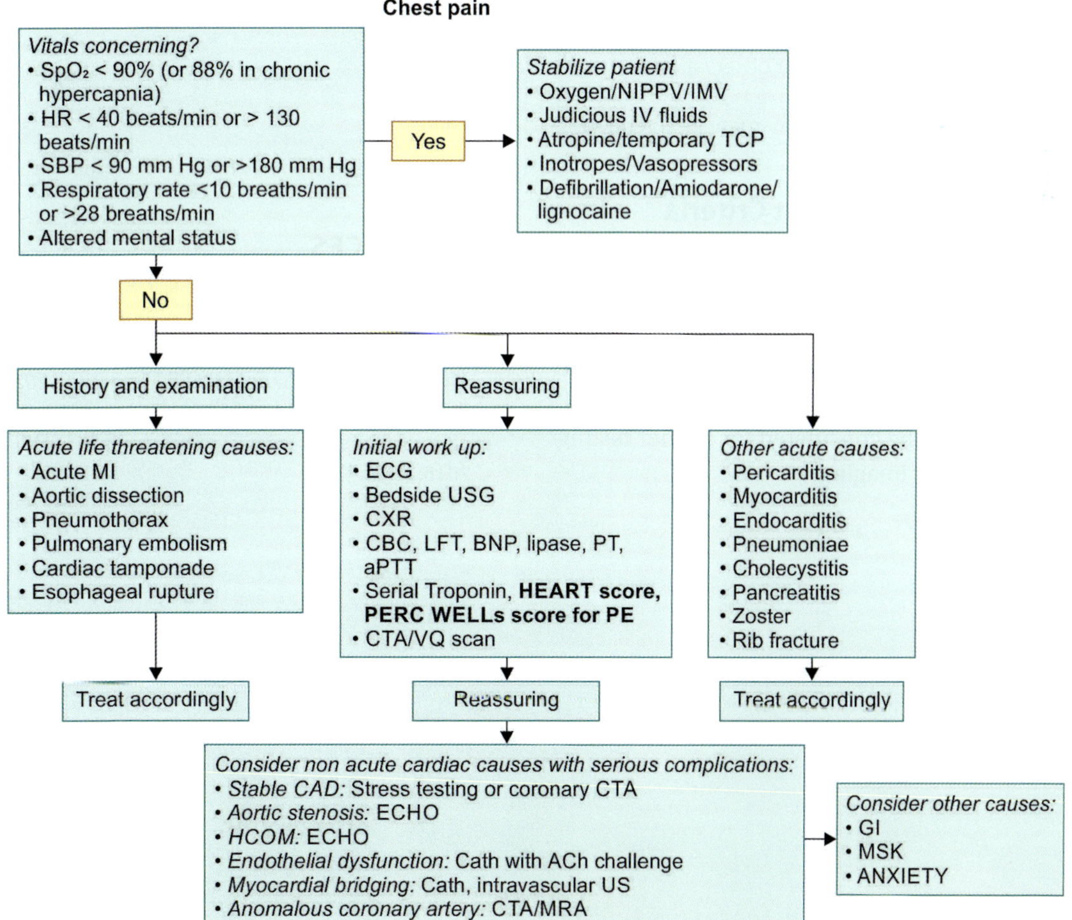

## SCORES

### HEART Score[3]

| HEART Score | | |
|---|---|---|
| History | • Slightly suspicious<br>• Moderately suspicious<br>• Highly suspicious | 0<br>1<br>2 |
| EKG | • Normal<br>• Nonspecific repolarization disturbance<br>• Significant ST deviation | 0<br>1<br>2 |
| Age | • <45<br>• 45–64<br>• >65 | 0<br>1<br>2 |
| Risk factors | • No known risk factors<br>• 1–2 risk factors<br>• >3 risk factors OR atherosclerotic disease | 0<br>1<br>2 |
| Initial troponin | • Less than upper limit of normal<br>• 1–3 × normal limit<br>• >3 × normal limit | 0<br>1<br>2 |
| | **Total:** | |
| *Total HEART Score:* Risk category and recommended management strategy.<br>*0–3:* Low risk, potential candidate for early discharge<br>*4–6:* Moderate risk, potential candidate for observation and further evaluation<br>*7–10:* High risk, candidate for urgent or emergent intervention | | |

### Pulmonary Embolism Rule-out Criteria (PERC Rule)

This rule is only valid in patients with a low clinical probability of PE (gestalt estimate < 15%). In patients with a low probability of PE who fulfill all eight criteria, the likelihood of PE is low and no further testing is required. All other patients should be considered for further testing with sensitive D-dimer or imaging.

- Age < 50 years
- Heart rate < 100 beats/min
- Oxyhemoglobin saturation ≥ 95%
- No hemoptysis
- No estrogen uses
- No prior DVT or PE
- No unilateral leg swelling
- No surgery/trauma requiring hospitalization within the prior 4 weeks

### Modified Wells Score

| *Features* | *Score (points)* |
|---|---|
| Clinical signs and symptoms of DVT | 3.0 |
| No alternative diagnosis | 3.0 |
| Heart rate > 100 beats/min | 1.5 |
| Immobilization ≥ 3 days or surgery in the previous 4 weeks | 1.5 |
| Previous DVT or PE | 1.5 |
| Hemoptysis | 1.0 |
| Malignancy with active treatment in the past 6 months or under palliative care Pretest clinical probability | 1.0 |
| PE unlikely | ≤4.0 |
| PE likely | >4.0 |

(PE: pulmonary embolism; DVT: deep vein thrombosis)

## REFERENCES

1. Johnson K, Ghassemzadeh S. Chest Pain. In: StatPearls. Treasure Island (FL): StatPearls Publishing; 2024.
2. Haghandish N. Approach to Chest pain Nasim Haghandish. Montreal, QC, Canada: McGill University; 2021.
3. Brady W, de Souza K. The HEART score: A guide to its application in the emergency department. Turk J Emerg Med. 2018;18(2):47-51.

CHAPTER 4

# Shortness of Breath

**Kindly scan the QR code below to access the online in an interactive format.**

CHAPTER 5

# Oliguria

## DEFINITION

Oliguria is defined as a urine output that is <1 mL/kg/h in infants, <0.5 mL/kg/h in children, and <400 mL daily in adults. It can be a sign of various underlying medical conditions, such as dehydration, kidney disease, or urinary tract obstruction. It is often an acute state.[1]

## ETIOLOGY

- Gastrointestinal losses—vomiting, diarrhea, bleeding, and external drainage
- Renal losses—effects of diuretics, osmotic diuresis, salt wasting nephropathies, and hypoaldosteronism
- Skin losses—sweat, burns, and other dermatological conditions
- Third space sequestration—intestinal obstruction, crush injury, fracture, and acute pancreatitis
- Physiological and pathological stimuli **(Flowchart 1)**[2]

## CLINICAL MANIFESTATIONS

| | | |
|---|---|---|
| Symptoms | • Lassitude<br>• Postural dizziness | Due to volume depletion |
| | • Vomiting<br>• Diarrhea<br>• Polyuria | As the underlying cause |
| Physical examination findings | • Decreased skin turgor<br>• Low arterial blood pressure<br>• Postural hypotension<br>• Reduced jugular venous pressure | |
| Laboratory abnormalities | • Elevated serum creatinine<br>• Elevated blood urea nitrogen<br>• Hypernatremia or hyponatremia<br>• Hyperkalemia or hypokalemia<br>• Metabolic acidosis or metabolic alkalosis | |

**Flowchart 1:** Physiological and pathological stimuli leading to oliguria.

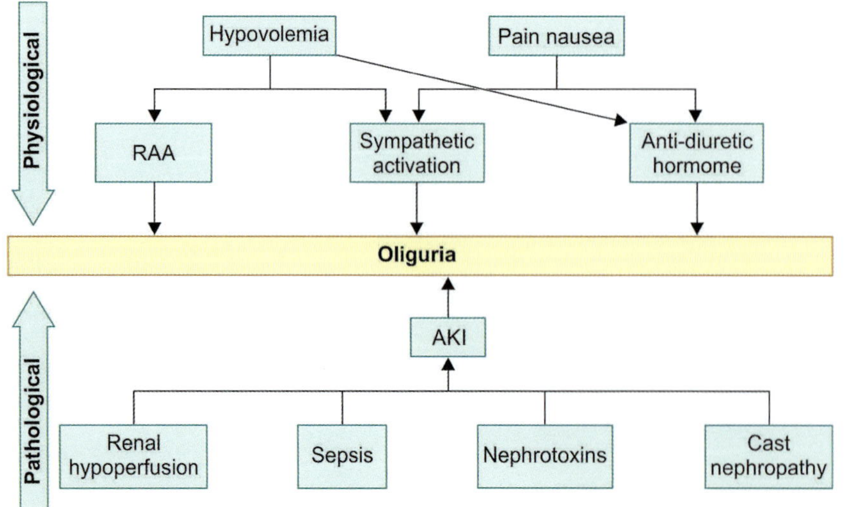

## WORKUP

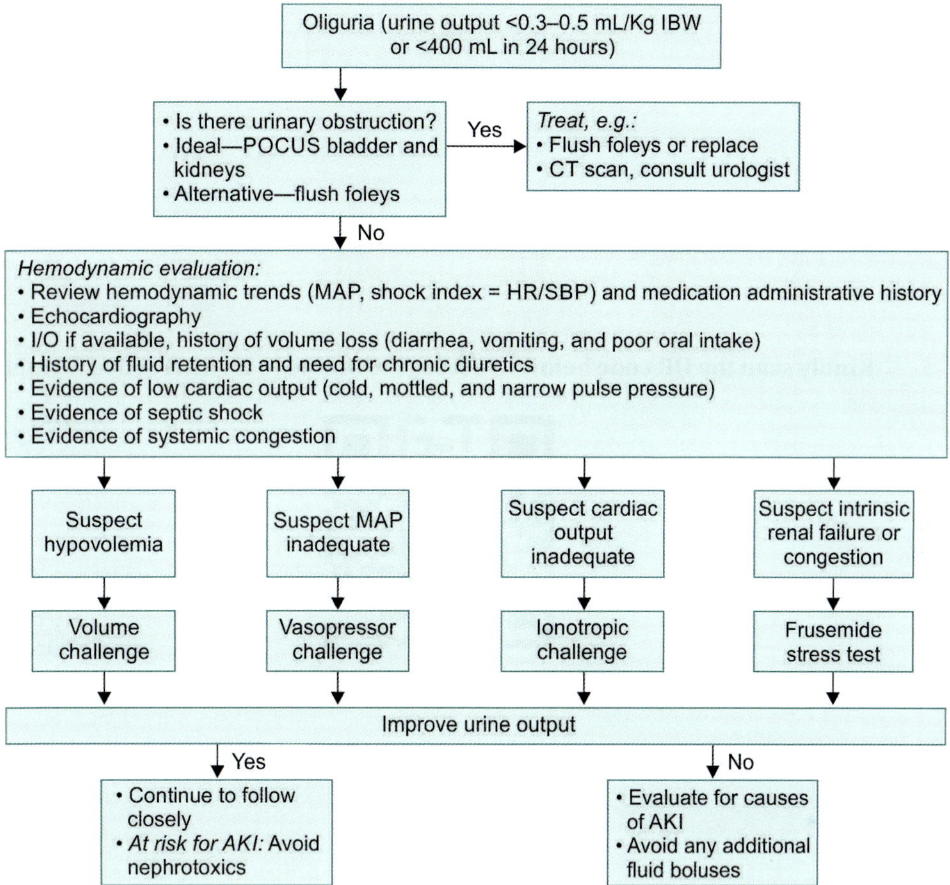


## REFERENCES

1. Devarajan P, Langman CB. (2022). Oliguria Workup Updated: Feb 28, 2022 MEDSCAPE Drugs and Diseases. [online] Available from https://emedicine.medscape.com/article/983156-workup?form=fpf [Last accessed February, 2025].
2. Klein SJ, Lehner GF, Forni LG, Joannidis M. Oliguria in critically ill patients: a narrative review. J Nephrol. 2018;31:855-62.

CHAPTER 6

# Rhabdomyolysis

**Kindly scan the QR code below to access the online in an interactive format.**

CHAPTER 7

# DIC

**Kindly scan the QR code below to access the online in an interactive format.**

CHAPTER

# 8 Altered Sensorium

**Kindly scan the QR code below to access the online in an interactive format.**

CHAPTER 9

# Anaphylaxis

**Kindly scan the QR code below to access the online in an interactive format.**

SECTION

# 2 System Wise Approach

# PART 1

# RESPIRATORY

***Editors:*** Vikram Damaraju, Manoj K Singh

***Associate Editors:*** Alpesh Parmar, Anusha Lakhinena, Avadh Vithlani, Jitendra G Kotadiya, Minesh V Patel, Neeta Bose, Parth Patel, Pradip Dabhi, Pujith Chandaluri, Ravirajsinh Gohil, Revathi Aiyer, Sri Lakshmi Tiruveedhula, Tushar Patel, Vipul P Parekh, Vitrag H Shah

CHAPTER 10

# Type 2 Respiratory Failure

## DEFINITION

pH ≤7.35 and $PaCO_2 \geq 6.5$ kPa with coexistent hypoxemia.

## MECHANISMS

- Decreased central respiratory drive
- Neuromuscular impairment
- Chest wall restriction

## ABG INTERPRETATION

| pH | Primary problem | Expected compensation | Condition |
|---|---|---|---|
| <7.35 | $pCO_2$ >45 mm Hg | $HCO_3$ increases 1 mmol/L for every 10 mm Hg increase in $PaCO_2$ above 40 mm Hg | Acute respiratory acidosis |
| <7.35 | $pCO_2$ >45 mm Hg | $HCO_3$ increases 3.5 mmol/L for every 10 mm Hg increase in $PaCO_2$ above 40 mm Hg | Chronic respiratory acidosis |

## NONINVASIVE VENTILATION[1]

| Indications for NIV | Contraindications for NIV | NIV setting | NIV monitoring |
|---|---|---|---|
| pH <7.35 and $pCO_2$ > 6.5 Kpa or<br>• *COPD:* RR >23/min Persistent even after bronchodilators and controlled oxygen therapy (COT)<br>• *Neuromuscular disease:* RR >20/min, VC <1 L<br>• *Obesity:* RR > 23/min or daytime $pCO_2$ >6 kPa and somnolence | *Absolute:*<br>• Severe facial deformity<br>• Facial burns<br>• Fixed upper airway obstruction<br>*Relative:*<br>• pH <7.15<br>• pH <7.25 with decreased/altered sensorium<br>*NIV is not indicated in Asthma and Pneumonia:* if RR worsens, consider IMV | • Full face mask<br>• EPAP 3 $cmH_2O$ (or higher if OSA is known or expected) IPAP 15 $cmH_2O$ Up titrate IPAP over the next 10–30 min to 20–30 $cmH_2O$ to achieve an increase in respiratory movements and to decrease RR *IPAP should not exceed 30, and EPAP should not exceed 8 $cmH_2O$<br>• Backup RR 16–20/min<br>• I:E in COPD—1:2 to 1:3; OHS, NM, CWD—1:1 to 1:2<br>• Inspiratory time COPD—0.8-1.2 sec; OHS, NM, CWD—1.2 to 1.5 sec; | • Oxygenation Target $SpO_2$ 88–92%<br>• Watch out for warning signs: pH <7.25 even after optimal NIV settings new onset confusion persistent RR > 25<br>• *Actions:*<br>– Check Synchronization, Mask fit, Exhalation port<br>– Check for the requirements of bronchodilators/ chest physiotherapy/ anxiolytics |

## POSSIBLE NEED FOR EPAP > 8 $cmH_2O$

- Severe obesity hypoventilation syndrome
- Lung recruitment in severe hypoxia
- To oppose iPEEP in severe airflow obstruction

## INDICATIONS FOR INVASIVE MECHANICAL VENTILATION

- Imminent respiratory arrest
- Severe respiratory distress
- Contraindications to NIV
- Persisting pH < 7.15 or worsening pH despite NIV
- GCS < 8

## INITIAL SETTINGS IN INVASIVE MECHANICAL VENTILATION[2]

| *Parameter* | *Obstructive disease* | *Restrictive disease* |
|---|---|---|
| Oxygenation | 88–92% (except in asthma when 92–96% is indicated) | 88–92% |
| Tidal volume (mL/kg) | 6–8 | 6 |
| Respiratory rate | 10–15 | 15–25 |
| I:E | 1:2–1:4 | 1:1–1:2 |
| Acid–base balance | pH 7.2–7.4 permissive hypercapnia is allowed when PIP >30 | pH 7.2–7.4 permissive hypercapnia is allowed when PIP >30 |

## WEANING FROM INVASIVE MECHANICAL VENTILATION

The following criteria need to be met before starting weaning:

- Adequate oxygenation: P/F > 200 mm Hg or 27 KPa
- $FiO_2$ < 0.5
- PEEP >10 $cmH_2O$
- Adequate alveolar ventilation (pH > 7.35 and $pCO_2$ > 6.5 kPa)
- Fluid balance optimization (positive fluid balance adversely affects weaning)

## RISK FACTORS FOR EXTUBATION FAILURE DURING WEANING FROM IMV

- Positive fluid balance
- Raised rapid shallow breathing index during spontaneous breathing trial
- Pneumonia or pulmonary disease is the cause requiring IMV
- Increased age
- Prolonged duration of IMV
- Anemia
- Increased severity of illness
- Low albumin
- Previous failed extubation
- Bulbar dysfunction

## REFERENCES

1. See KC. Approach to acute respiratory failure for frontline clinicians. Singapore Med J. 2022;63(12):740-5.
2. Davidson AC, Banham S, Elliott M, Kennedy D, Gelder C, Glossop A, et al. BTS/ICS guideline for the ventilatory management of acute hypercapnic respiratory failure in adults. Thorax. 2016;71(Suppl 2):ii1-35. Erratum in: Thorax. 2017;72(6):588.

CHAPTER 11

# Pneumothorax

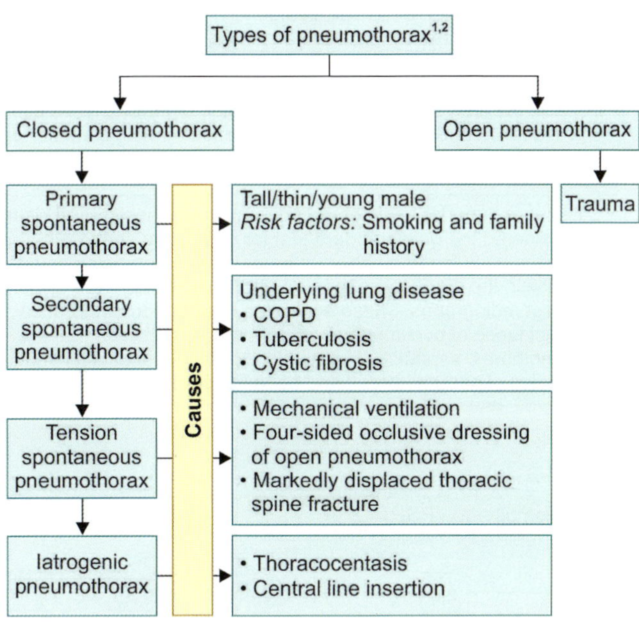


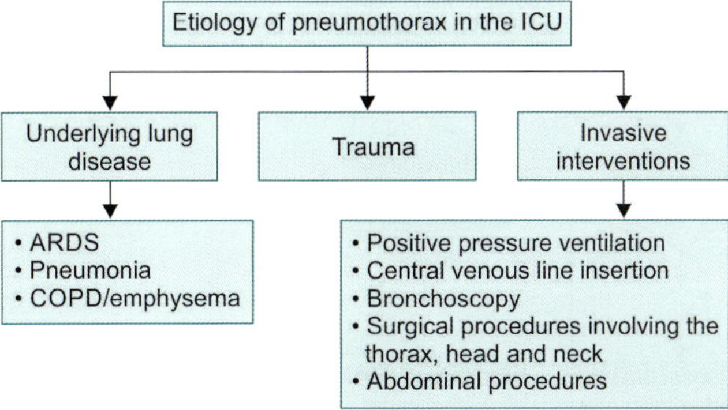

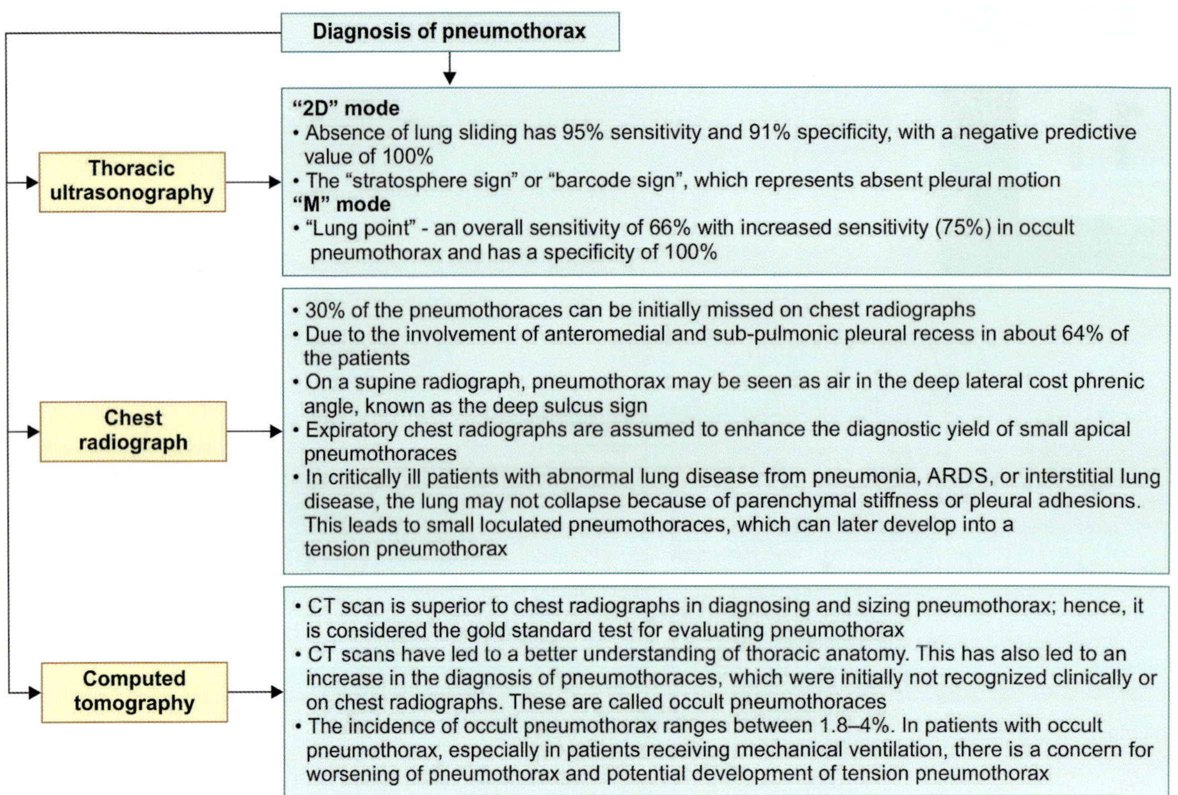
Diagnosis of pneumothorax
Thoracic ultrasonography
"2D" mode
• Absence of lung sliding has 95% sensitivity and 91% specificity, with a negative predictive value of 100%
• The "stratosphere sign" or "barcode sign", which represents absent pleural motion
"M" mode
• "Lung point" - an overall sensitivity of 66% with increased sensitivity (75%) in occult pneumothorax and has a specificity of 100%
Chest radiograph
• 30% of the pneumothoraces can be initially missed on chest radiographs
• Due to the involvement of anteromedial and sub-pulmonic pleural recess in about 64% of the patients
• On a supine radiograph, pneumothorax may be seen as air in the deep lateral cost phrenic angle, known as the deep sulcus sign
• Expiratory chest radiographs are assumed to enhance the diagnostic yield of small apical pneumothoraces
• In critically ill patients with abnormal lung disease from pneumonia, ARDS, or interstitial lung disease, the lung may not collapse because of parenchymal stiffness or pleural adhesions. This leads to small loculated pneumothoraces, which can later develop into a tension pneumothorax
Computed tomography
• CT scan is superior to chest radiographs in diagnosing and sizing pneumothorax; hence, it is considered the gold standard test for evaluating pneumothorax
• CT scans have led to a better understanding of thoracic anatomy. This has also led to an increase in the diagnosis of pneumothoraces, which were initially not recognized clinically or on chest radiographs. These are called occult pneumothoraces
• The incidence of occult pneumothorax ranges between 1.8–4%. In patients with occult pneumothorax, especially in patients receiving mechanical ventilation, there is a concern for worsening of pneumothorax and potential development of tension pneumothorax

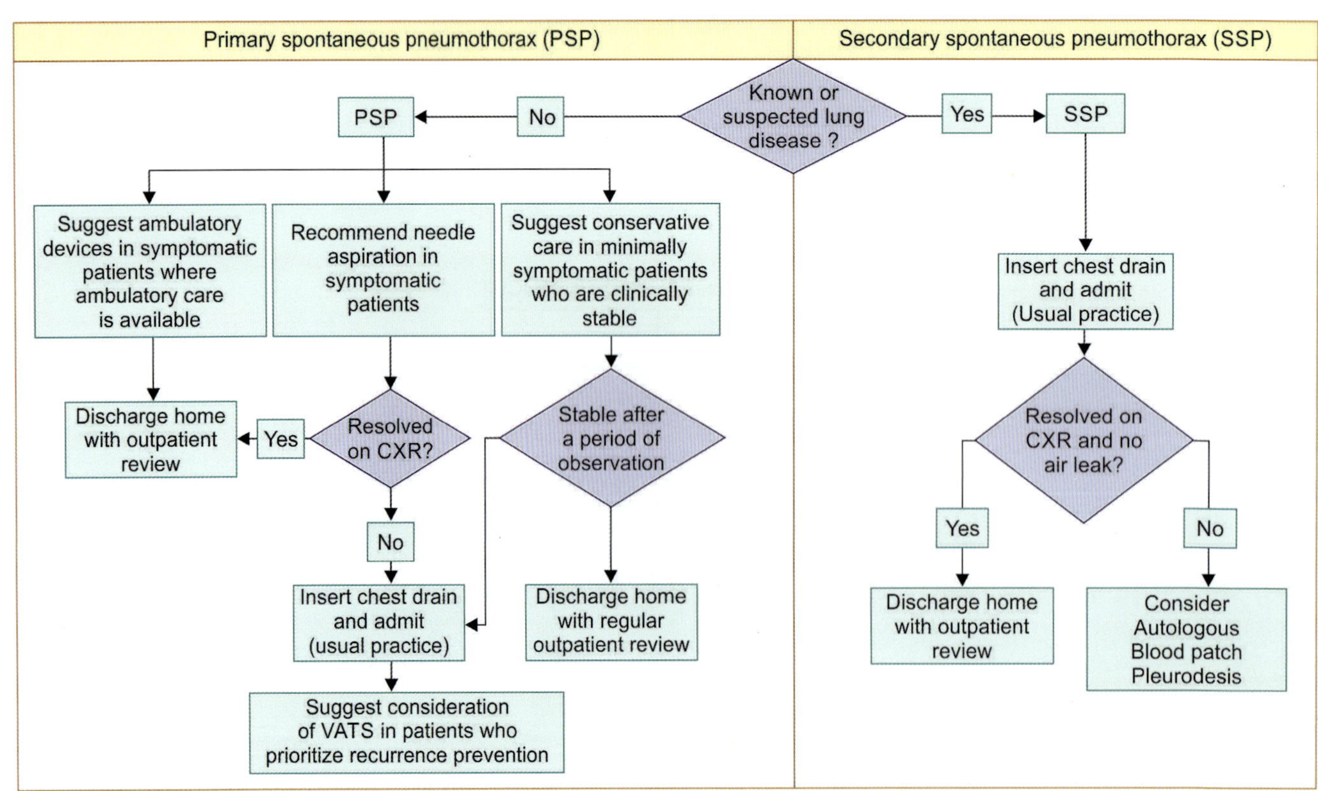
Primary spontaneous pneumothorax (PSP)
Secondary spontaneous pneumothorax (SSP)
Known or suspected lung disease ?
No
PSP
Yes
SSP
Suggest ambulatory devices in symptomatic patients where ambulatory care is available
Recommend needle aspiration in symptomatic patients
Suggest conservative care in minimally symptomatic patients who are clinically stable
Discharge home with outpatient review
Yes
Resolved on CXR?
Stable after a period of observation
No
Insert chest drain and admit (usual practice)
Discharge home with regular outpatient review
Suggest consideration of VATS in patients who prioritize recurrence prevention
Insert chest drain and admit (Usual practice)
Resolved on CXR and no air leak?
Yes
No
Discharge home with outpatient review
Consider Autologous Blood patch Pleurodesis

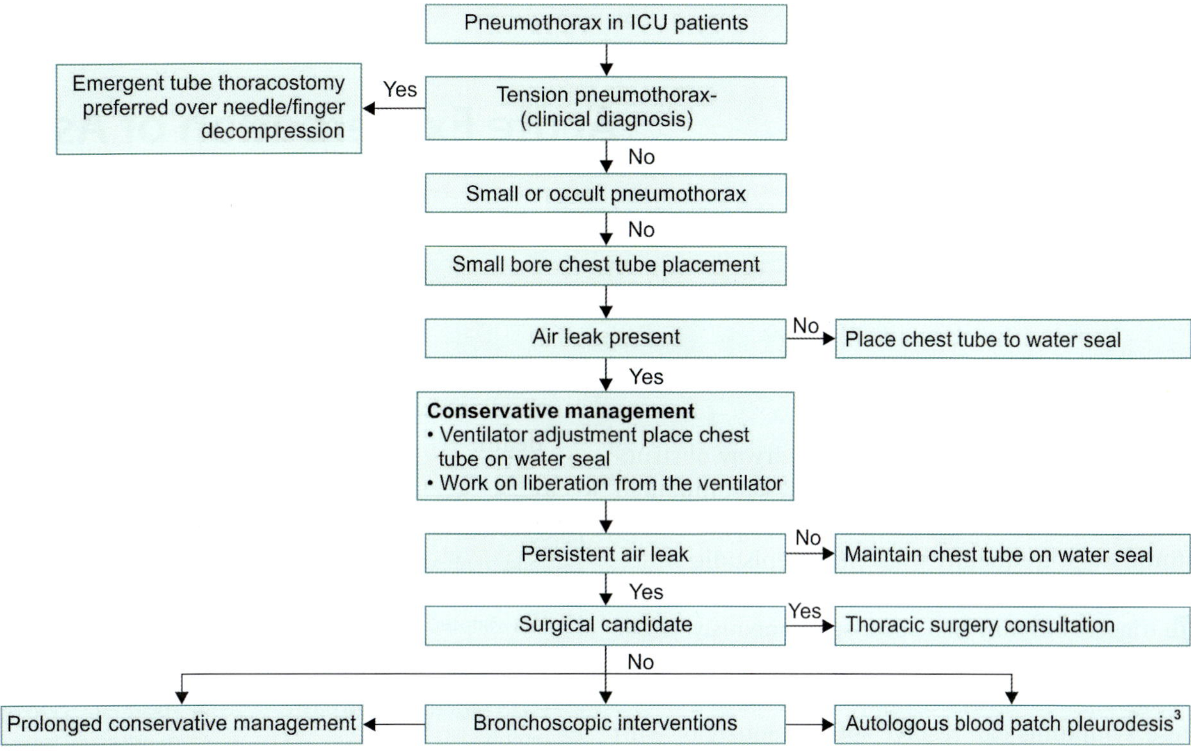


## REFERENCES

1. Thachuthara-George J. Pneumothorax in patients with respiratory failure in ICU. Joseph Thachuthara-George. J Thorac Dis. 2021;13(8):5195-204.
2. Walker S, Hallifax R, Ricciardi S, Fitzgerald D, Keijzers M, Lauk O, et al. Joint ERS/EACTS/ESTS clinical practice guidelines on adults with spontaneous pneumothorax. Eur Respir J. 2024;63(5):2300797.
3. Harcke HT, Pearse LA, Levy AD, Getz JM, Robinson SR. Chest wall thickness in military personnel: implications for needle thoracentesis in tension pneumothorax. Mil Med. 2007;172(120):1260-3.

CHAPTER 12

# Acute Exacerbation of Asthma

## INTRODUCTION

- Asthma is characterized by episodic airway obstruction and hyperresponsiveness, usually accompanied by airway inflammation.[1]
- Asthma most frequently presents as episodic shortness of breath, wheezing, and cough, which can occur with triggers but may also occur spontaneously. Other symptoms can include chest tightness and mucus production.[1]
- These symptoms can resolve spontaneously or with therapy. In some patients, wheezing and dyspnea can be persistent.[1]
- Episodes of acute bronchospasm, known as exacerbations, may be severe enough to require emergency medical care or hospitalization and may result in death.[1]

| *Mild to moderate* | *Severe* |
|---|---|
| • Talks in phrases or sentences<br>• Prefers sitting to lying<br>• Not agitated<br>• Respiratory rate 16 to 30 breaths/minute<br>• Heart rate 100 to 120 beats/minute<br>• $SpO_2$ >90%<br>• PEF >50% but <80% predicted or personal best | • Speaks in single words<br>• Sits hunched forward<br>• Agitated, diaphoretic<br>• Respiratory rate >30 breaths/minute<br>• Heart rate >120 beats/minute<br>• $SpO_2$ (on room air) <90%<br>• PEF ≤50% predicted or personal best |

| *Clinical course and treatment as per the severity of asthma*[3] | | | |
|---|---|---|---|
| ***Degree of severity*** | ***Symptoms and signs*** | ***Initial PEF (or $FEV_1$)*** | ***Clinical course*** |
| Mild | Dyspnea only with activity | PEF ≥70% of predicted or personal best | Usually treated at home. Prompt relief with SABA, possible short course of oral GC |
| Moderate | Dyspnea interferes with or limits usual activity | PEF 40–69% of predicted or personal best | Usually requires office or ER visit. Relief from frequent inhaled SABA. Oral systemic CS, some symptoms last for 1–2 days after starting treatment |
| Severe | Dyspnea at rest; interferes with conversation | PEF <40% of predicted or personal best | Usually, it requires an ER visit and likely hospitalization. Partial relief from frequent inhaled SABA. Oral systemic CS, some symptoms last for >3 days after treatment begins. Adjunctive therapies are helpful |
| *Subset:* Life-threatening | Too dyspneic to speak; perspiration | PEF <25% of personal or predicted best | Requires ER visit and hospitalization in ICU. No response to frequent inhaled SABA. Needs IV CS and adjunctive therapies |

## ALGORITHM FOR MANAGEMENT OF ASTHMA EXACERBATIONS IN ADULTS

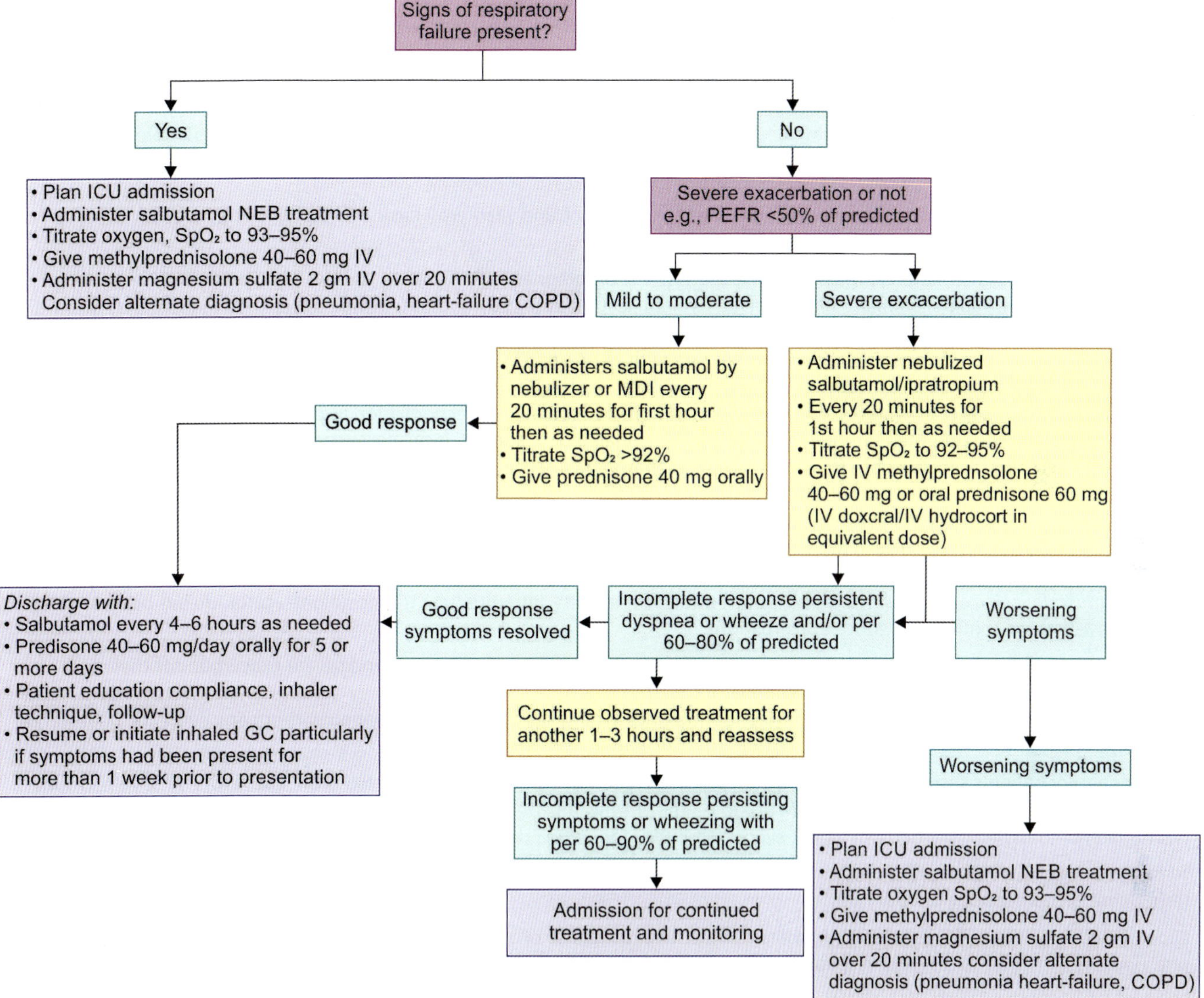


**Clinical red flags**

- Fragmented speech with brief pauses; excessive use of accessory muscles for respiration; inability to lie supine; severe diaphoresis; other significant symptoms that fail to improve with initial emergency treatment
- Life-threatening airway obstruction can still occur when these signs are NOT present
- Imminent respiratory arrest, cyanosis, lack of respiratory effort, and altered mental status.[4]

*Assessment*

- *PEFR:* PEFR <40% predicted (or <200 L/minute in most adults) indicates severe obstruction; patients of severe distress often fail to perform peak flow tests[2,4]
- *$SpO_2$:* Severe hypoxemia (e.g., $SpO_2$ ≤95% despite high flow $O_2$ treatment by nonrebreather mask) marks imminent respiratory arrest or possible severe complication (e.g., pneumothorax); continuous pulse oximetry monitoring is recommended[4]
- *ABG:* ABGs offer an assessment of hypercapnia: hypercapnia usually does not occur unless PEF is <25% of normal (generally <100 to 150 L/min)[4]
- *CXR:* Obtained if complications are suspected (e.g., pneumonia, pneumothorax) or the patient is high-risk (e.g., IV drug abuser, immunosuppressed, chronic obstructive pulmonary disease, heart failure)

*Contd…*

*Contd...*

*Standard treatments*

- *Inhaled beta agonist:* Give Salbutamol (short-acting beta agonist-SABA) 2.5 to 5 mg by nebulization every 20 minutes for three doses, then 2.5 to 5 mg every one to four hours as needed or 4 to 8 puffs given by metered dose inhaler (MDI) with spacer every 20 minutes for three doses, every one to four hours as needed. Alternatively, for severe exacerbations, 10 to 15 mg can be administered by continuous nebulization over one hour[4]
- *Long-acting beta agonists (LABA):* They have a ~12-hour duration of action. Formoterol has a quick onset comparable to the short-acting β2-agonists. Salmeterol has a slower onset of action. These agents can be used for prophylaxis of exercise-induced bronchospasm
- *Ultra-long-acting beta Agonists:* These agents (indacaterol, olodaterol, and vilanterol) have a 24-h effect. They are only used in combination with ICSs in the treatment of asthma

*Oxygen:* Oxygen supplementation to maintain $SpO_2$ ≥92% (>95% in pregnancy)[2,4]

- *Anticholinergics-Ipratropium bromide:* 500 μcg given by nebulization every 20 minutes for three doses OR 4 to 8 puffs by MDI with spacer every 20 minutes for three doses; then may administer additional doses hourly as needed for up to 3 hours[4]
- *Inhaled LAMA:* Long-acting muscarinic agents to be used with LABA and ICS
- *Theophylline,* an oral compound that increases cyclic AMP levels by inhibiting phosphodiesterase, is now rarely used for asthma due to its narrow therapeutic window, drug-drug interactions, and reduced bronchodilation as compared to other agents[1]
- *Inhaled corticosteroids:* Low/medium/high-dose, along with inhaled beta agonist, is the cornerstone of treatment
- *Systemic glucocorticoids:* Intravenous for patients with respiratory failure, give methylprednisolone 60 to 125 mg IV. For less severe asthma exacerbations, give prednisone 40 to 60 mg orally; alternatives include dexamethasone 6 to 10 mg IV or hydrocortisone 150 to 200 mg IV; glucocorticoids may be given IM or orally if IV access is unavailable[2,4]
  - *Oral* corticosteroids are also used to treat asthma exacerbations, frequently at a dose of 40–60 mg/d of prednisone or equivalent for 1–2 weeks[1]
  - *Intramuscular* corticosteroids in high-risk, poorly adherent patients, intramuscular triamcinolone acetonide has been used to achieve asthma control and reduce exacerbations[1]

*Magnesium sulfate:* Give 2 g (8 mmol) IV over 20 minutes for life-threatening exacerbations and severe exacerbations that are unimproved after one hour of intensive bronchodilator therapy[2,4]

There is no recommendation to give prophylactic antibiotics in all cases of acute exacerbation without any evidence of bacterial infection[2,4]

*Epinephrine:* For patients suspected of having an anaphylactic reaction or unable to use inhaled bronchodilators for severe asthma exacerbation, give epinephrine 0.3 to 0.5 mg IM (0.3 to 0.5 mL of 1 mg/mL [may be labeled 1:1,000] solution) into the mid-outer thigh (vastus lateralis muscle); if needed can repeat every 20 minutes for up to 3 doses; give epinephrine OR terbutaline but not both[4]

*Terbutaline:* May give 0.25 mg by SC injection every 20 minutes times 3 doses for patients unable to use inhaled bronchodilators; give terbutaline OR epinephrine but not both[4]

*Endotracheal intubation:* The decision to intubate during the initial phase of a severe asthma attack is clinical. Decreasing respiratory rate, depressed mental status, poor respiratory effort, or severe hypoxemia suggests the patient requires intubation

*Mechanical ventilation:* Directed to maintain adequate oxygenation and ventilation while minimizing elevations in airway pressures. This is achieved by using low tidal volumes (6 to 8 mL/kg), and low respiratory rates (10–12/min). In some patients, elevations in $PaCO_2$ must be tolerated to avoid barotrauma (i.e., permissive hypercapnia)[4]

## REFERENCES

1. In: Loscalzo J, Fauci A, Kasper D, Hauser S, Longo D, Jameson JL (Eds). Harrisons Principles of Internal Medicine, 21st edition. New York: McGraw Hill.
2. Global Initiative for Asthma. (2023). Global initiative for asthma: 2023 GINA Report, global strategy for asthma management and prevention. [Online] Available from https://ginasthma.org/2023-gina-main-report/ [Last accessed February, 2025].
3. Cloutier MM, Baptist AP, Blake KV, Brooks EG, Bryant-Stephens T, DiMango E, et al. 2020 focused updates to the asthma management guidelines: A report from the National Asthma Education and Prevention Program Coordinating Committee Expert Panel Working Group. J Allergy Clin Immunol. 2020;146(6):1217-70.
4. Cahill KN, Dixon AE, Zachrison KS. (2024). Acute exacerbations of asthma in adults: Emergency department and inpatient management. [Online] Available from https://www.uptodate.com/contents/acute-exacerbations-of-asthma-in-adults-emergency-department-and-inpatient-management/print [Last accessed February, 2025].

CHAPTER 13

# Acute Exacerbation of Chronic Obstructive Pulmonary Disease

## INTRODUCTION

In a patient with COPD, an exacerbation is an event characterized by dyspnea and/or cough and sputum that worsen over ≤14 days, which may be accompanied by tachypnea and/or tachycardia and is often associated with increased local and systemic inflammation caused by airway infection, pollution, or other insult to the airways.

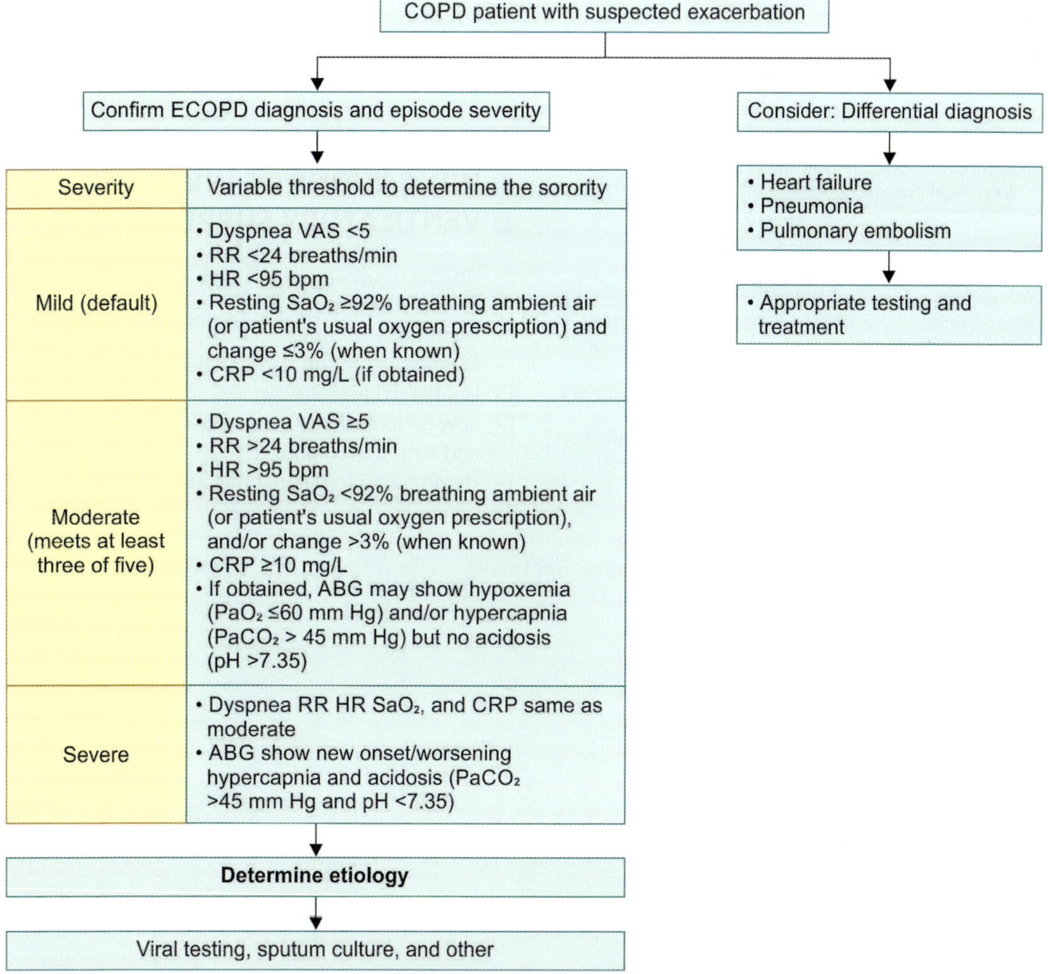


(ABG: arterial blood gas; CRP: C-reactive protein; $PaO_2$: arterial pressure of oxygen; RR: respiratory rate; $SaO_2$: oxygen saturation; VAS: visual analog dyspnea scale)

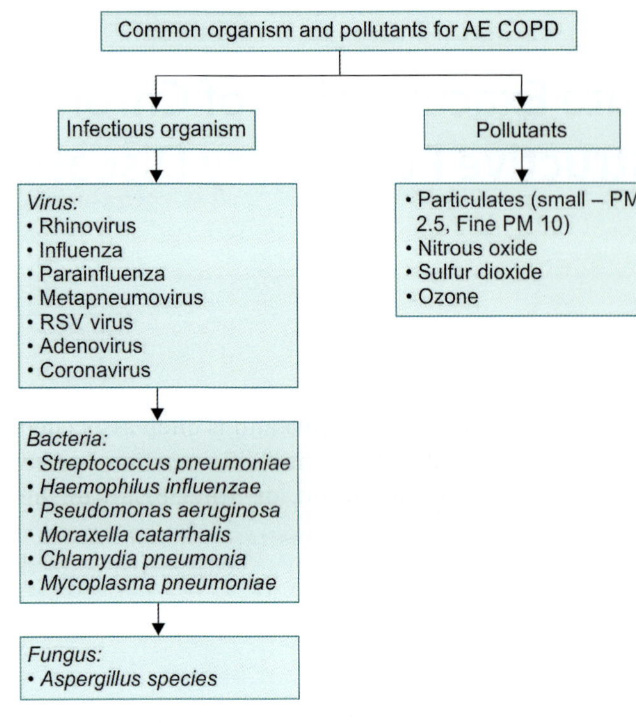


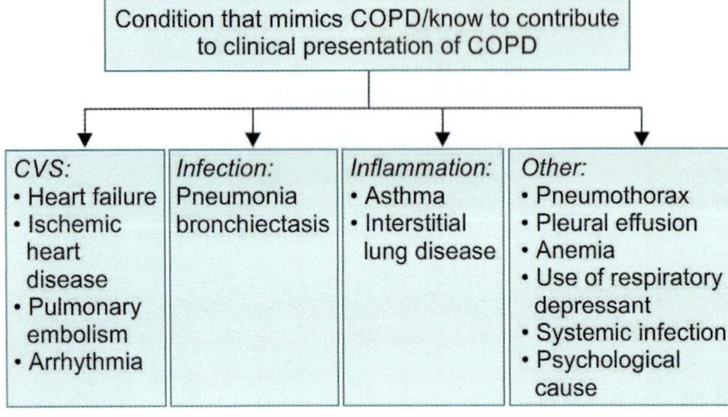


## MANAGEMENT OF SEVERE BUT NOT LIFE-THREATENING EXACERBATION

- $O_2$ therapy
- Bronchodilator
- Antibiotic/antiviral (based on suspicions)
- Corticosteroid
- Theophylline
- $MgSO_4$
- NIV
- Physiotherapy to clear secretion
- Mx of fluid balance (negative balance)
- Heparin/LMWH for VTE prophylaxis
- Management of associated conditions (pneumothorax, pleural effusion, PE, arrhythmia, HF, etc.)

## INDICATIONS OF NIV

- Respiratory acidosis ($PCO_2$ >45 and pH <7.35)
- Feature of respiratory insufficiency
- Use of accessory muscle
- Brief, fragmented speech
- Asynchronous bilateral chest and abdomen
- Persistent hypoxemia despite oxygen

## INDICATIONS OF INVASIVE VENTILATORY SUPPORT

- Unable to tolerate NIV
- Cardiac/respiratory arrest
- Altered sensorium
- Massive aspiration and persistent vomiting
- Unable to clear airway
- Severe hemodynamic instability without response to fluid and vasoactive agent
- Hemodynamically unstable arrhythmia

CHAPTER

# 14 Acute Respiratory Distress Syndrome

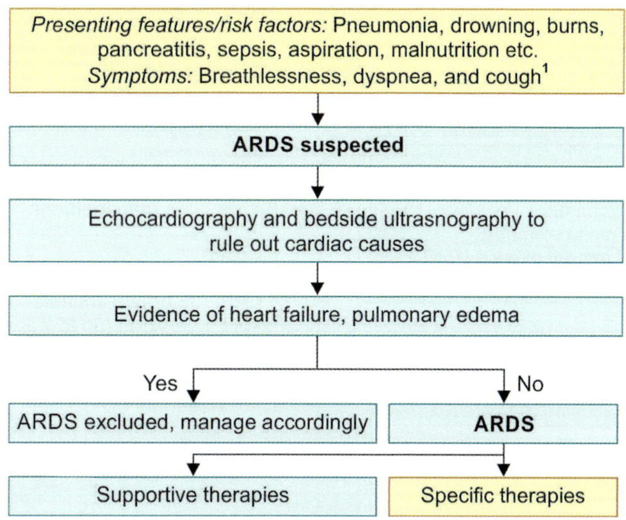


**Classification of ARDS[2-5]**

| *Parameter* | *AECC criteria* | *Berlin criteria* | *Possible short-term reviews* |
|---|---|---|---|
| Year | 1994 | 2012 | 2020s |
| Timing | Not specified (acute) | New or worsening within 7 days | |
| Chest imaging | Bilateral infiltrates on chest radiograph | Bilateral infiltrates on chest radiograph or CT | Ultrasound |
| Oxygenation | • $PaO_2/FiO_2$<br>• Acute lung injury <300 mm Hg<br>• ARDS <200 mm Hg | • $PaO_2/FiO_2$<br>• 200–300 mm Hg mild<br>• 100–200 mm Hg moderate<br>• <100 mm Hg Severe | $SpO_2/FiO_2$ ratio |
| PEEP | Not specified | Minimum PEEP 5 $cmH_2O$ (Continuous positive airway pressure in mild ARDS) | High flow nasal oxygen, no requirement for minimal PEEP |
| Origin of edema | Pulmonary artery wedge pressure ≤17 mm Hg | Not fully explainable by cardiac failure | |
| Biological markers | None | None | |

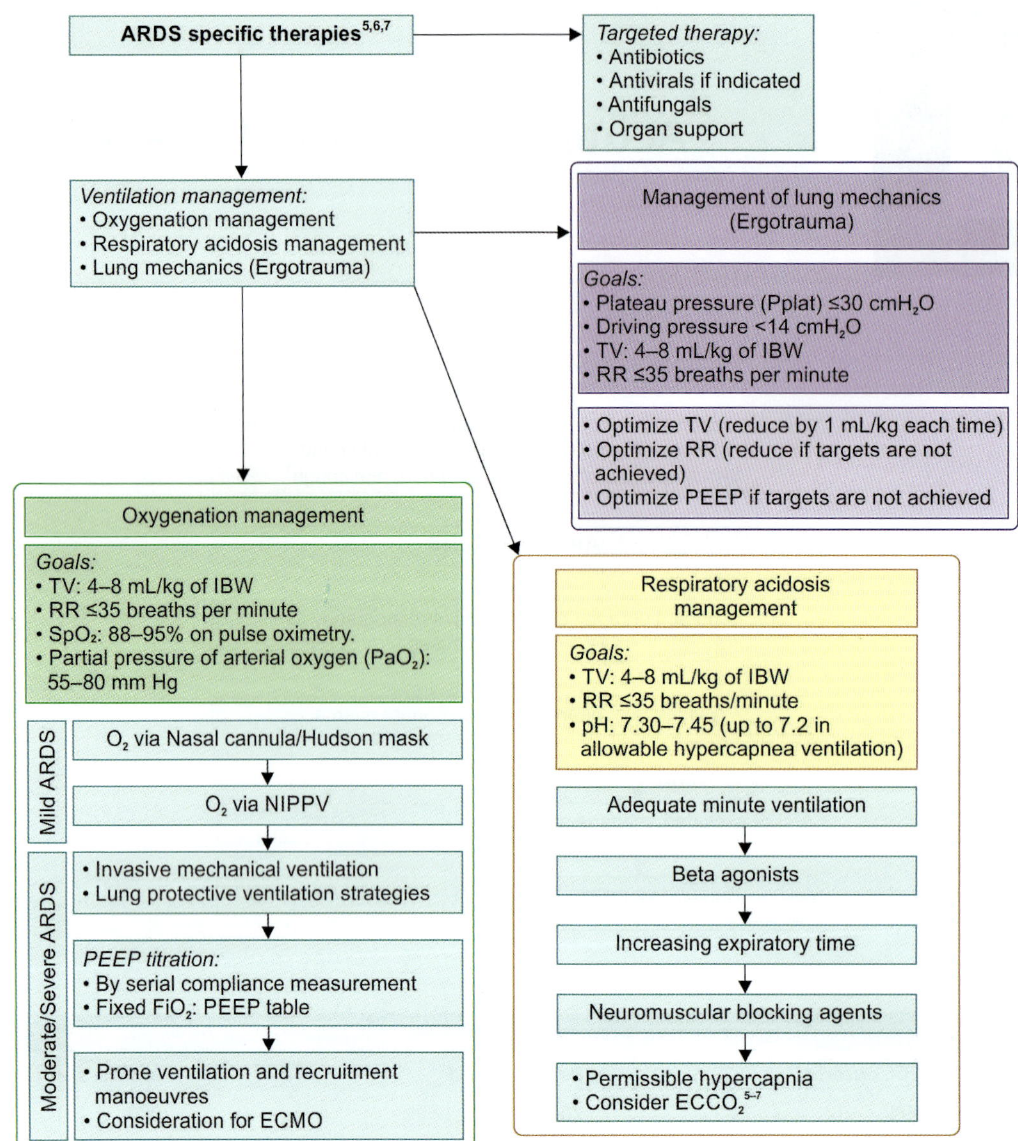
ARDS specific therapies[5,6,7]
Targeted therapy:
• Antibiotics
• Antivirals if indicated
• Antifungals
• Organ support
Ventilation management:
• Oxygenation management
• Respiratory acidosis management
• Lung mechanics (Ergotrauma)
Management of lung mechanics (Ergotrauma)
Goals:
• Plateau pressure (Pplat) ≤30 cmH2O
• Driving pressure <14 cmH2O
• TV: 4–8 mL/kg of IBW
• RR ≤35 breaths per minute
• Optimize TV (reduce by 1 mL/kg each time)
• Optimize RR (reduce if targets are not achieved)
• Optimize PEEP if targets are not achieved
Oxygenation management
Goals:
• TV: 4–8 mL/kg of IBW
• RR ≤35 breaths per minute
• SpO2: 88–95% on pulse oximetry.
• Partial pressure of arterial oxygen (PaO2): 55–80 mm Hg
Mild ARDS
O2 via Nasal cannula/Hudson mask
O2 via NIPPV
Moderate/Severe ARDS
• Invasive mechanical ventilation
• Lung protective ventilation strategies
PEEP titration:
• By serial compliance measurement
• Fixed FiO2: PEEP table
• Prone ventilation and recruitment manoeuvres
• Consideration for ECMO
Respiratory acidosis management
Goals:
• TV: 4–8 mL/kg of IBW
• RR ≤35 breaths/minute
• pH: 7.30–7.45 (up to 7.2 in allowable hypercapnea ventilation)
Adequate minute ventilation
Beta agonists
Increasing expiratory time
Neuromuscular blocking agents
• Permissible hypercapnia
• Consider ECCO2[5–7]

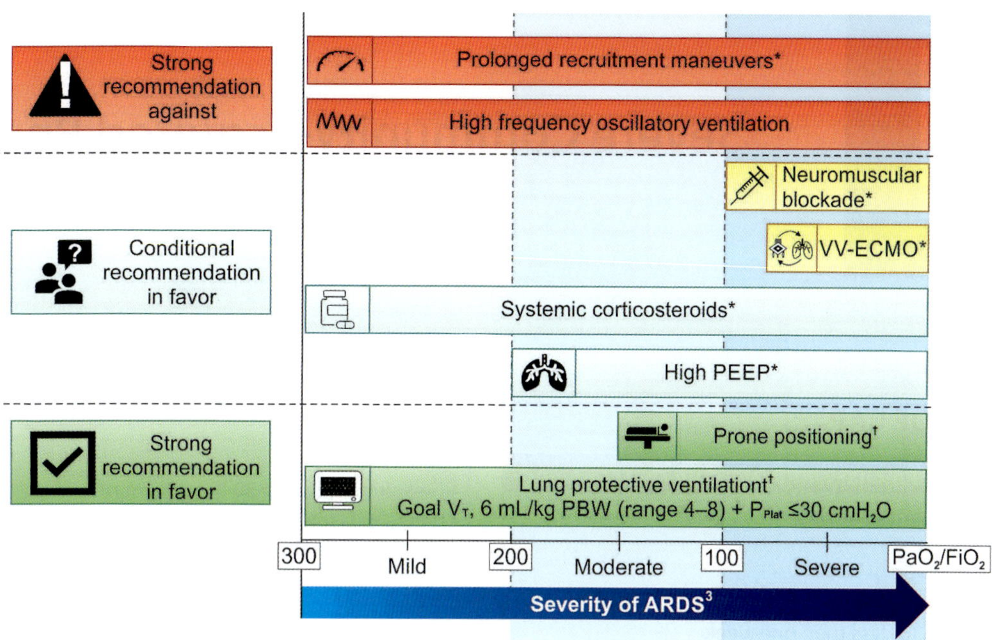


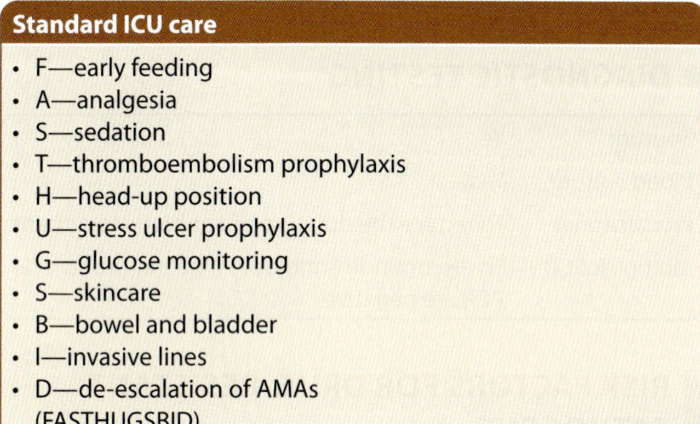

**Standard ICU care**

- F—early feeding
- A—analgesia
- S—sedation
- T—thromboembolism prophylaxis
- H—head-up position
- U—stress ulcer prophylaxis
- G—glucose monitoring
- S—skincare
- B—bowel and bladder
- I—invasive lines
- D—de-escalation of AMAs (FASTHUGSBID)

## REFERENCES

1. In: Chawla R, Todi S (Eds). ICU protocols: a stepwise approach, ISCCM. Singapore: Springer Verlag; 2020.
2. Diamond M, Peniston HL, Sanghavi DK, et al. Acute Respiratory Distress Syndrome. [Updated 2024 Jan 31]. In: StatPearls [Internet]. Treasure Island (FL): StatPearls Publishing; 2025 https://www.ncbi.nlm.nih.gov/books/NBK436002/
3. Qadir N, Sahetya S, Munshi L, et al. An Update on Management of Adult Patients with Acute Respiratory Distress Syndrome. Am J Respir Crit Care Med. 2024; 209(1):24-36.
4. Grasselli G, Calfee CS, Camporota L, et al; European Society of Intensive Care Medicine Taskforce on ARDS. ESICM guidelines on acute respiratory distress syndrome: definition, phenotyping and respiratory support strategies. Intensive Care Med. 2023;49(7):727-59.
5. Fan E, Sorbo LD, Goligher EC, et al. An Official American Thoracic Society/European Society of Intensive Care Medicine/Society of Critical Care Medicine Clinical Practice Guideline: Mechanical Ventilation in Adult Patients with Acute Respiratory Distress Syndrome. Am J Respir Crit Care Med. 2017;195(9):1253-63.
6. Griffiths MJD, McAuley DF, Perkins GD, Barrett N, Blackwood B, Boyle A, et al. Guidelines on the management of acute respiratory distress syndrome. BMJ Open Resp Res. 2019;6(1):e000420.
7. Papazian L, Aubron C, Brochard L, Chiche JD, Combes A, Dreyfuss D, et al. Formal guidelines: management of acute respiratory distress syndrome. Ann Intensive Care. 2019;9(1):69.

CHAPTER 15

# Severe Community-acquired Pneumonia

## DEFINITION OF CAP[1]

**Newly recognized pulmonary infiltrate(s) on chest imaging**

*Respiratory Symptoms (at least one)*
- Cough
- Expectoration
- Dyspnea
- Pleuritic chest pain for less than one week

*Other Signs or Findings (at least one)*
- Abnormal lung sounds (rhonchi or crackles)
- Fever (≥100.4 °F)
- Leukocytosis (above normal limits for laboratory)
- Hypoxia (< 90%)

**CURB 65 score**

| ***Symptom*** | ***Points*** |
|---|---|
| Confusion | 1 |
| BUN >7 mmol/L (19 mg/dL) | 1 |
| Respiratory rate ≥30 | 1 |
| BP: S <90 mm Hg, D ≤60 mm Hg | 1 |
| Age ≥65 years | 1 |
| **Total Score** | **Management** |
| **0–1** | Outpatient |
| **2** | In Patient |
| **3+** | ICU |

## SEVERE COMMUNITY-ACQUIRED PNEUMONIA DEFINITION[2]

**One major criterion OR three or more minor criteria**

*Major criteria*
- Septic shock with the need for vasopressors
- Respiratory failure requiring mechanical ventilation

*Contd...*

*Contd...*

*Minor criteria*
- Respiratory rate (>30 breaths/min)
- $PaO_2/FiO_2$ ratio (<250)
- Multilobar infiltrates (>2 lobes)
- Confusion/disorientation
- Uremia (blood urea nitrogen level >20 mg/dL)
- Leukopenia (white blood cell count <4,000 cells/mL)
- Thrombocytopenia (platelet count <100,000/mL)
- Hypothermia (core temperature <36°C)
- Hypotension requiring aggressive fluid resuscitation

## DIAGNOSTIC TESTING[2]

| | |
|---|---|
| Sputum | Yes |
| Blood culture | Yes |
| Procalcitonin | To reduce the duration of antibiotic treatment |
| Multiplex PCR | To discontinue antibiotics if bacterial and viral PCR are negative |

## RISK FACTORS FOR DRUG-RESISTANT PATHOGENS

**Prior colonization with *Pseudomonas aeruginosa* or methicillin-resistant *Staphylococcus aureus***

*Contact with the healthcare environment in the past 90 days:*
- Prior hospitalization
- Recent intensive care unit care
- Hemodialysis
- Nursing home residence
- Home wound care
- Home intravenous antibiotic therapy

*Specific host disease risk factors:*
- Immunosuppression
- Bronchiectasis

*Contd...*

*Contd...*

- Diabetes
- Cerebrovascular disease
- Chronic respiratory disease
- Overall poor functional status

*Specific therapies:*

- Corticosteroids and other immunosuppressive therapies
- Gastric acid suppression
- Tube feeding
- Broad-spectrum antibiotics

## TREATMENT: STANDARD REGIMEN[2,3]

| | |
|---|---|
| β-lactam PLUS atypical coverage | • Ampicillin/sulbactam 1.5–3 g IV q6h<br>• Ceftriaxone 2g IV q24h<br>• Cefotaxime 1–2 g IV q8h |
| | • Azithromycin 500 mg IV/PO q24h<br>• Clarithromycin 500 mg IV/PO q12h<br>• Doxycycline 100 mg IV/PO q12h<br>• Levofloxacin 750 mg IV/PO q24h<br>• Moxifloxacin 400 mg IV/PO q24h |

## RECENT HOSPITALIZATION AND PARENTERAL ANTIBIOTICS IN THE LAST 90 DAYS

| | |
|---|---|
| MRSA coverage | • Vancomycin, per hospital guidelines<br>• Linezolid 600 mg IV/PO q12h |
| β-lactam PLUS atypical coverage | • Piperacillin/tazobactam 4.5 g IV q6h<br>• Cefepime 2 g IV q8h<br>• Ceftazidime 2 g IV q8h<br>• Imipenem 500 mg IV q6h<br>• Meropenem 1000 mg IV q8h |
| | • Azithromycin 500 mg IV/PO q24h<br>• Clarithromycin 500 mg IV/PO q12h<br>• Doxycycline 100 mg IV/PO q12<br>• Levofloxacin 750 mg IV/PO q24h<br>• Moxifloxacin 400 mg IV/PO q24h |

## HISTORY OF MRSA COLONIZATION OR INFECTION AT ANY SITE WITHIN 1 YEAR OR MRSA NASAL PCR POSITIVE

| | |
|---|---|
| MRSA coverage | • Vancomycin per hospital guidelines<br>• Linezolid 600 mg IV/PO q12h |

## HISTORY OF *P. AERUGINOSA* COLONIZATION OR INFECTION AT ANY SITE WITHIN 1 YEAR (OR) ADVANCED STRUCTURAL LUNG DISEASE

| | |
|---|---|
| β-lactam PLUS atypical coverage | • Piperacillin/tazobactam 4.5 g IV q6h<br>• Cefepime 2 g IV q8h<br>• Ceftazidime 2 g IV q8h<br>• Imipenem 500 mg IV q6h<br>• Meropenem 1000 mg IV q8h |
| | • Azithromycin 500 mg IV/PO q24h<br>• Clarithromycin 500 mg IV/PO q12h<br>• Doxycycline 100 mg IV/PO q12<br>• Levofloxacin 750 mg IV/PO q24h<br>• Moxifloxacin 400 mg IV/PO q24h |

| | |
|---|---|
| Allergy to β-lactams | levofloxacin 750 mg IV/PO q24h +/– aztreonam 2g IV q8h +/– MRSA coverage |

| | |
|---|---|
| *Oseltamivir* | As empirical during the influenza season/ influenza confirmed by PCR |
| *High-flow nasal oxygen (HFNO)* | Acute hypoxemic respiratory failure does not need immediate intubation |
| *Non-invasive mechanical ventilation (NIV)* | Persistent hypoxemic respiratory failure not needing immediate intubation, irrespective of HFNO |
| *Steroids* | • If shock is present<br>• Does not apply to patients with viral sCAP (influenza, SARS, and MERS), uncontrolled diabetes, and corticosteroid treatment for other reasons<br>• Methylprednisolone (0.5 mg/kg every 12 h for 5 days) |

## REFERENCES


1. Martin-Loeches I, Torres A, Nagavci B, Aliberti S, Antonelli M, Bassetti M, et al. ERS/ESICM/ESCMID/ALAT guidelines for the management of severe community-acquired pneumonia. Intensive Care Med. 2023;49(6):615-32.
2. Metlay JP, Waterer GW, Long AC, Anzueto A, Brozek J, Crothers K, et al. Diagnosis and Treatment of Adults with Community-acquired Pneumonia. An Official Clinical Practice Guideline of the American Thoracic Society and Infectious Diseases Society of America. Am J Respir Crit Care Med. 2019;200(7):e45-e67.
3. Niederman MS, Torres A. Severe community-acquired pneumonia. Eur Respir Rev. 2022;31(166):220123.

CHAPTER 16

# Bronchopleural Fistula

## DEFINITIONS

| *Terms* | *Description* |
|---|---|
| Alveolar-pleural fistula (APF) | Air leak from lung parenchyma into the pleural cavity |
| Bronchopleural fistula (BPF) | Air leak from an abnormal communication between the airways and the pleural cavity |
| Persistent air leak (PAL) | If the air leak persists for >5–7 days, it is termed PAL |

## CERFOLIO CLASSIFICATION OF AIR LEAKS

| *Grade* | *Description* |
|---|---|
| Grade 1, FE | During any forced expiration, only |
| Grade 2, E | Expiration only |
| Grade 3, I | Inspiration only |
| Grade 4, c | Continuous bubbling present in the air leak chamber during both inspiration and expiration |

## CAUSES AND RISK FACTORS FOR PAL

| *Aspect* | *Description* |
|---|---|
| Surgical causes | Pneumonectomy, lobectomy, Lung Volume reduction surgery |
| Nonsurgical causes | Spontaneous pneumothorax, necrotizing pneumonia, mechanical ventilation, thoracentesis, transthoracic needle biopsy or aspiration, pulmonary tuberculosis |
| Risk factors | COPD, smoking, diabetes, steroid use, low $FEV_1$, low DLCO, upper lobe emphysema, pleural adhesions |

## COMPLICATIONS OF PAL

- Inadequate lung expansion
- Ventilation/perfusion mismatch
- Infection of the pleural cavity
- Increased hospitalization rates and mortality

## DIAGNOSIS AND LOCALIZATION OF PAL

| *Aspect* | *Description* |
|---|---|
| Computed tomography Scan | Assess air leak locations (central or peripheral) and fissure integrity (FI exceeding 90% indicates minimal collateral ventilation and predicts response to bronchoscopic management) |
| Methylene blue injection | Identifies fistula location via retrograde (through the pleural cavity and identifying dye through bronchoscopy) or anterograde (dye instilled through bronchoscopy; however, cannot determine its exact location) |
| Sequential balloon occlusion by flexible bronchoscopy | Detects air leak reduction using sequential (Fogarty) balloon occlusion of main bronchus to lobar to segmental to subsegmental bronchus. The test is considered positive if the leak diminishes by >50% |
| Pressure transducer catheter (Chartis system) | A catheter is equipped with an inflatable balloon and pressure transducer. By analyzing the airflow from the occluded lobe, it can evaluate collateral ventilation status |

## TREATMENT

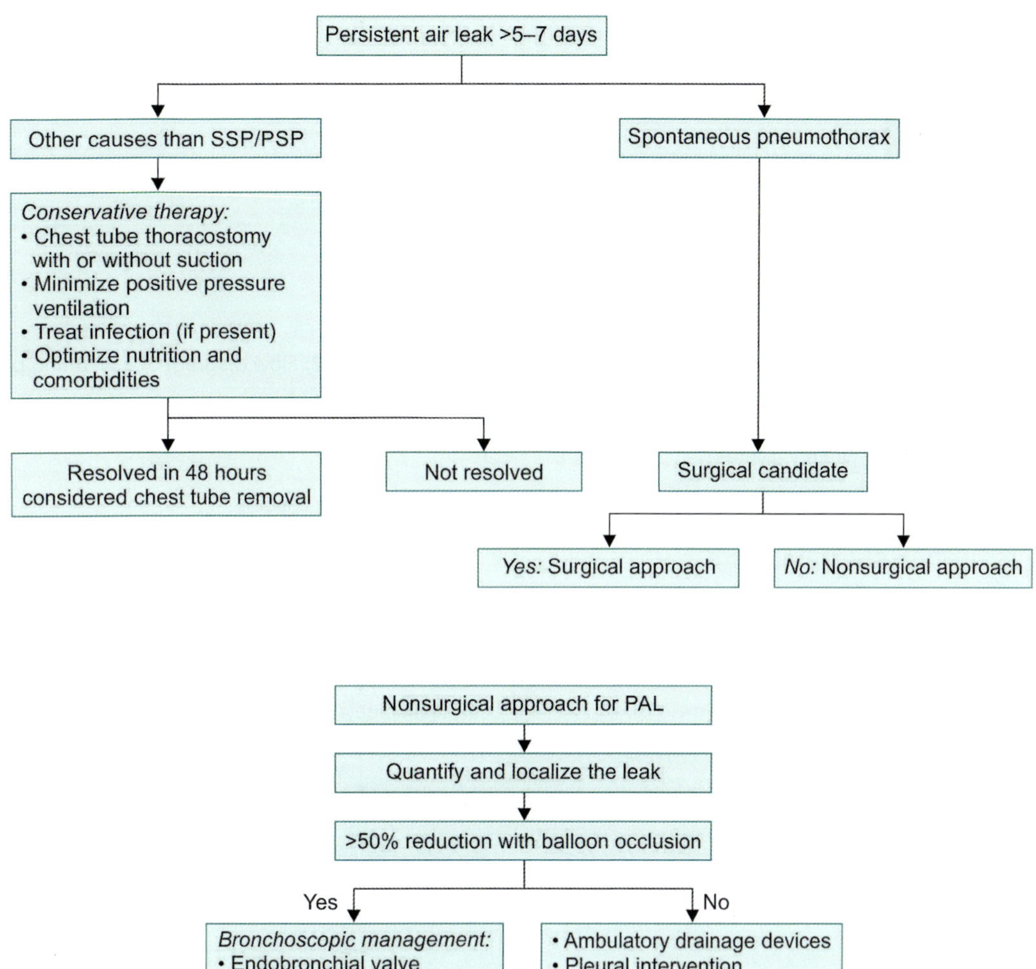


## SUGGESTED READING

1. Bashour Si, Ost De. An Update On Bronchopleural Fistulae Following Cancer-Related Surgery. Curr Opin Pulm Med. 2023;29(4):223-31.
2. Grotberg JC, Hyzy Rc, De Cardenas J, Co IN. Bronchopleural Fistula In The Mechanically Ventilated Patient: A Concise Review. Crit Care Med. 2021;49(2):292-301.
3. Jin L, Li Y. Bronchoscopic Interventions For Bronchopleural Fistulas. Ther Adv Respir Dis. 2023;17: 17534666231164541.
4. Ruenwilai P. Bronchoscopic Management In Persistent Air Leak: A Narrative Review. J Thorac Dis. 2024;16(6): 4030-42.

CHAPTER 17

# Weaning

**Flowchart 1:** Continuum of the care of mechanically ventilated patient.

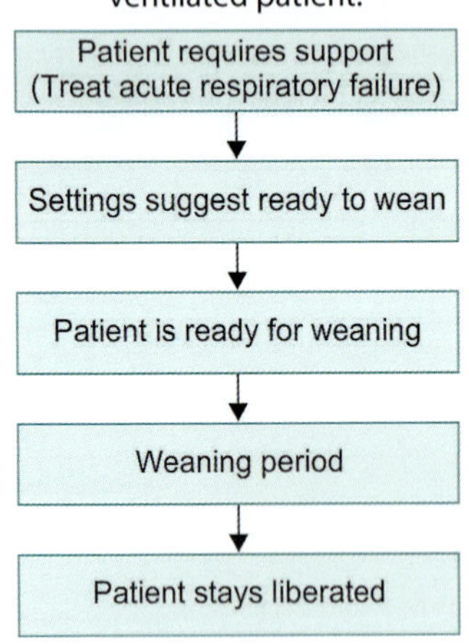


**Flowchart 2:** Flow diagram of a weaning protocol.

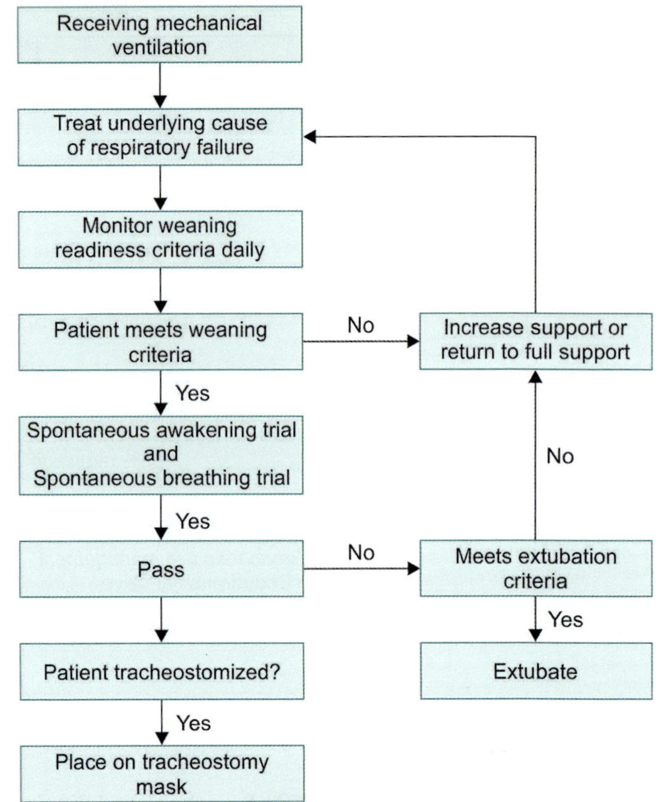


**BOX 1:** Criteria for readiness for SBT (weaning).

*Required criteria*

- The cause of the respiratory failure has improved
- $PaO_2/FiO_2$ ≥150 or $SpO_2$ ≥90% on $FiO_2$ ≤40% and positive end-expiratory pressure (PEEP) ≤5 $cmH_2O$
- pH >7.25
- Hemodynamic stability (no or low-dose vasopressor medications)
- Able to initiate an inspiratory effort

*Additional criteria (optional criteria)*

- Hemoglobin ≥7 mg/dL
- Core temperature ≤38–38.5 °C

**BOX 2:** A Mnemonic for screening for readiness to wean.

- **A**im of the ventilation met with alert and afebrile
- **B**reathing indices within acceptable limits and no distress
- **C**irculation: Hemodynamically stable
- **D**rugs: No sedative or NMBA drug effect
- **E**lectrolytes: No sodium, potassium, calcium, magnesium, or phosphate disturbances
- **F**luid status: Not dehydrated, not edematous
- **G**lucose-Euglycemia, no hypo- or hyperglycemia
- No **H**allucinations/no delirium and co-operative patient
- No **I**mpending procedures or transfers

**BOX 3:** Protocol for preparation and procedure for weaning.

*Preparation:*
- Inform the patient (if conscious) about
- The steps of the weaning process and what is expected of him or her
- Regarding the procedure in detail (first, remove the ventilator and then remove the Endotracheal tube)
- Probable difficulty in breathing through the tube

*Reassurance:*
- Use ventilator cards, which help intubated patients to communicate (like a signboard)
- Suctioning equipment, Oxygen therapy devices, oral and nasal airways, and intubation tray should be on standby (including equipment for difficult intubation)

*Procedure:*
- Once preparation is done, keep the patient in a comfortable propped position
- Pre-oxygenation (increase $FiO_2$ by 10–20% except in COPD patients)
- Do thorough endotracheal, nasogastric, and oral suctioning
- Plan the mode of weaning: low-pressure support or T-piece
- Take patient off the ventilator if weaning is planned through T-piece OR switch over to low-pressure support mode (Pressure support 6–8 $cmH_2O$ above PEEP and PEEP 5 $cmH_2O$)

**BOX 4:** Parameters to be observed during weaning.

*Patient's clinical status:*
- Breathlessness or respiratory distress
- Profuse diaphoresis
- Use of accessory muscles of respiration
- Paradoxical breathing
- Bronchospasm
- Altered mental status

*Monitoring parameters:*
- HR watch for tachycardia, arrhythmia
- BP watch for accelerated hypertension
- $SpO_2$ watch for desaturation
- $CO_2$ watch for increasing $ETCO_2$
- ABG after 30–120 minutes
- Weaning index-preferably RSBI

**TABLE 1:** Comparison of various weaning indices.

| *Index* | *Cut off value* | *Equation/measurement* | *Remarks* |
|---|---|---|---|
| Respiratory rate | <30/min | | Simple: Part of a routine monitoring |
| Tidal volume (Vt) | >5 mL/kg | By spirometer if the patient is on a T-piece; By ventilator expiratory parameters if the patient is on PSV | Part of routine monitoring requires a spirometer (in some instances) |
| Forced vital capacity (FVC) | >15 mL/kg | Same as tidal volume | Difficult to measure in all patients |
| Minute ventilation | <15 L/min | Vt x RR | Easy to measure |

*Contd...*

*Contd…*

| *Index* | *Cut off value* | *Equation/measurement* | *Remarks* |
|---|---|---|---|
| Rapid shallow breathing index (RSBI) | <105 breaths/min/L | Frequency (RR)/Vt | Most studied: Easy to measure; Simple to measure; High sensitivity but less specificity |
| Maximum inspiratory pressure (Pimax) | <-30 $cmH_2O$ (normal: –90 to 120 $cmH_2O$) | Breathing with ventilator valves closed (Pimax maneuver) | Requires patient's cooperation |
| P0.1/Pimax | >0.3<br>P0.1 is the pressure at the airway opening 0.1s after the start of inspiratory flow | P0.1/Pimax | Complex<br>No added advantage |
| P0.1 x f/VT | <300 | | Less studied |
| Dynamic compliance, rate, oxygenation, max inspiratory pressure (CROP index) | >13 | (Cdyn × Pimax × ($PaO_2$/$PAO_2$)/f | Complex |
| Dynamic compliance, oxygenation, rate, effort (CORE index) | >8 | Cdyn × (Pimax/P0.1) × ($PaO_2$/$PAO_2$)/f | Complex |
| Weaning index (WI) | <50 | RSBI × EI × VDI<br>(EI: peak pressure/negative inspiratory force; VDI: MV/10) | Complex |
| Integrative weaning index (IWI) | >25 | (CRS × $SaO_2$)/(f/VT)<br>(CRS = static compliance of the respiratory system) | Very complex and Labor intensive |
| Heart rate, acidosis, consciousness, oxygenation, respiratory rate (HACOR) | ≥5 | Predicts weaning failure | Complex and more validated for predicting NIV failure |
| Diaphragmatic RSBI | 1.767 | RR/diaphragmatic displacement (in millimeters) and expressed as breath/minute/millimeter | Predicts weaning failure<br>Requires expertise<br>Require larger studies to validate |
| Minute ventilation recovery time | | Calculated before and 30 minutes after SBT | Simple but inaccurate;<br>Multiple confounding factors |

**BOX 5:** Classification of patients according to the weaning process.

- *Simple weaning:* Patients who proceed from initiation of weaning to successful extubation on the first attempt without difficulty
- *Difficult weaning:* Patients who fail initial weaning up to three SBTs or as long as 7 days from the first SBT to achieve successful weaning
- *Prolonged weaning:* Patients who fail at least three weaning attempts or require >7 days of weaning after the first SBT

## SUGGESTED READING


1. Boles JM, Bion J, Connors A, Herridge M, Marsh B, Melot C, et al. Weaning from mechanical ventilation. Eur Respir J. 2007;29(5):1033-56.
2. Haas CF, Loik PS. Ventilator Discontinuation Protocols. Respiratory Care. 2012;57(10):1649.

CHAPTER 18

# Ventilator-associated Pneumonia/ Hospital-acquired Pneumonia/ Healthcare-associated Pneumonia

| *Term* | *Definition*[1] |
|---|---|
| *Classification by site of acquisition* | |
| Community-acquired pneumonia (CAP) | An acute infection of the pulmonary parenchyma acquired outside of healthcare settings |
| Nosocomial pneumonia | An acute infection of the pulmonary parenchyma acquired in hospital settings, which encompasses hospital-acquired pneumonia and ventilator-associated pneumonia |
| Hospital-acquired pneumonia (HAP) | Pneumonia acquired ≥ 48 hours after hospital admission; includes both HAP and VAP |
| Ventilator-associated pneumonia (VAP) | Pneumonia acquired ≥ 48 hours after endotracheal intubation |
| Healthcare-associated pneumonia (HCAP) | Retired term, which referred to pneumonia acquired in health care facilities (e.g., nursing homes, hemodialysis centers) or after recent hospitalization |

## SURVEILLANCE DEFINITION OF VENTILATOR-ASSOCIATED EVENTS[2]

Patient has a baseline period of stability or improvement on the ventilator, defined by ≥2 calendar days of stable or decreasing daily minimum $FiO_2$ or PEEP values. The baseline period is defined as the two calendar days immediately preceding the first day of increased daily minimum PEEP or $FiO_2$

↓

*After a period of stability or improvement on the ventilator, the patient has at least one of the following indicators of worsening oxygenation:*
- Minimum daily $FiO_2$ values increase ≥0.2 (20 points) over the daily minimum $FiO_2$ in the preceding two calendar days (the baseline period), for >2 calendar days
- Minimum daily PEEP values increase ≥3 $cmH_2O$ over the daily minimum PEEP in the preceding two calendar days (the baseline period), for ≥2 calendar days

↓

Ventilator-associated complication (IVAC)

↓

*On or after calendar day 3 of mechanical ventilation and within 2 calendar days before or after the onset of worsening oxygenation, the patient meets both of the following criteria:*
- Temperature >38°C or <36°C, OR white blood cell count ≥12,000 cells/$mm^3$ or ≤4,000 cells/$mm^3$
- A new antimicrobial agentis" is started, and is continued for 24 calendar days See VAE surveillance protocol (available at: http://www.cdc.gov/nhan/acute-care-hospital/var/index.html) for eligible agents

↓

Contd...

*Contd...*

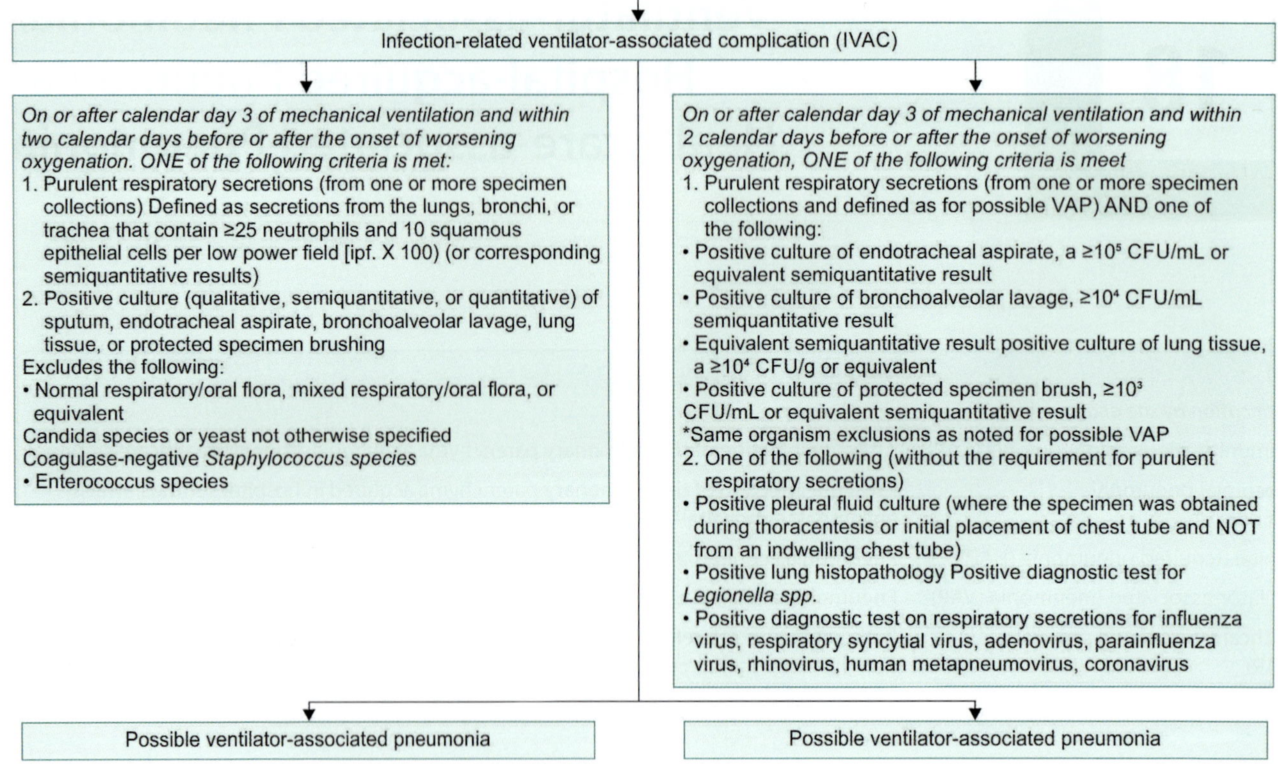


## DIAGNOSTIC STRATEGIES[2]

No Gold standard strategies are available.

- Clinical strategy
- Invasive strategy
- CPIS score-based strategy

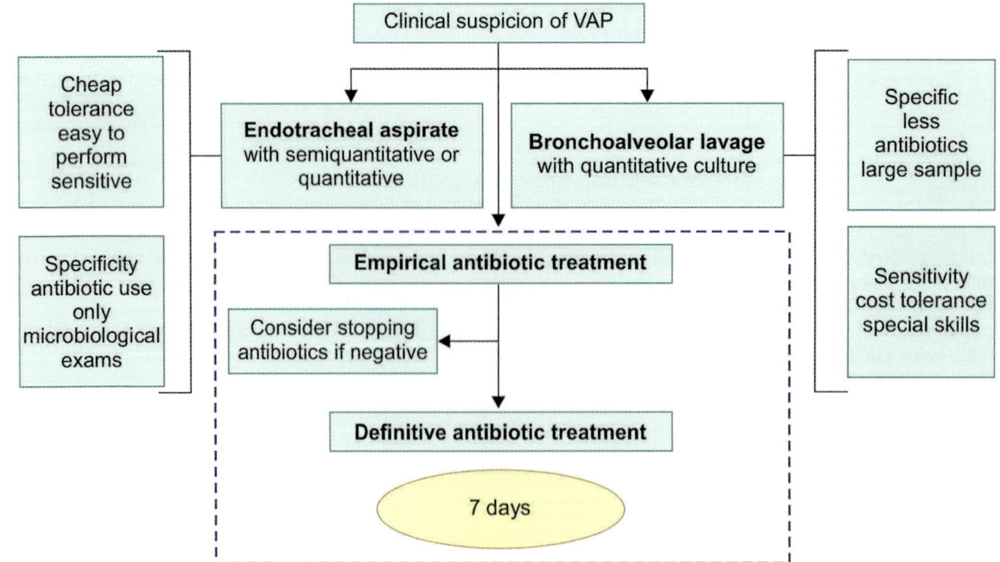

## CLINICAL STRATEGY

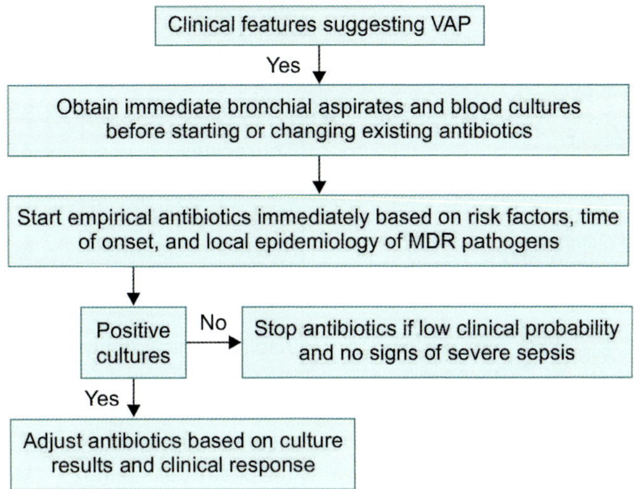


## INVASIVE STRATEGY

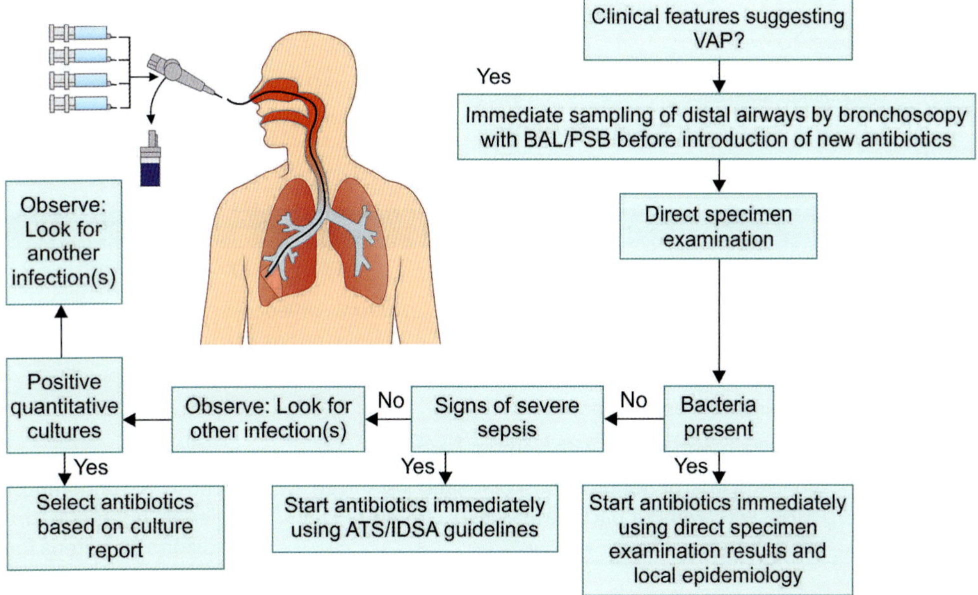

## CPIS SCORE-BASED STRATEGY

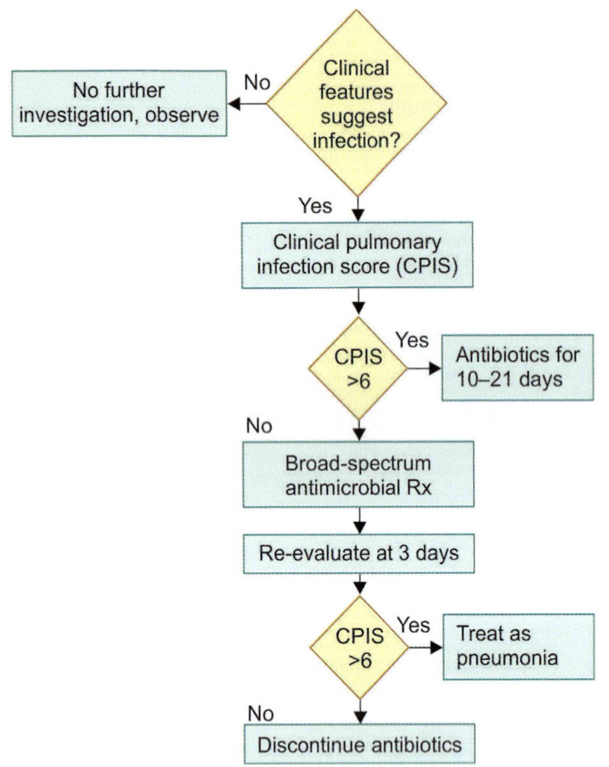


**TABLE 1:** Clinical pulmonary infection score used in this study.

| *Parameter* | *Result* | *Score* |
|---|---|---|
| Temperature (°C) | • 36.5–38.4<br>• 38.5–38.9<br>• ≤36 or ≥239 | 0<br>1<br>2 |
| Leukocytes (cells/mm$^3$) | • 4,000–11,000<br>• <4,000 or >11,000<br>• ≥500 band cells | 0<br>1<br>2 |
| Tracheal secretions (subjective) | • None<br>• Mild/nonpurulent<br>• Purulent | 0<br>1<br>2 |
| Radiographic findings on chest X-ray | • No infiltrates<br>• Diffuse/patchy infiltrates<br>• Localized infiltrate | 0<br>1<br>2 |
| Culture result (respiratory sampling) | • No/mild growth<br>• Moderate/florid growth<br>• Moderate/florid growth and pathogen consistent with Gram stain | 0<br>1<br>2 |
| Oxygenation status ($PaO_2/FiO_2$ ratio) | • 240 or ARDS<br>• 240 and absence of ARDS | 0<br>2 |

Clinical difference: VAP vs VAT

| *Variables* | *VAP* | *NAT* |
|---|---|---|
| Clinical signs and symptoms | Temperature (38°C) or leukocyte count >12,000/mL, or leucopenia <4,000/mL. tat least one of these) plus new onset of purulent endotracheal secretions or change in sputum | |
| Radiology: Chest radiograph or CT scan | New and progressive or persistent infiltrate, or consolidation, or cavitation | NO new infiltrate |
| Microbiology criteria | Gram-stain with PMNLs with/without bacteria | |
| FOB | Bronchoscopic or nonbronchoscopic samples, smear: PMNLs with/without bacteria; BAL≥ $10^4$ cfu/mL, or PSB ≥ $10^3$ cfu/mL | Bronchoscopic or nonbronchoscopic samples are not required; if done, do not fulfill diagnostic criteria for VAP |

## TREATMENT PROTOCOL[3]

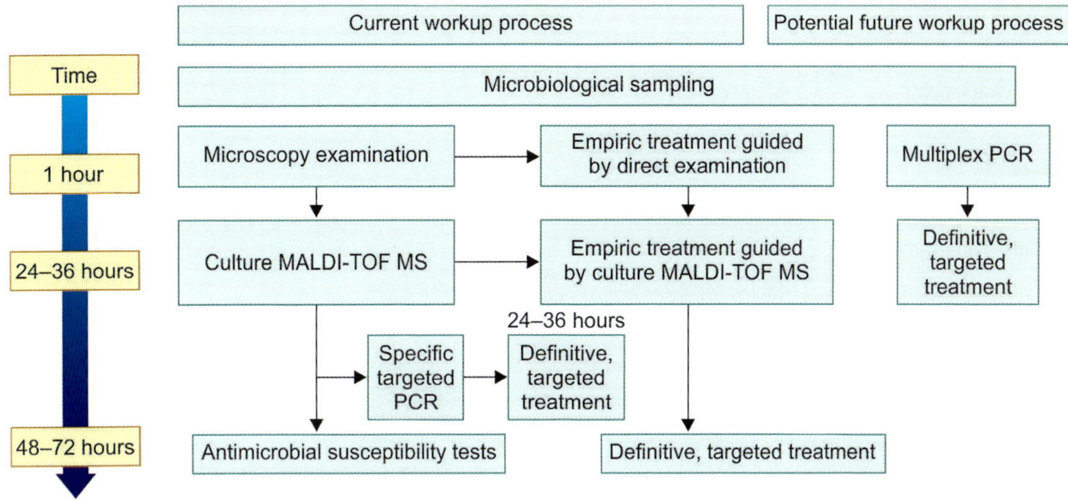


## EMPIRIC TREATMENT PROTOCOL FOR VENTILATOR-ASSOCIATED PNEUMONIA

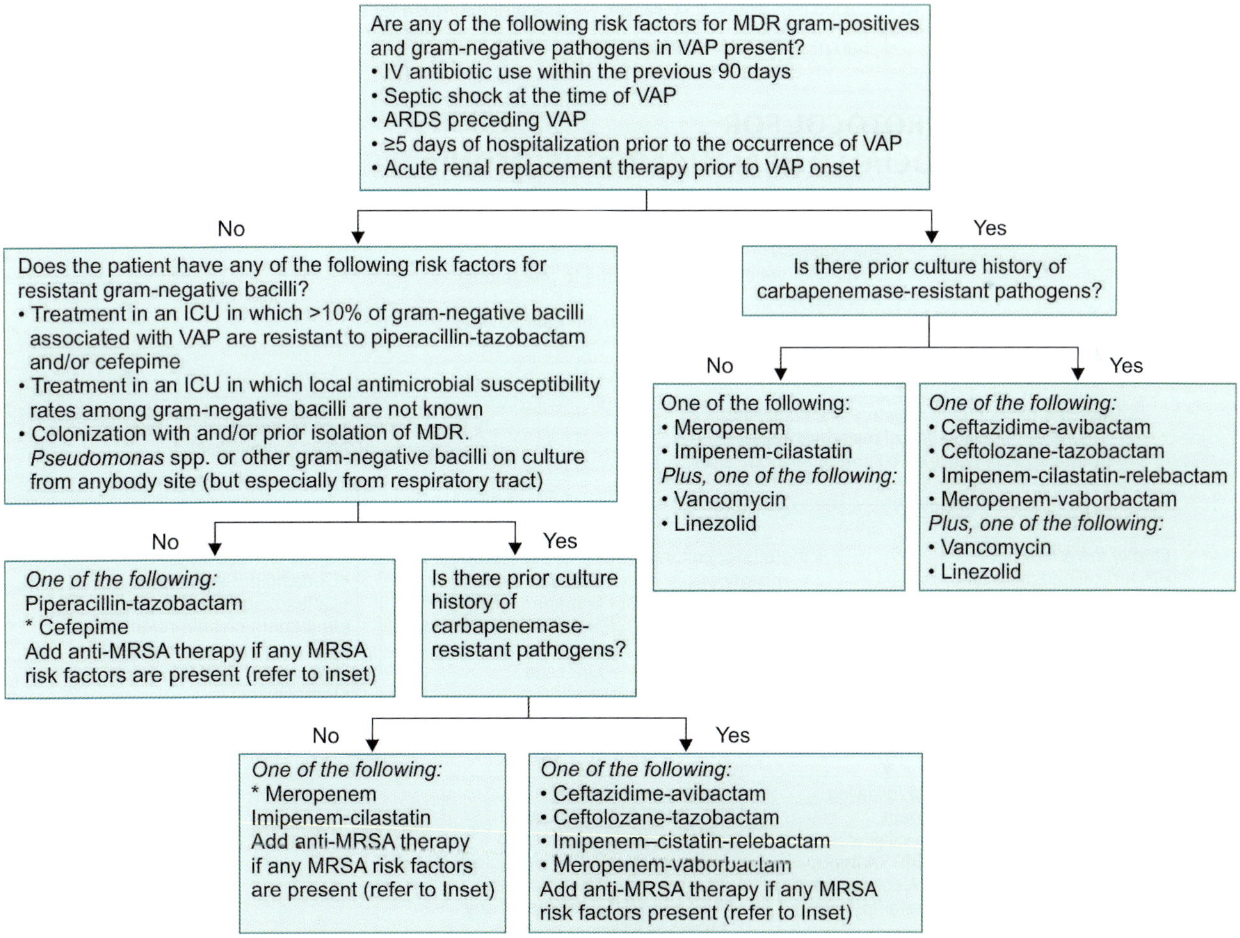

Are any of the following risk factors for MDR gram-positives and gram-negative pathogens in VAP present?
- IV antibiotic use within the previous 90 days
- Septic shock at the time of VAP
- ARDS preceding VAP
- ≥5 days of hospitalization prior to the occurrence of VAP
- Acute renal replacement therapy prior to VAP onset

**No →** Does the patient have any of the following risk factors for resistant gram-negative bacilli?
- Treatment in an ICU in which >10% of gram-negative bacilli associated with VAP are resistant to piperacillin-tazobactam and/or cefepime
- Treatment in an ICU in which local antimicrobial susceptibility rates among gram-negative bacilli are not known
- Colonization with and/or prior isolation of MDR. *Pseudomonas* spp. or other gram-negative bacilli on culture from anybody site (but especially from respiratory tract)

- **No →** *One of the following:*
  Piperacillin-tazobactam
  * Cefepime
  Add anti-MRSA therapy if any MRSA risk factors are present (refer to inset)
- **Yes →** Is there prior culture history of carbapenemase-resistant pathogens?
  - **No →** *One of the following:*
    * Meropenem
    Imipenem-cilastatin
    Add anti-MRSA therapy if any MRSA risk factors are present (refer to Inset)
  - **Yes →** *One of the following:*
    - Ceftazidime-avibactam
    - Ceftolozane-tazobactam
    - Imipenem–cistatin-relebactam
    - Meropenem-vaborbactam

    Add anti-MRSA therapy if any MRSA risk factors present (refer to Inset)

**Yes →** Is there prior culture history of carbapenemase-resistant pathogens?

- **No →** One of the following:
  - Meropenem
  - Imipenem-cilastatin

  *Plus, one of the following:*
  - Vancomycin
  - Linezolid
- **Yes →** *One of the following:*
  - Ceftazidime-avibactam
  - Ceftolozane-tazobactam
  - Imipenem-cilastatin-relebactam
  - Meropenem-vaborbactam

  *Plus, one of the following:*
  - Vancomycin
  - Linezolid

*Contd...*

*Contd...*

| Inset | |
|---|---|
| Dosing of preferred antibiotics | |
| Piperacillin-tazobactam | 4.5 g IV every 6 hours |
| Cefepime | 2 g IV every 8 hours |
| Meropenem 1 | 1 g IV every 8 hours |
| Imipenem-cilastatin 1 | 500 mg IV every 6 hours |
| Ceftazidime-avibactam | 2.5 g IV every 8 hours |
| Ceftolozane-tazobactam | 3 g IV every 8 hours |
| Imipenem-cilastatin-relebactam | 1.25 g IV every 6 hours |
| Meropenem-vaborbactam | 4 g IV every 8 hours |
| *Add anti-MRSA therapy if the patient has one of the following risk factors for MRSA:*<br>• Treatment in a unit in which >10 to 20% of *S. aureus* isolates associated with VAP are methicillin-resistant Treatment in a unit in which the prevalence of MRSA is not known<br>• Colonization with and/or prior isolation of MRSA on culture from anybody site (but especially the respiratory tract) | |
| *Anti-MRSA therapy consists of one of the following:* | |
| Vancomycin | • Generally, 15–20 mg/kg every 8–12 hours for most patients with normal kidney function<br>• Interval adjustments should be based on AUC-guided (preferred) or trough-guided serum concentration monitoring. The vancomycin loading dose is based on actual body weight; the dose is rounded to the nearest 250 mg increment and not exceeding 2000 mg. Within this range, we use a higher dose for critically ill patients |
| Linezolid | 600 mg IV every 12 hours |

## EMPIRIC TREATMENT PROTOCOL FOR NONVENTILATOR-ASSOCIATED HEALTHCARE PNEUMONIA

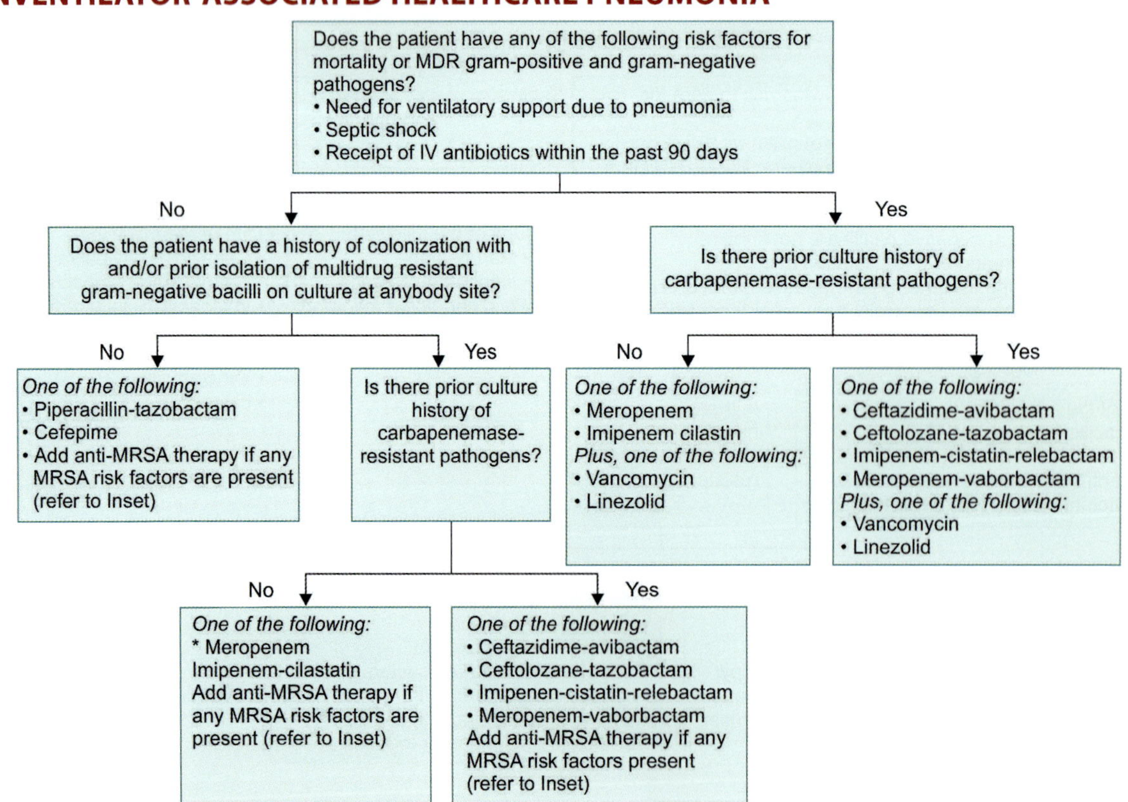


*Contd...*

*Contd...*

| Inset | |
|---|---|
| Dosing of preferred antibiotics | |
| Piperacillin-tazobactam | 4.5 g IV every 6 hours |
| Cefepime | 2 g IV every 8 hours |
| Meropenem | 1 g IV every 8 hours |
| Imipenem-cilastatin | 500 mg IV every 6 hours |
| Ceftazidime-avibactam | 2.5 g IV every 8 hours |
| Ceftolozane-tazobactam | 3 g IV every 8 hours |
| Imipenem-cilastatin-relebactam | 1.25 g IV every 6 hours |
| Meropenem-vaborbactam | 4 g IV every 8 hours |
| *Add anti-MRSA therapy if the patient has one of the following risk factors for MRSA:*<br>• Treatment in a unit in which >10 to 20% of *S. aureus* isolates associated with VAP are methicillin resistant<br>• Treatment in a unit in which the prevalence of MRSA is not known<br>• Colonization with and/or prior isolation of MRSA on culture from anybody site (but especially the respiratory tract) | |
| *Anti-MRSA therapy consists of one of the following:* | |
| Vancomycin | • Generally, 15–20 mg/kg every 8–12 hours for most patients with normal kidney function<br>• Interval adjustments should be based on AUC-guided (preferred) or trough-guided serum concentration monitoring. The vancomycin loading dose is based on actual body weight; the dose is rounded to the nearest 250 mg increment and not exceeding 2,000 mg. Within this range, we use a higher dose for critically ill patients |
| Linezolid | 600 mg IV every 12 hours |

## PREVENTIVE STRATEGIES IN VENTILATOR-ASSOCIATED PNEUMONIA

| *Category* | *Rationale* | *Intervention* | *Quality of evidence* |
|---|---|---|---|
| Essential practices | Good evidence that the intervention decreases the average duration of mechanical ventilation, length of stay, mortality, and/or costs. The benefits likely outweigh the risks | • Avoid intubation and prevent reintubation<br>• Use high-flow nasal oxygen or noninvasive positive pressure ventilation (NIPPV) as appropriate whenever safe and feasible | High |
| | | • Minimize sedation<br>• Avoid benzodiazepines in favor of other agents<br>• Use a protocol to minimize sedation<br>• Implement a ventilator liberation protocol | Moderate |
| | | Maintain and improve physical conditioning | Moderate |
| | | Elevate the head of the bed to 30 to 45° | Low |
| | | Provide oral care with toothbrushing but without chlorhexidine | Moderate |
| | | Provide early enteral vs. parenteral nutrition | High |
| | | Change the ventilator circuit only if it is visibly soiled or malfunctioning (or per manufacturers' instructions) | High |

*Contd...*

*Contd...*

| *Category* | *Rationale* | *Intervention* | *Quality of evidence* |
|---|---|---|---|
| Additional approaches | Good evidence that the intervention improves outcomes in some populations, but may confer some risk in others | Use selective oral or digestive decontamination in countries and ICUs with low prevalence of antibiotic-resistant organisms | High |
| | May lower VAP rates, but insufficient data to determine the impact on duration of mechanical ventilation, length of stay, or mortality | Utilize endotracheal tubes with subglottic secretion drainage ports for patients expected to require >48–72 hours of mechanical ventilation | Moderate |
| | | Consider early tracheostomy | Moderate |
| | | Consider postpyloric rather than gastric feeding for patients with gastric intolerance or at high risk for aspiration | Moderate |
| Generally, not recommended | Inconsistently associated with lower VAP rates and no impact or negative impact on duration of mechanical ventilation, length of stay, or mortality | Oral care with chlorhexidine | Moderate |
| | | Probiotics | Moderate |
| | | Ultrathin polyurethane endotracheal tube cuffs | Moderate |
| | | Tapered endotracheal tube cuffs | Moderate |
| | | Automated control of endotracheal tube cuff pressure | Moderate |
| | | Frequent cuff-pressure monitoring | Moderate |
| | | Silver-coated endotracheal tubes | Moderate |
| | | Kinetic beds | Moderate |
| | | Prone positioning | Moderate |
| | | Chlorhexidine bathing | Moderate |
| | No impact on VAP rates, average duration of mechanical ventilation, length of stay, or mortality | Stress-ulcer prophylaxis | Moderate |
| | | Monitoring residual gastric volumes | Moderate |
| | | Early parenteral nutrition | Moderate |
| No recommendation | No impact on VAP rates or other patient outcomes, unclear impact on costs | Close endotracheal suctioning | Moderate |

## REFERENCES


1. www.uptodate.com. Treatment of hospital-acquired and ventilator-associated pneumonia in adults. [Online] Available from https://www.uptodate.com/contents/treatment-of-hospital-acquired-and-ventilator-associated-pneumonia-in-adults [Last accessed February, 2025].
2. Centers for Disease Control and Prevention. Ventilator-associated-pneumonia. [Online] Available from https://www.cdc.gov/ventilator-associated-pneumonia/about/index.html [Last accessed February, 2025].
3. Torres A, Niederman MS, Chastre J, Ewig S, Fernandez-Vandellos P, Hanberger H, et al. Summary of the international clinical guidelines for the management of hospital-acquired and ventilator-acquired pneumonia. ERJ Open Res. 2018;4(2):00028-2018.

CHAPTER

# 19

# Massive Hemoptysis

| ***Life-threatening hemoptysis***[A1,2] | | | |
|---|---|---|---|
| Hemoptysis that results in significant airway obstruction, abnormal gas exchange or hemodynamic instability | | | |
| Approximate volumes: 150 mL (about half a cup) in 24 hours or a bleeding rate of 100 mL/hour | | | |
| All admission to ICU | | | |
| | *Initial Assessment*[B]<br>• Assess ABC—Airway, breathing, circulation<br>• X-ray chest—to identify the site and cause of bleeding<br>• CBC, PT INR, APPT, routine biochemistry, blood group-cross-match | Not Stable | *Stabilize patient*[C]<br>• Secure airway/oxygen support (avoid NIV) achieve hemodynamic stability<br>• Correct bleeding diathesis<br>• Position of the patient; bleeding site dependent |
| | Stable | | |
| | *CT Chest*[E]<br>Any finding suggests the source of bleeding that is likely amenable to embolization is there or not? | No | *Flexible bronchoscopy*[D]<br>To localize bleeding source and reduce bleeding (Iced saline, topical epinephrine, balloon blocker) |
| | Yes | | |
| | • Thoracic aortogram f/by selective bronchial and systemic angiography<br>• Is the bleeding source identified and amenable to embolization? | Yes | Is the patient stabilized? |
| | No | | No |
| Yes | • Perform pulmonary angiography<br>• Is the bleeding source found? | No | • Consider advance bronchoscopy<br>• Balloon tamponade, Laser, APC, Stent |
| | Yes | | |
| *Embolization* | | | |
| | Rebleeding? | | |
| Yes | No | | |
| Repeat endovascular embolization and/or refer to surgery[F] | Continue observation and/or plan definitive treatment | | |

*Contd...*

*Contd...*

| | *"Life-threatening" or "Massive" Hemoptysis*[3-5] |
|---|---|
| A | • A specific volume of blood is required to define "massive," which is inconsistent across literature and difficult to estimate from the history given by patients as usually overestimated by them<br>• Assessment of the seriousness of hemoptysis requires the patient's cardiopulmonary reserve and his general condition<br>• As low as 100 mL of blood can cause asphyxia and death, as documented in the literature, and hence, "life-threatening hemoptysis" is a more appropriate term to define this serious condition |
| B | • Initial evaluation and management will often need to occur concurrently<br>• Respiratory auscultation may be misguided as the finding might be bilateral due to the spillage of blood to the opposite site<br>• Physical signs like a bruise and telangiectasis might direct etiology<br>• For detecting the site of bleeding, the X-ray chest (35%) is inferior to the CT Chest (70–88.5%). Hence, the chest CT should be done first if it is easily available and the patient is stable |
| C | • When intubation is required, the largest possible size ET tube, preferably eight sizes or more, should be considered as the risk of a blockade is high with smaller sizes<br>• NIV with a full-face mask should be avoided due to the risk of asphyxia, NIV with a nasal mask may be optional<br>• Lung isolation techniques are not always necessary but can be performed in those with limited cardiopulmonary reserve or severe hypoxemia as a measure to protect the nonbleeding lung<br>• Single lung ventilation by placing an ET tube into the main bronchi of non-bleeding lung or by placement of bronchial blockers to the bleeding side. It is typically employed after bronchoscopy when the bleeding side is known<br>• Double lumen tube is now less preferred to the above option as complexity associated with placement as well in maintenance of it |
| D | • Flexible bronchoscopy is the preferred first-line modality in an unstable patient<br>• Though rigid bronchoscopy has the advantage of better ventilation and airway control, flexible bronchoscopy is preferred by most bronchoscopists as most of the cases can be managed with flexible bronchoscopy and limitations of RIGID bronchoscopy, like limited centers have its availability and training for it<br>• Bronchoscopy is helpful diagnostically and can be combined with local therapies to temporize the bleeding (e.g., iced saline, local vasoconstrictors, bronchial blocker/balloon) |
| E | • CT chest is a first-line modality in a stable patient with life-threatening hemoptysis<br>• Bronchiectasis, cavitary lesion, fibrosis, fibrocavitory disease, atelectasis, pleural thickening, fungal ball, tumor, or vascular opacity are findings to suggest possible sources of bleeding and guide to proceed for angiography<br>• For patients with preexisting bilateral lung disease and/or aspiration of blood into non-bleeding segments, localization of the bleeding site may be difficult |
| F | • Repeat endovascular embolization is preferred over urgent surgery<br>• Thoracic vascular injury, leaking thoracic aneurysm with bronchial communication, and hydatid cyst are cases where urgent surgery is best option |

## REFERENCES


1. Ibrahim WH. Massive haemoptysis: the definition should be revised. Eur Respir J. 2008;32(4):1131-2.
2. Kathuria H, Hollingsworth HM, Vilvendhan R, Reardon C. Management of life-threatening hemoptysis. J Intensive Care. 2020;8:23.
3. Sopko DR, Smith TP. Smith, Bronchial artery embolization for hemoptysis. Semin Intervent Radiol. 2011;28(1):48-62.
4. Ingbar DH, Dincer HE. Evaluation and management of life-threatening hemoptysis. [Online] Available from https://www.uptodate.com/contents/evaluation-and-management-of-life-threatening-hemoptysis. [Last accessed February, 2025].
5. Radchenko C, Alraiyes AH, Shojaee S. A systematic approach to the management of massive hemoptysis. J Thorac Dis. 2017;9(Suppl 10):S1069-86.

CHAPTER

# 20 Pneumonia in an Immunocompromised Host

**TABLE 1:** Differential diagnoses according to radiological pattern.

| *Radiological pattern* | *Differential diagnoses* |
|---|---|
| Nodular lesions | • Bacterial pneumonia<br>• Aspergillosis<br>• Nocardiosis<br>• Mucormycosis |
| Micronodules | • Bacterial pneumonia<br>• Viral pneumonia<br>• Mycobacteria |
| Cavitation | • Mycobacteria<br>• Histoplasma<br>• Bacterial pneumonia (*S. aureus*) |
| Excavated nodules | • Bacterial pneumonia<br>• Nocardiosis<br>• Actinomyces<br>• Fungal (*Aspergillus, Mucor*) |
| Septal thickening | Atypical bacterial pneumonia |
| Ground glassing | • Pneumocystis<br>• Viral pneumonia<br>• Atypical bacterial pneumonia |
| Consolidation | • Bacterial pneumonia<br>• Tuberculosis<br>• Aspergillosis |
| Pleural effusion | • Bacterial pneumonia<br>• Tuberculosis |

**TABLE 2:** Types of immune defect and causes.

| *Defect* | *Type of defect* | *Cause* | *Organism* |
|---|---|---|---|
| Innate immunity | Deficiency or dysfunction of macrophages, monocytes, dendritic cells, neutrophils, NK cells, complement, pulmonary epithelium | • SOT (solid organ transplant)<br>• Steroids<br>• Neutropenia<br>• MDS (myelodysplastic syndrome)<br>• AML (Acute myeloid leukemia)<br>• HSCT (Hematopoietic stem cell transplant) – Allogenic | • Bacterial pneumonia<br>• Mycobacteria<br>• Respiratory and systemic viruses<br>• Aspergillus<br>• Mucor<br>• Nocardia<br>• Toxoplasma |

*Contd...*

*Contd...*

| Defect | Type of defect | Cause | Organism |
|---|---|---|---|
| Cell-mediated immunity | T-cell dysfunction or deficiency | • SOT<br>• Steroids<br>• Acute T-cell leukemia<br>• Hairy cell leukemia<br>• T lymphoma<br>• Chemotherapy | • Bacterial pneumonia<br>• Mycobacteria<br>• Respiratory and Systemic Viruses<br>• Toxoplasma<br>• Opportunistic infections<br>• Pneumocystis<br>• Cryptococcus |
| Humoral immunity | • B-cell dysfunction or deficiency<br>• Hypogammaglobulinemia | • Splenectomy<br>• Asplenism<br>• CVID (combined variable immune deficiency)<br>• CLL (chronic lymphoid leukemia)<br>• Complement deficiency<br>• Anti-CD-20 | • Bacterial pneumonia<br>• *S. pneumonia*<br>• *Neisseria meningitidis*<br>• *Haemophilus influenzae* |

**TABLE 3:** Most common organisms causing ICHP and their evaluation.

| Organisms | Evaluation |
|---|---|
| *Bacteria – encapsulated organisms*<br>*(Streptococcus, Hemophilus, Neisseria)*<br>*Pseudomonas, Klebsiella, MRSA*<br>*Mycobacterium tuberculosis*<br>*Non-tuberculous Mycobacteria*<br>*Legionella* | • Sputum/Blood/BAL – culture<br>• BAL PCR<br>• Urine antigen<br>• Tissue culture in extrapulmonary involvement<br>• Sputum/BAL/Tissue – AFB and CBNAAT |
| • *Viruses – HSV, CMV, VZV, Adeno*<br>• *RNA viruses (Influenza, Para influenza viruses, Rhinovirus, Human Meta Pneumovirus)* | • PCR – BAL, blood, tissue<br>• Tissue culture<br>• Serology<br>• Histopathology |
| *Fungal – Aspergillus, Nocardia, Mucor, Pneumocystis jiroveci, Cryptococcus, Blastomyces, Histoplasma* | • Blood/Sputum/ BAL – staining, culture, PCR<br>• BAL/Serum Galactomannan<br>• Serum/urine antigen<br>• Tissue culture<br>• Histopathology |
| *Parasites: Toxoplasma gondi and Strongyloides stercoralis* | Blood/BAL/pleural/peritoneal fluid PCR |

## SUGGESTED READING


1. Azoulay E, Russell L, Van De Louw A, Metaxa V, Bauer P, Povoa P, et al. Diagnosis of severe respiratory infections in immunocompromised patients. Intensive Care Med. 2020;46(2):298-314.
2. Cheng GS, Crothers K, Aliberti S, Bergeron A, Boeckh M, Chien JW, et al. Immunocompromised Host Pneumonia: Definitions and Diagnostic Criteria: An Official American Thoracic Society Workshop Report. Ann Am Thorac Soc. 2023;20(3):341-53.

CHAPTER 21

# Pleural Effusions in Intensive Care Unit

## INTRODUCTION

Pleural effusions are commonly identified in critically ill patients. By itself, pleural effusions are an uncommon indication for ICU admission. There may be an underlying systemic illness or pleural disease.

## ASSOCIATED MEDICAL CONDITIONS IN INTENSIVE CARE UNIT[1-3]

| | *Transudates* | *Exudates* |
|---|---|---|
| Common | • Left heart failure<br>• Nephrotic syndrome<br>• Cirrhosis of liver<br>• Ascites<br>• Peritoneal dialysis<br>• Lung atelectasis | • Parapneumonic<br>• Pulmonary embolism<br>• Malignancy<br>• Collagen vascular disease |
| Uncommon | • Pulmonary embolism<br>• Hypoalbuminemia<br>• Myxedema<br>• Iatrogenic | • Pancreatitis<br>• Uremia<br>• Drug-induced Iatrogenic |

## ASSOCIATED SURGICAL CONDITIONS IN INTENSIVE CARE UNIT

- Subphrenic and other abdominal collections
- Blunt or penetrating thoracic trauma
- Aortic dissection or aneurysm
- Esophageal injury
- Postoperatively after cardiothoracic surgery
- Urinothorax
- Chylothorax

## MANAGEMENT[2-4]

- Chest X-ray easily misses an effusion in the ICU, ultrasound picks up almost all effusions, and a CT scan is the gold standard. However, a CT chest is not always feasible in an intubated patient in ICU. CT scans point towards a specific etiology like LV failure or malignancy and help in decision-making on pleural drainage
- USG is portable, simple point-of-care testing at the bedside. There is no radiation exposure. Also helps in the characterization of the internal complexity of effusion. It can help in diagnostic or therapeutic interventions. The sensitivity and specificity of identifying an effusion depends on the user. Ultrasound-guided thoracocentesis reduces complications like pneumothorax
- Diagnostic thoracocentesis can often help in changing the management of the patient
- Small bilateral effusions attributable to fluid overload can be observed. Asymptomatic effusions in the first 48 hours following a major thoracic or abdominal surgery can be observed
- *Diagnostic thoracocentesis:* If there is a suspected infection, malignancy, uncertain diagnosis or, clinical deterioration, or persistent/enlarging effusion causing symptoms or gas-exchange abnormalities
- Therapeutic thoracocentesis can lead to improvement in oxygenation and end-expiratory lung volume. Therapeutic thoracocentesis should be done if there is a benefit from the intervention clinically

## APPROACH TO PLEURAL EFFUSIONS IN INTENSIVE CARE UNIT

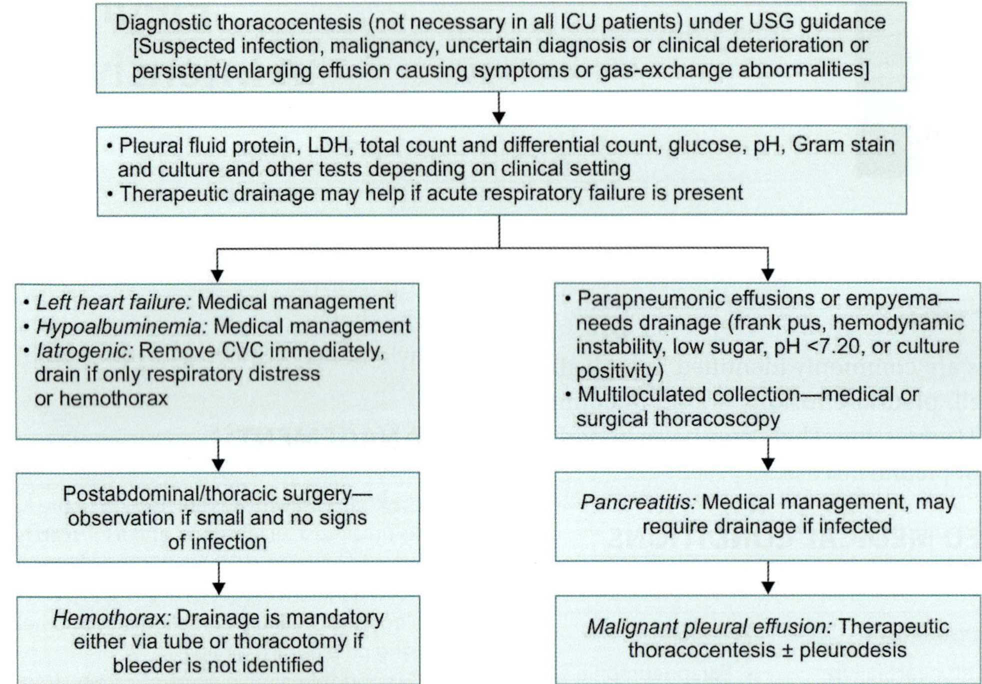


## REFERENCES


1. Fartoukh M, Azoulay E, Galliot R, Le Gall JR, Baud F, Chevret S, et al. Clinically documented pleural effusions in medical ICU patients: how useful is routine thoracentesis? Chest. 2002;121(1):178-84.
2. Vetrugno L, Bignami E, Orso D, Vargas M, Guadagnin GM, Saglietti F, et al. Utility of pleural effusion drainage in the ICU: an updated systematic review and META-analysis. J Critic Care. 2019;52:22-32.
3. Bediwy AS, Al-Biltagi M, Saeed NK, Bediwy HA, Elbeltagi R. Pleural effusion in critically ill patients and intensive care setting. World J Clin Cases. 2023;11(5):989-99.
4. Fysh ET, Smallbone P, Mattock N, McCloskey C, Litton E, Wibrow B, et al. Clinically significant pleural effusion in intensive care: a prospective multicenter cohort study. Critical Care Explorations. 2020;2(1):e0070.

CHAPTER

# 22 Algorithm for Dyspnea in ER: USG-based Approach

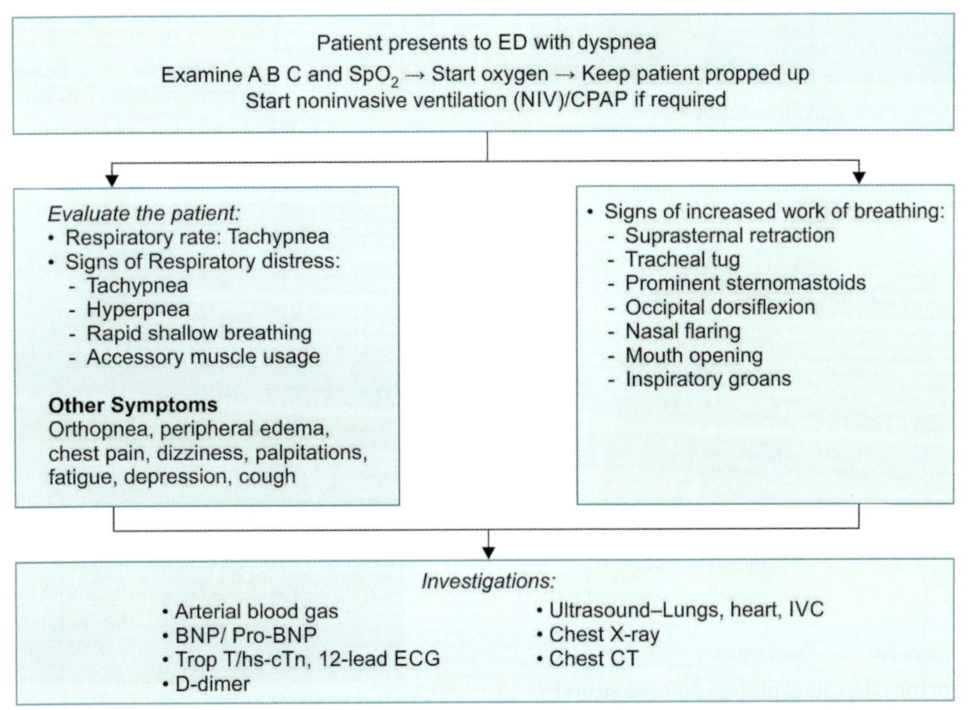


## RELEVANCE OF ULTRASOUND IN A PATIENT WITH DYSPNEA

Ultrasound use at the bedside is increasing and being performed routinely in the intensive care units and the emergency departments.[1-3] Patients presenting with acute dyspnea are common at the emergency room and need to be managed urgently. The modality of lung ultrasound can aid the physician in making a differential diagnosis rapidly and can be very useful for timely management of such patients.

Being portable and radiation-free, a real-time examination of lungs is feasible, US is comparable to chest radiography and may have higher sensitivity and similar specificity for detection of pleural effusion, pneumonia, pneumothorax, and pulmonary edema.[4-7]

Lung US is predominantly an artifact-based imaging modality, typically visualizing only abnormalities touching the pleural line.

## REQUIREMENTS FOR US EXAMINATION

*Probes* ***(Fig. 1):*** Curvilinear or phased-array 5–9-MHz probes. Linear 7–12-MHz probes offer the best resolution of superficial structures and are useful in children.

Examine from cephalic to caudal direction on the anterior, lateral, and posterior chest wall bilaterally (6 areas) with patient in both the supine and upright position **(Figs. 2 to 4)**. Keep probe perpendicular to the

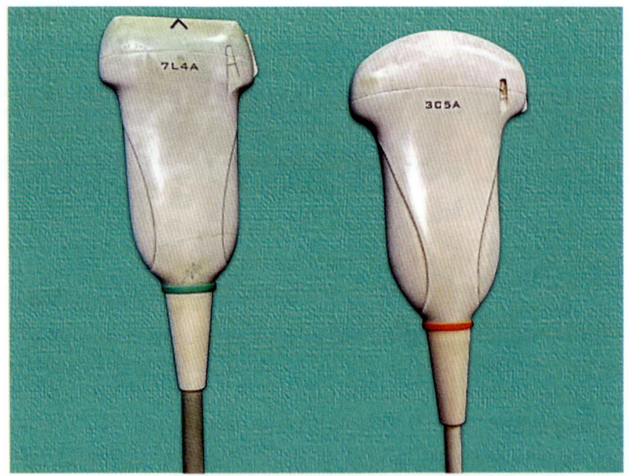

**Fig. 1:** Linear and curvilinear probes.

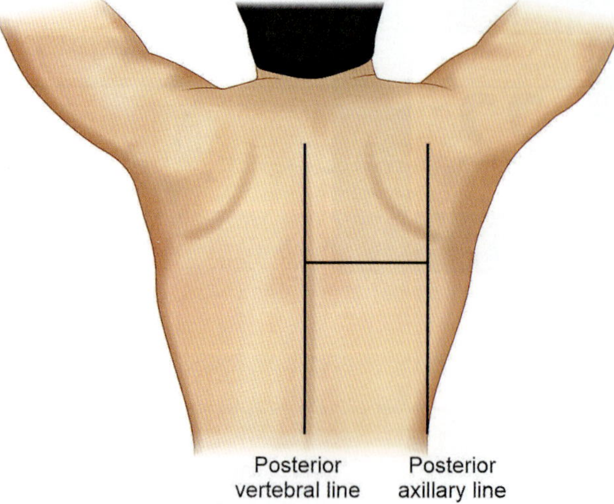

**Fig. 4:** Posterior chest wall.

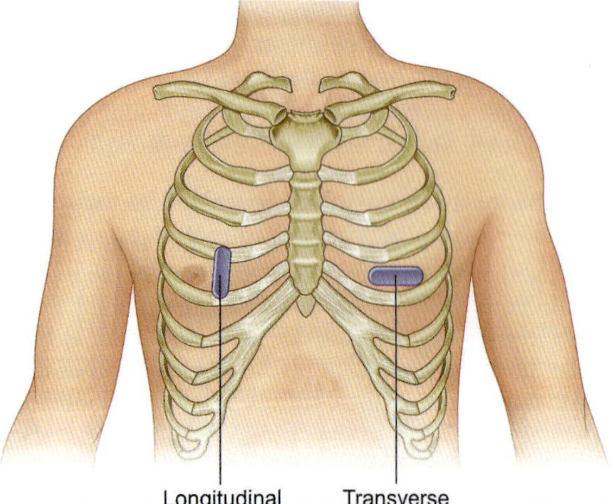

**Fig. 2:** Placement of the ultrasound probe—transverse and sagittal views of anterior chest wall.

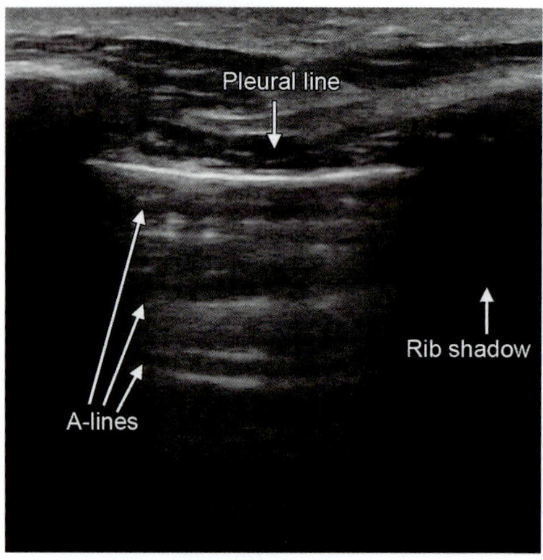

**Fig. 5:** A-lines ultrasound image.

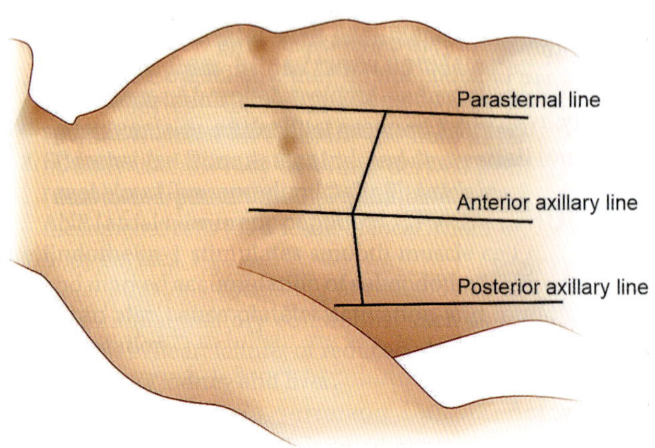

**Fig. 3:** Lateral chest wall.

skin to ensure perpendicular orientation to the pleural line to produce the requisite artifacts for interpretation and the marker pointing toward head end.[8,9]

*Look for the following findings:*

- *Pleural line:* It is the hyperechoic line that represents the junction of the visceral and the parietal pleura.
- *A-lines* ***(Figs. 5 and 6)****:* Repetitive horizontal artifacts seen parallel to the pleural line, which are essentially reverberation artifacts of the hyperechoic pleural line. The black knobby shadows are the rib shadows and between them are the intercostal spaces, where A-lines can be appreciated.
- *B-lines* ***(Figs. 7 and 8)****:* With the thickening of the interstitium, hyperechoic vertical artifacts arising from

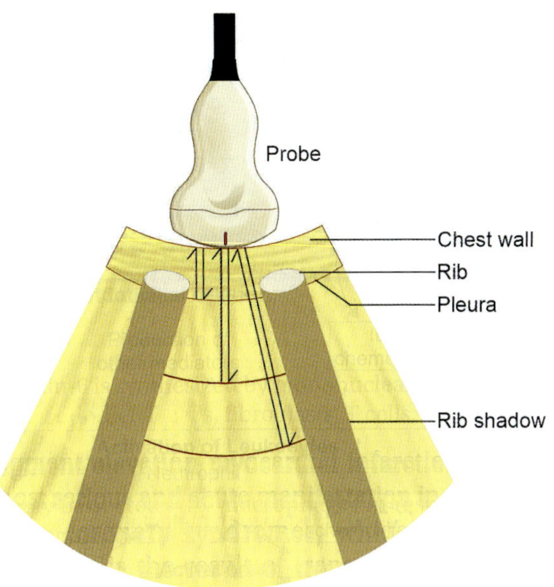


**Fig. 6:** A-lines—schematic image.

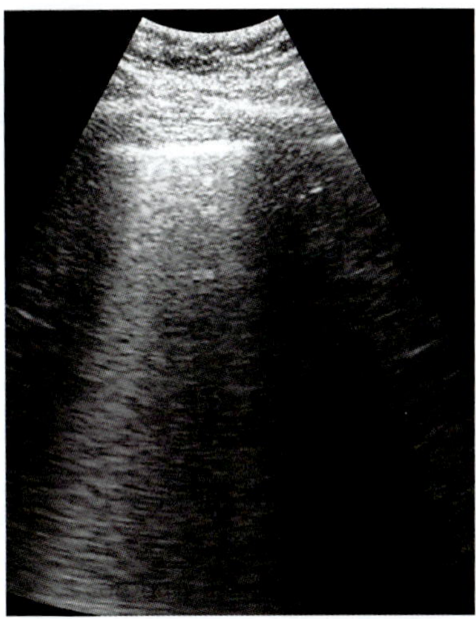

**Fig. 7:** B-lines—ultrasound image.

the pleural line are seen, which cut across to the bottom of the image, wiping out the normal A-lines. They are also known as comet-tail artifact.[1,8] This appearance is seen in secondary to fibrosis or fluid. Lesser than 2 lines per interspace may be normal.[2,10]

As per the BLUE-protocol, lung scan has to be performed bilaterally and at three areas: the mid-subclavicular line, the point just crural to the nipple; at the point at which the posterior axillary line crosses the horizontal nipple line (PLAPS point-posterolateral alveolar and/or pleural Syndrome).[11]

- *Lung sliding:* This is a twinkling visible at the pleural line, which happens due to the respiration causing

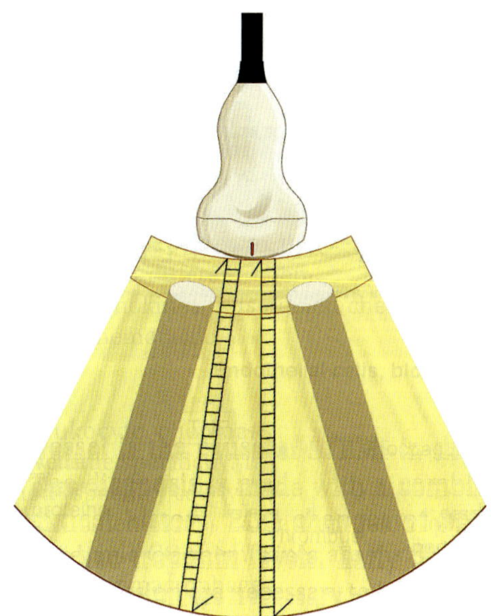

**Fig. 8:** B-lines—schematic image.

the sliding of visceral and parietal pleura against each other seen as a glistening motion of the pleural line. Absence of lung sliding' in the presence of A-lines and "lung point" indicates pneumothorax (81% sensitive and 100% specific).
- *Lung point:* In case of pneumothorax, the visceral and parietal pleura are separated and the normal sliding is lost in that area. There is a point of transition between the pneumothorax and normal lung, where on one side, lung sliding is absent and in the other side it is visible. If this is identified it is 100% specific for pneumothorax.[12]
- *M-mode imaging:* In a normal lung, above the pleural line there are smooth horizontal lines and beneath the pleural line, due to lung motion there is a sandy/granular appearance, which is known as 'seashore' sign. In case of a pneumothorax, there is no lung movement below the pleura, hence the whole picture appears as uninterrupted horizontal lines, which is known as the 'bar code sign', this being diagnostic **(Fig. 9)**.
- *Pleural effusion:* Seen as an anechoic area between parietal and visceral pleura along with sinusoid sign, which occurs due to movement of the pleura to and fro from the chest wall during breathing, forming a sinusoidal waveform, best seen in the M-mode (dynamic sign) **(Fig. 10)**.

Simple effusions are usually present in the posterior dependent lung.[1,5,8] Complexities arising due to chronic effusions, malignant effusions, hemithorax, and empyema, appear more heterogeneous depending on the amount of

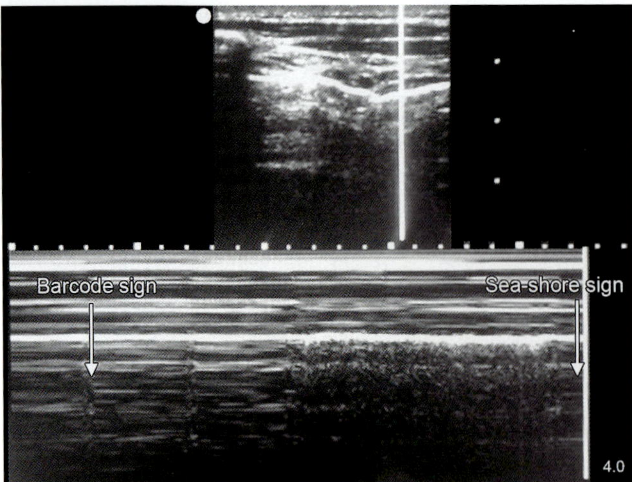


**Fig. 9:** Barcode and sea-shore sign.

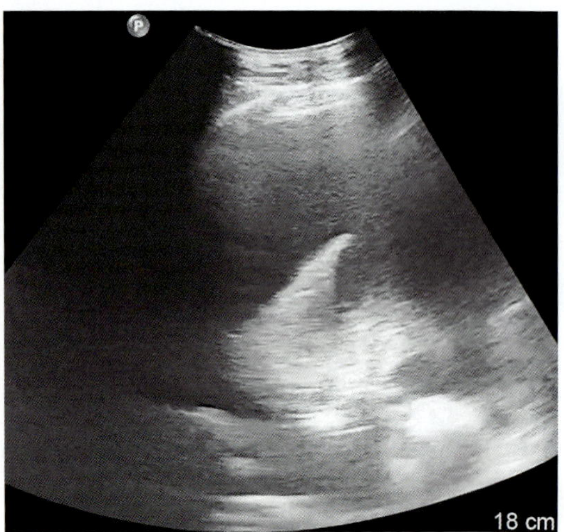


**Fig. 10:** Pleural effusion with atelectatic lung.

debris or septations or pleural thickening. In case of a large effusion, there is a wider acoustic window, sometimes vertebral bodies can be visualized, this is the *spine sign*.

- Acute interstitial syndrome (AIS), defined as B-pattern with at least three B-lines in two lung zones bilaterally. This interstitial pattern showing multiple B-lines along with some irregularity of the pleural line usually develops as a first step in the loss of aeration.
- *Consolidation:* Focal B-lines with tissue-like echo-texture (hepatization) and dynamic air broncho-grams (hyperechoic punctiform images). This pattern develops as a result of loss of aeration. Increasing density and echogenicity indicates increasing severity of the condition.
- *Pneumonia:* It appears as solid 'liver' like appearance on the ultrasound, this is also known as *hepatization.* Lungs become congested due to presence of fluid or cells and the A-lines disappear. Initially there may be presence of B-lines. If air bronchograms are present, they are manifested as hyperechoic foci within the consolidated lung. Sometimes, the consolidated abnormal lung and the aerated normal lung can be seen divided by an irregular hyperechoic line, this is known as *shred sign.*

## CHEST ULTRASOUND FINDINGS AND CLINICAL ENTITIES

| | *A-lines* | *B-lines* | *Lund sliding* | *Lung point* | *Pleural effusion* |
|---|---|---|---|---|---|
| Normal | Present | Rare | Present | Absent | Absent |
| Pulmonary edema | Absent | Present (many) | Present | Absent | May be present |
| Interstitial syndrome | Absent | Present – number according to intensity | Present | Absent | Absent |
| Pneumothorax | Present/ Absent | Rules out Pneumothorax | Rules out Pneumothorax | Characteristic of Pneumothorax | Absent |
| Pneumonia | Absent | Present (many) | Present | Absent | |
| Fibrosis | Absent | Present | Absent | Absent | Absent |

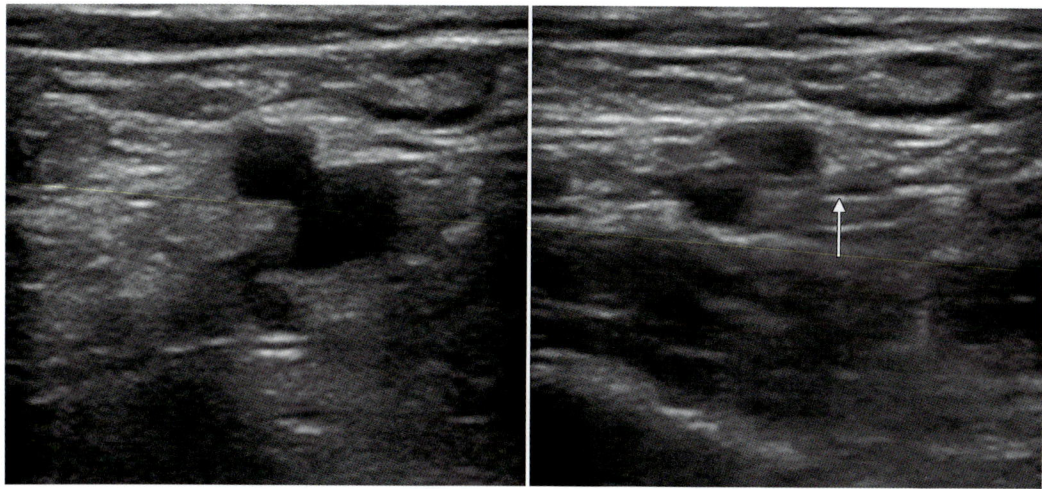

**Fig. 11:** Vein collapsing on compression indicating no clots.

Apart from the lungs, cardiac ultrasound is evaluated:

- Left ventricular function and size
- Right ventricular function and size
- Subxiphoid view—for the IVC diameter, which is visualized 2 cm caudal to the hepatic vein inlet. Collapsibility during inspiration is noted by placing the probe in the long axis with M mode.[13] A maximum diameter of ≥2 cm along with <50% collapsibility was indicative of plethoric IVC and on the other hand a maximal diameter of ≤2 cm and >50% collapsibility was considered collapsible.
- Parasternal long and short-axis views—left ventricular ejection fraction is estimated by wall contraction and thickening.[14]
- Mitral valve E-point septal separation (EPSS) indicates status of the left ventricular function—it is the distance measured from the anterior mitral valve leaflet and the ventricular septum in early diastole measured in M mode. Left ventricular systolic function is graded as normal (EF > 50%), moderate dysfunction (EF 30–50%), or severe dysfunction (EF <30%) based on eyeballing and EPSS measurement.

Next, scan Lower extremity vasculature for thrombosis. Diagnosis can be done by direct visualization within the veins, by compressing the veins (non-compressibility indicating a clot) and by using the Color Doppler Augmentation (on squeezing the distal part of the leg, if there is a homogenous increase in venous flow, it indicates no occlusive thrombus in between) **(Fig. 11)**.

Scanning is to be done starting with the common femoral vein (CFV), Great Saphenous Vein, Bifurcation of CFV into Femoral Vein and Deep Femoral Vein, Popliteal Vein and Trifurcation of the Popliteal Vein (Anterior Tibial Vein, Posterior Tibial Vein and Peroneal Vein).

## ALGORITHM FOR USG-BASED APPROACH: PATIENT PRESENTING WITH SEVERE DYSPNEA

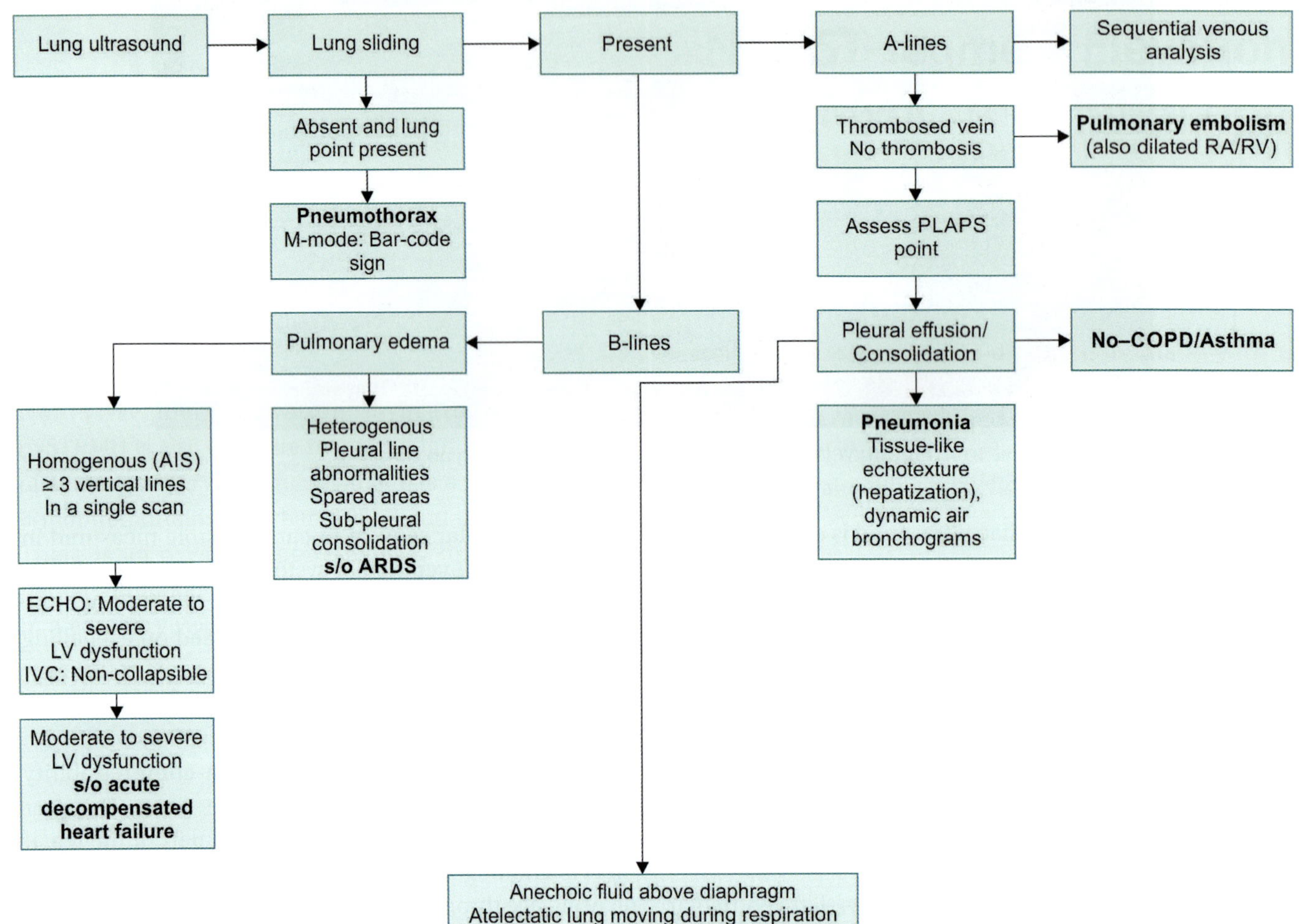


Lung ultrasound s/o pulmonary edema indicates acute heart failure based on diffuse B-lines, also termed alveolar interstitial syndrome (AIS), although this is highly sensitive, but this can be found in noncardiogenic pulmonary edema, bilateral pneumonia, pulmonary fibrosis, acute respiratory distress syndrome and lung cancer. Additional scanning of the IVC for collapsibility and diameter variation with inspiration, indicating high CVP can supplement for diagnosis of Acute heart failure, but this also lacks specificity (elevated CVP can be seen in cardiac tamponade, pulmonary embolism, and valvular heart disease). Ultrasound scanning protocol including lung, cardiac, and IVC together can diagnose acute heart failure with near 100% specificity.[15]

The algorithm approach with help of lung ultrasound in a patient with dyspnea can help in reaching a working diagnosis and accurately differentiate conditions like acute heart failure, pneumothorax, pneumonia, ARDS, etc. This approach helps an emergency physician to diagnose various conditions at the bedside to supplement his/her clinical acumen.

## REFERENCES

1. Lichtenstein DA. Lung ultrasound in the critically ill. Ann Intensive Care. 2014;4(1):1.
2. Lichtenstein DA. Current Misconceptions in Lung Ultrasound: A Short Guide for Experts. Chest. 2019;156(1):21-5.
3. Saraogi A. Lung ultrasound: Present and future. Lung India. 2015;32(3):250-7.
4. Ebrahimi A, Yousefifard M, Mohammad Kazemi H, Rasouli HR, Asady H, Moghadas Jafari A, et al. Diagnostic Accuracy of Chest Ultrasonography versus Chest Radiography for Identification of Pneumothorax: A Systematic Review and Meta-Analysis. Tanaffos. 2014;13(4):29-40.

5. Lichtenstein D, Goldstein I, Mourgeon E, Cluzel P, Grenier P, Rouby JJ. Comparative diagnostic performances of auscultation, chest radiography, and lung ultrasonography in acute respiratory distress syndrome. Anesthesiology. 2004;100(1):9-15.
6. Maw AM, Hassanin A, Ho PM, McInnes MDF, Moss A, Juarez-Colunga E, et al. Diagnostic Accuracy of Point-of-Care Lung Ultrasonography and Chest Radiography in Adults With Symptoms Suggestive of Acute Decompensated Heart Failure: A Systematic Review and Meta-analysis. JAMA Netw Open. 2019;2(3):e190703.
7. Ye X, Xiao H, Chen B, Zhang S. Accuracy of Lung Ultrasonography versus Chest Radiography for the Diagnosis of Adult Community-Acquired Pneumonia: Review of the Literature and Meta-Analysis. PLoS One. 2015;10(6):e0130066.
8. Gargani L, Volpicelli G. How I do it: lung ultrasound. Cardiovasc Ultrasound. 2014;12(1):25.
9. Buonsenso D, Musolino AM, Gatto A, Lazzareschi I, Curatola A, Valentini P. Lung ultrasound in infants with bronchiolitis. BMC Pulm Med. 2019;19(1):159.
10. Neto FMJ, Rahal AJ, Vieira FA, da Silva PS, de Gusmao Funari MB. Advances in lung ultrasound. Einstein (Sao Paulo). 2016;14(3):443-8.
11. Lichtenstein DA, Meziere GA. Relevance of lung ultrasound in the diagnosis of acute respiratory failure*: the BLUE protocol. Chest. 2008;134:117-25.
12. Lichtenstein D, Meziere G, Biderman P, Gepner A. The "lung point": an ultrasound sign specific to pneumothorax. Intensive Care Med. 2000;26(10):1434-40.
13. Wallace DJ, Allison M, Stone MB. Inferior vena cava percentage collapse during respiration is affected by the sampling location: an ultrasound study in healthy volunteers. Acad Emerg Med. 2010;17:96-9.
14. Moore CL, Rose GA, Tayal VS, Sullivan DM, Arrowood JA, Kline JA. Determination of left ventricular function by emergency physician echocardiography of hypotensive patients. Acad Emerg Med. 2002;9:186-93.
15. Russell FM, Ehrman RR, Cosby K, Ansari A, Tseeng S, Christain E, et al. Acute Heart Failure in Patients With Undifferentiated Dyspnea: A Lung and Cardiac Ultrasound (LuCUS) Protocol. Acad Emerg Med. 2015;22:182-91.

# PART 2

# CARDIOVASCULAR/HEMODYNAMICS

***Editors:*** Natesh Prabu R, Jacob George Pulinilkunnathil

***Associate Editors:*** M Srivatsa Nagachandan, Vaishnavi R, Rahul Baby Joseph, Mathew Antony, Nishanth Baliga, Sandhya S, Kandaswamy N, Divya Dinakar, Priyanka KJ, Hemalatha RV, Vadhan Prasanna S, Thomas Isaiah Sudarsan

CHAPTER

# 23 ST-segment Elevation Myocardial Infarction

## INTRODUCTION

ST-segment elevation myocardial infarction (STEMI) is the most serious and acute manifestation in the spectrum of acute coronary syndromes, which needs prompt treatment. It is the result of transmural ischemia and is associated with significant morbidity and mortality. Though it can be due to occlusive or non-occlusive causes of coronary artery disease, a complete thrombotic occlusion by an atherosclerotic plaque in an epicardial coronary vessel is the cause of STEMI in the majority of cases. The diagnosis is made with a combination of positive clinical history, ECG changes of STEMI, and elevated cardiac troponin levels. Early diagnosis and immediate reperfusion are necessary to limit the ischemia and infarct size, which helps to reduce the risk of post-STEMI complications and heart failure. Reperfusion strategies depend on both hospital and patient-related factors.

**TABLE 1:** Significant ECG changes for STEMI.

| |
|---|
| New ST elevation at the J-point in at least two contiguous leads:<br>1. ≥2.5 mm in men <40 years } In V2–V3<br>≥2 mm in men >40 years } In V2–V3<br>≥1.5 mm in women regardless of age<br>2. ≥1 mm in the other leads (in the absence of left ventricular hypertrophy or left bundle branch block)<br>J point |
| ST-segment elevation in V3R and V4R → ongoing RV ischemia |
| ST-segment depression in leads V1–V3 and/or ST-segment elevation in V7–V9 → posterior coronary artery occlusion |
| ST depression ≥1 mm in ≥6 surface leads (inferolateral ST depression) and ST-segment elevation in aVR and/or V1 → multi-vessel ischemia or left main coronary artery obstruction |
| **New onset left bundle branch block** |

**TABLE 2:** MINOCA presenting as STEMI.

- Central chest pain is classically retrosternal, crushing, heavy, severe, and diffuse in nature
- Described by the patient as 'pressing' or 'squeezing'
- May occur at rest or on activity or wax and wane in intensity
- Sometimes radiating to the left arm, neck, or jaw AND associated symptoms of nausea, vomiting dyspnea, light-headedness, palpitations, syncope, anxiety, or impending sense of doom

(MINOCA: myocardial infarction with non-obstructive coronary artery)

**Flowchart 1:** Algorithm for management of ST-elevation myocardial infarction.

*If necessary:*
- Supplemental oxygen
- Nitrates
- Analgesics
- Beta-blockers

- Antiplatelets
- Anticoagulant

PCI facility available within 2 hours

Yes → Coronary angiography to look for obstruction → Coronary artery

- Obstructed → Percutaneous coronary intervention within 2 hours → Emergency coronary artery bypass surgery if unfavorable anatomy for PCI
- Not obstructed → MINOCA → Medical therapy and risk factor optimization

No → Symptoms of ischemia >12 hours

- Yes → Fibrinolysis not recommended → Evidence of ongoing ischemia
  - No → Non-urgent PCI
  - Yes → Transfer to a PCI facility within 24 hours → Coronary angiography to look for obstruction
- No → Contraindications to fibrinolysis
  - Yes → Transfer to a PCI facility within 24 hours
  - No →
    - Fibrinolysis with tenecteplase/alteplase/reteplase
    - Streptokinase in resource-limited settings

    → Transfer to a PCI facility within 24 hours

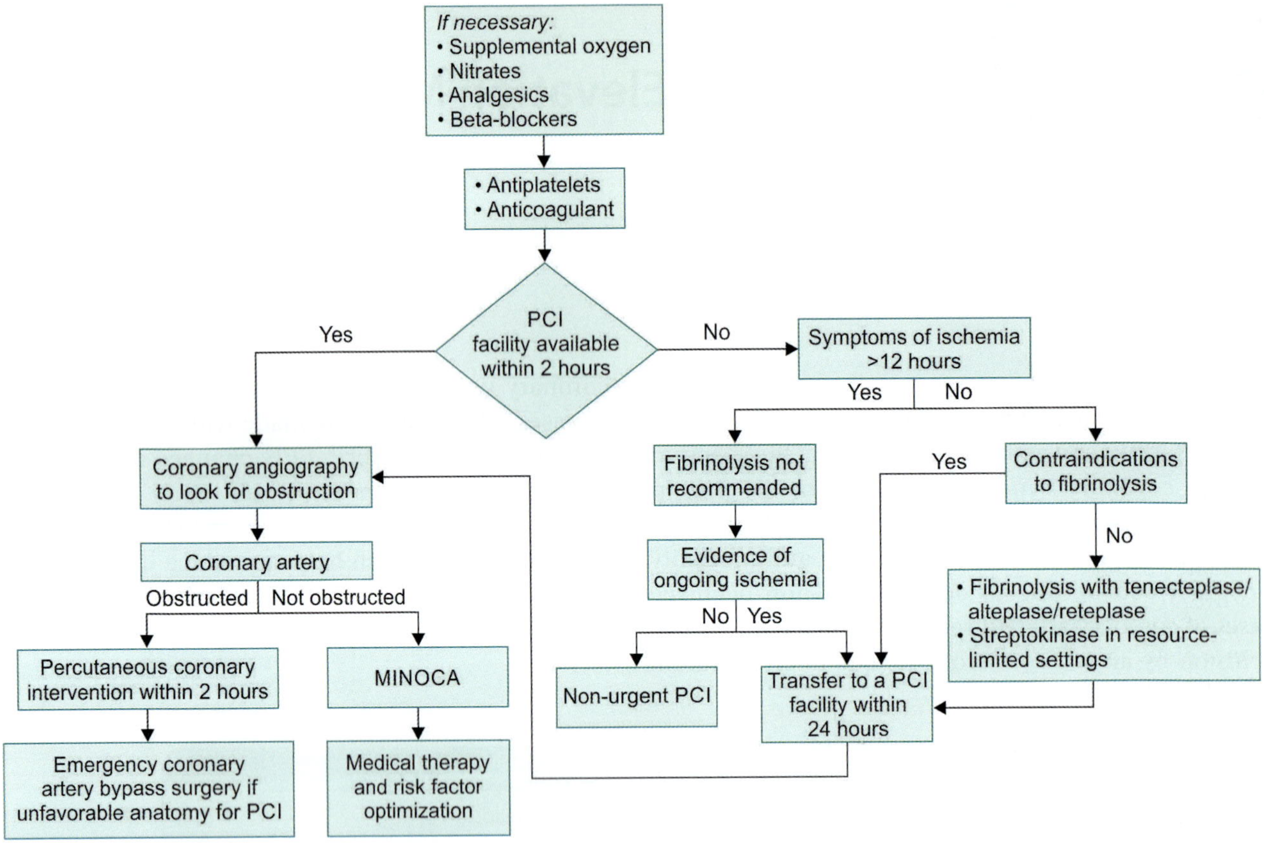

(MINOCA: myocardial Infarction with non-obstructive coronary artery; PCI: percutaneous coronary intervention; STEMI: ST-elevation myocardial infarction)

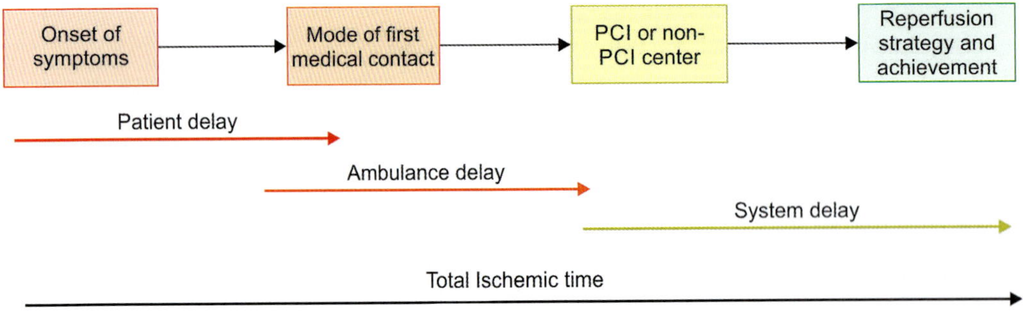


**Fig. 1:** Total ischemic time and sources of delay.

## REPERFUSION STRATEGIES FOR STEMI

| Primary PCI | Thrombolysis | Post-thrombolysis PCI |
|---|---|---|
| • Within 90–120 minutes of pain onset<br>• Wire crossing time 60 minutes<br>• First-line reperfusion strategy for STEMI | • Can be done from 3 hours to 12 hours of pain onset<br>• Lytic time 10 minutes | • Rescue PCI for failed thrombolysis<br>• Pharmacoinvasive strategy PCI after 3–24 hours of thrombolysis |

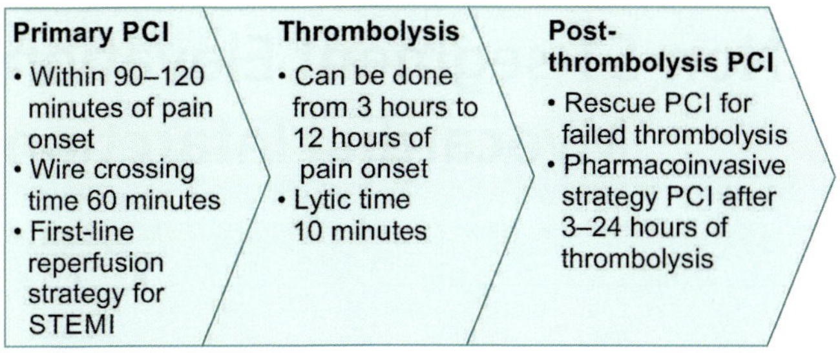

**Fig. 2:** Reperfusion strategies for STEMI. (PCI: percutaneous coronary intervention; STEMI: ST-elevation myocardial infarction)

## CONTRAINDICATIONS TO THROMBOLYSIS

**TABLE 3:** Contraindications to thrombolysis.

| *Absolute contraindications* | *Relative contraindications* |
|---|---|
| • Previous ischemic or hemorrhagic stroke <6 months<br>• CNS – AVM<br>• Aortic dissection<br>• Active bleeding or bleeding diathesis, excluding menstruation<br>• Significant closed-head trauma or facial trauma within 3 months | • TIA < 6 months<br>• Pregnancy<br>• BP >180/110 mm Hg<br>• Prolonged CPR (>10 minutes) patients<br>• Major surgery within 3 weeks<br>• Active peptic ulcer<br>• Current use of anticoagulant that has produced an elevated INR >1.7 |

(BP: blood pressure; CNS-AVM: central nervous system arteriovenous malformations; INR: international normalized ratio; TIA: transient Ischemic attack)

**TABLE 4:** Indications for emergency coronary artery bypass graft (CABG) in patients with MI.

- Vascular anatomy is not amenable to PCI
- Cardiogenic shock
- Mechanical complications like free wall/papillary muscle rupture
- Failed PCI with ongoing ischemia

(PCI: percutaneous coronary intervention)

**TABLE 5:** Initial antiplatelet therapy.

***Aspirin to all patients***

- *Patients treated with primary PCI:* Ticagrelor loading dose of 180 mg or prasugrel loading dose of 60 mg
- Patients at high risk of bleeding or those for whom prasugrel or ticagrelor cannot be used: clopidogrel 600 mg
- *Patients treated with fibrinolytics:* Clopidogrel loading dose 300 mg if age ≤75 years

*Contd…*

*Contd…*

***Aspirin to all patients***

- If the age is ≥75 years, give loading dose of 75 mg
- *Patients not receiving reperfusion therapy:* Ticagrelor loading dose 180 mg

(PCI: percutaneous coronary intervention)

**TABLE 6:** Initial anticoagulant therapy.

- *Patients treated with primary PCI:* Consider UFH in patients who receive a potent oral antiplatelet agent (ticagrelor or prasugrel)
- For those patients who receive clopidogrel, consider bivalirudin
- *Patients treated with fibrinolysis:* Enoxaparin is for patients not at high bleeding risk, and fondaparinux is for those at high bleeding risk
- For those patients in whom PCI is possible or likely after fibrinolytic therapy, UFH is used
- *Patients not receiving reperfusion therapy:* Enoxaparin or UFH

(PCI: percutaneous coronary intervention)

## COMPLICATIONS AFTER STEMI

| Mechanical | Arrhythmic | Ischemic |
|---|---|---|
| Ventricular septal rupture | Atrial fibrillation is most common | Heart failure |
| Septal rupture | Inadequate perfusion due to ischemia leads to ventricular tachyarrhythmias | Postinfarction pericarditis |
| Papillary muscle rupture | | Left ventricular thrombus |

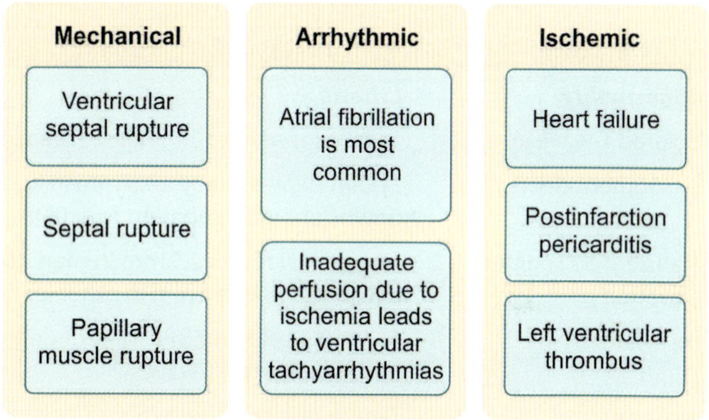

**Fig. 3:** Complications after STEMI.

## SUGGESTED READING


1. Bhatt DL, Lopes RD, Harrington RA. Diagnosis and treatment of acute coronary syndromes: A Review. JAMA. 2022;327(7):662-75.
2. Byrne RA, Rossello X, Coughlan JJ, Barbato E, Berry C, Chieffo A, et al. 2023 ESC guidelines for the management of acute coronary syndromes. Eur Heart J. 2023;44(38):3720-826.
3. Gulati M, Levy PD, Mukherjee D, Amsterdam E, Bhatt DL, Birtcher KK, et al. 2021 AHA/ACC/ASE/Chest/Saem/SCCT/SCMR guideline for the evaluation and diagnosis of chest pain: A report of the American College of Cardiology/American Heart Association Joint Committee on Clinical Practice Guidelines. Circulation. 2021;144(22):e368-454.

CHAPTER 24

# Non-ST-segment Elevation Myocardial Infarction

## INTRODUCTION

Non-ST-segment elevation myocardial infarction (NSTEMI) is also an acute manifestation in the spectrum of acute coronary syndromes that has a relatively lower 6-month mortality rate than STEMI and unstable angina. There is an oxygen supply–demand mismatch due to partial thrombotic occlusion by an atherosclerotic plaque in a coronary vessel or due to transient occlusion of the vessel like vasospasm. The diagnosis is made with a combination of positive clinical history, electrocardiogram (ECG) changes of NSTEMI, and elevated cardiac troponin levels. Medical management is imperative, with further work-up for evaluation and definitive treatment planned.

## ECG ABNORMALITIES IN PATIENTS WITH NON-ST-SEGMENT ELEVATION ACUTE CORONARY SYNDROME

**TABLE 1:** ECG abnormalities in patients with non-ST-segment elevation acute coronary syndrome.

| ***Abnormality*** | ***Criteria*** |
|---|---|
| Isolated T-wave inversion | T-wave inversion >1 mm in ≥5 leads including, I, II, aVL, and V2–V6 |
| ST segment depression | J point depressed by ≥0.5 mm in leads V2 and V3 or ≥1 mm in all other leads followed by a horizontal or downsloping ST-segment for ≥0.08s in ≥1 leads (except aVR) |
| Transient ST-segment elevation | J point elevation ≥2.5 mm in men <40 years, ≥2 mm in men >40 years, ≥1.5 mm in women regardless of age in V2–V3 or ≥1 mm in other leads lasting for <20 minutes |
| De-winter ST-T | 1–3 mm upsloping ST-segment depression at the J point in leads V1–V6 that continue into tall, positive, and symmetrical T-waves |
| Wellen's | *Type A:* Isoelectric or minimally elevated J point (<1 mm) + biphasic T-wave in leads V2 and V3<br>*Type B:* Symmetric and deeply inverted T waves in leads V2 and V3, occasionally in leads V1, V4, V5, and V6 |

**TABLE 2:** Criteria for urgent versus early invasive angiography in NSTEMI.

| ***Criteria for urgent/immediate PCI in NSTEMI*** | ***Criteria for the early invasive strategy of invasive angiography ± PCI within 24 h of NSTEMI*** |
|---|---|
| Hemodynamic instability | A confirmed diagnosis of NSTEMI based on hs-cTn algorithms |
| Recurrent or ongoing chest pain refractory to medical treatment | Dynamic ST-segment or T-wave changes |
| Acute HF presumed secondary to ongoing myocardial ischemia | Transient ST-segment elevation |
| Life-threatening arrhythmias or cardiac arrest after presentation | A GRACE risk score >140 |
| Mechanical complications | |
| Recurrent dynamic ECG changes suggestive of ischemia | |

(GRACE: Global Registry of Acute Coronary Events; NSTEMI: non-ST-elevation myocardial infarction; PCI: percutaneous coronary intervention)

**Flowchart 1:** Algorithm for management of non-ST elevation myocardial infarction (NSTEMI).

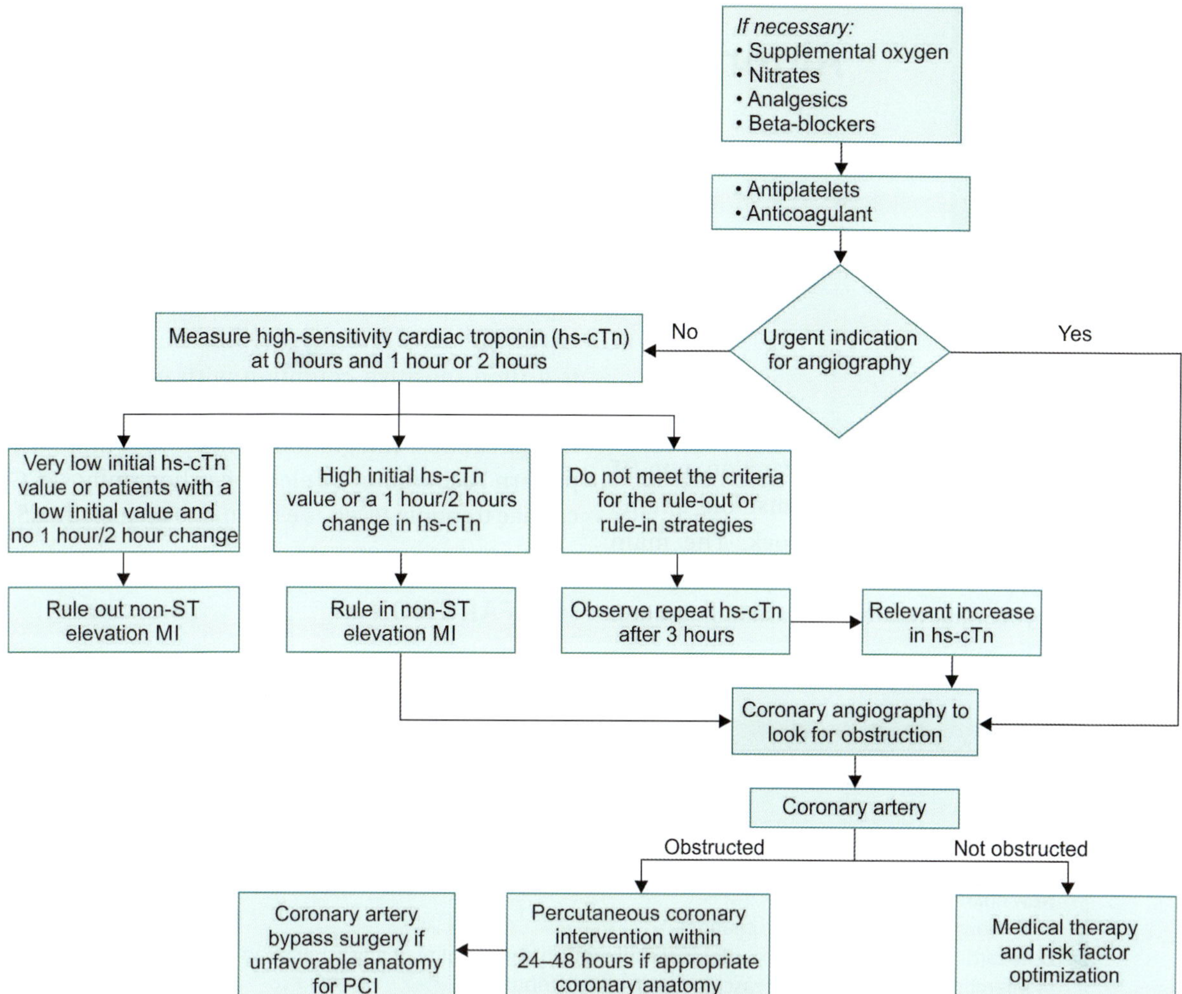


(hs-cTn: high-sensitivity cardiac troponin)

## SUGGESTED READING

1. Bhatt DL, Lopes RD, Harrington RA. Diagnosis and Treatment of Acute Coronary Syndromes: A Review. JAMA. 2022;327(7):662-75.
2. Byrne RA, Rossello X, Coughlan JJ, Barbato E, Berry C, Chieffo A, et al. 2023 ESC Guidelines for the management of acute coronary syndromes. Eur Heart J. 2023;44(38):3720-826.
3. Gulati M, Levy PD, Mukherjee D, Amsterdam E, Bhatt DL, Birtcher KK, et al. 2021 AHA/ACC/ASE/Chest/Saem/SCCT/SCMR guideline for the evaluation and diagnosis of chest pain: A report of the American College of Cardiology/American Heart Association Joint Committee on Clinical Practice Guidelines. Circulation. 2021;144(22):e368-454.

CHAPTER 25

# Algorithm for Acute Coronary Syndrome Evaluation and Unstable Angina

## INTRODUCTION

Acute coronary syndrome (ACS) is a spectrum of diseases ranging from ST-elevation myocardial infarction, non-ST elevation myocardial infarction, and unstable angina (UA) with or without cardiogenic shock. The main pathophysiology in ACS is the demand-supply mismatch of oxygen to the myocardial tissue. Myocardial infarction is a time-sensitive condition with early diagnosis and treatment resulting in markedly better benefits and less complications. Integration of history, symptoms, signs, pattern recognition of electrocardiography (ECG), and cardiac troponin levels is essential to diagnose ACS.

## UNIVERSAL DEFINITION OF MYOCARDIAL INFARCTION

**BOX 1:** Universal definition of myocardial infarction (MI)

↑ High sensitivity troponin I above the 99th percentile of the upper reference limit (>20% variation)

+

one of the following criteria

- Ischaemic symptoms
- New changes in ECG
- ECG showing dynamic Q-wave changes
- Echocardiography showing new regional wall motion abnormality or any other imaging evidence of infarction around a specific vascular territorial distribution
- Angiography or autopsy reveals coronary thrombus

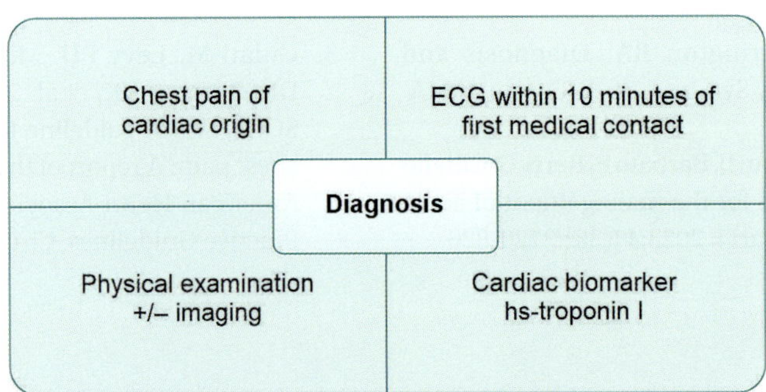


**Fig. 1:** Pillars of diagnosis of acute coronary syndrome.

*Chest pain-equivalent symptoms:* Dyspnea, epigastric pain, and pain in the left or right arm or neck/jaw.

## DIAGNOSTIC WORKUP FOR A CASE OF SUSPECTED ACUTE CORONARY SYNDROME

**Flowchart 1:** Diagnostic workup for acute coronary syndrome.

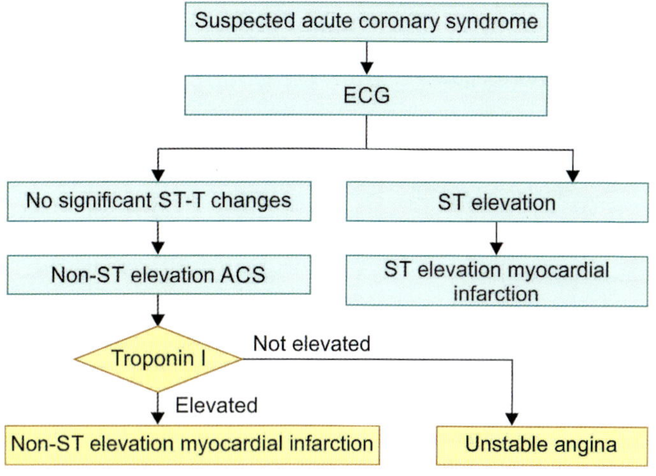


(ACS: acute coronary syndrome, ECG: electrocardiogram)

## SUPPORTIVE INVESTIGATIONS IN DEFINITIVE DIAGNOSIS OF ACUTE CORONARY SYNDROME

**TABLE 1:** Supportive investigations in definitive diagnosis of acute coronary syndrome.

| ***Investigation*** | ***Utility*** |
|---|---|
| Chest X-ray | Rule out non-cardiac origin causes of chest pain |
| Echocardiography | • Identify regional wall motion abnormalities<br>• Exclude mechanical complications<br>• Look for alternate diagnoses |
| Coronary angiography | The gold standard for diagnosing obstructed coronary arteries |
| Coronary CT angiography | To rule out NSTEMI if ECG and cTn values are inconclusive |
| Cardiac magnetic resonance imaging | Assess the viability and perfusion of myocardium in the setting of diagnostic uncertainty |

(NSTEMI: non-ST-elevation myocardial infarction, PCI: percutaneous coronary intervention)

**BOX 2:** Echocardiography in acute coronary syndrome.

*Echocardiography in acute coronary syndrome*
- High sensitivity but a relatively lower specificity
- Useful to identify signs suggestive of ongoing ischemia or prior MI
- Useful to suggest alternative etiologies for chest pain like acute aortic disease, RV signs in pulmonary embolism
- Assess LV ejection fraction, diastolic dysfunction, and RV function
- Assess regional wall motion abnormalities
- Detect mechanical complications after MI

*Poor prognostic factors in echocardiography*
- Left atrial enlargement
- Mitral regurgitation
- Left ventricular longitudinal strain
- Right ventricular dysfunction
- Increased pulmonary artery pressures

(LV: left ventricle; MI: myocardial infarction; RV: right ventricle)

## DIFFERENTIAL DIAGNOSIS OF ACUTE CORONARY SYNDROME

| *Cardiac* | *Vascular* | *Pulmonary* |
|---|---|---|
| • Hypertensive crisis<br>• Arrhythmia<br>• Myocarditis/pericarditis<br>• Takutsubo cardiomyopathy<br>• Coronary spasm MINOCA (≤50% stenosis) | • Aortic dissection<br>• Aneurysm<br>• Stroke | • Pneumonia<br>• Pulmonary embolism<br>• Pleuritis<br>• Pneumothorax |
| *Gastrointestinal* | *Musculoskeletal* | *Other* |
| • Peptic ulcer<br>• Pancreatitis<br>• Cholecystitis | • Muscle injury<br>• Trauma<br>• Costochondritis<br>• Cervical spine pathologies | • Anxiety disorder<br>• Herpes zoster |

**Fig. 2:** Differential diagnosis of acute coronary syndrome.

## UNSTABLE ANGINA

Unstable angina involves reduced perfusion of myocardial tissue, either due to decreased supply like partial intraluminal plaque or thrombosis, vasospasm, and elevated blood pressure, or increased demand, like arrhythmias, fever, thyrotoxicosis, and anemia. Most often, a combination of multiple factors can provoke UA. The diagnosis is made with a combination of the positive clinical history of prolonged chest pain >20 minutes at rest, no ST-segment elevation in ECG, and no dynamic elevation of cardiac troponin levels.

**Flowchart 2:** Algorithm for management of unstable angina.

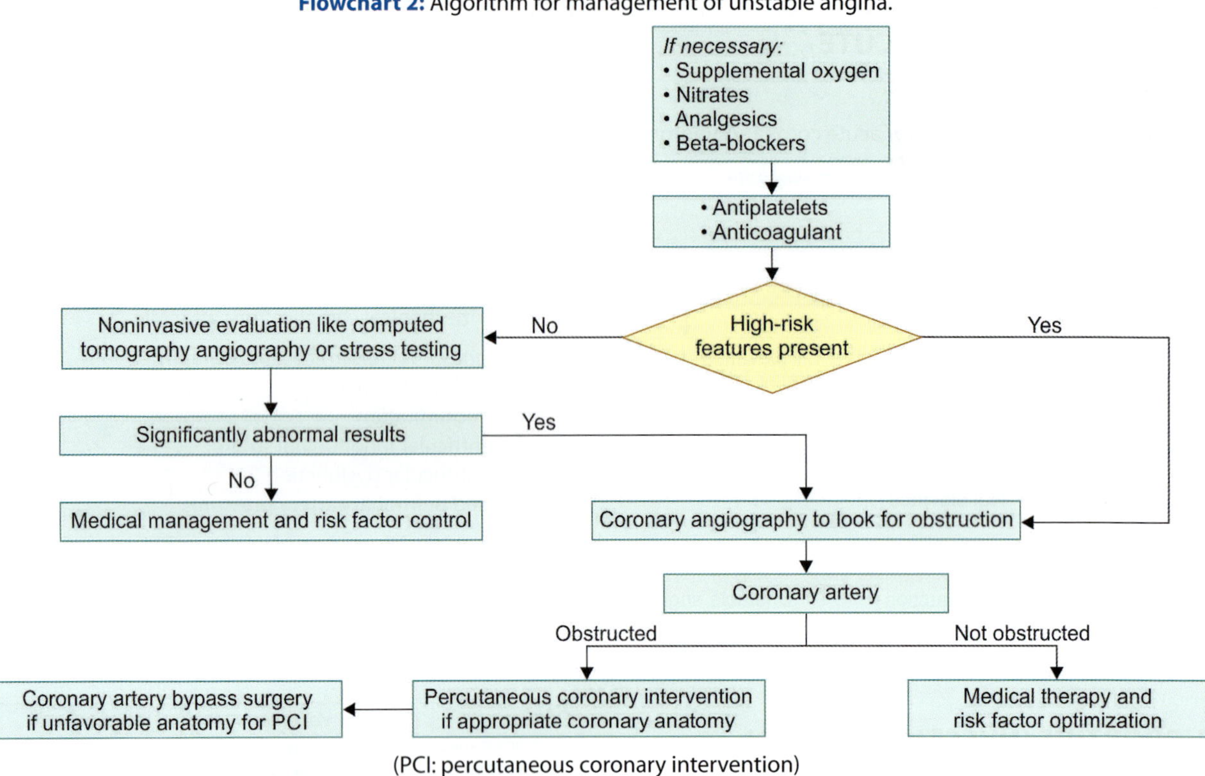


(PCI: percutaneous coronary intervention)

**BOX 3:** Presentations of angina that suggest acute coronary syndrome.

- Rest angina, which is usually more than 20 minutes in duration
- New onset angina that markedly limits physical activity
- Increasing angina that is more frequent, longer in duration, or occurs with less exertion than previous angina

**BOX 4:** High-risk features in unstable angina which needs coronary angiography.

- Heart failure
- Hemodynamic instability
- Dynamic ECG changes
- Worsening chest discomfort

## SUGGESTED READING

1. Bhatt DL, Lopes RD, Harrington RA. Diagnosis and Treatment Of Acute Coronary Syndromes: A Review. JAMA. 2022;327(7):662-75.
2. Byrne RA, Rossello X, Coughlan JJ, Barbato E, Berry C, Chieffo A, et al. 2023 ESC Guidelines for the management of acute coronary syndromes. Eur Heart J. 2023;44(38): 3720-826.
3. Gulati M, Levy PD, Mukherjee D, Amsterdam E, Bhatt DL, Birtcher KK, et al. 2021 AHA/ACC/ASE/Chest/Saem/SCCT/SCMR guideline for the evaluation and diagnosis of chest pain: A report of the American College of Cardiology/American Heart Association Joint Committee on Clinical Practice Guidelines. Circulation. 2021;144(22): e368-454.

CHAPTER 26

# New-onset Atrial Fibrillation

## INTRODUCTION

Incidence of Atrial fibrillation (AF) in the critically ill has been reported to be from 4%- 15% in most intensive care units. Incidence can go up to 40% in patients with septic shock.[1]

Pathophysiology of new onset atrial fibrillation (NOAF) in critically ill patients is usually due to an arrhythmogenic substrate combined with a trigger. Remodeling of the atria can exist due to chronic conditions like heart failure, fibrosis, activation of the Renin-angiotensin system(RAS), chronic inflammation, etc. Remodeling of atria can be structural, electrical, or both. The presence of a trigger in critical illness can set the heart muscle fibers to produce electrical remodeling ion channel expressions, causing persistent abnormal automaticity, self-sustaining action potentials, and re-entrant circuits. In the absence of substrate, if only a trigger is present, then AF is usually self-terminating. The triggers in critical illness are different from the community setting in that illness causes rapid atrial remodeling in the myriads of multiple triggers present in this environment. Higher levels of inflammatory markers have been shown to increase the incidence of AF by increasing the infiltration into muscles and oxidative stress to the myocytes. Treatment of just the triggers can reverse the AF without the requirement of any long-term therapies.

**Flowchart 1** shows the various pathophysiology mechanisms.

**Flowchart 1:** Pathophysiology of NOAF mecha-nisms.

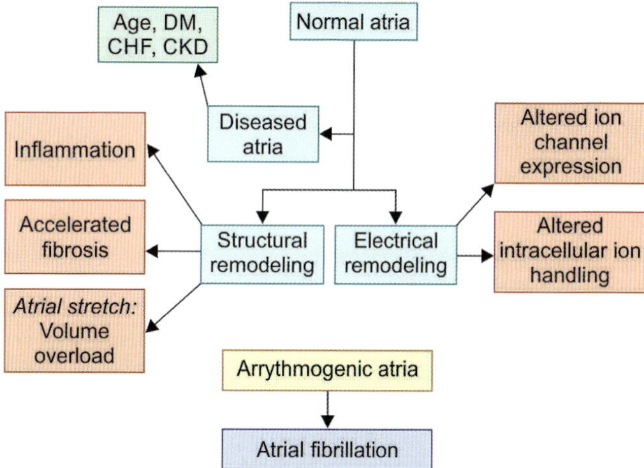


(CHF: congestive cardiac failure; CKD: chronic kidney disease; DM: diabetes mellitus)

## CLINICAL APPROACH

Consider the following:

- Is the hemodynamic instability caused due to the rate change?
- Are there any potential stimuli? Arrhythmogenic vasopressors?
- Are there any reversible triggers? Electrolytes, hypoxia, fluid overload?

Answering the above questions can help in a systematic way can help in the timely and effective treatment of AF. The approach to management is outlined in **Flowchart 2**.

**Flowchart 2:** The approach to management is outlined in new onset atrial fibrillation (NOAF).

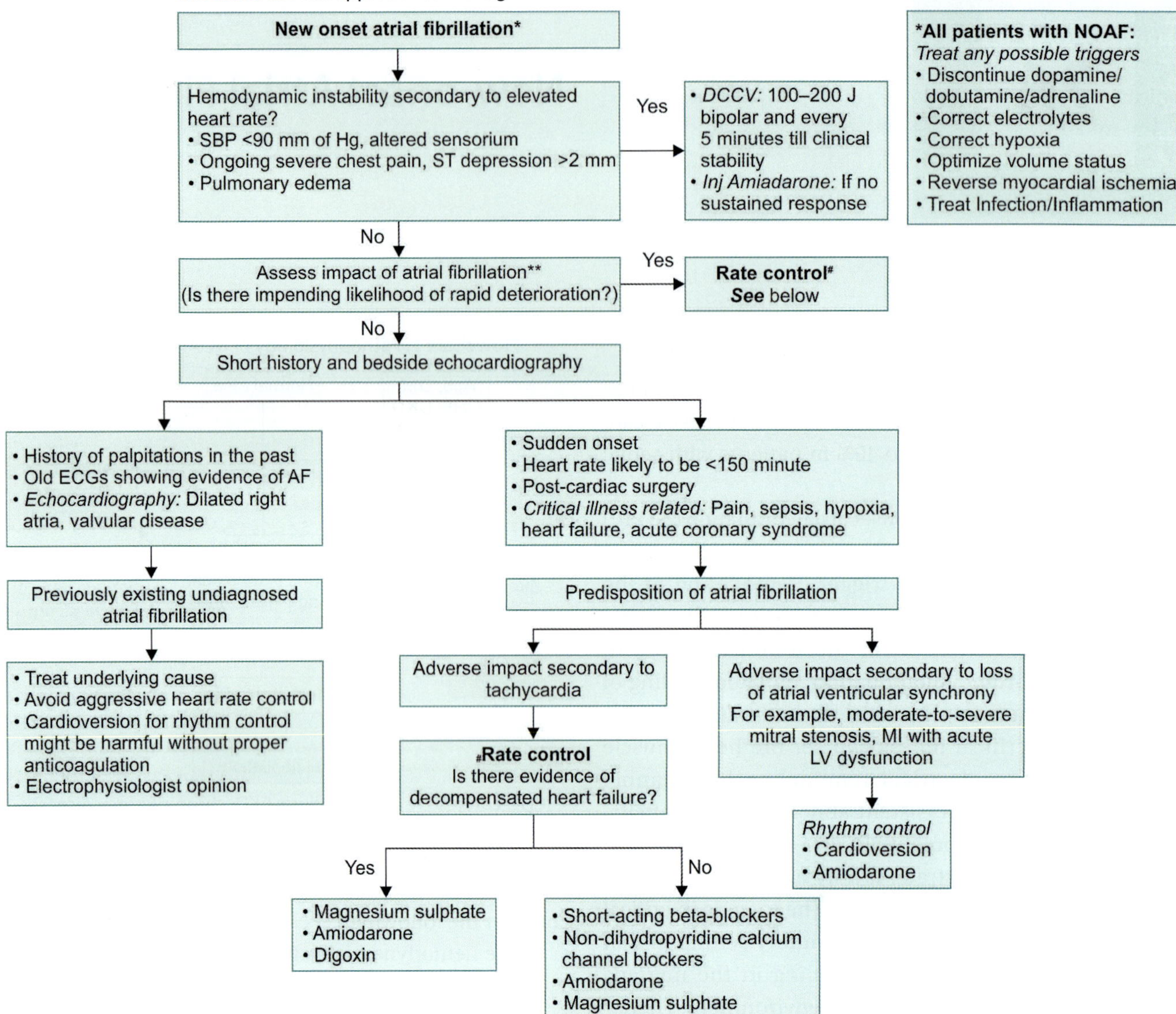


**If AF can eggravate heart failure, myocardial ischemia, embolic stroke or organ failure that can lead to rapid deterioration.
(SBP: systolic blood pressure; DCCV: direct current cardioversion; ECG: electrocardiogram)

International treatment guidelines for AF concentrate on the community management of AF and not on the population of critically ill.[2] Valvular heart disease chronic hypertension plays less of a role in the ICU compared to the community. Most expert consensus or practice guidelines recognize that none of the guidelines are based on robust evidence and are mostly based on observational studies.[3] Risk vs. benefit of certain therapies like beta blockers and calcium channel antagonists can have adverse effects on critically ill patients due to their negative ionotropic effects, which could worsen hypotension and organ dysfunction. Digoxin could be less effective in the setting of a high sympathetic tone and vasopressors.

There is a variation of practice for the control of AF in different critical care units around the world. Most ICUs do not have a set protocol for management, and the choice of drug or therapy is based on conventional practices or on the experience of the physicians. In a subgroup of sepsis, when all types of drugs were studied, beta-blockers were associated with the lowest mortality.[4]

## ROLE OF ANTICOAGULATION

Risks of cardioembolic stroke are higher among patients with AF. However, critically ill patients with various complications may require an interruption of anticoagulation or invasive procedures. Guidelines also mention starting of anticoagulation before starting DCCV. Studies done on patients with sepsis who received anticoagulation versus no anticoagulation showed no increase in the risk of stroke but an increase in the risk of bleeding in the anticoagulation group.[5] Currently, there are no guidelines for anticoagulation in new-onset AF in sepsis or other critically ill patients. Considering the complex nature of the illness and the increased risk of bleeding with no real potential benefit of anticoagulation, it may be advisable to not routinely administer anticoagulation. Patients receiving anticoagulation for thromboprophylaxis can be continued.

## ROLE OF ELECTROPHYSIOLOGICAL STUDIES AND ABLATION

The 2023 American Heart Association (AHA) guidelines recommend electrophysiological studies for patients with acute onset AF before 30 years of age to look for re-entrant pathways that would require pathway ablation (grade IIb). In patients with preexisting chronic and resistant atrial fibrillation, there is a role for ablation once the patient is stable to prevent progression into ventricular tachycardia (VT).[2] If Wolff-Parkinson-White (WPW) syndrome is present, drugs like amiodarone, which block the AV node, can precipitate a VT. Ablation can be considered early in such patients.

## LONG-TERM OUTCOMES

New onset AF has a higher risk of mortality even after adjusting for multiple confounders and competing risks with a Hazards ratio of 2.10.[6] It has also shown to be an independent risk factor for mortality that can be used instead of SOFA.[7] Presence of NOAF in critical illness increases the risk of recurrent AF and then increases the risk of overall cardiac mortality: ischemic stroke, heart failure, and death. Aberrant pathway ablation might be required on an emergency basis if this is suspected.

## REFERENCES


1. Johnston BW, Chean CS, Duarte R, Hill R, Blackwood B, McAuley DF, et al. Management of new onset atrial fibrillation in critically unwell adult patients: a systematic review and narrative synthesis. Br J Anaesth. 2022;128(5):759-71.
2. Joglar JA, Chung MK, Armbruster AL, Benjamin EJ, Chyou JY, Cronin EM, et al. 2023 ACC/AHA/ACCP/HRS Guideline for the Diagnosis and Management of Atrial Fibrillation: A Report of the American College of Cardiology/American Heart Association Joint Committee on Clinical Practice Guidelines. Circulation. 2024;149(1):e1-156.
3. Andreasen AS, Wetterslev M, Sigurdsson MI, Bove J, Kjærgaard J, Aslam TN, et al. New-onset atrial fibrillation in critically ill adult patients-an SSAI clinical practice guideline. Acta Anaesthesiol Scand. 2023;67(8):1110-7.
4. Walkey AJ, Evans SR, Winter MR, Benjamin EJ. Practice Patterns and Outcomes of Treatments for Atrial Fibrillation During Sepsis: A Propensity-Matched Cohort Study. Chest. 2016;149(1):74-83.
5. Walkey AJ, Quinn EK, Winter MR, McManus DD, Benjamin EJ. Practice Patterns and Outcomes Associated With Use of Anticoagulation Among Patients With Atrial Fibrillation During Sepsis. JAMA Cardiol. 2016;1(6):682-90.
6. Klein Klouwenberg PMC, Frencken JF, Kuipers S, Ong DSY, Peelen LM, Van Vught LA, et al. Incidence, Predictors, and Outcomes of New-Onset Atrial Fibrillation in Critically Ill Patients with Sepsis. A Cohort Study. Am J Respir Crit Care Med. 2017;195(2):205-11.
7. Chen AY, Sokol SS, Kress JP, Lat I. New-Onset Atrial Fibrillation Is an Independent Predictor of Mortality in Medical Intensive Care Unit Patients. Ann Pharmacother. 2015;49(5):523-7.

CHAPTER 27

# New-onset Ventricular Arrhythmia

## INTRODUCTION

Cardiac rhythm abnormalities occur frequently in the ICU, which can occur either as a primary cause for ICU admission or as a complication of acute illness. The reported prevalence of supraventricular or ventricular arrhythmias in ICU varies between 44 and 90%. Click or tap here to enter text. Ventricular arrhythmias (VA) cover a wide range of conditions, from premature ventricular complexes (PVCs) to ventricular fibrillation (VF). The symptoms can vary greatly, from no symptoms at all to sudden cardiac arrest. Although VA occurs less frequently than supraventricular arrhythmias, it is associated with a significantly higher in-hospital mortality.

## CLASSIFICATION OF VENTRICULAR ARRHYTHMIAS

**Flowchart 1:** Classification of ventricular arrhythmias.

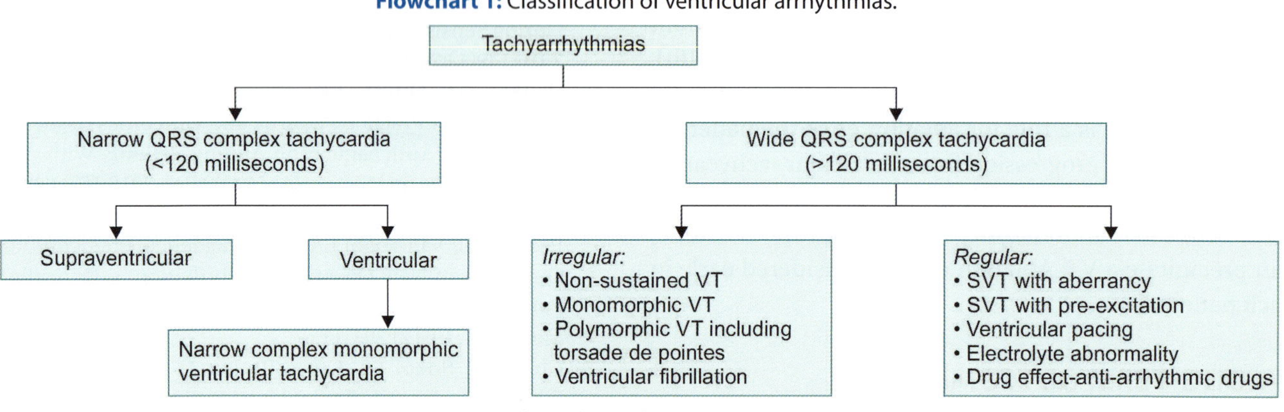


(SVT: supraventricular tachycardia; VT: ventricular tachycardia)

## ELECTROCARDIOGRAPHY IN DIAGNOSIS OF VENTRICULAR ARRHYTHMIAS

**Flowchart 2:** Electrocardiography (ECG) in the diagnosis of ventricular arrhythmias.

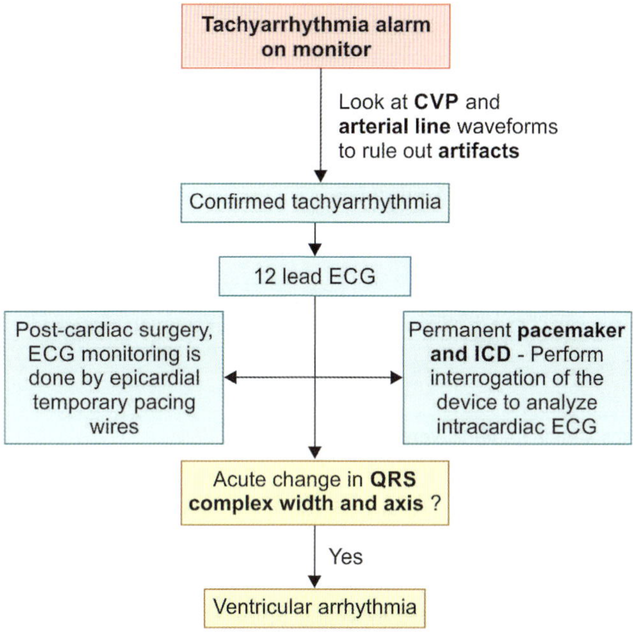


(CVP: central venous pressure; ICD: implantable cardioverter-defibrillator)

## DIAGNOSTIC ALGORITHM

### Supraventricular Tachycardia (SVT) Versus SVT with Aberrancy

**Flowchart 3:** Diagnostic algorithm—SVT versus SVT with aberrancy.

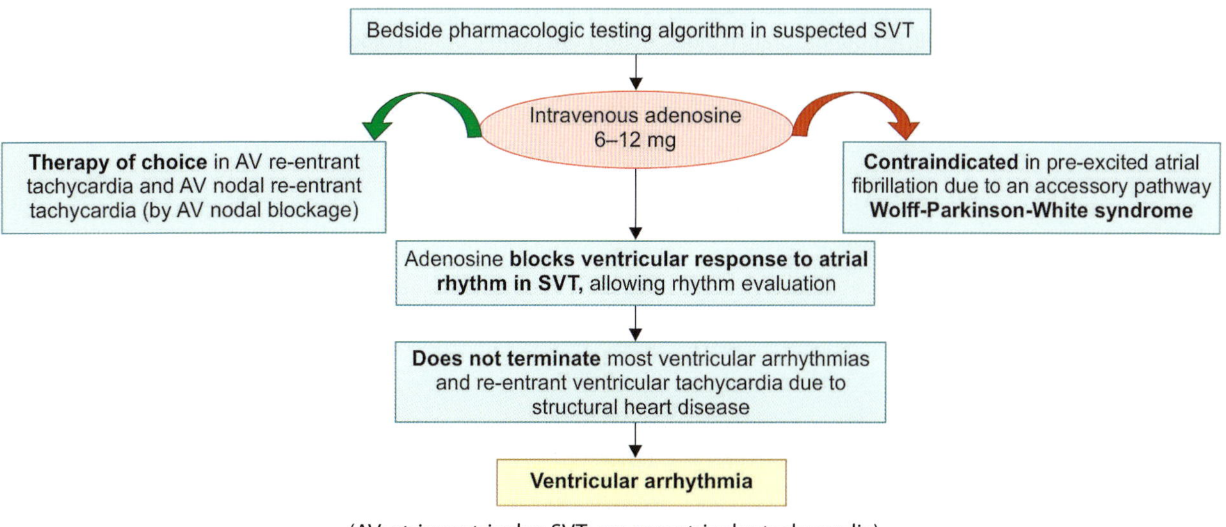


(AV: atrioventricular; SVT: supraventricular tachycardia)

## DIAGNOSTIC ALGORITHM

### Ventricular Arrhythmia

**Flowchart 4:** Diagnostic algorithm of ventricular arrhythmias.

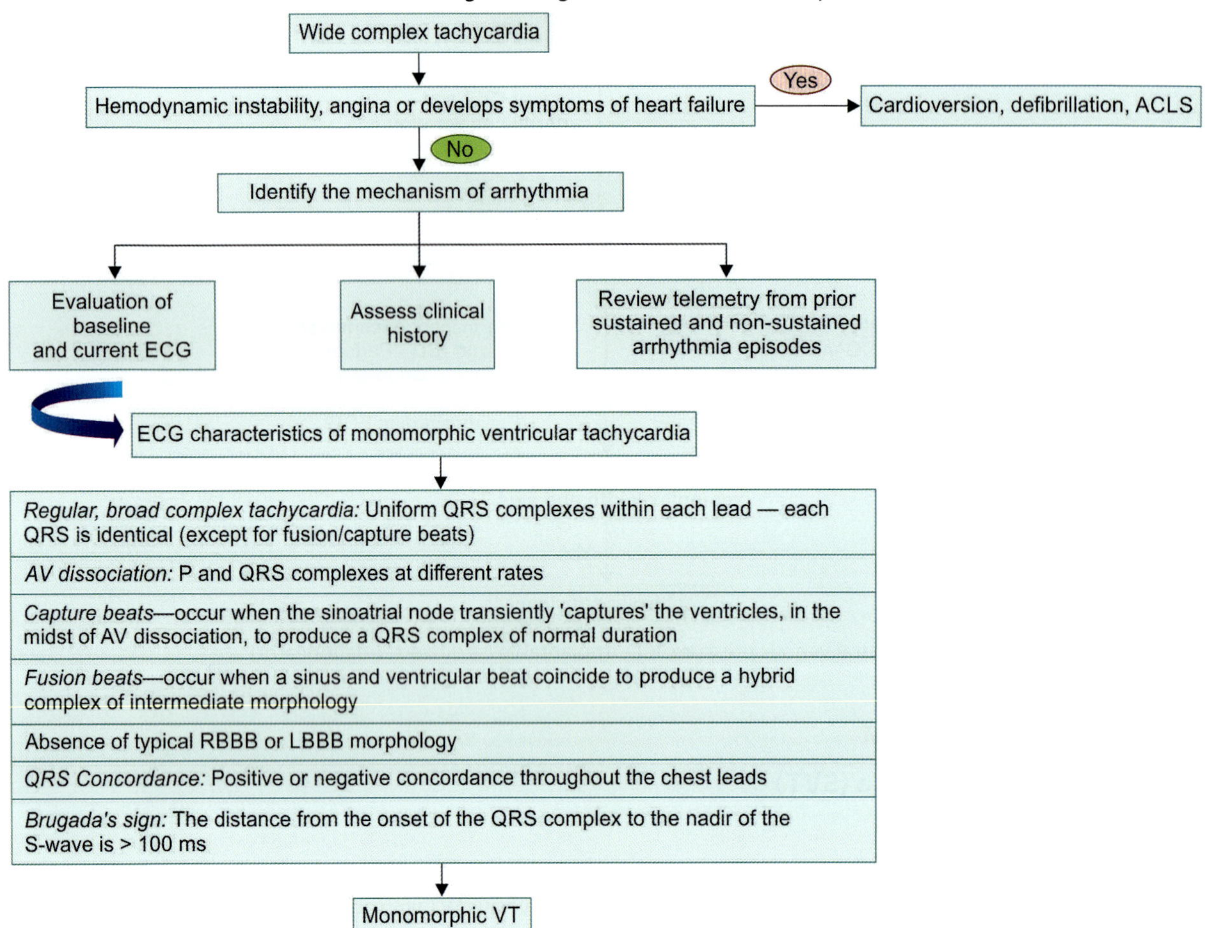


(AV: atrioventricular; LBBB: left bundle branch block; RBBB: right bundle branch block; VT: ventricular tachycardia)

## MANAGEMENT ALGORITHM

### Ventricular Arrhythmias

**Flowchart 5:** Management algorithm—ventricular arrhythmias (VA).

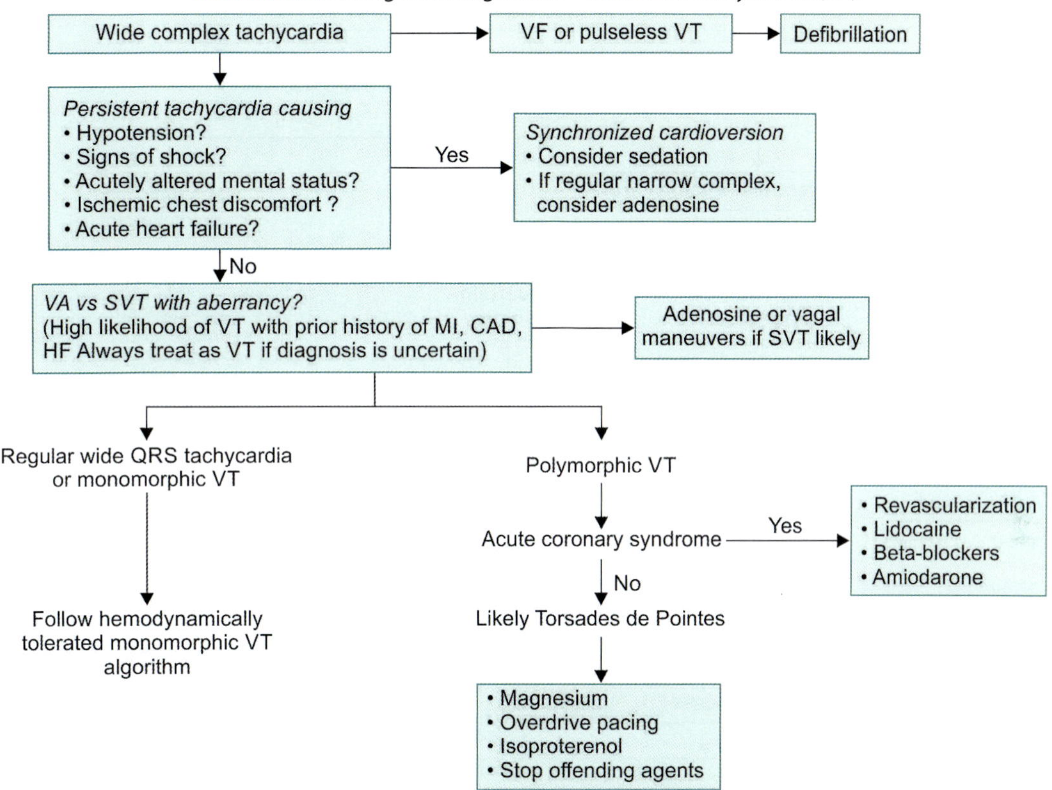


(SVT: supraventricular tachycardia; VT: ventricular tachycardia)

## Hemodynamically Stable Monomorphic Ventricular Tachycardia

**Flowchart 6:** Management algorithm for hemodynamically stable monomorphic ventricular tachycardia (VT).

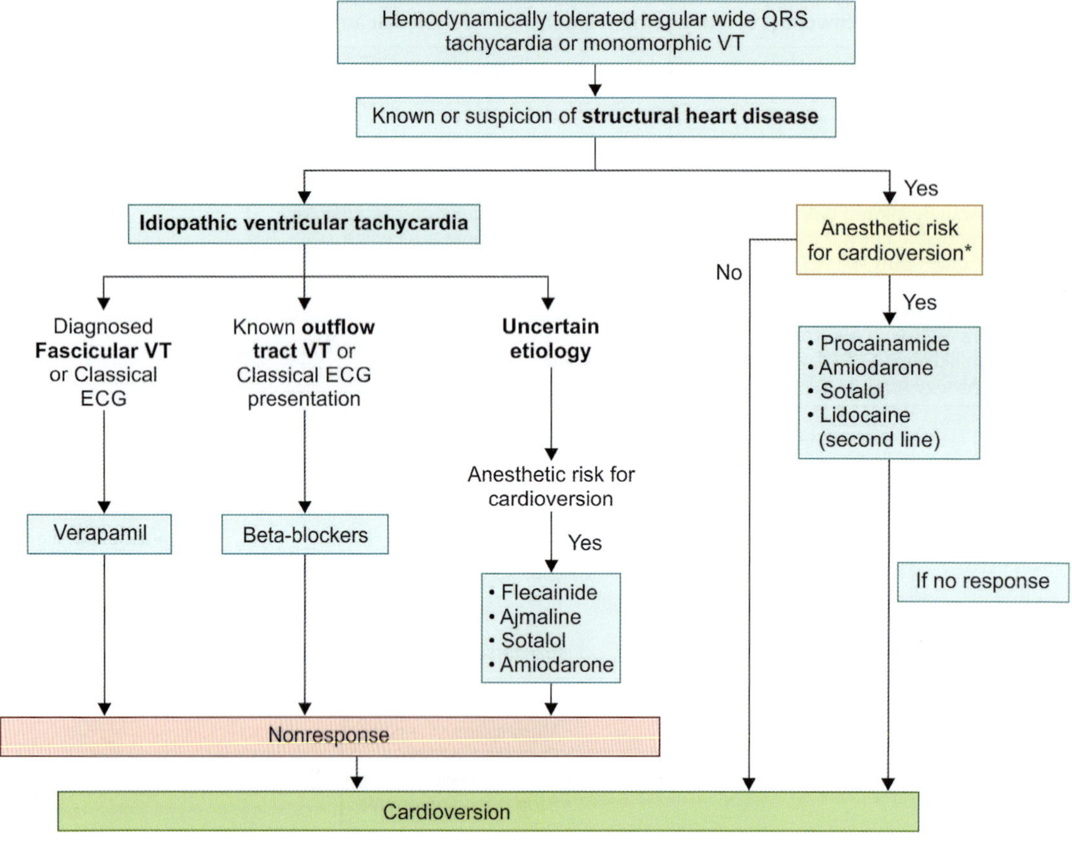


*Benefit of cardioversion should be weighed against risks related to anesthesia/sedation.

## SPECIAL CONSIDERATIONS

### Electrical Strom

An electrical storm is defined as three or more episodes of sustained VT, VF, or appropriate shocks from an ICD within 24 hours. The common causes to consider are ischemia, acute Heart Failure, and hyperactivation of a scar-related or automatic VT. The incidence ranges from 2 to 10% in patients with implantable cardioverter-defibrillators. Although most patients have structural heart disease, a search for inciting factors such as electrical abnormalities, drugs, ischemia, cardiomyopathy, and thyrotoxicosis must be actively sought.

- Initial treatment of choice is *amiodarone*, along with a *non-selective beta-blocker* such as propranolol.
- If ischemia is believed to be a contributing factor, patients should be rapidly transferred to the cardiac catheterization laboratory for possible *revascularization.*
- Often, these patients need intubation and general anesthesia using *propofol and intravenous opioids to lower sympathetic tone*, which could act as a substrate for recurring arrhythmias.
- For patients whose potential substrate is amenable to catheter-based therapies, treatment consists of an acute electrophysiology investigation combined with provisional *catheter ablation.*
- In cases that are refractory treatment, *cardiac sympathetic denervation, and stellate ganglion block* may be explored.
- In refractory electrical storms, early *biventricular mechanical circulatory support* may be regarded as a transitional measure toward more definitive therapy to mitigate the risk of adverse neurological outcomes.

### Pregnancy

The pregnant patient exhibits an elevated risk of both supraventricular and ventricular arrhythmias attributable to neurohormonal alterations associated with pregnancy, characterized by heightened sympathetic outflow and enhanced activation of the renin-angiotensin-aldosterone system. The incidence of supraventricular tachycardias during pregnancy is elevated (24 per 100,000 pregnancies), although the relative incidence of ventricular tachycardia and ventricular fibrillation is low (2 per 100,000). Amniotic fluid embolism, peripartum cardiomyopathy, obstetric hemorrhage, and obstetric infection are all etiologies of ventricular arrhythmias specific to pregnancy.

In patients with ventricular tachyarrhythmia, the management parallels that of nonpregnant individuals. Patients may undergo electrical cardioversion with minimal risk to the pregnancy, as negligible energy is transmitted to the fetus.

Key considerations encompass (1) monitoring fetal heart rate during any acute tachyarrhythmia, (2) acknowledging the high-risk nature of the pregnant airway when sedating a patient for cardioversion, (3) preventing aortocaval compression by positioning the patient in the left lateral decubitus position after the 20th week of gestation, and (4) recognizing that in cardiac arrest, delivery is integral to the resuscitation process, necessitating perimortem cesarean delivery if there is no return of spontaneous circulation within 4 minutes. Patients may undergo acute pharmacological cardioversion utilizing class Ia (procainamide) and class III (amiodarone) agents, noting that procainamide is classified as a US Food and Drug Administration pregnancy category C drug, while amiodarone is categorized as category D. However, amiodarone may be considered when the therapeutic benefits surpass the associated risks, particularly in cases of acute ventricular tachyarrhythmia.

## CONCLUSION

Ventricular arrhythmias frequently occur in the ICU and are linked to considerable morbidity, mortality, and healthcare expenses. A practical approach to understanding the underlying mechanisms and pathophysiology-guided approach to treatment improves outcomes.

## SUGGESTED READING

1. Al-Khatib SM, Stevenson WG, Ackerman MJ, Bryant WJ, Callans DJ, Curtis AB, et al. 2017 AHA/ACC/HRS Guideline for Management of Patients With Ventricular Arrhythmias and the Prevention of Sudden Cardiac Death: Executive Summary: A Report of the American College of Cardiology/American Heart Association Task Force on Clinical Practice Guidelines and the Heart Rhythm Society. JACC. 2018; 138(13):e210-71.
2. Drew BJ, Ackerman MJ, Funk M, Gibler WB, Kligfield P, Menon V, et al. Prevention of torsade de pointes in hospital settings: a scientific statement from the American Heart Association and the American College of Cardiology Foundation. J Am Coll Cardiol. 2010;55(9):934-47.
3. Klinkhammer B, Glotzer TV. Management of Arrhythmias in the Cardiovascular Intensive Care Unit. Crit Care Clin. 2024;40(1):89-103.
4. Kupari M, Koskinen P. Alcohol, cardiac arrhythmias and sudden death. Novartis Found Symp. 1998;216:68-79; discussion 79-85.
5. Senaratne JM, Sandhu R, Barnett CF, Grunau B, Wong GC, van Diepen S. Approach to Ventricular Arrhythmias in the Intensive Care Unit. J Intensive Care Med. 2021;36(7): 731-48.
6. Smith J, Johnson R, Patel A. Management of Ventricular Arrhythmias Worldwide: A Comparison of the Latest ESC, AHA/ACC/HRS, and CCS/CHRS Guidelines. J Cardiac Electrophysiol. 2023;34(2):150-64.
7. Zeppenfeld K, Tfelt-Hansen J, de Riva M, Winkel BG, Behr ER, Blom NA, et al. 2022 ESC Guidelines for the management of patients with ventricular arrhythmias and the prevention of sudden cardiac death. Eur Heart J. 2022;43(40):3997-4126.

CHAPTER

# 28

# Symptomatic Bradyarrhythmias

## INTRODUCTION

Symptomatic bradycardia is a common and potentially life-threatening condition encountered in the intensive care unit (ICU). It requires prompt recognition and intervention to prevent further hemodynamic deterioration and end-organ damage. The diagnosis of the etiology of such cases is a challenge in the ICU since most of the patients have multiple comorbidities and are subjected to various pharmacological and physiological stressors. The etiology may range from intrinsic cardiac conduction abnormalities to extrinsic factors, such as medication and metabolic derangements. Moreover, the clinical presentation can vary widely, from subtle cognitive changes to overt cardiovascular collapse. The treatment is focused on the urgency of treatment, potential causes, and resources available.

**TABLE 1:** Definitions and classification of bradyarrhythmia.

| *Type* | *Subtypes* | *Definition/description* | *Salient features* |
|---|---|---|---|
| Sinus Bradycardia | N/A | It is a rhythm originating from the sinus node due to inappropriate impulse generation, generating less than 60 beats per minute (bpm)[1] | • Rate - < 60 BPM<br>• Rhythm - Regular<br>• Presence of a 'P' wave before every 'QRS' complex<br>• Normal P axis - Upright P in Leads II |
| Junctional Bradycardia | N/A | Whenever the SA node fails to produce an impulse, the cells of the atrium and conduction system start taking over the pacemaker activity. When the pacemaker activity is taken over by cells superior to the AV node, it is known as a junctional rhythm.[1] | • Rate <40 BPM<br>• P-waves may be inverted or absent.<br>• Narrow QRS Complex (except when associated with bundle branch blocks) |
| Atrioventricular Blocks | | Atrioventricular blocks are caused due to abnormal impulse conduction | |
| | First-degree AV Block | | • "P" precedes the QRS complexes<br>• QRS duration is normal (narrow QRS)<br>• Fixed prolonged PR interval (> 0.21 sec)[2,3] |
| | Second-degree Mobitz - I | | • Progressive prolongation of the PR interval leading to a non-conducted P wave<br>• The PR interval is the longest immediately before a drop beat<br>• It is generally a benign rhythm, causing minimal hemodynamic instability<br>• There is a low risk of progression to a complete heart block |

*Contd...*

*Contd...*

| *Type* | *Subtypes* | *Definition/description* | *Salient features* |
|---|---|---|---|
| | Second-degree Mobitz - II | | • Constant PR Interval<br>• Intermittent non-conducted P-waves<br>• Usually associated with hemodynamic instability, progression to complete heart block, and sudden cardiac death |
| | Complete heart block | Complete atrioventricular dissociation | • Fixed P-P intervals<br>• Fixed R-R intervals<br>• Variable P-R intervals |

(N/A not available, QRS: QRS complex in the electrocardiogram; -P-R interval: the interval between P and R wave in the electrocardiogram; R-R interval: the interval between R and R-wave in the electrocardiogram; P-P interval: the interval between P and P-wave in the electrocardiogram)

**TABLE 2:** Etiology.

| | |
|---|---|
| Sinus bradycardia (Mnemonic *HARD*) | **H**ypoxia, hypothermia |
| | **A**cute myocardial infarction (RCA infarct) |
| | **R**aised intracranial pressure |
| | **D**rugs: Beta-blockers, calcium channel blockers (CCB), digitalis, dexmedetomidine, propofol, fentanyl. |
| Atrioventricular blocks (Mnemonic *MAMO*) | **M**etabolic: hypoxia, Acidosis, hyperkalemia, hypothermia, hypothyroidism |
| | **A**utoimmune: systemic lupus erythematosus, Rheumatoid Arthritis, sarcoidosis |
| | **M**edications: Digoxin, antiarrhythmics. |
| | **O**thers: Myocarditis, Amyloidosis, (HOCM) |

(RCA: right coronary artery; CCB: calcium channel blockers; HOCM: hypertrophic cardiomyopathy)

**TABLE 3:** Investigations.

| *No.* | *Routine tests* | *Special tests* |
|---|---|---|
| 1. | Complete blood count | Echocardiography (cardiomyopathies) |
| 2. | Electrolytes (potassium and magnesium) | 24-hour Holter |
| 3. | Renal function test (uremia) | Cardiac enzymes (acute MI) |
| 4. | Liver function tests (ammonia) | CT Brain (raised ICP) |
| 5. | Thyroid function test | Rheumatology evaluation (SLE, RA) |
| 6. | Arterial blood gas analysis (hypoxia, acidosis) | |

(MI: myocardial infarction; ICP: intracranial pressure; SLE: systemic lupus erythematosus; RA: rheumatoid arthritis; CT: computer tomography)

Patients with bradyarrhythmias may present with a wide range of symptoms, from being asymptomatic to experiencing life-threatening hemodynamic instability. In critically ill patients, especially those on sedatives or mechanical ventilation, symptoms of bradyarrhythmias may be masked, and the condition is often identified through routine cardiac monitoring or when hemodynamic instability becomes apparent. Evaluating such patients would include looking for inciting events and correctable causes and identifying irreversible conditions to prognosticate and prepare the patient for a pacemaker.

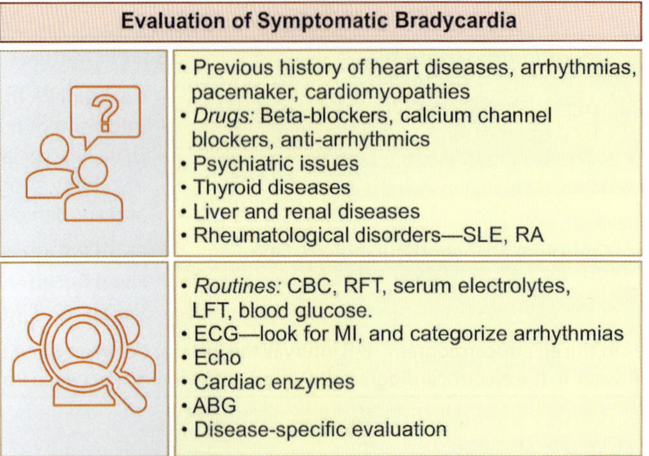


**Fig. 1:** Evaluation. (SLE: systemic lupus erythematosus; RA: rheumatoid arthritis; CT: computer tomography; ABG: arterial blood gas; ECHO: echocardiography; ECG: electrocardiography; LFT: liver function test)

**Flowchart 1:** Approach to symptomatic bradyarrhythmia.

**Symptomatic bradycardia (HR <60 bpm)**

- Evaluate and correct inciting causes—electrolytes, MI, drugs, metabolic, hypothermia
- Stop drugs—beta-and calcium-channel blockers, class I and III antiarrhythmics

→ ABCDE approach

→ Hemodynamic instability

- **Yes**
  - • IV Atropine (0.04 mg/kg) • Adrenaline infusion (titrate according to response)
  - • Repeat atropine (max—3 mg) • Transcutaneous pacing
  - Transvenous pacing
  - Decide on permanent pacing (depends on reversibility of etiology)
- **No**
  - 12-lead ECG and identifying type of block
  - Risk of progression to complete heart block
    - Yes (Mobitz-II, 3rd degree) → Transvenous pacing
    - No (Sinus bradycardia, 1st degree, 2nd degree Mobitz-I) → Treat etiology observe

Management of bradyarrhythmias in the ICU depends on the underlying cause, the patient's symptoms, and the degree of hemodynamic compromise. Treatment strategies include

1. Reversing Underlying Cause
2. Pharmacologic Therapy
3. Temporary/permanent pacing.

**TABLE 4:** Drugs used in the management of symptomatic bradyarrhythmias.

| ***Drugs*** | ***Points to note*** |
|---|---|
| Atropine | • Dose – 0.04 mg/kg repeat every 3-5 min<br>• Lower doses – risk of paradoxical bradycardia[4,5]<br>• Maximum dose – 3 mg<br>• Caution in – transplanted heart,[6] acute MI,<br>• May not work in - drug overdose, Mobitz – 2, complete heart block |
| Adrenaline | • Dose – 5-8 mcg/kg/min<br>• Preferred in hemodynamic instability<br>• Drug of choice in transplanted (denervated heart) |
| Isoproterenol/ isoprenaline | • Excellent drug for bradycardia<br>• Pure beta agonist – hence the possibility of hypotension (beta-2 activity causes peripheral vasodilation)<br>• Its infusion may be tried in bradycardia resistant to adrenaline<br>• Cost and availability limit its use |
| Calcium gluconate | • Dose – 60 mg/kg IV over 5 min every 10-20 min up to 3-4 times<br>• Max 3-4g/dose (30-40 ml of 10% solution)<br>• Used in beta-blocker and calcium channel blocker toxicity<br>• Off-label use in cardiac arrest due to hyperkalemia, hypocalcemia, and hypermagnesemia.[7,8] |
| IV Glucagon | • Off-label use in beta and calcium channel blocker toxicity in severe refractory cardiogenic shock<br>• Dose = 50-150 mcg/kg over 1min loading dose f/b 3–5 mg/h IV |
| Dopamine | • In hemodynamically unstable patients, it can be tried<br>• At high doses—predominantly vasoconstrictor, which may be undesirable<br>• To consider switching to adrenaline once available |
| Dobutamine | • Can be a great drug in normotensive or hypertensive patients<br>• Vasodilator—hence can lead to hypotension |
| Theophylline | • Can increase the heart rate but can cause serious arrhythmia. Hence, it is not used commonly<br>• Can be used in postcardiac transplant patients and spinal cord injury<br>• PDE inhibitors increase intracellular cAMP concentrations |

**TABLE 5:** Pacemaker.

| | |
|---|---|
| Types | 1. Temporary:<br>A. Transcutaneous<br>B. Transvenous<br>2. Permanent |
| Indications | • Symptomatic bradycardia<br>• Unexplained syncope with significant sinus node abnormalities<br>• Second-degree Mobitz type II, Third-degree AV block with or without symptoms<br>• Symptomatic second-degree Mobitz type I<br>• Asystole >3 sec, or escape rhythm <40/min or originating below AV node<br>• Atrial fibrillation with bradycardia<br>• Muscular dystrophies with conduction system predilection<br>• In acute MI:<br>– Second-degree AV Block with bundle branch block<br>– Complete heart block (persistent/ transient)[9] |
| Contraindication | • Local infection at the implantation site<br>• Active systemic infection<br>• Severe bleeding tendencies (relative contraindication)<br>• Active anticoagulation therapy (relative contraindication) |

*Contd...*

*Contd...*

| | |
|---|---|
| Complications | *Acute:*<br>• Infection<br>• Hematoma<br>• Pneumothorax<br>• Cardiac perforation<br>• Lead dislodgement<br>*Chronic:*<br>• Infection<br>• Lead failure<br>• Pacemaker syndrome |

## CONCLUSION

Bradyarrhythmias in the ICU represent a complex clinical challenge, requiring rapid identification and treatment to prevent deterioration in critically ill patients. A systematic approach to diagnosing and managing these arrhythmias, including addressing reversible causes, pharmacologic support, and pacing when necessary, is critical to improving patient outcomes. Close monitoring and individualized care, based on the underlying etiology and patient-specific factors, remain key components of effective management in this high-risk population.

## REFERENCES

1. Lattell J, Upadhyay GA. Bradyarrhythmias and Physiologic Pacing in the ICU. J Intensive Care Med. 2022;37(5):595-610.
2. Hafeez Y, Grossman SA. Sinus Bradycardia. In: StatPearls [Internet]. Treasure Island (FL): StatPearls Publishing; 2024.
3. Ufberg JW, Clark JS. Bradydysrhythmias and atrioventricular conduction blocks. Emerg Med Clin North Am. 2006;24(1):1-9.
4. Kashou AH, Goyal A, Nguyen T, et al. Atrioventricular Block. In: StatPearls [Internet]. Treasure Island (FL): StatPearls Publishing; 2024.
5. Das G. Therapeutic review. Cardiac effects of atropine in man: an update. Int J Clin Pharmacol Ther Toxicol. 1989;27(10):473-7.
6. Bernheim A, Fatio R, Kiowski W, Weilenmann D, Rickli H, Brunner-La Rocca HP. Atropine often results in complete atrioventricular block or sinus arrest after cardiac transplantation: an unpredictable and dose-independent phenomenon. Transplantation. 2004;77(8):1181-5.
7. Vallentin MF, Granfeldt A, Meilandt C, Povlsen AL, Sindberg B, Holmberg MJ, et al. Effect of Intravenous or Intraosseous Calcium vs Saline on Return of Spontaneous Circulation in Adults With Out-of-Hospital Cardiac Arrest: A Randomized Clinical Trial. JAMA. 2021;326(22):2268-76.
8. Chakraborty A, Patel P, Can AS. Calcium Gluconate. In: StatPearls [Internet]. Treasure Island (FL): StatPearls Publishing; 2024.
9. Dalia T, Amr BS. Pacemaker Indications. In: StatPearls [Internet]. Treasure Island (FL): StatPearls Publishing; 2024.

CHAPTER 29

# Cardiac Tamponade

## INTRODUCTION

Cardiac tamponade is a life-threatening, slow, or rapid compression of the heart due to the pericardial accumulation of fluid, pus, blood, clots, or gas as a result of inflammation, trauma, rupture of the heart, or aortic dissection.

## CLINICAL FEATURES

### Symptoms

- Dyspnea
- Chest pain
- Syncope
- Presyncope

### Signs

- *Becks Triad:*
  - Hypotension
  - Elevated JVP
  - Muffled Heart sounds
- *Tachycardia:* Measure to increase stroke volume
- *Pulsus Paradoxus:*
  - 10 mm Hg decrease in systolic Blood pressure with inspiration
  - Clinically seen as a disappearance of Korotkoff's sound during inspiration during auscultatory measurement of BP
- *Kussmaul sign:* No decrease in JVP with inspiration

## PATHOPHYSIOLOGY

- The rapidity of the filling of pericardial space determines the severity of the symptoms, not the volume
- In *Acute cases*, e.g. trauma, a volume of 50-150 ml is sufficient to cause tamponade
- In *Chronic cases*, the pericardium can dilate to accommodate a volume of up to 2 L before tamponade occurs

### Pathophysiology of Shock in Cardiac Tamponade

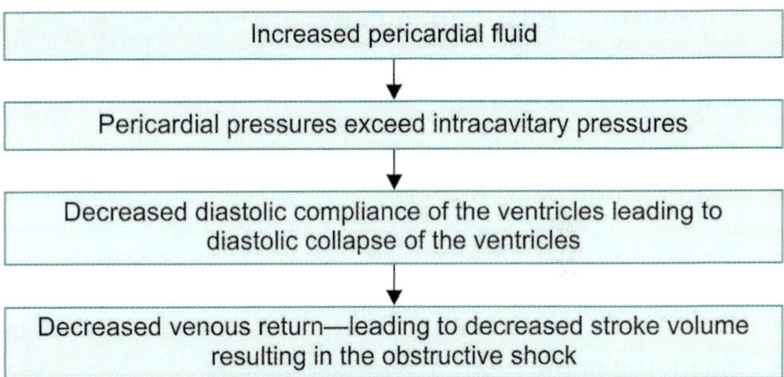


### Pathophysiology of Pulsus Paradoxus

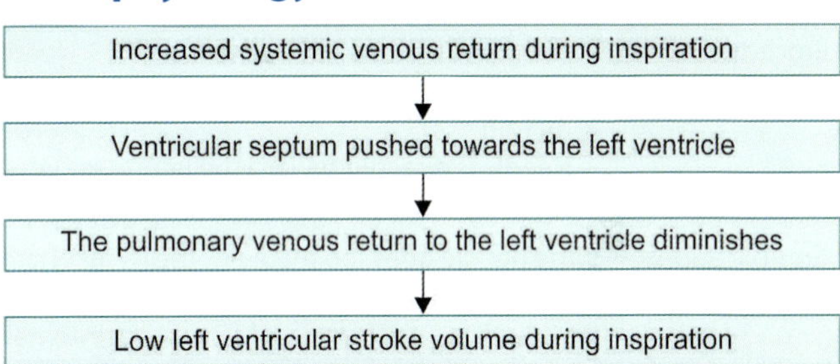


Normally, the right ventricle bulges outwardly during inspiration to accommodate the increased venous return, but due to the raised pericardial pressures, the above phenomenon occurs and accentuates the fall in systolic BP during inspiration to greater than 10 mm Hg.

## CAUSES

| *Common* | *Uncommon* |
|---|---|
| • Tubercular<br>• Pericarditis<br>• Trauma<br>• Iatrogenic (Peri operative)<br>• Malignancy | • Bacterial<br>• Aortic dissection<br>• Connective tissue disease<br>• Radiation-induced<br>• Post myocardial infarction<br>• Uremia<br>• Pneumopericardium |

## DIAGNOSIS

Though the cardiac tamponade is a clinical diagnosis. The following tools may be useful for diagnosing tamponade.

### Electrocardiogram Findings

- Sinus tachycardia
- Low voltage complexes Nonspecific
- Electrical Alterans:
  - Beat-to-beat variation in the QRS appearance
  - Due to the back-to-back swinging motion of the heart
  - Along with sinus tachycardia is a highly specific sign of Cardiac tamponade

### Chest X-ray Findings

- Cardiomegaly with relatively less plethora of lung fields
- Water bottle heart on X-ray

### Two-dimensional Echo Findings

- Pericardial effusion may be small in an acute effusion
- Swinging of the heart in a large effusion
- *Right atrial collapse*—occurs in late diastole. Significant if it occurs >1/3 of the cycle. Not very specific
- *Right ventricular collapse*—occurs in early diastole. More specific
- *Left atrial collapse* is very specific
- *Left ventricular collapse* is not seen commonly due to the muscular nature of the wall of the LV
- *IVC distension:* Present in most patients but may be absent in hypovolemic patients
- *Hepatic venous Flow reversal*

## MANAGEMENT OF CARDIAC TAMPONADE

- Fluid boluses and Vasopressors may be used as one arrangement till the pericardiocentesis to be done
- It is better to avoid positive pressure ventilation if possible
- If cardiac tamponade is the cause of hemodynamic instability, rapid relief of signs and symptoms are seen after pericardiocentesis
- Urgent pericardiocentesis is warranted.

### Pericardiocentesis Procedure

| | *Subxiphoid* | *Parasternal* | *Apical* |
|---|---|---|---|
| Procedure | • Needle to be inserted between Xiphisternum and the left costal margin<br>• Needle is directed toward the left shoulder | • Needle to be inserted at the 5th intercostal space at the upper border of the lower rib<br>• Perpendicular to the skin | • 1–2 cm lateral to the apex<br>• Within 5th, 6th or 7th intercostal space<br>• At the upper border of the rib |
| Complications | If the needle goes too medially, the chance of entering the right atrium | If >1 cm away from the sternal border, then chance of trauma to the internal mammary artery | • Puncture to the left ventricle<br>• Pneumothorax |

- The USG-guided procedure has less complications
- Rapidly remove 60–80 mL
- Maximum remove 500 mL to avoid pericardial decompression syndrome

## SUGGESTED READING


1. Imazio M, Maria De Ferrari G. Cardiac tamponade: an educational review. Eur Heart J Acute Cardiovasc Care. 2021;10(1):102-9.
2. Imazio M, Mayosi BM, Brucato A, et al. Triage and management of pericardial effusion. J Cardiovasc Med (Hagerstown). 2010;11:928-35.
3. Ristic AD, Imazio M, Adler Y, et al. Triage strategy for urgent management of cardiac tamponade: a position statement of the European Society of Cardiology Working Group on Myocardial and Pericardial Diseases. Eur Heart J. 2014;35: 2279-84.

CHAPTER **30**

# Pulmonary Thromboembolism

## PULMONARY EMBOLISM

- Important cause of morbidity and mortality
- Incidence 23 – 69/100,000/year
- Acute onset of right ventricular failure due to pressure overload associated with hypoxia

## CLASSIFICATION

| *Massive* | *Submassive* | *Mild* |
|---|---|---|
| Sustained hypotension Systolic Blood pressure < 90 mm Hg for more than 15 minutes or requiring inotropic support | Acute PE without hypotension, but evidence of right ventricular dysfunction / myocardial necrosis | Pulmonary embolism with no hypotension or features of RV strain |

### Classification Based on Mortality Risk

#### *Risk Factors*

- *Immobilization:* Recent travel for >4 hrs duration, immobilization following recent surgery, trauma to lower limb, or stroke
- *Underlying Malignancy:* GI malignancy, Ca pancreas, etc
- *Medications:* Oral contraceptive Pills, Chemotherapeutic agents such as Paclitaxel, Bevacizumab, antipsychotic drugs
- *Inherited causes:* Factor V Leiden mutation, Antithrombin III deficiency, Protein C and Protein S deficiency, APLA, Hyperhomocysteinemia

## PATHOPHYSIOLOGY

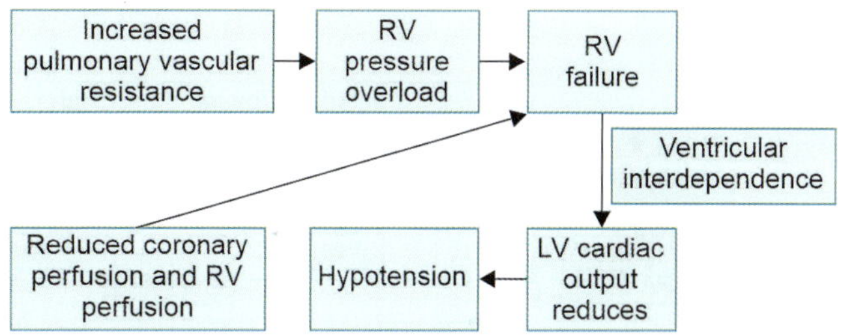


- *Clinical prediction tools:* Wells score and revised Geneva score
- *If low risk for PE:* apply PERC score and can exclude PE in the emergency department

#### *Investigations*

- *ABG:* Increased alveolar-arterial oxygen gradient, respiratory alkalosis

**Classification of patients with acute PE based on early mortality risk.**

| *Mortality risk* | *Shock/Hypotension* | *sPESI ≥1* | *Sign of RV dysfunction on imaging* | *Elevated cardiac biomarkers (TropI or BNP)* |
|---|---|---|---|---|
| High | + | + | + | + |
| Intermediate high | – | + | + | + |
| Intermediate low | – | + | Either signs of RV dysguntion or elevated cardiac biomarkers | |
| Low | – | – | – | – |

(BNP: brain natriuretic peptide; PE: PE = pulmonary embolism; RV = right ventricular; sPESI: simplified pulmonary embolism severity index)

- *Chest X-ray:* Palla's sign - Enlarged descending pulmonary artery
- Hampton's hump - Peripheral wedge-shaped opacity
- Westermark's sign - Focal oligemia
- Chang sign- dilated right or left descending pulmonary artery
- A normal chest X-ray in a hypoxic patient is more suggestive of PE.
- *ECG:* Sinus tachycardia (most common), S1Q3T3 pattern, new onset RBBB, right axis deviation, T-wave inversions in leads V1–4
- *D-dimer:* D-dimer should be used only in patients with low to intermediate clinical probability of PE.

If the D-dimer assay is negative, no treatment is indicated in low to intermediate-risk cases. If positive, CTPA should be performed for a definitive diagnosis.

- Age-adjusted D-dimer (age × 10 mcg/L) for patients older than 50 years should be considered to identify low-risk patients.
- CT pulmonary angiography - identifies thrombus in the pulmonary circulation and also identifies clot burden and RV strain.
- Pulmonary angiography - Gold standard test - now being replaced by CT angiography.

## Echo

- RV enlargement in parasternal long-axis view/apical 4-chamber view
- Flattened interventricular septum in PSAX view
- 60/60 sign - Pulmonary acceleration time (PAT): Less than 60 milliseconds and Tricuspid regurgitation (TR) jet gradient: Less than 60 mm Hg
- McConnell sign in apical 4-chamber view
- Tricuspid annular Systolic plane Excursion in A4 chamber view <16
- Mobile right heart thrombus/a thrombus in transit

## ALGORITHM FOR A SUSPECTED CASE OF PULMONARY EMBOLISM

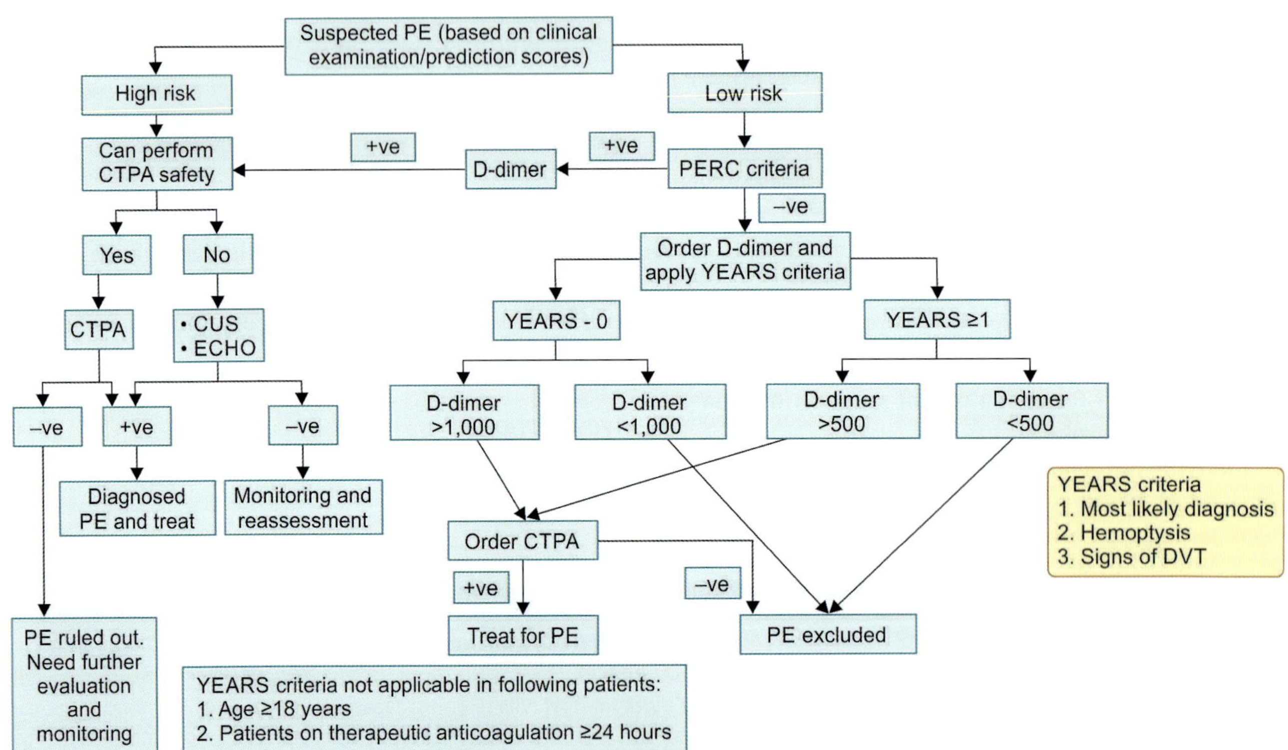


(CUS: compression ultrasound; CTPA: CT pulmonary angiography; PERC: pulmonary embolism rule out criteria)

## MANAGEMENT OF PULMONARY EMBOLISM

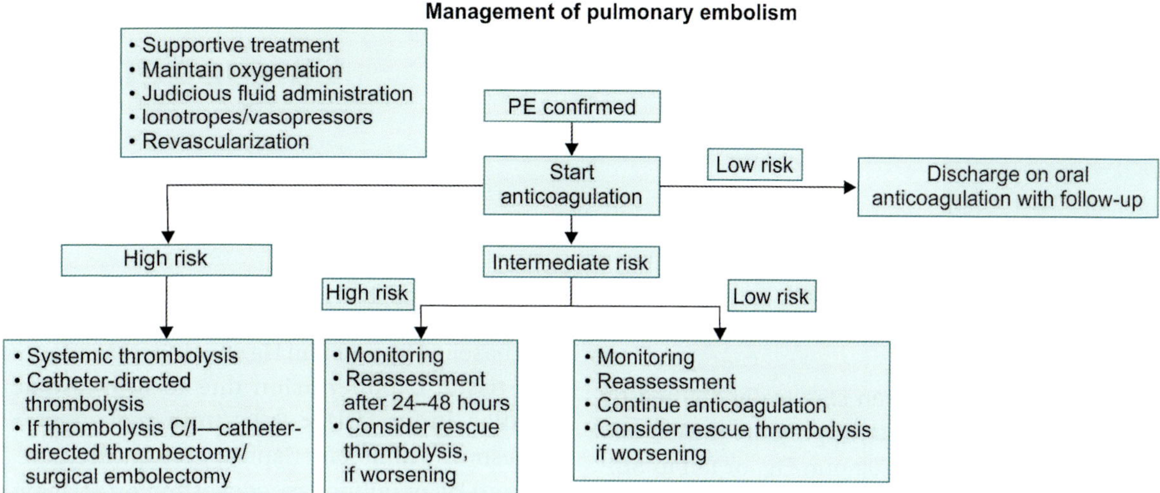


### Anticoagulant of Choice

- Unfractionated heparin - Target aPTT 1.5-2.5 times the normal
- Low molecular weight heparin 1 mg/kg of enoxaparin
- Fondaparinux
- Rivaroxaban and Apixaban can also be started for anticoagulation
- Duration - for provoked PE - at least 3 months
- Unprovoked PE - Life long
- Malignancy associated PE - lifelong

### Thrombolysis

For massive PE only

- Agents - Streptokinase (250,000 IU loading dose over half an hour followed by 100,000 IU/h over 12 hours)
- Urokinase (4400 IU/kg over 10 minutes followed by 4000 IU/kg over 12-24 hours), Alteplase (100 mg over 2 hours)
- Thrombolysis in intermediate risk. Pulmonary embolism is not recommended by guidelines, although some studies have looked into it.

## SUGGESTED READING

1. Huisman MV, Barco S, Cannegieter SC, et al. Pulmonary embolism. Nat Rev Dis Primers. 2018;4:18028.
2. Kahn SR, Wit K. Pulmonary Embolism. N Engl J Med 2022;387:45-57.
3. Balakrishna AM, Reddi V, Belford PW, et al. Intermediate-Risk Pulmonary Embolism: A Review of Contemporary Diagnosis, Risk Stratification and Management. Medicina (Kaunas). 2022;58(9):1186.

CHAPTER

# 31 Cardiogenic Shock

## DEFINITION

Cardiogenic shock (CS) has been classically defined by sustained hypotension [mean arterial pressure (MAP) <65, Systolic blood pressure (SBP) < 90 mm Hg, or fall in SBP from baseline by > 40 mm Hg or vasopressor dependency)] *with* tissue hypoperfusion due to low cardiac output (Cardiac Index (CI) < 2.2 L/min/$m^2$) *and/or* due to congestion (Pulmonary Capillary Wedge Pressure (PCWP) > 15 mm Hg or pulmonary congestion on imaging).[1]

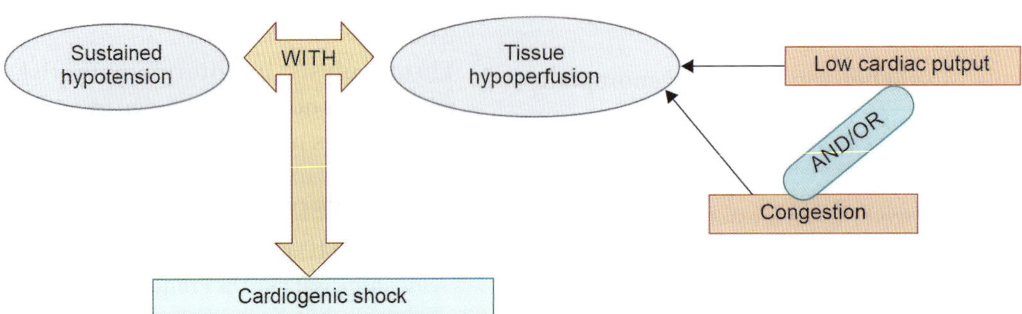


**Fig. 1:** Classical definition of cardiogenic shock.

## DIAGNOSIS OF CARDIOGENIC SHOCK

**Flowchart 1:** Algorithm for diagnosis of Cardiogenic Shock.[2]

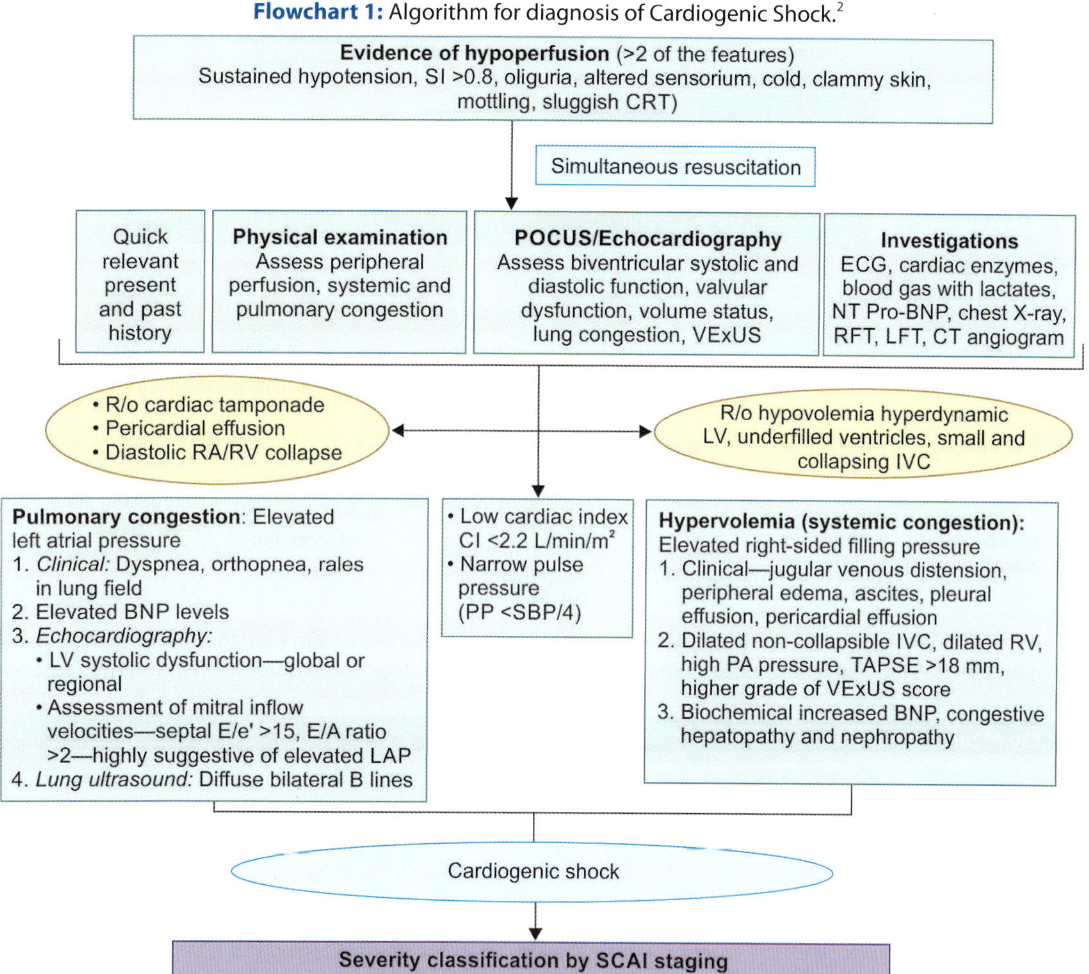


(SI: shock index; CRT: capillary refill time; POCUS: point-of-care ultrasonography; VEXUS: venous excess ultrasound; ECG: electrocardiogram; NT-proBNP: N-terminal prohormone of brain natriuretic peptide; RFT: renal function test; LFT: liver function test; CT: computed tomogram; R/o: rule out; RA: right atrium; RV: Right ventricle; LV: left ventricle; IVC: inferior vena cava; LAP: left atrial pressure; CI: cardiac index; SBP: systolic blood pressure; PP: pulse pressure; TAPSE: tricuspid annular plane systolic excursion)

The effects of shock are initially reversible, but it rapidly becomes irreversible, resulting in multiorgan failure and death. Hence, early detection and intervention are critical for improving a patient's chance of survival.

**How severe is this cardiogenic shock?**

The severity of cardiogenic shock can be classified based on SCAI stages (A-E), whose characteristics are shown in **Figure 2**. Cardiac arrest, even if brief, can significantly worsen a patient's clinical course unexpectedly. The (A) modifier is applied to patients who have encountered cardiac arrest, irrespective of its duration, who undergo treatment with chest compressions or direct current (DC) cardioversion.

## ETIOLOGY

The most frequent cause of cardiogenic shock is acute myocardial infarction **(Table 1)**.

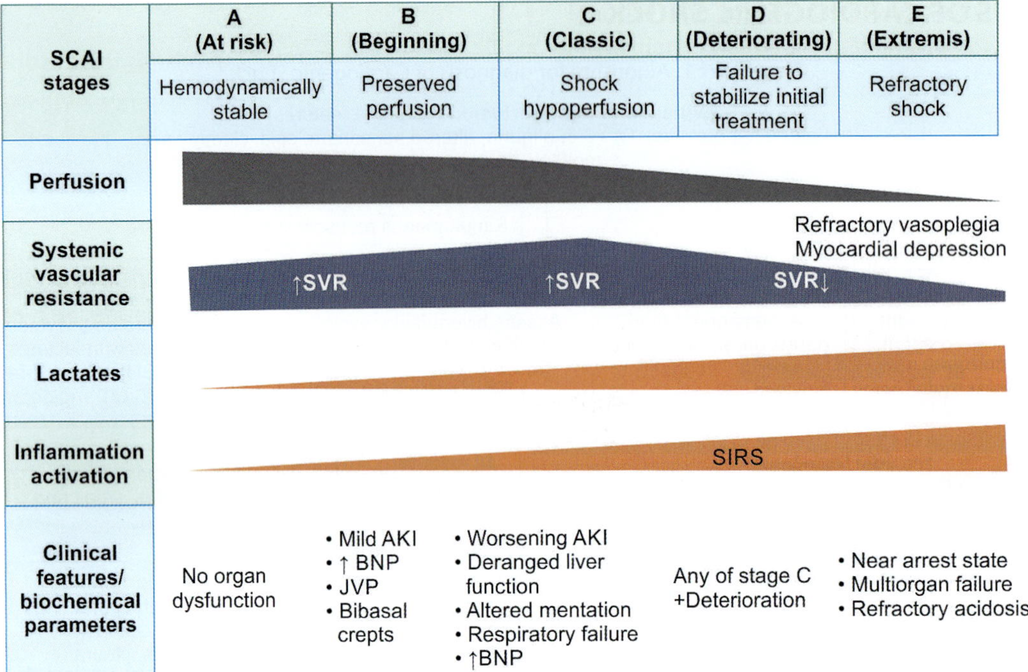


**Fig. 2:** Characteristics of SCAI (Society of Cardiovascular Angiography and Interventions) and its stages.[3] (AKI: acute kidney injury; BNP: brain natriuretic peptide; JVP: jugular venous pulse; SIRS: systemic inflammatory response syndrome; SVR: systemic vascular resistance)

**TABLE 1:** Etiology of cardiogenic shock.

| ***Myocardial*** | ***Nonmyocardial*** |
|---|---|
| I. Acute myocardial infarction<br>1. > 40 % loss of left ventricular mass<br>2. Right ventricular infarction<br>3. Mechanical complications<br>a. Papillary muscle rupture<br>b. Ventricular septal rupture<br>c. Free wall rupture | Valvular<br>1. Native valve<br>a. Stenosis<br>b. Acute regurgitation<br>c. Valvular obstruction<br>2. Prosthetic valve<br>a. Valve obstruction<br>b. Leaflet failure or restriction<br>c. Mechanical failure<br>d. Valve dehiscence |
| II. Acute decompensated heart failure<br>1. Chronic heart failure with decompensation<br>2. Acute failure - first presentation<br>a. Dilated cardiomyopathy<br>b. Myocarditis<br>c. Stress-induced cardiomyopathy (Takotsubo cardiomyopathy)<br>d. Peripartum cardiomyopathy (PPCM)<br>e. Endocrine disorders | Electrical<br>1. Atrial arrhythmia with rapid ventricular rate<br>2. Ventricular tachycardia<br>3. Bradycardia |
| III. Postcardiotomy shock | Extracardiac/obstructive<br>1. Cardiac tamponade<br>2. Pulmonary embolism |
| IV. Miscellaneous<br>1. Dynamic outflow tract obstruction<br>2. Post cardiac arrest, stunning<br>3. Myocardial depression in the setting of shock or SIRS<br>4. Myocardial contusion in chest trauma | Others<br>1. Toxidromes (CCB, Betablocker, Aluminium phosphide poisoning)<br>2. Hypothermic myocardial depression |

(SIRS: systemic inflammatory response syndrome; CCB: calcium channel blocker)

## Phenotyping the Cardiogenic Shock

1. Forrester classification for hemodynamic phenotyping
2. Type of cardiac involvement: Biventricular, Left ventricular predominant, right ventricular predominant.
3. Based on machine learning: Not congested, Cardiorenal and Cardiometabolic.[5]

**TABLE 2:** Hemodynamic classification of cardiogenic shock based on perfusion and filling pressures.[4]

| | | ***Filling pressures*** | |
|---|---|---|---|
| | | ***↓/↔ PCWP/RAP (Dry lungs)*** | ***↑ PCWP/RAP (Wet lungs)*** |
| ***Peripheral Perfusion*** | ↓ SVR (Warm peripheries) | Vasodilatory Shock (↑ CI) | Mixed Cardiogenic-Vasodilatory Shock (↓ CI) |
| | ↑SVR (Cold Peripheries) | Euvolemic Cardiogenic Shock (↓ CI) | Classic Cardiogenic Shock (↓Ci) |

(SVR: Systemic vascular resistance; CI: Cardiac Index; PCWP: pulmonary capillary wedge pressure; RAP: Right atrial pressure)

## Management of Confirmed Cardiogenic Shock[6]

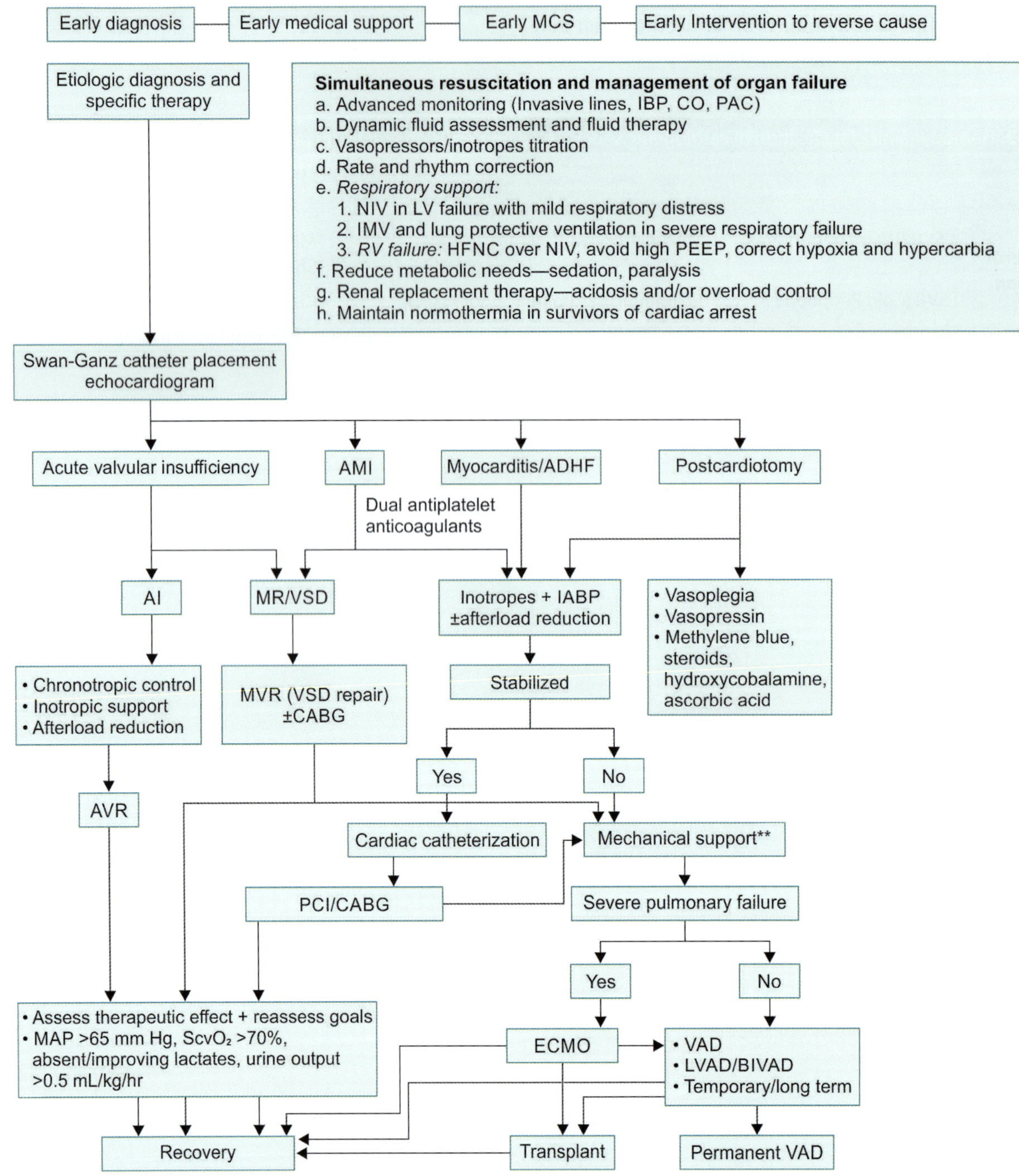


*Note:*

- Immunosuppressants can be considered in selected cases of Heart failure
- iNO/ systemic pulmonary vasodilators – in RV predominant CS
- CCB, betablockers – High dose insulin Euglycemic therapy, calcium, vasopressors, glucagon, lipid emulsion, hemodialysis for hydrophilic drugs, temporary pacing

## *Proposed Vasoactive Treatment Strategy

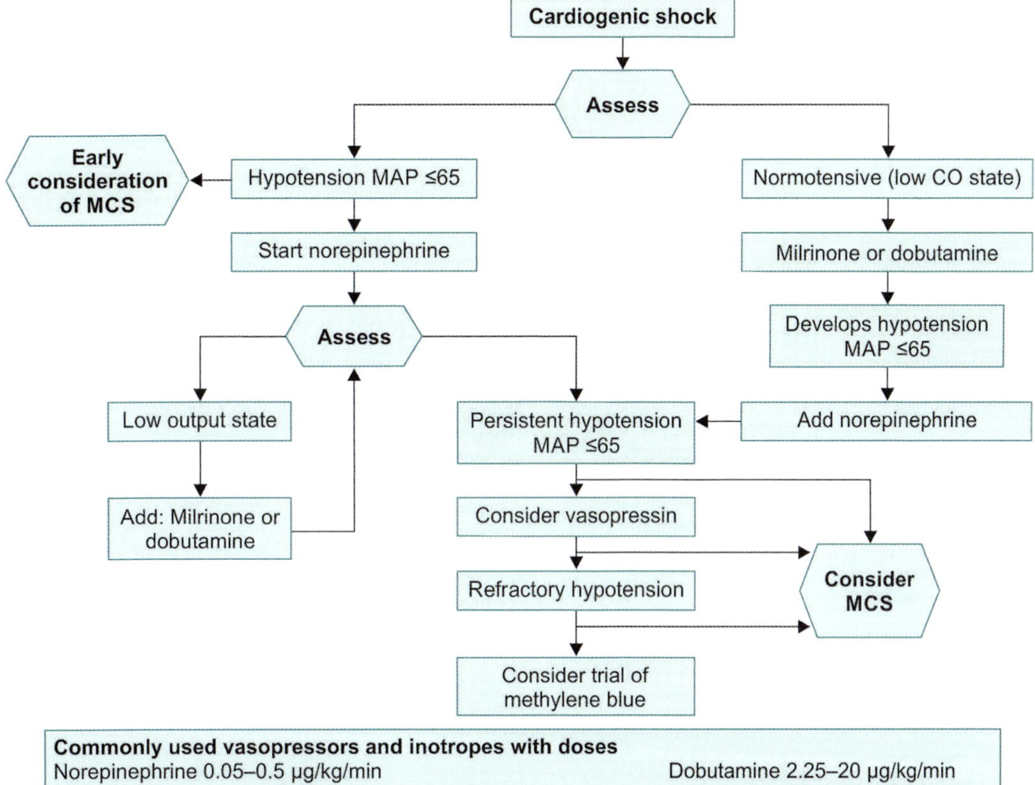


**Commonly used vasopressors and inotropes with doses**

Norepinephrine 0.05–0.5 μg/kg/min
Epinephrine 0.01–0.2μg/kg/min
Vasopressin 0.02–0.04 U/min
Dopamine Low: 2–5 μg/kg/min, Intermediate: 5–10 μg/kg/min, High: 10–20 μg/ kg/min
Dobutamine 2.25–20 μg/kg/min
Milrinone 0.125–0.75 μg/kg/min
Levosimendan 0.05–2 μg/kg/min

## **Selection of Appropriate Mechanical Support Based on Cardiac Flow

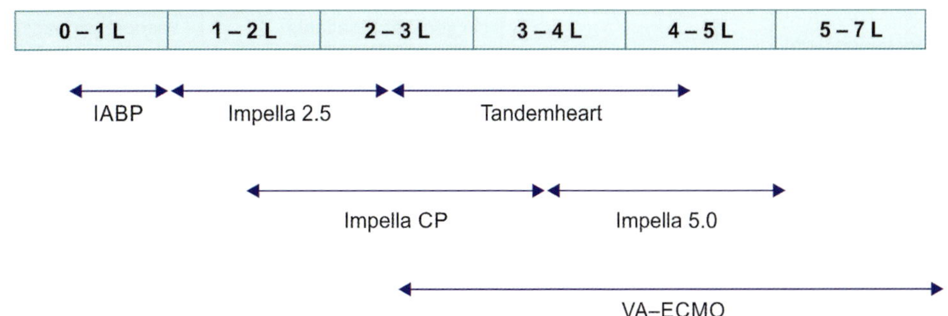

## SUMMARY OF MANAGEMENT OF CARDIOGENIC SHOCK

**Flowchart 2:** Algorithm for diagnosis of Cardiogenic Shock.[4,7]

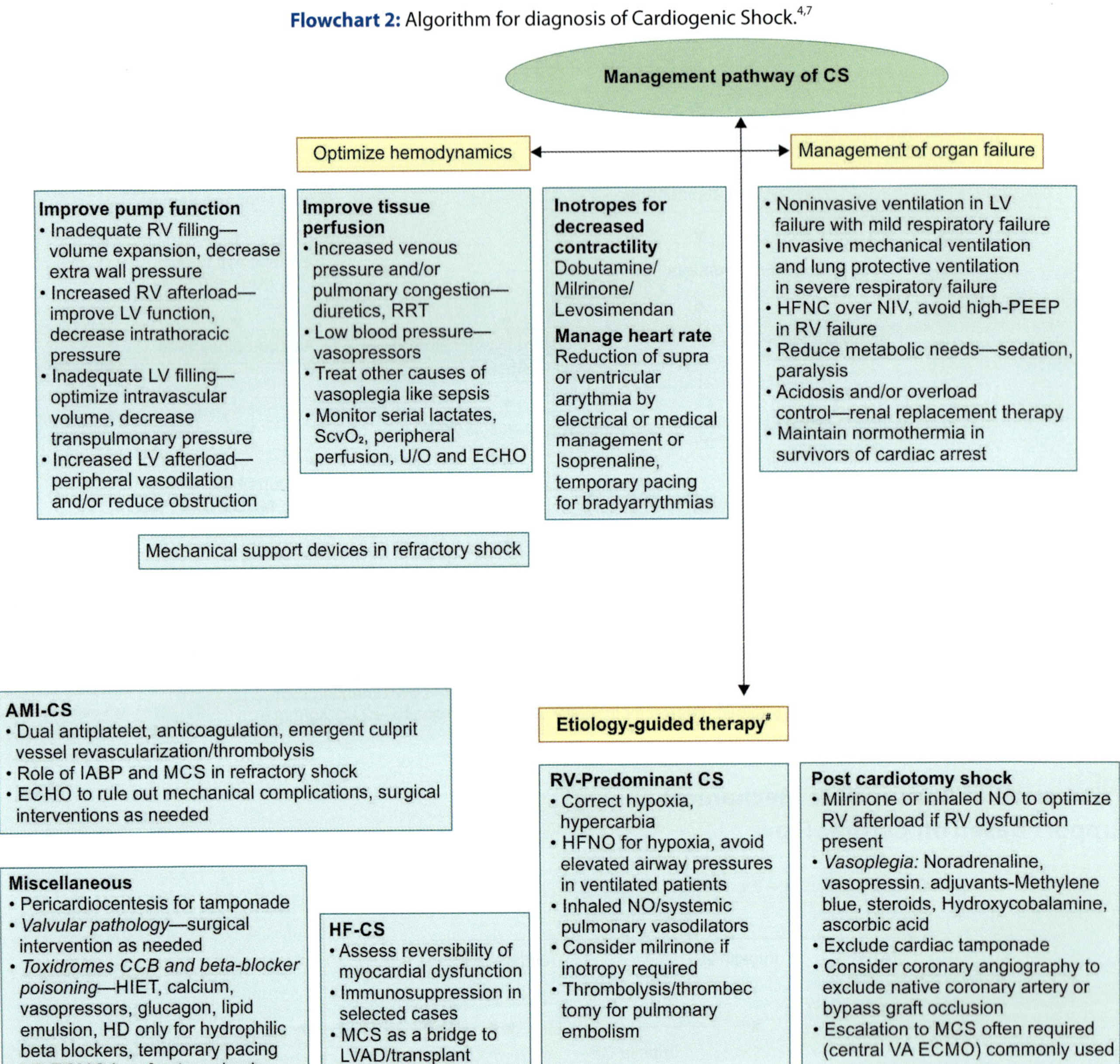


(RV: right ventricle; LV: left ventricle; RRT: renal replacement therapy; $ScvO_2$: central venous oxygen saturation; U/O: urine output; ECHO: echocardiogram; HFNC: high flow nasal cannula; NIV: Non-invasive ventilation; PEEP: positive end-expiratory pressure; AMI: acute myocardial infarction; CS: cardiogenic shock; HF: heart failure; CCB: calcium channel blocker; HIET: high dose insulin euglycemic therapy; HD: hemodialysis; VA-ECMO: veno arterial extracorporeal membrane oxygenation; MCS: mechanical circulatory support; NO: nitric oxide; LVAD: left ventricular assist device.

#Etiology of cardiogenic shock (Table 2)

Mechanical Circulatory Support devices present notable benefits compared to vasopressor therapy, offering substantial cardiovascular assistance without heightened risks of myocardial ischemia and potentially reducing myocardial oxygen demand. Implementing support devices at an early stage is a crucial therapeutic measure. Available MCS are Impella RP, Tandem Heart RA-PA, VA ECMO, IABP, Impella (2.5, CP, 5.0, 5.5), and Tandem heart LA - FA.[8]

## CONCLUSION

Cardiogenic shock is often challenging to diagnose when there are mixed components of shock. Identifying the primary cause and appropriate treatment is most important in the management of CS. Invasive monitoring and classification of CS help determine the need for appropriate hemodynamic support. Early initiation of MCS is useful in reducing cardiac pressure, augmenting cardiac output, and thus mitigating or preventing organ failures.

## REFERENCES

1. Hochman JS, Sleeper LA, Webb JG, Sanborn TA, White HD, Talley JD, et al. Early revascularization in acute myocardial infarction complicated by cardiogenic shock. SHOCK Investigators. Should We Emergently Revascularize Occluded Coronaries for Cardiogenic Shock. N Engl J Med. 1999;341(9):625-34.
2. Lahouti S. (2023). Cardiogenic shock. [Online] Available from https://recapem.com/cardiogenic-shock/ [Last accessed February; 2025].
3. Naidu SS, Baran DA, Jentzer JC, Hollenberg SM, van Diepen S, Basir MB, et al. SCAI SHOCK Stage Classification Expert Consensus Update: A Review and Incorporation of Validation Studies: This statement was endorsed by the American College of Cardiology (ACC), American College of Emergency Physicians (ACEP), American Heart Association (AHA), European Society of Cardiology (ESC) Association for Acute Cardiovascular Care (ACVC), International Society for Heart and Lung Transplantation (ISHLT), Society of Critical Care Medicine (SCCM), and Society of Thoracic Surgeons (STS) in December 2021. J Am Coll Cardiol. 2022;79(9):933-46.
4. Sarma D, Jentzer JC. Cardiogenic Shock: Pathogenesis, Classification, and Management. Crit Care Clin. 2024;40(1):37-56.
5. Zweck E, Thayer KL, Helgestad OKL, Kanwar M, Ayouty M, Garan AR, et al. Phenotyping Cardiogenic Shock. J Am Heart Assoc. 2021;10(14):e020085.
6. van Diepen S, Katz JN, Albert NM, Henry TD, Jacobs AK, Kapur NK, et al. Contemporary Management of Cardiogenic Shock: A Scientific Statement from the American Heart Association. Circulation. 2017;136(16):e232-68.
7. Laghlam D, Benghanem S, Ortuno S, Bouabdallaoui N, Manzo-Silberman S, Hamzaoui O, et al. Management of cardiogenic shock: a narrative review. Ann Intensive Care. 2024;14:45.
8. Tehrani BN, Truesdell AG, Psotka MA, Rosner C, Singh R, Sinha SS, et al. A Standardized and Comprehensive Approach to the Management of Cardiogenic Shock. JACC Heart Fail. 2020;8(11):879-91.

CHAPTER 32

# Sudden Cardiac Death

## DEFINITION

- Sudden natural death is presumed to be of a cardiac cause that occurs within 1 hour of onset of symptoms in witnessed cases and within 24 hours of last being seen alive when it is unwitnessed.
- 15–20% of all deaths in the western world
- If the patient is revived, then the event is called sudden cardiac arrest

## SYMPTOMS

- Chest pain
- Dyspnea
- Palpitations
- Retrograde amnesia may occur

## ETIOLOGY

### Coronary Artery Disease

- Atherosclerotic
- *Nonatherosclerotic:* Coronary arteritis, anomalous origin of the coronary artery from Pulmonary artery.

### Cardiomyopathy

- Hypertrophic
- Dilated

### Congenital Cardiac Diseases

- Tetralogy of Fallot
- Aortic stenosis
- Transposition of great arteries

### Primary Electrical Disease

- Congenital long QT syndrome
- Brugada syndrome
- Wolff–Parkinson–White syndrome
- Levs and Lenegre's disease

### Medication

- Haloperidol
- Azithromycin
- Erythromycin
- Cotrimoxazole
- Diuretics

### Autonomic Nervous System

Infarcted areas are just like denervated hearts in being supersensitive to catecholamines.

## PATHOPHYSIOLOGY

### Mechanisms of Ventricular Arrhythmia

#### *Automaticity*

Certain tissues are in an already partially depolarized state closer to the action potential, which can result in automatic activity, e.g., Infarcted tissues.

#### *Triggered Activity*

After depolarization coinciding with the refractory period of the cardiac action, i.e.., during or after repolarization leads to triggered activity, e.g., hypokalemia, digoxin toxicity

### Reentry

When the excitation current encounters refractoriness in its normal pathway, it may choose a more excitatory pathway, e.g., around an infarcted area and re-enter through the normal pathway

### Risk Factors

- Age 45-75 years
- Early morning - Cortisol surges as the light hits the retina

- Excessive physical activity in untrained individuals
- Family history of sudden cardiac death
- Males > Females
- Smoking
- Caffeine
- Commotio cordis

## APPROACH TO THE MANAGEMENT OF POSTCARDIAC ARREST PATIENT

Postcardiac arrest care → Treatment of correctable causes → Evaluation of cause of sudden cardiac arrest → Primary and secondary prevention

## POSTCARDIAC ARREST CARE

- Target systolic BP> 90 mm Hg
- Mean BP > 65 mm Hg
- Targeted temperature monitoring
- Avoid Hypoxia, Hyper and hypoglycemia, Hyperthermia, Hypercarbia
- Neuro-prognostication 72 hours after rewarming the patient if targeted temperature monitoring is used

## TREATMENT OF REVERSIBLE CAUSES

- Hypokalemia
- Bradycardia
- Ischemia
- Coronary spasm
- Thrombosis
- Fever,
- Acute starvation
- Dieting.
- Drug-induced arrhythmias

## EVALUATION OF SUDDEN CARDIAC ARREST

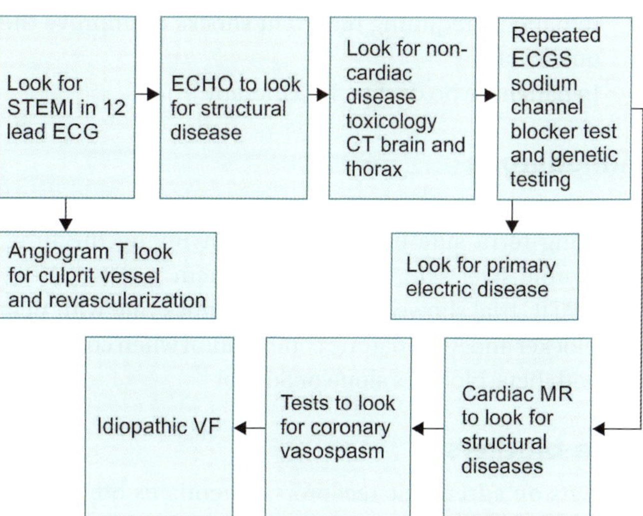


## PRIMARY PREVENTION OF SUDDEN CARDIAC DEATH

### ICD Placement

#### *Primary Prevention*

- In patients with LVEF ≤ 35 % and NYHA Class II -III despite optimal medical management for 3 months
- With expected survival for >1 year with good functional status

#### *Secondary Prevention*

- ICD should be used for patients with sudden cardiac arrest survivors with sustained ventricular arrhythmia when all the reversible causes have been treated or ruled out.
- AVID, CASH, and CIDS trials show some benefits of the ICD compared to Antiarrhythmics in reducing total mortality and reduction in SCD.

## ANTIARRHYTHMICS DRUGS

Not an alternative to ICD. Prevents recurrent shocks or inappropriate shocks secondary to supraventricular arrhythmias

### Indications

- In those who are not candidates for ICD
- In patients requiring recurrent shocks to improve the quality of life
- In patients who decline ICD therapy

### Amiodarone

- Effective antiarrhythmic
- Long-term side effects present involving the lung, thyroid, liver, skin, and nervous system
- OPTIC trial showed reduced ICD shock rate with Beta blocker and Amiodarone combination when compared with beta-blockers alone or Sotalol

### Beta-blockers

- Acts on adrenergic receptors, potentiates other Class I and III
- Removes sympathetic stimulation
- Especially useful in MI, Heart failure, Congenital long QT syndrome
- And Heart Failure
- The AVID trial showed mortality reduction in people discharged with a beta blocker.

### Sotalol

- Decreases ICD shocks compared to placebo
- Worsens heart failure
- Decreases VT threshold

### Catheter Ablation

- In patients requiring recurrent shocks to improve the quality of life
- In patients who decline ICD therapy
- In those who are not candidates for ICD
- Particularly useful for patients with VT
- By due to re-entrant pathology
- VT in postinfarct state at the borders of the infarct

## EVALUATION OF VICTIM OF CARDIAC ARREST

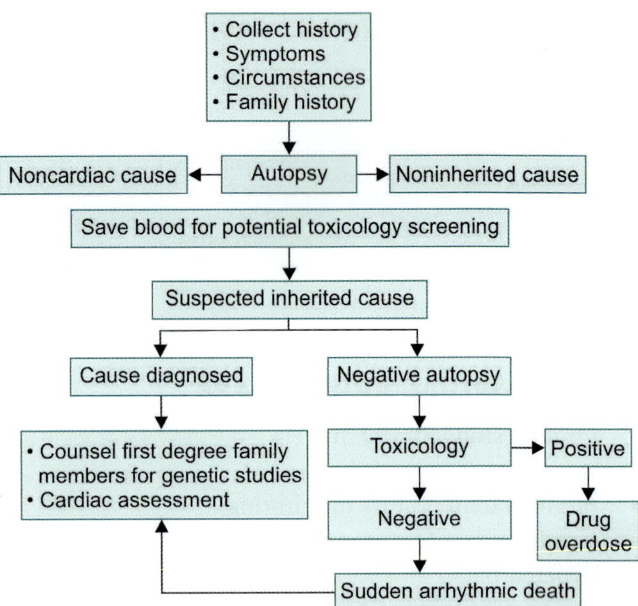


## SUGGESTED READING

1. Kumar A, Avishay DM, Jones CR, Shaikh JD, Kaur R, Aljadah M, et al. Sudden cardiac death: epidemiology, pathogenesis and management. Rev Cardiovasc Med. 2021;22(1):147-58.
2. Kuriachan VP, Sumner GL, Mitchell LB. Sudden Cardiac Death. Curr Probl Cardiol. 2015;40(4):133-200.
3. Parakh, Neeraj. Sudden cardiac death. Journal of the Practice of Cardiovascular Sciences; 2015.

# CHAPTER 33

# Pulmonary Hypertension

Defined as a mean pulmonary artery pressure >20 mm Hg. Precapillary PH is defined by an increase in pulmonary vascular resistance of wood units (WU) and is secondary to pulmonary pathology while, postcapillary PH, has a low pulmonary vascular resistance <3 WU and is due to diseases of the left side of the heart.

*Classified into five groups:*

| | |
|---|---|
| Group 1 | *Pulmonary arterial hypertension:*<br>• Idiopathic<br>• Heritable<br>• Drug or toxin-induced<br>• Pulmonary vino-occlusive disease<br>• Associated with<br>• Connective tissue disease<br>• Portal hypertension<br>• HIV<br>• Congenital heart disease<br>• Schistosomiasis |
| Group 2 | *Due to left heart disease:*<br>• Heart failure<br>• Valvular heart disease |
| Group 3 | *Due to lung disease or hypoxia:*<br>• Obstructive<br>• Restrictive<br>• Mixed<br>• Hypoxia, apart from lung disease |
| Group 4 | *Due to pulmonary artery obstruction:*<br>• Chronic thromboembolic pulmonary hypertension<br>• Other causes |
| Group 5 | *Due to unclear or multifactorial mechanisms:*<br>• Systemic and metabolic disorders<br>• Hematological disorders<br>• Complex congenital heart disease |

## PATHOPHYSIOLOGY

- Pulmonary vasculature is a low-pressure system
- *Thromboxane:* Increases Pulmonary vascular resistance

*Nitric oxide and prostacyclin* decrease pulmonary vascular resistance

A high thromboxane levels and low nitric oxide and prostacyclin levels lead to elevated Pulmonary pressures

- RV failure

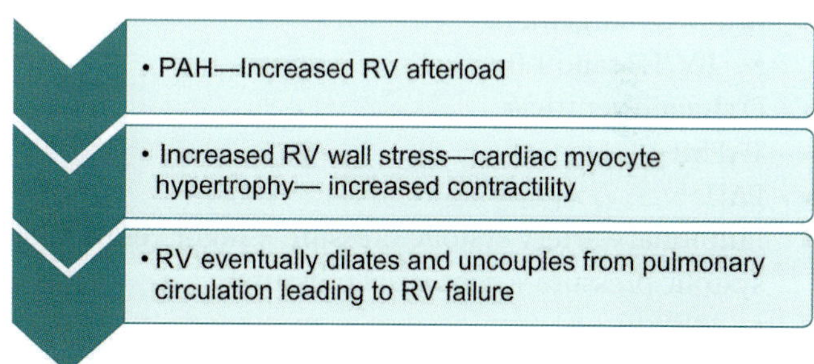


- RV affecting LV

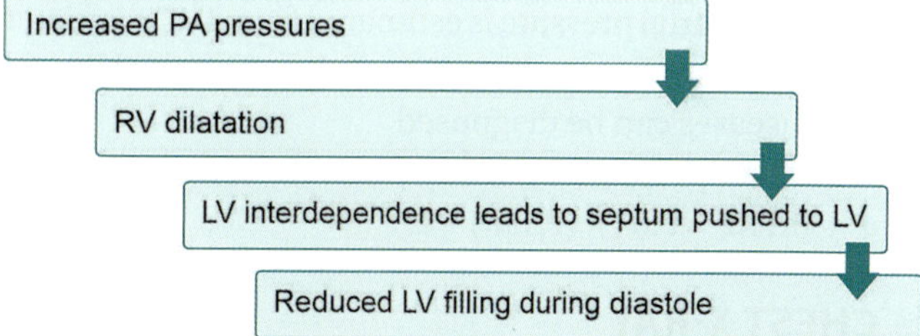


## CLINICAL FEATURES

- Shortness of breath
- Pedal edema
- Abdominal distension
- *Syncope:* Decreased cardiac output during increased physical activity
- Orthopnea
- Palpitations
- Hemoptysis

Symptoms of both the disease—causing PAH and PH per se are seen

## SIGNS

- Prominent P2
- Increased Jugular venous pulsation
- Ascites
- Hepatomegaly
- Pedal edema

## DIAGNOSIS

- ECG
- RV strain pattern
- RAD
- RBBB
- Non-specific ST T changes
- Sinus Tachycardia

## TWO-DIMENSIONAL ECHO

- RA, RV enlargement
  - RV/LV ratio 1.0
- D shaped ventricle
- TAPSE < 1.4 cm
- PAH
- Pulmonary artery systolic pressure = Right ventricular systolic pressure + right atrial pressure
  - *RVSP:*
  - Tricuspid regurgitation (continuous wave Doppler) - Peak velocity of the regurgitant jet can be obtained
  - RVSP = 4 × (TR velocity) $^2$ + Right atrial Pressure
  - Right atrial pressure is estimated from IVC diameter
  - Valvular heart diseases and congenital heart diseases can be diagnosed
  - Mean pulmonary artery pressure is calculated as mPAP = 0.61 × (PASP) + 2.

## CHEST X-RAY

- Prominent pulmonary arteries/oligemic lung fields
- Pleural effusion
- The right border of the heart is prominent
- Reduced retrosternal space noted in lateral X-ray
- Hyper inflated lungs
- Flattened Diaphragm

## VENTILATION PERFUSION SCANNING

- Sensitive screening tool for diagnosing CTEPH and pulmonary Embolism
- Normal V/Q scan rules out the above conditions
- CT Thorax and Pulmonary Angiogram
- CT Thorax helps in evaluating lung parenchyma and detecting diseases such as Interstitial Lung Diseases and Emphysema, which may suggest obstructive lung disease
- Pulmonary edema ground glass opacities.
- Kerley b lines may suggest left heart etiology.

## COMPUTED TOMOGRAPHY PULMONARY ANGIOGRAM

- Aorta pulmonary ratio can be measured.
- Pulmonary Embolism and CTEPH can be detected with specificity.

## RIGHT HEART CATHETERIZATION

- Gold standard for diagnosing Pulmonary Hypertension
- Invasive in technique
- Preferred only in specific conditions
  - If etiology is unknown
  - If left heart contribution is unclear
  - If lung pathology does not completely explain the etiology
  - Suspected pulmonary vascular diseases
  - Suspected mixed etiologies

## MANAGEMENT OF PULMONARY HYPERTENSION

| ***RV preload*** | ***RV contractility*** | ***RV afterload*** |
|---|---|---|
| • Careful optimization required<br>• Avoid overload to prevent septal shift to the left side and hypotension<br>• A passive leg raise test may be useful to assess for fluid responsiveness<br>• Not useful in tachycardia and arrhythmias | • Inotropes<br>– Milrinone<br>– Increases RV contractility<br>– Decreases RV afterload by causing vasodilatation<br>• Dobutamine<br>– Increases RV contractility<br>– Decreases RV afterload by causing vasodilatation<br>– Both the above medications may require vasopressors as they may cause systemic vasodilatation and a drop in blood pressures | • Vasopressors<br>– *Vasopressin:* Causes systemic vasoconstriction and relative decrease in pulmonary afterload<br>– *Noradrenaline:* Causes both systemic and pulmonary vasoconstriction yet is beneficial by causing RV – PA coupling due to its inotropic effects<br>– Should be reduced<br>– Correct Hypoxia and Hypercarbia<br>– Prostacyclin<br>- IV Treprostinil<br>- IV epoprostenol<br>- Chance of systemic hypotension<br>- Inhaled forms act only on the pulmonary circulation<br>– Inhaled Nitric Oxide<br>- Reduces RV afterload and PA pressures effectively<br>- Rebound Pulmonary hypertension may occur if discontinued<br>- No effect on Mortality<br>• PDE5 inhibitor<br>• Sildenafil and Tadalafil are in use<br>• Acts by causing CGMP-mediated vasodilation<br>• Selexipag is an oral prostacyclin receptor agonist used in management of pulmonary hypertension. Selexipag reduces PVR and also the relative risk of composite morbidity/mortality events by 40% when used alone or in combination with other agents |

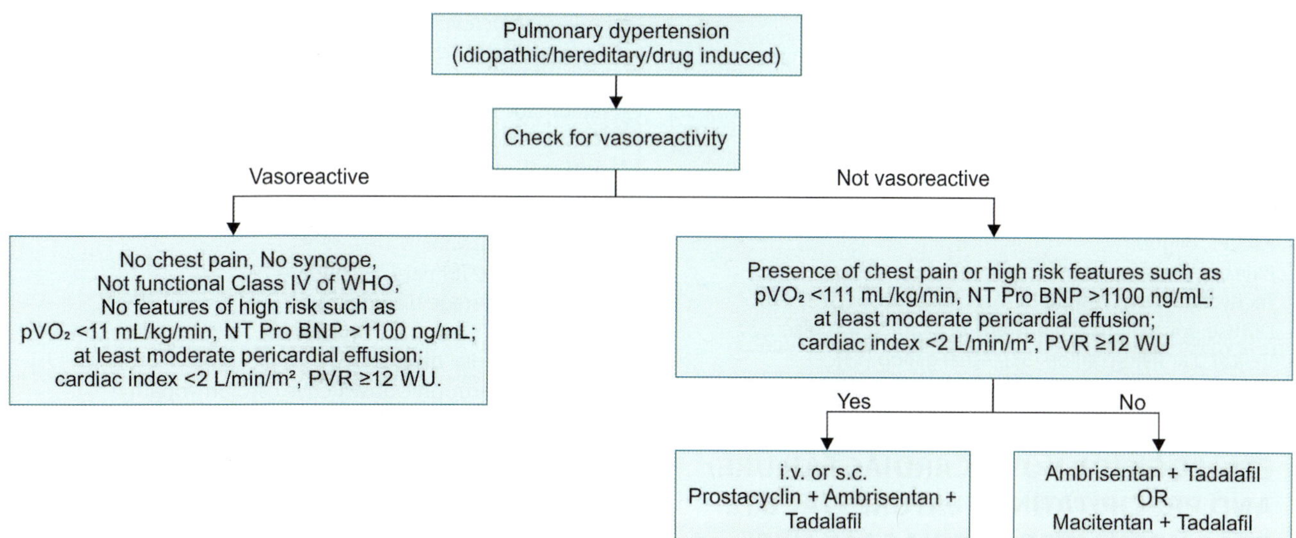


(NT-proBNP: N-terminal pro-B-type natriuretic peptide; $pVO_2$: peak volume oxygen consumption; PVR: pulmonary vascular resistance; WHO-FC: World Health Organization Functional Class; WU: wood unit)

## SUGGESTED READING

1. Jain D, Isser HS. Pulmonary hypertension - Diagnosis and management. Journal of Current Cardiology, (2025). https://doi.org/10.4103/JCC.JCC_34_24
2. Hassoun PM. Pulmonary arterial hypertension. N Engl J Med 2021;385:2361-76.
3. Maron BA. Revised definition of pulmonary hypertension and approach to management:A clinical primer. J Am Heart Assoc. 2023;12:e029024.

CHAPTER 34

# Cardiac Failure

## INTRODUCTION

Acute cardiac failure is a life-threatening disorder characterized by a syndrome related to decreased cardiac output or increased filling pressure (Pulmonary and/or Systemic venous congestion). It frequently requires emergent pharmacological and at times mechanical supportive treatment for stabilization in the intensive care unit (ICU).

## SIGNS AND SYMPTOMS OF HEART FAILURE

*Symptoms:*
- Prior history of heart failure or myocardial injury
- Dyspnea on exertion, orthopnea or paroxysmal nocturnal dyspnea (PND)
- Fatigue
- Syncope, altered sensorium in elderly
- Increasing edema, weight or abdominal girth

*Signs:*
- Elevated jugular venous pressure
- Peripheral edema
- Ascites, oliguria
- Rales, hypoxia or tachypnea
- Tachycardia, arrhythmia
- Diffuse point of maximal intensity of apical impulse
- Ventricular filling gallop (S3), Atrial gallop (S4)
- Cold and clammy extremities

## ETIOLOGY (DE NOVO CARDIAC FAILURE) AND PRECIPITATING FEATURES (ACUTE DECOMPENSATED CARDIAC FAILURE)

*Precipitating cause:*
- Acute coronary syndrome (ACS) and complications
- Hypertension, Dissection

*Contd...*

*Contd...*

- Arrhythmia
- Structural heart disease (Mitral and Aortic valve incompetency due to infective endocarditis)
- Peripartum, Stress cardiomyopathy
- Infections (Systemic, Pulmonary)
- Dietary or drug noncompliance
- Drugs (NSAIDS, alcohol, Steroids)
- Other comorbidities, i.e., Malignancy, CKD, enemia
- Heat stress, Pregnancy, surgery
- Thyroid disorders

(NSAIDS: nonsteroidal anti-inflammatory drugs, CKD: chronic kidney disease)

*Systolic dysfunction:*
- Coronary artery disease (Infarction, Ischemia)
- Hypertensive heart disease
- Rheumatic heart disease (Pressure: Aortic stenosis)
- Nonischemic Dilated cardiomyopathy: Familial, infective, postviral, toxic, metabolic.
- Intra or extracardiac shunting (Chronic)

*Diastolic dysfunction:*
- Hypertrophic: Primary, Secondary
- Infiltrative Storage disorder
- Fibrosis
- Endomyocardial disorders
- HOCM (Hypertrophic obstructive cardiomyopathy)

*Pulmonary:*
- Cor Pulmonale
- Pulmonary vascular disorders

*High output heart failure:*
- Anemia
- Hyperthyroidism
- Beri-Beri
- Av- shunting

## DIAGNOSTIC ALGORITHM OF HEART FAILURE

**Flowchart 1**

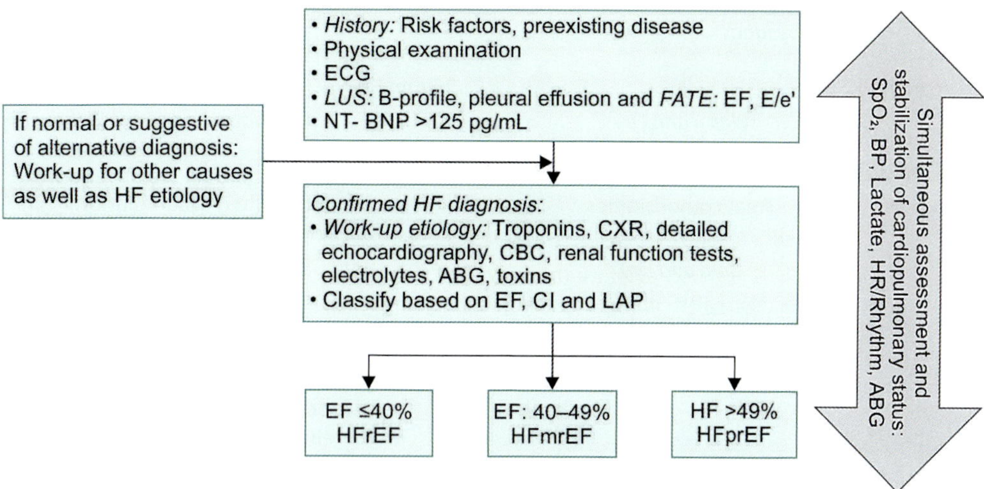


(ECG: electrocardiogram; LUS: lung ultrasound; FATE: focused assessment by transthoracic echocardiography; EF: ejection fraction; NT-BNP: N-terminal of brain natriuretic peptide; HF: heart failure; ABG: arterial blood gas; CBC: complete blood count; CI: cardiac index; LAP: left atrial pressure; HFrEF: heart failure with reduced EF; HFmrEF: heart failure with mildly reduced EF; HFpEF: herat failure with preserved EF)

## EMERGENT MANAGEMENT OF HEART FAILURE

**Flowchart 2:** Indicated in patients with Inadequate response to standard oxygen therapy, severe hypoxemia with $SpO_2$ <90% or $PaO_2/FiO_2$ <200 mm Hg, worsening hypercapnia ($PaCO_2$ >45 mm Hg) or acidosis (pH <7.3 but >7.1) associated with respiratory muscle fatigue, respiratory distress with tachypnea (Respiratory rate >24 breaths/min)

| Monitoring | Symptom relief | Drug therapy |
|---|---|---|
| • Heart rate, BP (invasive arterial if SBP <100 mm Hg), $SpO_2$, ECG, RR, clinical, ABG, lactate<br>• Monitor for worsening renal, liver (ischemic/congestive) and other end organ dysfunction during therapy | • Opioids, nitrates (if SBP >100 mm Hg), oxygen therapy if $SpO_2$ <95%<br>• Respiratory support: Noninvasive ventilation (NIV)/ HFNC or endotracheal intubation with MV(ETT-MV) as indicated, provides afterload reduction | • Vascular insufficiency with fluid redistribution: Vasodilators +/– diuretics<br>• Cardiac insuffiency with fluid congestion: Diuretics<br>• Cardiogenic shock (1–2%): Vasopressors(shock with dry lungs) with lonodilators, MC |

(RR: respiratory rate; SBP: systolic blood pressure; ETT- MV: endotracheal intubation with mechanical ventilation; HFNC: high flow nasal cannula)

## MANAGEMENT OF HEART FAILURE WITH PRESERVED EJECTION FRACTION IN INTENSIVE CARE UNIT

The emergent management of patients in HF with EF> 50% (HFprEF) in the ICU is similar to those of patients with HFrEF (***See* Flowchart 3**). The cornerstone of management is decongestion with diuretics in those with evidence of fluid overload along with treatment of hypertension, CAD, AF, anemia, and CKD. Role of vasodilators. ACE inhibitors, ARBs, and nitrates do not have a proven role in HFPEF management except in patients with HFmrEF. SGLT2 inhibitors have a role in reducing long-term mortality in patients with HFprEF. There is no role for digoxin, inotropes or vasodilators, or MCS in these patients.

## MANAGEMENT BASED ON CLINICAL PRESENTATION (NOHRIA–STEVENSON CLASSIFICATION)

| | *Dry lungs* → | *Congestion at rest Wet lungs with oedema*[1] |
|---|---|---|
| *PCWP:* | *0 mm Hg* — *18 mm Hg* | *35 mm Hg* |
| Perfusion (Cardiac index (L/m/m$^2$)) Warm peripheries → Cold peripheries[2]<br>3.5 | *Warm and Dry*<br>Rx:<br>Escalation of disease-modifying therapy (HFrEF)<br>Treat comorbidities | *Warm and Wet (Most common)*<br>Rx:<br>• Vasodilators (if fluid redistribution)<br>• Diuretics (if fluid accumulation)<br>• Consider renal replacement therapy |
| 2.2<br>0.5 | *Cold and Dry*<br>Rx:<br>Fluid challenge (if fluid-responsive)<br>Inotropic agent | *Cold and Wet*<br>*(Cardiogenic shock)*<br>Rx:<br>• Vasodilator (If SBP is sufficiently high, i.e., without hypotension)<br>• Vasopressor and inotropes (if refractory hypotension)<br>• Diuretics (when perfusion is restored and signs of increased preload)<br>• MCS (if shock refractory to drugs) |

[1]Orthopnea, paroxysmal nocturnal dyspnea, pulmonary rales, S3 gallop, increase in systolic pulmonary arterial pressure, increase in jugular venous pressure, hepatojugular reflux, hepatomegaly, edema, ascites

[2]Narrow pulse pressure, cold extremities, mental change, sleepiness, Cheyne-Stokes respiration, hypotension, renal dysfunction, decrease in diuresis, hyponatremia, acidosis.

(SBP: systolic blood pressure; MCS: mechanical circulatory support; CI: cardiac index; PCWP: pulmonary capillary wedge pressure)

**Flowchart 3**

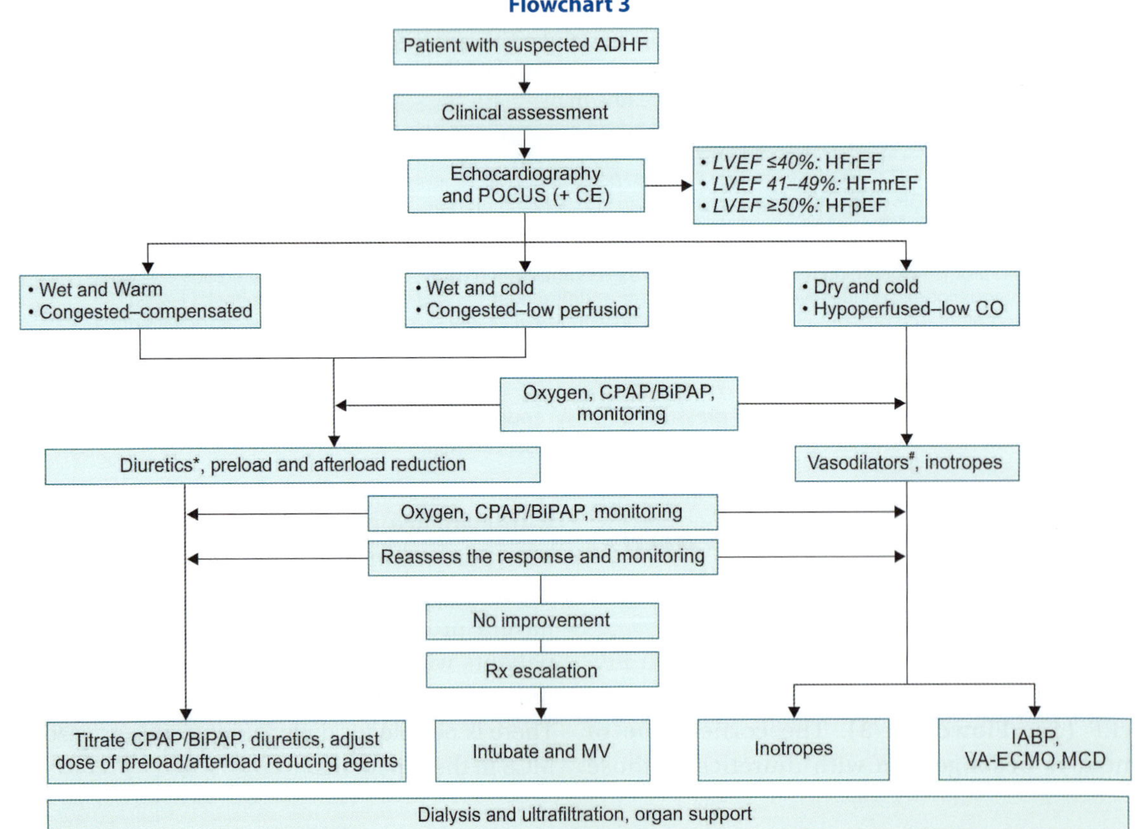


(Rx: treatment; VA-ECMO: venoarterial extracorporeal membrane oxygenation; IABP: intra-arterial balloon counterpulsation; MV: mechanical ventilation; CPAP: continuous positive airway pressure; BiPAP: biphasic positive airway pressure; CO: cardiac output)

## CONCLUSION

Acute heart failure is a dynamic disease state where progress in critical care has not matched the progress in the management of chronic heart failure. Time-limited urgent management based on pathophysiological phenotype helps prognostication and initiation of appropriate therapeutic interventions as outlined above and has been known to reduce mortality. Clinical evaluation, biomarkers, and POCUS/FATE are usually requisite enough to guide management, monitoring, and response in most cases except those in cardiogenic shock, RV involvement, and in patients with mixed types of shock in which case invasive monitoring might be indicated. Following the acute phase guideline directed medical therapy should be instituted while transitioning to ward care to prevent recurrent admissions and adverse outcomes.

## SUGGESTED READING


1. Arrigo M, Jessup M, Mullens W, Reza N, Shah AM, Sliwa K, et al. Acute heart failure. Nat Rev Dis Primers. 2020; 6(1):16.
2. Falco L, Martucci ML, Valente F, Verrengia M, Pacileo G, Masarone D. Pathophysiology-Based Management of Acute Heart Failure. Clin Pract. 2023;13(1):206-18.
3. Marini M, Manfredi R, Battistoni I, Francioni M, Vittoria Matassini M, Pongetti G, et al. Acute heart failure: differential diagnosis and treatment. Eur Heart J Suppl. 2023;25(Suppl C):C276-82.
4. Njoroge JN, Teerlink JR. Pathophysiology and Therapeutic Approaches to Acute Decompensated Heart Failure. Circ Res. 2021;128(10):1468-86.
5. Williams S, Kalakoutas A, Olusanya S, Schrage B, Tavazzi G, Carnicelli AP, et al. The management of heart failure cardiogenic shock: an international RAND appropriateness panel. Crit Care. 2024;28(1):105.

CHAPTER

# 35 Right Heart Failure

## INTRODUCTION

*Acute right ventricular dysfunction (RVD)* is defined as one of the following:

- Acute occurrence of right ventricular (RV) systolic dysfunction and dilatation seen on transthoracic echocardiography (TTE)
- A rise in natriuretic peptides in the absence of left ventricular (LV) impairment or, renal impairment, or
- RV strain patterns on electrocardiography (ECG)

*Acute right ventricular failure (RVF)* is defined as acute RVD plus low cardiac output (CO) and hypoperfusion resulting in multi-organ dysfunction or failure.

RVF is a result of failure of the RV to provide enough blood flow to the pulmonary circulation to accomplish adequate LV filling.

## ETIOLOGY OF RIGHT VENTRICULAR FAILURE

| *Excessive preload:* | *Excessive afterload:* |
|---|---|
| • Tricuspid regurgitation<br>• Pulmonic regurgitation<br>• Secondary to decompensated left heart failure<br>• Intracardiac left to right shunt<br>• Extracardiac arteriovenous shunts | • Mechanical obstruction (pulmonary embolism, pulmonic stenosis, congenital heart disease)<br>• Precapillary pulmonary hypertension<br>• Lung disease and hypoxia<br>• Postcapillary pulmonary hypertension (left heart disease) |
| *Decreased inotropy:* | *Decreased lusiotropy:* |
| • Myocardial infarction<br>• Myocarditis<br>• Post LVAD or cardiac surgery<br>• Nonischemic cardiomyopathies, including Arrhythmogenic RV cardiomyopathy<br>• Systemic sclerosis<br>• ? obesity | • Myocardial fibrosis<br>• Sarcomere stiffening<br>• Infiltrative cardiomyopathies<br>• Constrictive pericarditis |

## PATHOPHYSIOLOGY OF RIGHT VENTRICULAR FAILURE

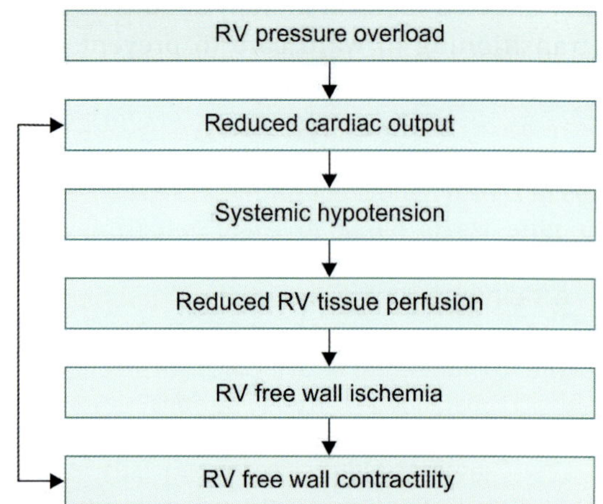


## DIAGNOSIS AND EVALUATION

| | |
|---|---|
| History | • *Symptoms of RHF:* Dyspnea, early satiety, abdominal fullness, lower extremity edema, right-upper-quadrant tenderness, exercise intolerance, fatigue<br>• *Past history:* CAD, LVF, VALVULAR HEART DISEASE, COPD, VTE/PE, CTD, HIV<br>• *Personal history:* tobacco, illicit drug, or anorexigen use<br>• *Family history:* PAH, LVF, Sudden cardiac death |
| Physical examination | Elevated JVP, right ventricular heave, loud (P2), tricuspid regurgitation murmur, enlarged and pulsatile liver, hepatojugular reflux, ascites, lower-extremity edema |
| ECG | Right atrial dilatation, right ventricular hypertrophy, right-axis deviation |
| ECHO | • Enlarged RV (more than aortic root/Left atria on (PLAX view)<br>• Enlarged RV (LV/RV ratio < 1 in apical four-chamber)<br>• Flattened interventricular septum (PSAX) |

*Contd...*

*Contd...*

| | |
|---|---|
| | • RV fractional area change <35% (4C VIEW)<br>• Tricuspid annular plane systolic excursion <16 mm (M-mode of 4C view)<br>• RV/LV basal ratio >1 with Mc Connell sign- (4C view)<br>• Distended IVC with reduced collapsibility (subcostal)<br>• 60/60 sign—acceleration time of pulmonary ejection < 60 milliseconds and mildly elevated (<60 mm Hg) peak systolic gradient at Tricuspid valve<br>• Right heart mobile thrombus in cases of thromboembolism |
| Other | Natriuretic peptide, cardiac MRI, Right heart catheterization |

## EVALUATION

- Identification and severity assessment of RV failure
- Identification of underlying cause/ trigger
- Differentiation between acute cor pulmonale and other causes

## TREATMENT

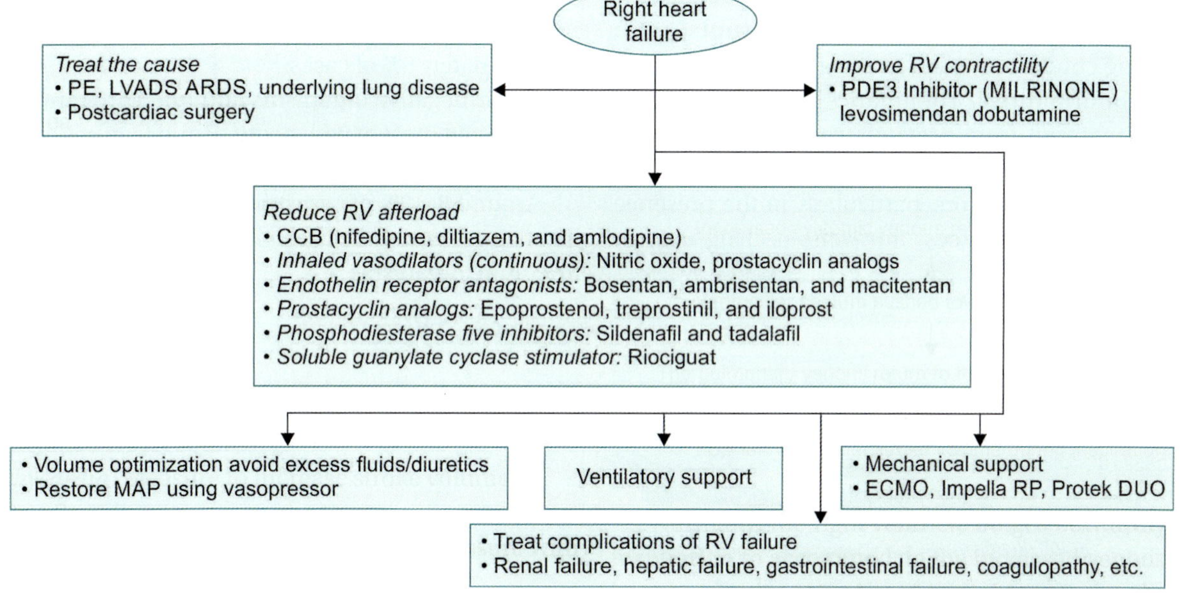


## SUGGESTED READING

1. Harjola VP, Mebazaa A, Čelutkienė J, Bettex D, Bueno H, Chioncel O, Konstantinides S, et al. Contemporary management of acute right ventricular failure: a statement from the Heart Failure Association and the Working Group on Pulmonary Circulation and Right Ventricular Function of the European Society of Cardiology. Eur J Heart Fail. 2016;18:226-41.
2. Levitt CV, Williams CA, Ahari J, Pourmand A. Approach to Decompensated Right Heart Failure in the Acute Setting. J Clin Med. 2024;13:869.
3. Monteagudo-Vela M, Tindale A, Monguió-Santín E, Reyes-Copa G, Panoulas V. Right ventricular failure: Current strategies and future development. Front Cardiovasc Med. 2023;10:998382.

CHAPTER

# 36

# Native Valve Infective Endocarditis

## INTRODUCTION

Native valve endocarditis (NVE) is characterized by microbial colonization and inflammation of the endocardial surface of the heart, most commonly affecting the cardiac valves, leading to valvular dysfunction, heart failure, and progressive/recurrent systemic signs of infection with distant organ metastasis and dysfunction.

NVE predominantly affects individuals with predisposing conditions, such as congenital or acquired valvular abnormalities, rheumatic heart disease, or prosthetic material from previous cardiac procedures. However, it can also occur in individuals without apparent cardiac risk factors, particularly in the presence of invasive medical devices, intravenous drug use, or immunosuppression.

## MICROBIOLOGY

Approximately 80% of cases of NVE are attributed to Gram-positive organisms like *Staphylococcus aureus*, Coagulase negative Staphylococci, Streptococci, and Enterococci ≈ 10%. HACEK organisms are fastidious gram-negative bacilli (*Haemophilus* species [except H. influenzae], *Aggregatibacter* species, *Cardiobacterium hominis*, *Eikenella corrodens*, and *Kingella kingae*) that account for approximately 5% of cases.

Gram-negative organisms and fungi are rare causes of NVE but can present with acute IE and features of systemic toxicity and septic shock.

Around 8–10% of cases may be culture-negative, often due to prior antibiotic use or infections caused by difficult-to-culture organisms.

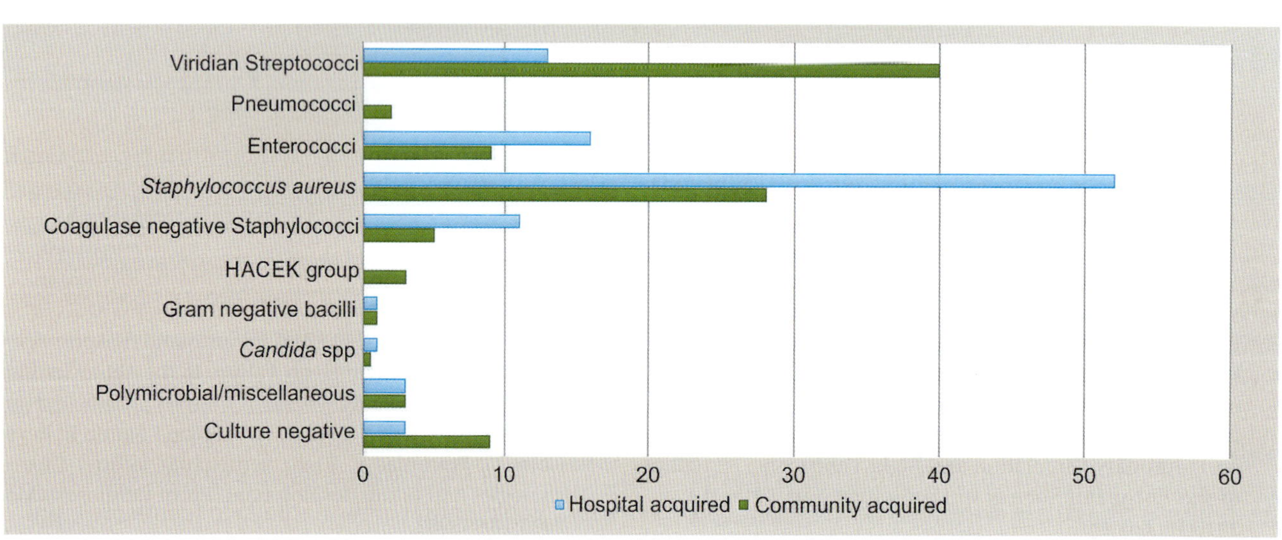

## RISK FACTORS

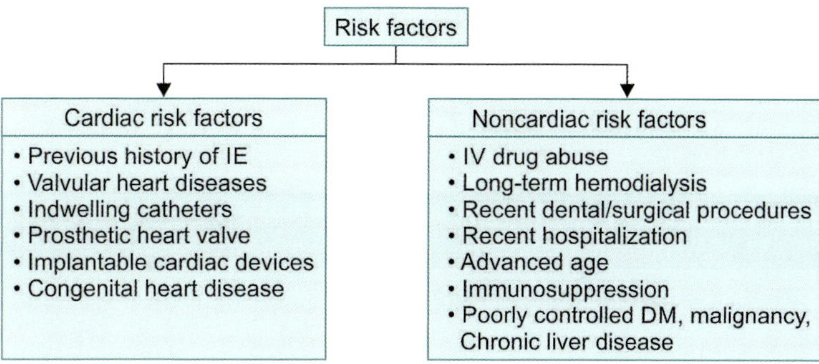


## PATHOGENESIS

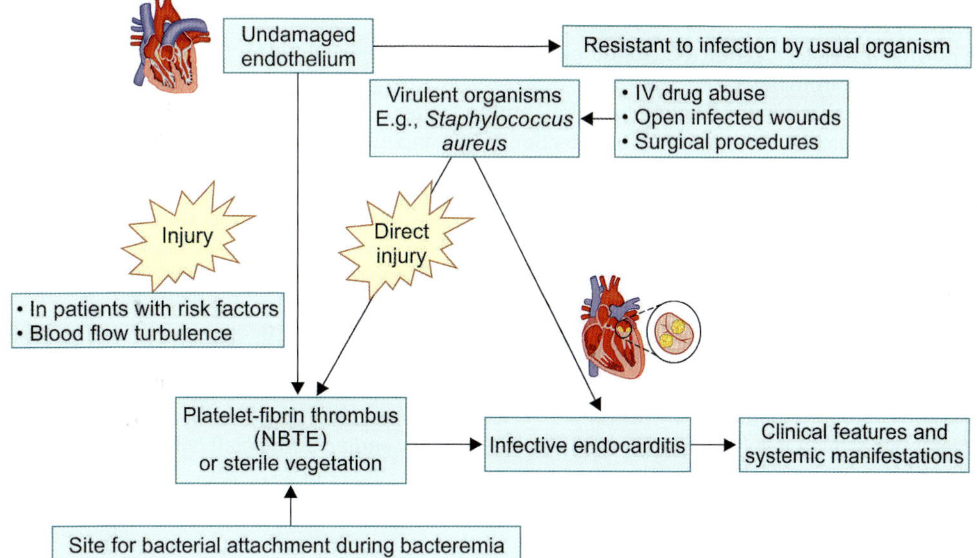


## CLINICAL FEATURES

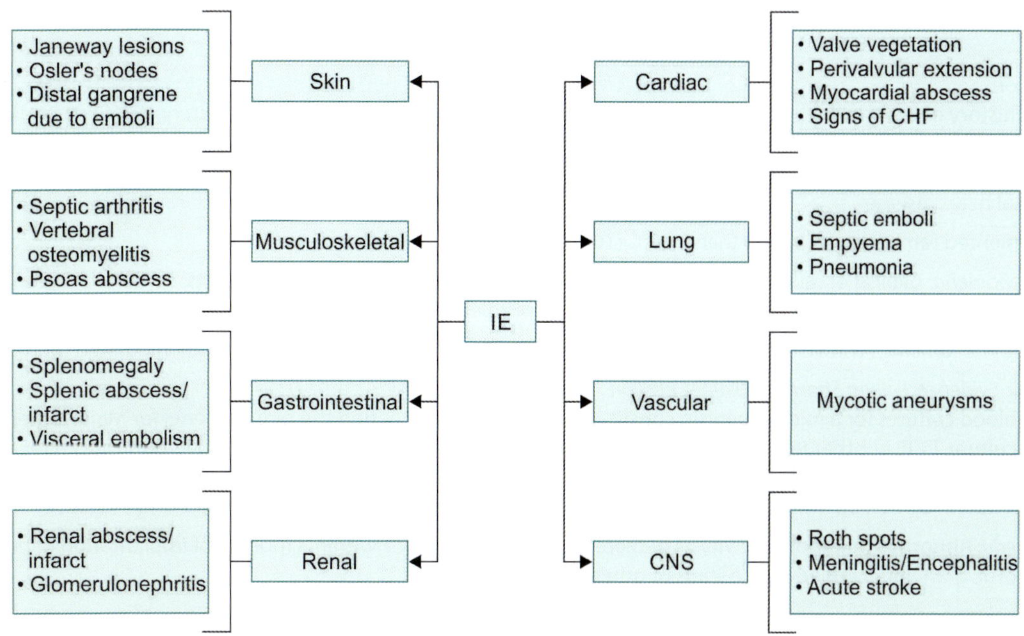

Classically described signs of IE, such as Osler nodes (tender, purple cutaneous nodules), Janeway lesions (non-tender, erythematous macules and papules on the palms and soles), and Roth spots (retinal hemorrhages with pale centers), are highly suggestive of the disease. However, these findings are relatively rare, occurring in only 5–10% of cases and typically in left-sided endocarditis.

## DIAGNOSIS

**2023 Duke-International Society for Cardiovascular Infectious Diseases Criteria for Infective Endocarditis: Updating the Modified Duke Criteria.**

***Major criteria***

A. *Microbiologic Major Criteria:*
   1. Positive blood cultures
      i. Microorganisms that commonly cause IE[a] isolated from 2 or more separate blood culture sets (Typical) Or
      ii. Microorganisms that occasionally or rarely cause IE isolated from 3 or more separate blood culture sets (Nontypical)
   2. Positive laboratory tests
      i. Positive polymerase chain reaction (PCR) or other nucleic acid-based technique for *Coxiella burnetii*, *Bartonella* species, or *Tropheryma whipplei* from blood Or
      ii. *Coxiella burnetii* antiphase I immunoglobulin G (IgG) antibody titer >1:800, Or isolated from a single blood culture Or
      iii. Indirect immunofluorescence assays (IFA) for detection of IgM and IgG antibodies to *Bartonella henselae* or *Bartonella quintana* with immunoglobulin G (IgG) titer ≥1:800

B. *Imaging Major Criteria:*
   1. Echocardiography and cardiac computed tomography (CT) imaging
      i. Echocardiography and/or cardiac CT showing vegetation, valvular/leaflet perforation, valvular/leaflet aneurysm, abscess, pseudoaneurysm, or intracardiac fistula Or
      ii. Significant new valvular regurgitation on echocardiography as compared with previous imaging. Worsening or changing of preexisting regurgitation is not sufficient. Or
      iii. New partial dehiscence of prosthetic valve as compared with previous imaging
   2. Positron emission computed tomography with 18F-fluorodeoxyglucose ([18F]FDG PET/CT imaging)
      Abnormal metabolic activity, involving a native or prosthetic valve, ascending aortic graft (with concomitant evidence of valve involvement), intracardiac device leads or other prosthetic material

C. *Surgical Major Criteria:* Evidence of IE documented by direct inspection during heart surgery neither Major Imaging Criteria nor subsequent histologic or microbiologic confirmation

**2023 Duke-International Society for Cardiovascular Infectious Diseases Criteria for Infective Endocarditis: Updating the Modified Duke Criteria**

***Minor criteria***

A. Predisposition
   - Previous history of IE
   - Prosthetic valve
   - Previous valve repair
   - Congenital heart disease
   - More than mild regurgitation or stenosis of any etiology
   - Endovascular intracardiac implantable electronic device (CIED)
   - Hypertrophic obstructive cardiomyopathy
   - Injection drug use

B. *Fever:* Documented temperature greater than 38.0°C (100.4°F)

C. *Vascular Phenomena:* Clinical or radiological evidence of arterial emboli, septic pulmonary infarcts, cerebral or splenic abscess, mycotic aneurysm, intracranial hemorrhage, Janeway lesions, purulent purpura

D. *Immunologic Phenomena:* Positive rheumatoid factor, Osler nodes, Roth spots, or immune complex-mediated glomerulonephritis

E. *Microbiologic Evidence, Falling Short of a Major Criterion*
   1. Positive blood cultures for a microorganism consistent with IE but not meeting the requirements for Major Criterion Or
   2. Positive culture, PCR, or other nucleicacid basedtest (amplicon or shotgun sequencing, in situ hybridization) for an organism consistent with IE from a sterile body site other than cardiac tissue, cardiac prosthesis, or arterial embolus; or a single finding of a skin bacterium by PCR on a valve or wire without additional clinical or microbiological supporting evidence.

F. *Imaging Criteria:* Abnormal metabolic activity as detected by [18F]FDG PET/CT within 3 months of implantation of prosthetic valve, ascending aortic graft, intracardiac device leads or other prosthetic material

G. *Physical Examination Criteria*

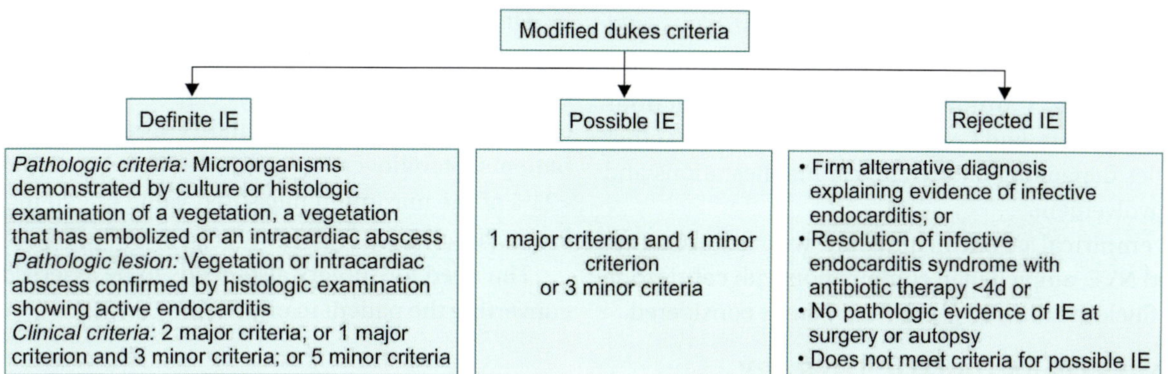


## INVESTIGATIONS

### Blood Culture

At least three sets of blood cultures from different venipuncture sites should be sent, irrespective of the timing of fever, with a minimum of 10 ml in each bottle, and the first and last cultures should be at least 1 hour apart.

When blood cultures are negative, additional tests to identify the causative organism include serology for Coxiella, Bartonella, Chlamydia, Legionella, Mycoplasma, and Brucella (in patients with relevant exposure risks).

### Imaging

Transthoracic echocardiography (TTE) is a helpful first-line investigation for suspected endocarditis, but its sensitivity is limited, around 55% for native valves and even lower for prosthetic valves. In situations where TTE is inconclusive and when the clinical suspicion is high, TEE is the next imaging of choice.

PET/CT (positron emission tomography-computed tomography) and 18F-fluorodeoxyglucose (a radiotracer used in PET/CT imaging) are increasingly being utilized presently in cases of suspected IE and could be considered in cases with high clinical suspicion. Other imaging studies, like CT/MRI, may be done to look for silent visceral/neurological embolization.

## DIAGNOSTIC PATHWAY FOR SUSPECTED NATIVE VALVE ENDOCARDITIS

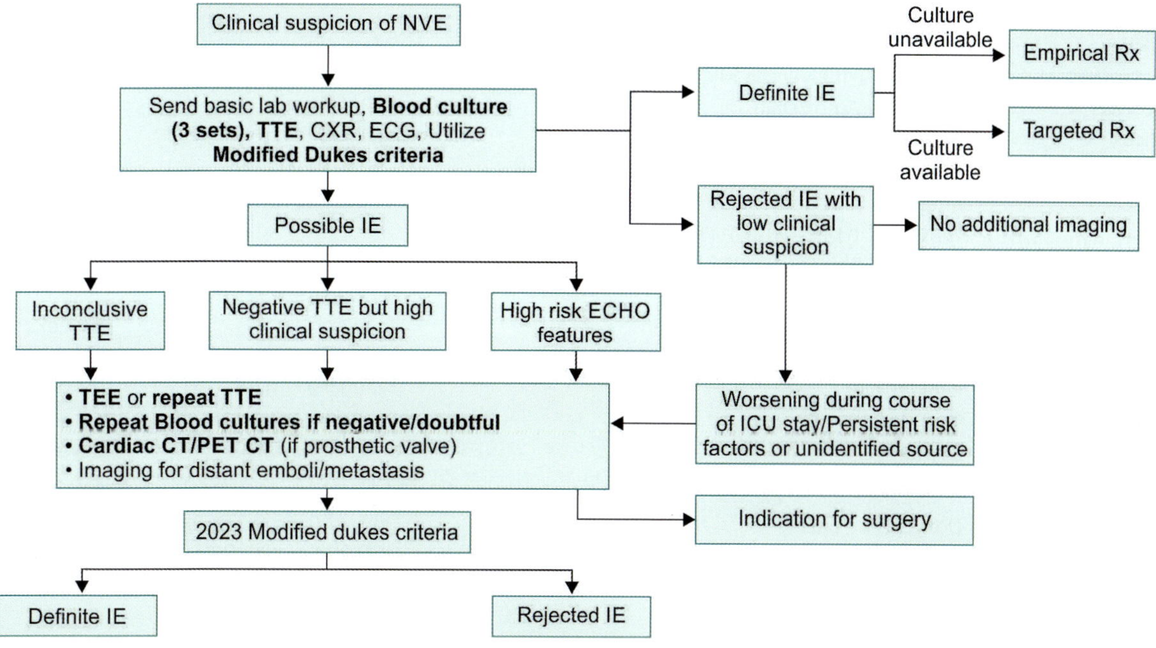

## MANAGEMENT

IE must be managed by a multidisciplinary team consisting of Cardiologists, Cardiothoracic surgeons, Infectious disease specialists, and Critical Care, with access to other specialties depending on the clinical manifestations and organ involvement.

For empirical cover, in patients with community-acquired NVE, ampicillin in combination with ceftriaxone or with flucloxacillin and gentamicin can be considered.

Once the clinical condition of the patient is stable and the patient has received at least 10 days of IV therapy, OPAT or step-down outpatient oral antibiotic treatment is a safe alternative to in-hospital IV treatment in selected patients. Stability criteria include No fever >2 days, CRP <25% of the maximum measured value or <20 mg/L, and leucocytes $<15 \times 10^9$/L.

The need for surgery also needs to be assessed before converting the patient to oral therapy or OPAT.

## PHASES OF ANTIBIOTIC THERAPY

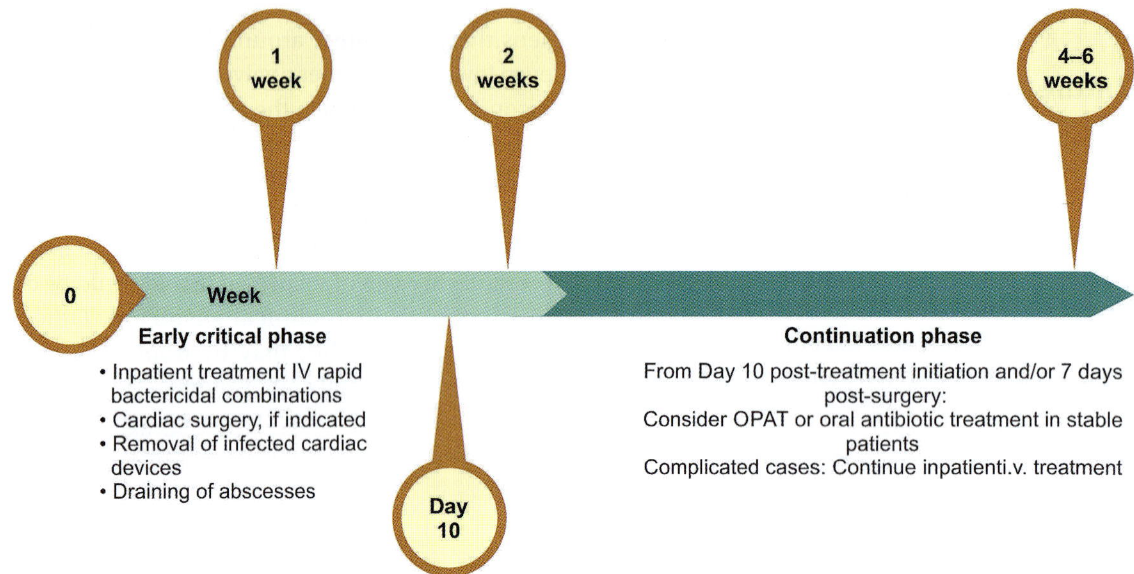


## SUGGESTED ANTIBIOTIC REGIMENS FOR TARGETED THERAPY

| *Organism* | *Antibiotic* | *Dose* | *Duration* |
|---|---|---|---|
| Viridian Streptococci, *Streptococcus gallolyticus* | • Penicillin G (If Penicillin MIC ≤0.12 μg/mL)<br>• Ampicillin/Amoxicillin<br>• Ceftriaxone<br>• Vancomycin (If Penicillin MIC >0.12/Allergy) | • 2-3 mU IV Q4H<br>• 2g IV Q4H<br>• 2g IV OD<br>• 15 mg/kg IV q12h | 4 weeks |
| Enterococci | • Ampicillin plus gentamicin<br>• Vancomycin plus gentamicin<br>• Ampicillin plus ceftriaxone (E. faecalis, Risk of AG nephrotoxicity) | • Ampi 2g IV Q4H<br>• Genta 1 mg/kg Q8H<br>• Vanco 15 mg/kg IV q12h<br>• Ceftriaxone 2g IV BD | 4–6 weeks<br>6 weeks<br>6 weeks |
| MSSA - NVE | • Nafcillin, oxacillin, or flucloxacillin<br>• Cefazolin<br>• Vancomycin | • 2g IV q4h<br>• 2g IV q8h<br>• 15 mg/kg IV q12h | 6 weeks<br>6 weeks<br>6 weeks |
| MRSA - NVE | • Vancomycin<br>• Daptomycin | • 15 mg/kg IV q8-12h<br>• 8–10 mg/kg OD | 6 weeks<br>6 weeks |
| HACEK Organisms | Ceftriaxone | 2g OD | 4 weeks |
| *Coxiella burnetii*—NVE | • Doxycycline plus<br>• Hydroxychloroquine (200 mg PO q8h) | • Doxy 100 mg PO Q12H<br>• HCQ 200 mg PO Q8H | At least 18 weeks |
| *Bartonella* spp. | • Doxycycline plus<br>• Gentamicin | • Doxy 100 mg PO Q12H<br>• Genta 1 mg/kg IV q8h | 6 weeks<br>2 weeks |

## SURGICAL TREATMENT

The main reasons to consider surgery in Acute IE include uncontrolled infection, difficult-to-treat organisms, signs of heart failure, and risk of embolization. Despite the high risk for surgery in these patients, current evidence suggests that surgical treatment may generate a survival advantage of up to 20% in the first year.

## INDICATIONS FOR SURGERY

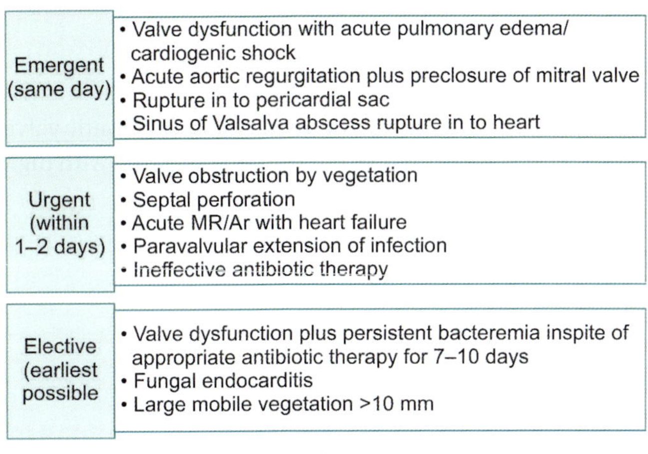

| | |
|---|---|
| Emergent (same day) | • Valve dysfunction with acute pulmonary edema/ cardiogenic shock<br>• Acute aortic regurgitation plus preclosure of mitral valve<br>• Rupture in to pericardial sac<br>• Sinus of Valsalva abscess rupture in to heart |
| Urgent (within 1–2 days) | • Valve obstruction by vegetation<br>• Septal perforation<br>• Acute MR/Ar with heart failure<br>• Paravalvular extension of infection<br>• Ineffective antibiotic therapy |
| Elective (earliest possible | • Valve dysfunction plus persistent bacteremia inspite of appropriate antibiotic therapy for 7–10 days<br>• Fungal endocarditis<br>• Large mobile vegetation >10 mm |

## CONCLUSION

Native valve infective endocarditis (NVE) is a challenging condition with diverse presentations and significant complications. Early recognition and accurate diagnosis, supported by updated criteria like Duke-ISCVID, are critical for effective management. Treatment requires a combination of targeted antimicrobial therapy and timely surgical intervention when needed. Despite advancements, NVE remains associated with high morbidity and mortality, highlighting the importance of prevention and vigilant care in at-risk individuals.

## SUGGESTED READING


1. Delgado V, Ajmone Marsan N, de Waha S, Bonaros N, Brida M, et al. ESC Scientific Document Group. 2023 ESC Guidelines for the management of endocarditis. Eur Heart J. 2023;44(39):3948-4042.
2. Fowler VG, Durack DT, Selton-Suty C, Athan E, Bayer AS, Chamis AL, et al. The 2023 Duke-International Society for Cardiovascular Infectious Diseases Criteria for Infective Endocarditis: Updating the Modified Duke Criteria. Clin Infect Dis. 2023;77(4):518-26.
3. Li M, Kim JB, Sastry BKS, Chen M. Infective endocarditis. Lancet. 2024;404(10450):377-92.
4. Nappi F. Native Infective Endocarditis: A State-of-the-Art-Review. Microorganisms. 2024;12(7):1481.

CHAPTER 37

# Prosthetic Valve Endocarditis

## INTRODUCTION

Prosthetic valve endocarditis (PVE) is an infection of the endovascular structure that occurs on parts of a prosthetic valve or on the reconstructed native valve of the heart. It accounts for 20% of infective endocarditis and is associated with high morbidity and mortality.

Based on the time of the disease acquirement, this disease is classified into three types:

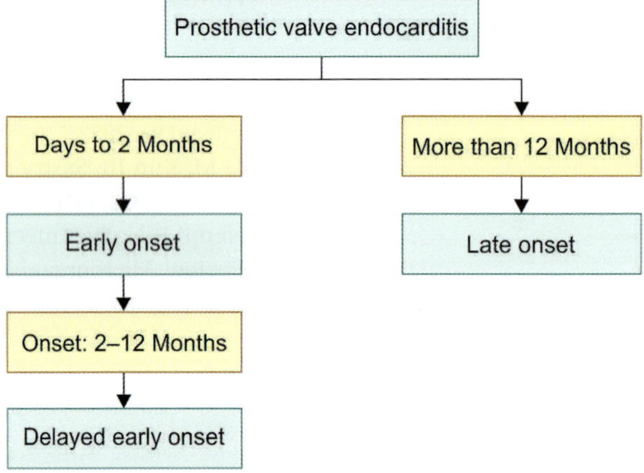

## RISK FACTORS

Prosthetic aortic valve has more predilection for PVE compared to other valves.

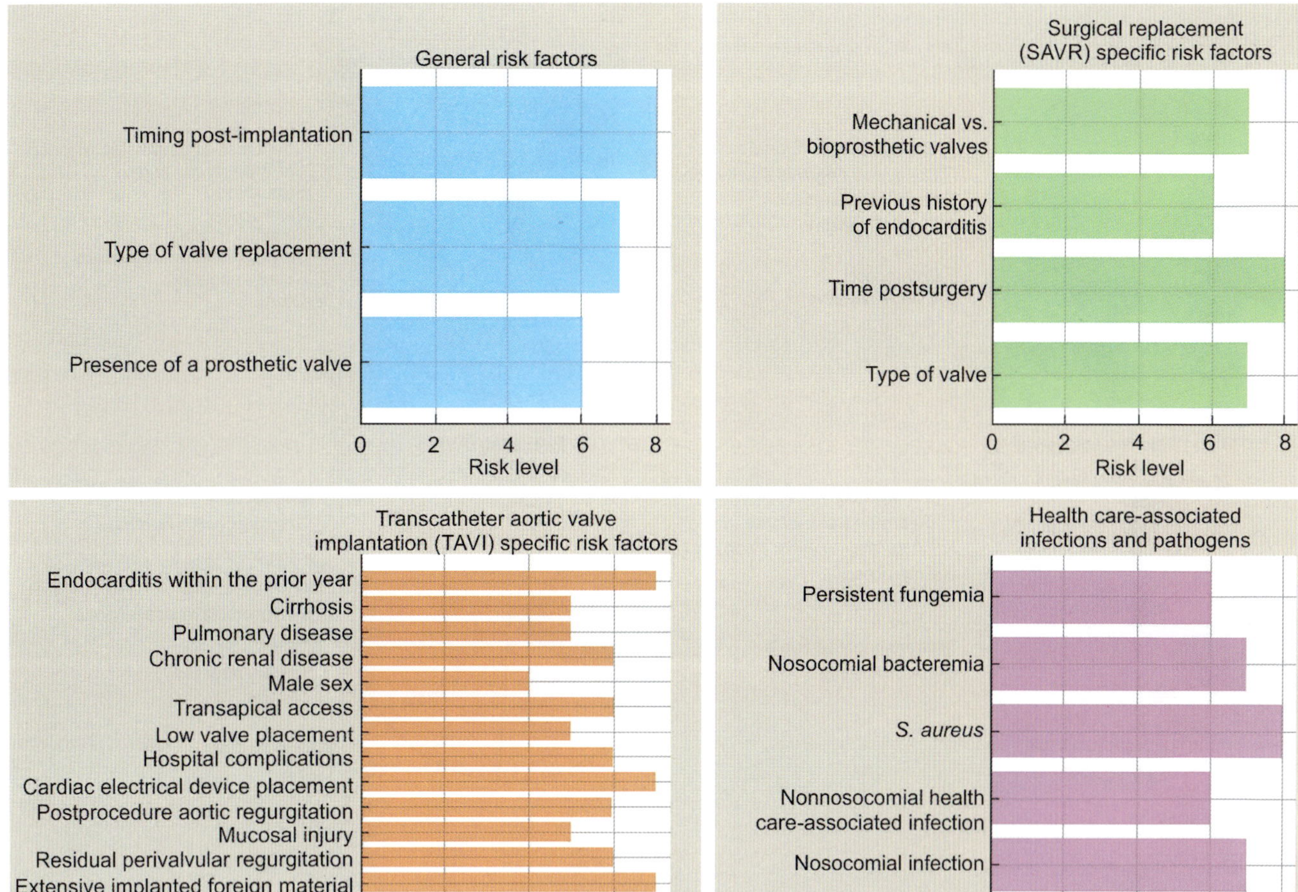

## MICROBIOLOGY

Delayed onset nosocomial infection is a blend of infections at the time of surgery or during surgical admission and community acquired infections.

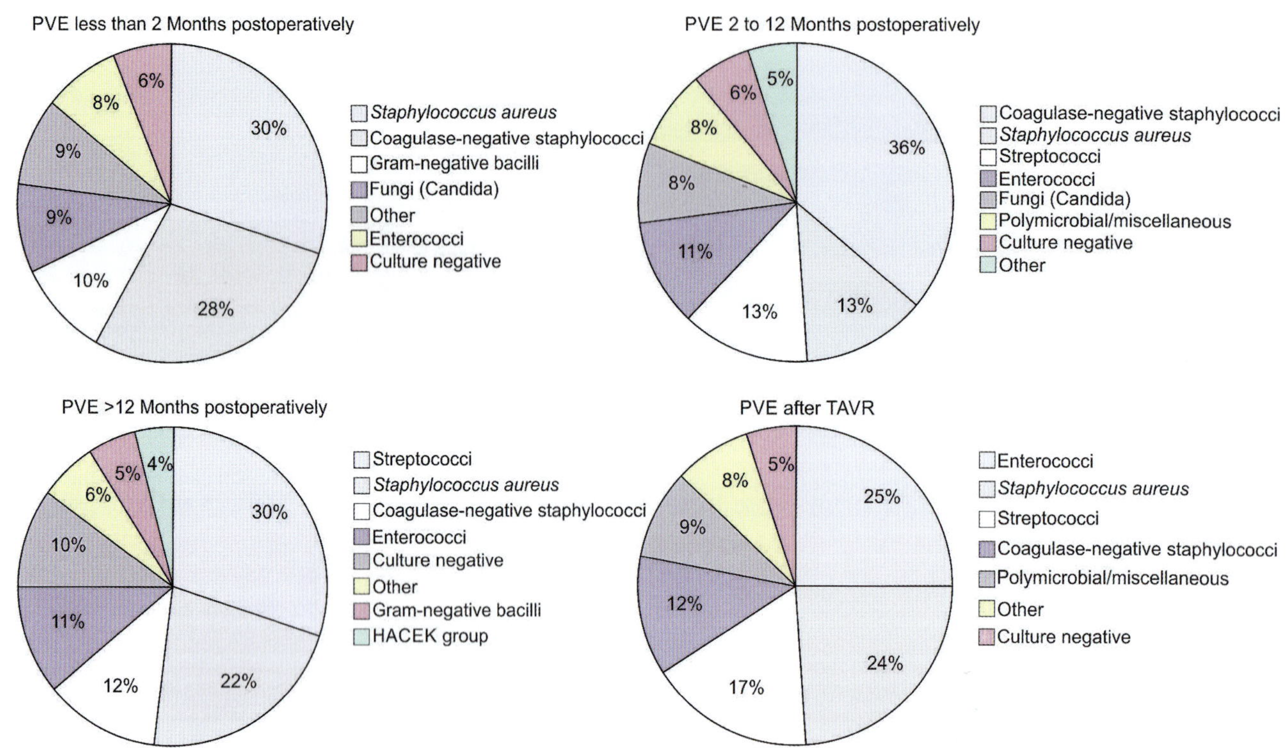

## CLINICAL MANIFESTATION

Most of the clinical symptoms post valve replacement are nonspecific, high degree suspicion is important.

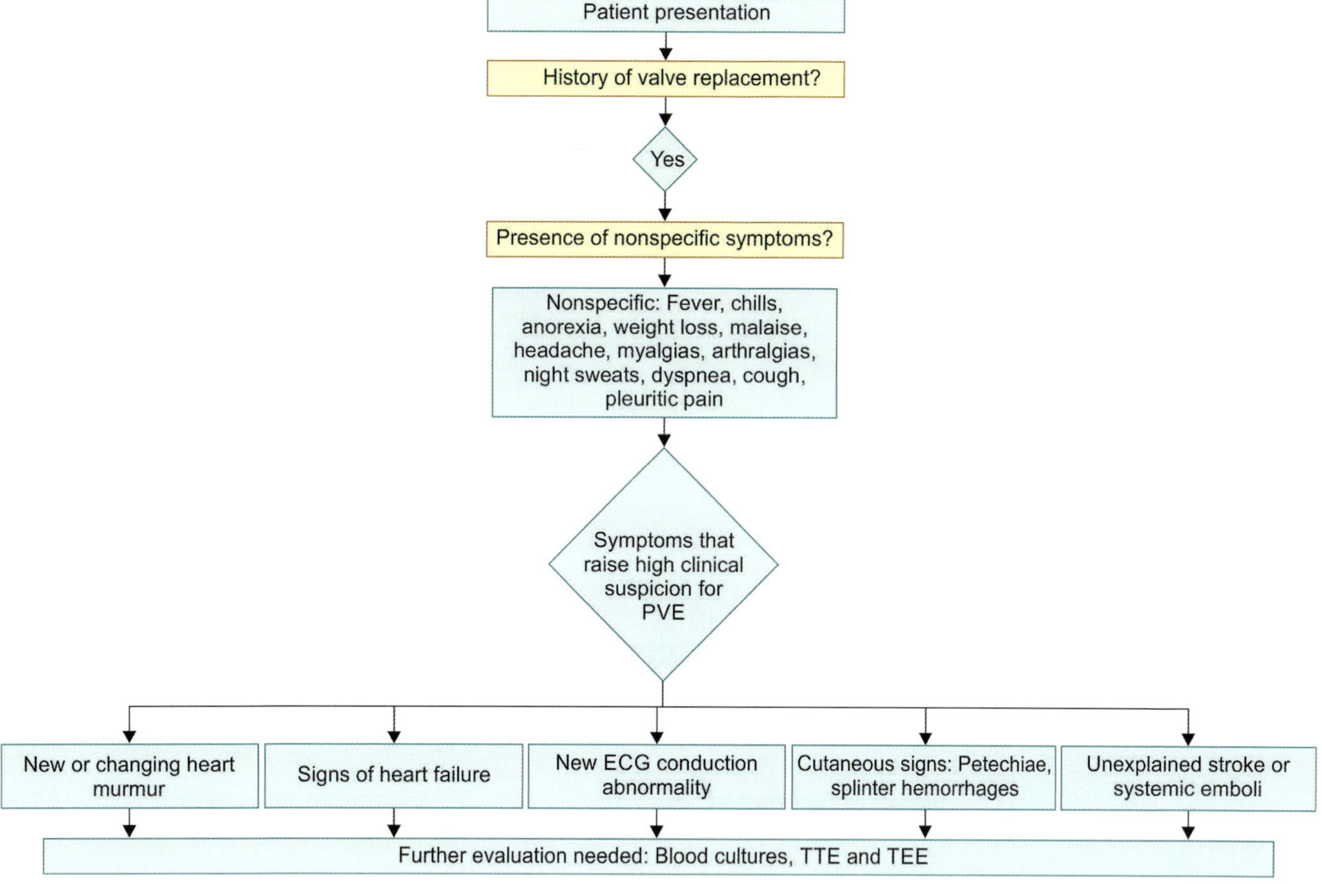

## EVALUATION

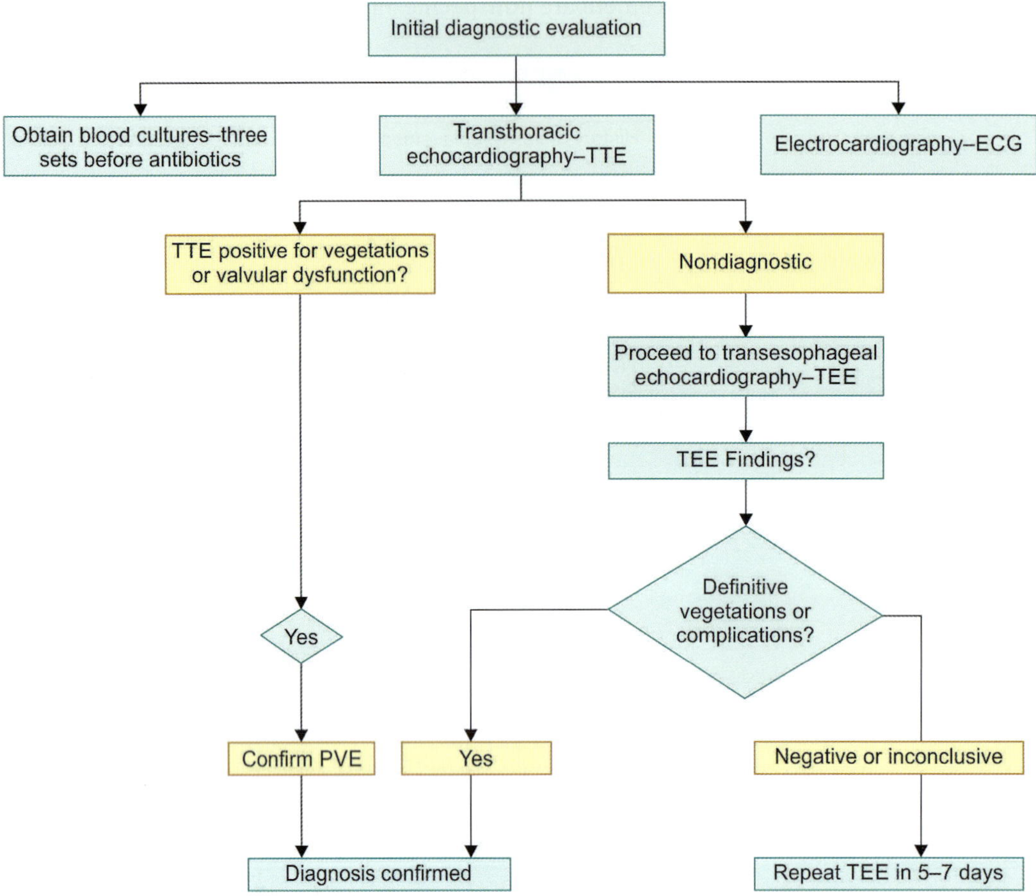


Prosthetic valve endocarditis is more difficult to recognize than native valve endocarditis.

## PERSISTENT NEGATIVE TEE

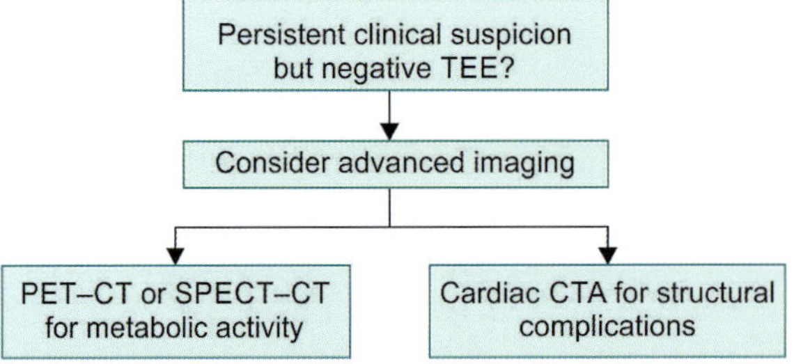

## ASSESSMENT FOR COMPLICATION

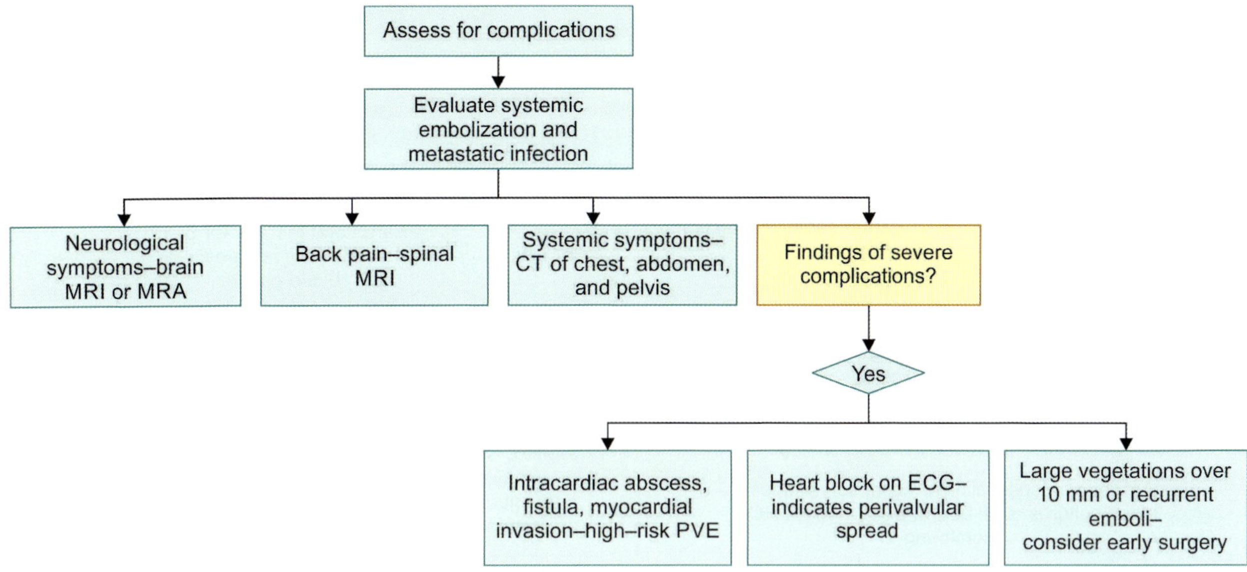


## SPECIAL SITUATION: TAVR

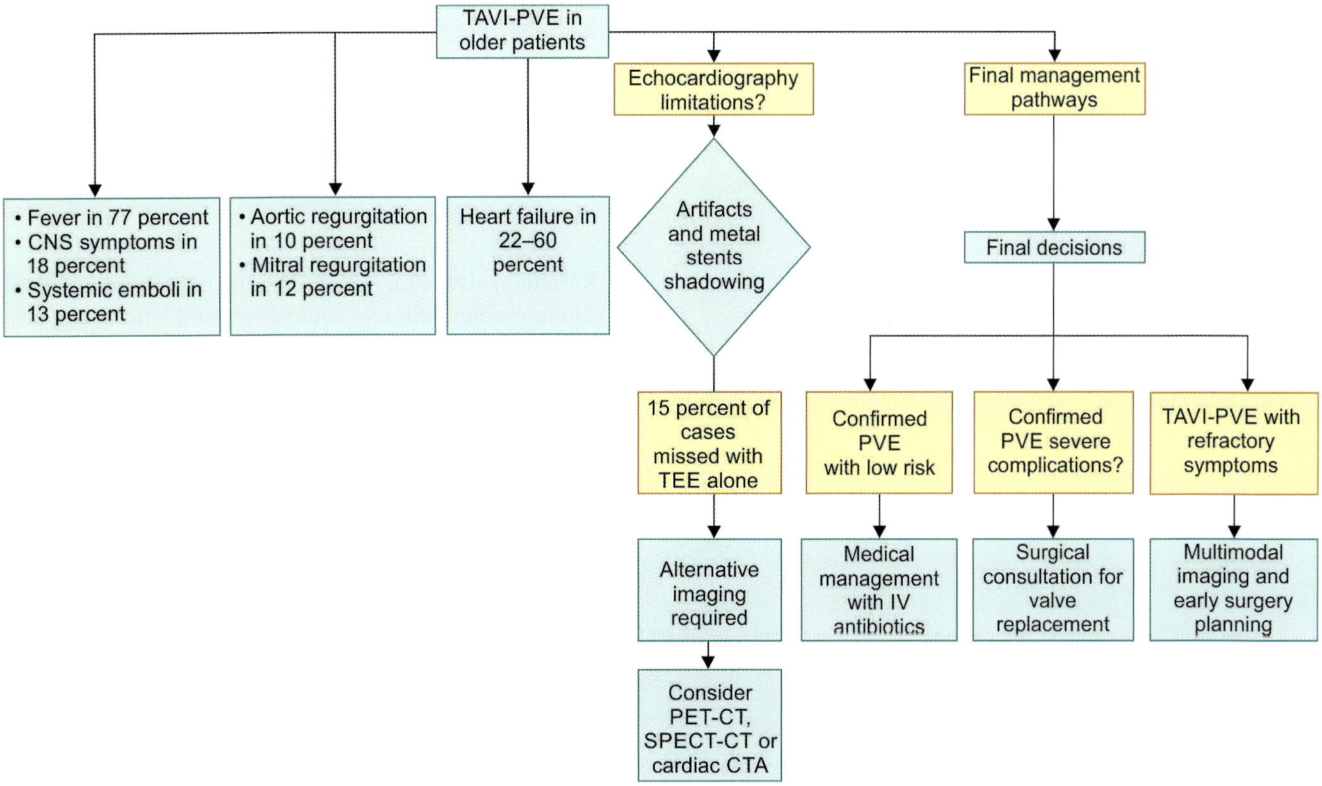

TAVI-PVE in older patients

- Fever in 77 percent
- CNS symptoms in 18 percent
- Systemic emboli in 13 percent

- Aortic regurgitation in 10 percent
- Mitral regurgitation in 12 percent

Heart failure in 22–60 percent

Echocardiography limitations?

Artifacts and metal stents shadowing

15 percent of cases missed with TEE alone

Alternative imaging required

Consider PET-CT, SPECT-CT or cardiac CTA

Final management pathways

Final decisions

Confirmed PVE with low risk → Medical management with IV antibiotics

Confirmed PVE severe complications? → Surgical consultation for valve replacement

TAVI-PVE with refractory symptoms → Multimodal imaging and early surgery planning

## MANAGEMENT: BASED ON CULTURE REPORT AVAILABILITY

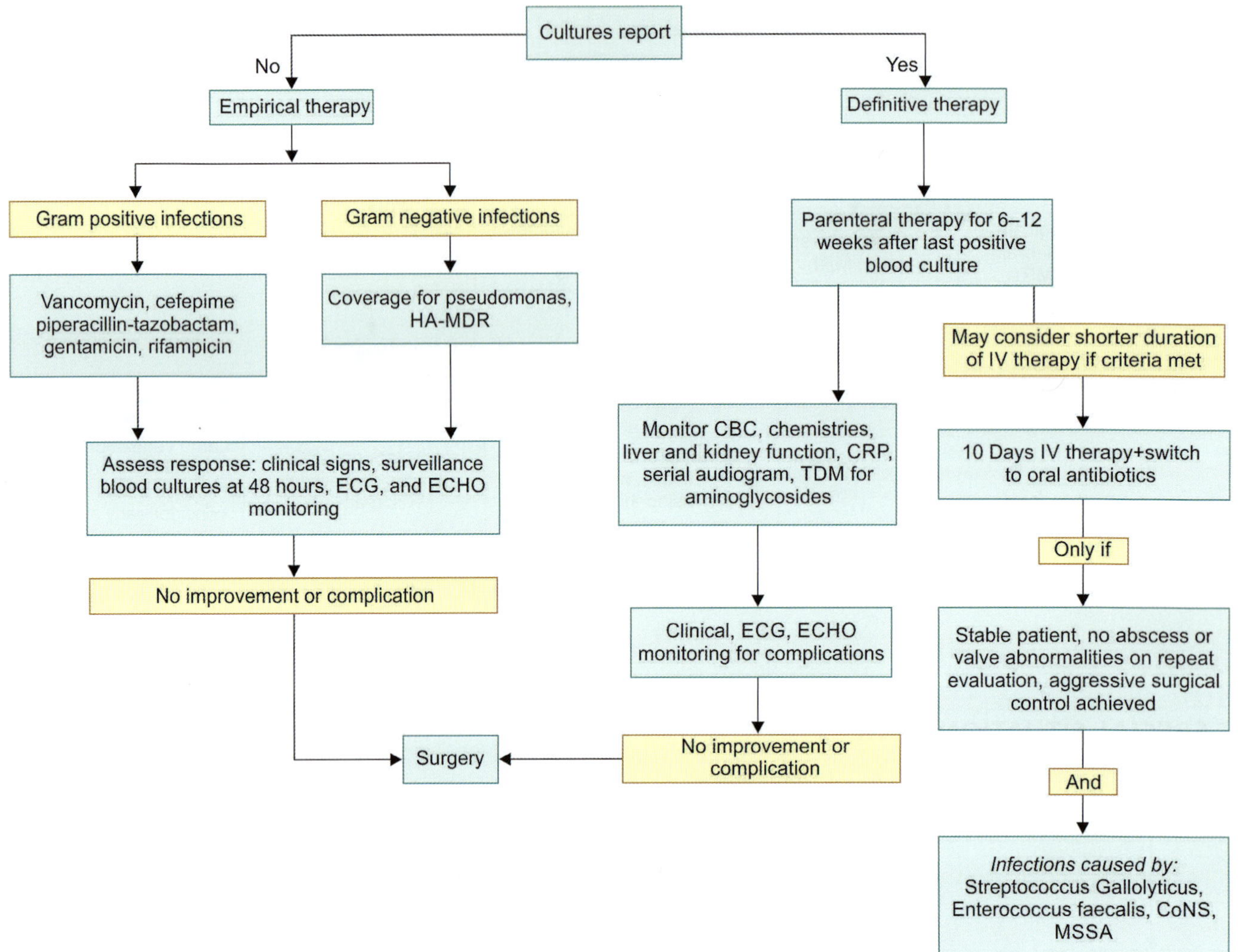


## SUGGESTED READING

1. Delgado V, Ajmone Marsan N, de Waha S, Bonaros N, Brida M, Burri H, et al. ESC Guidelines for the management of endocarditis. ESC Clinical Practice Guidelines. Eur Heart J 2023;44(39):3948-4042.
2. Karchmer AW, Chu VH. Prosthetic valve endocarditis: Epidemiology, clinical manifestations, and diagnosis. Available from https://www.uptodate.com/contents/prosthetic-valve-endocarditis-epidemiology-clinicalmanifestations-and-diagnosis [Last accessed February, 2025].

CHAPTER 38

# Hypertensive Crisis

## INTRODUCTION

Markedly elevated in patient blood pressure with systolic blood pressure >180 or diastolic blood pressure >110–120 mm Hg with or without target organ dysfunction.

(*Please note:* Historical terms such as hypertensive crisis (markedly elevated BP, e.g., SBP/DBP >180/110–120 mm Hg, with or without new or worsening target-organ damage) and hypertensive urgency (markedly elevated BP without evidence of new or worsening target-organ damage) fail to acknowledge the nuances of treatment decisions and, through the use of subjective emotive language such as crisis and urgency, may encourage unnecessary antihypertensive treatment).

## CLASSIFICATION

| | | Hypertension | |
|---|---|---|---|
| Markedly in patient elevated BP (SBP >180 OR DBP >110–120 mm Hg) | | | NOT MARKEDLY ELEVATED IN PATIENT BP (SBP<180 and DBP <110 mm Hg) |
| New or worsening target organ damage | | No | |
| Cerebral/cardiovascular/hematologic/ renovascular/ophthalmologic systems | Yes | | |
| Symptomatic markedly elevated BP (acute hypertension mediated organ damage-a hmod) | | ASYMPTOMATIC MARKEDLY ELEVATED BP (Uncontrolled Hypertension-U HTN) | |

## RISK FACTORS

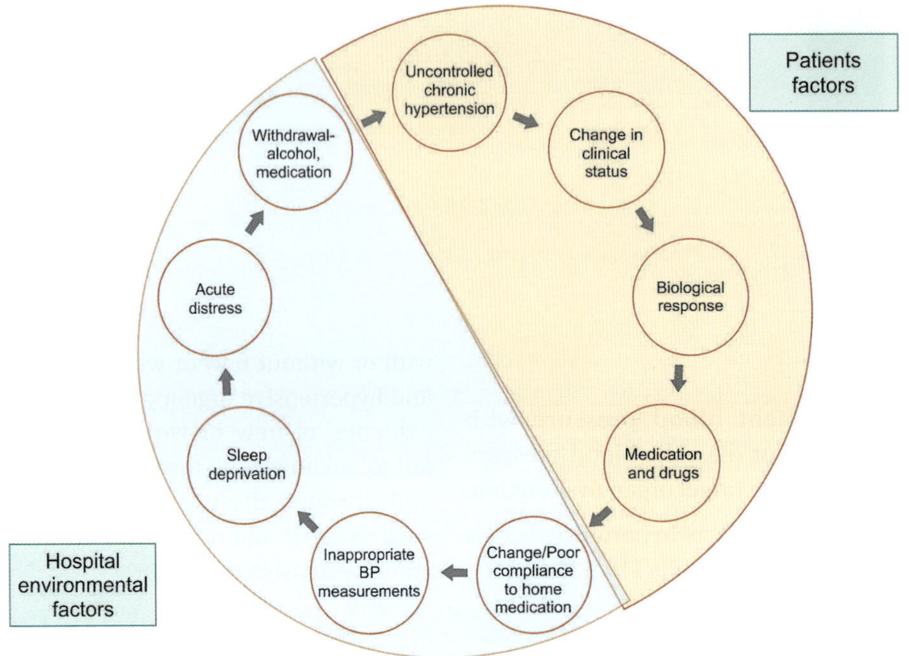


## CLINICAL PRESENTATION

The most frequent clinical presentations of Hypertensive Emergency are stroke (38% from all), followed by pulmonary oedema (35%) and coronary syndromes (25%).

## APPROACH TO MANAGEMENT OF MARKEDLY ELEVATED BLOOD PRESSURE

| | | | | | |
|---|---|---|---|---|---|
| • POCUS: Volume status, increased ONSD, Acute AR, Dissection flap in ascending Aorta/abdominal aorta, B lines.<br>• Chemistries: ? AKI<br>• Complete Blood Count: ?<br>• Schistocytes<br>• ECG and Troponin<br>• Urine analysis and Urine<br>• Toxicology screen<br>• Pregnancy evaluation and USG abdomen | | | • Markedly elevated BP (SBP >180 mm Hg or >DBP 110–120 mm Hg)<br>• Clinical History and Examination, pocus, Labs, ECG, CT, MRI<br>• Known cause of Hypertension | | |
| | | | | | Known causes: Pre-eclampsia/Aortic dissection/Scleroderma renal crisis/ Sympathomimetic intoxication/ Hyperthyroidism/Uncontrolled Pain/ Urinary obstruction/Stroke/post MI |
| | | | TARGET ORGAN DAMAGE | | |
| | | | yes | No | |
| Brain | Heart | Arteries | Kidney | Retina | Evaluate and Treat using specific stratergies unique to the underlying condition |
| TARGET ORGAN SPECIFIC BP CONTROL | | | | | |

## ORGAN-SPECIFIC BLOOD PRESSURE CONTROL

| | | | |
|---|---|---|---|
| | Acute Stroke | • 130 <SBP<180<br>• MAP decline 15% in 1 HR | |
| 1. Brain | Hypertensive Encephalopathy (PRES) | MAP decline 20 to 25% in 1 HR | • Labetalol<br>• Esmolol<br>• Nicardipine |
| | Cerebral Hemorrhage | MAP decline 15% | |
| | Acute Heart Failure | • SBP <180 or<br>• MAP decline 25% | |
| 2. Heart | Acute pulmonary oedema | Immediate SBP <140 | • Nitroglycerin<br>• Nitroprusside<br>• Labetalol<br>• Esmolol<br>• Clevidipine |
| | Acute coronary svndrome | Immediate SBP <140 | |
| 3. Arteries | Acute Aortic dissection | Immediate SBP < !20 | • Nitroglycerin<br>• Nitroprusside<br>• Labetalol<br>• Esmolol<br>• Clevidipine |
| | • Preeclampsia.<br>• Eclampsia and HEELP | Immediate SBP <160 and DBP <105 | • Labetalol<br>• Nicardipine<br>• Magnesium sulphate<br>• Hydralazine |
| 4. Rctina | Grade III-IV Keith-Wagener-Barker Hypertensive Retinopathy | • SBP<180<br>• MAP Decline by 15% | |
| 5. Kidney | • AKI<br>• Thrombotic microangiopathy | MAP Decline 20-25% over several hours | • Labetalol<br>• Nicardipine<br>• Magnesium sulphate<br>• Hydralazine |

## SUGGESTED READING


1. Balahura AM, Moroi ȘI, Scafa-Udriște A, Weiss E, Japie C, Bartoş D, et al. The Management of Hypertensive Emergencies-Is There a "Magical" Prescription for All? J Clin Med. 2022;11(11):3138.
2. Bress AP, Anderson TS, Flack JM, Ghazi L, Hall ME, Laffer CL, et al. The Management of Elevated Blood Pressure in the Acute Care Setting: A Scientific Statement From the American Heart Association. Hypertension. 2024;81(8):e94-106.
3. Holland M, Lewis PS. An audit and suggested guidelines for in-patient blood pressure measurement. J Hypertens. 2014;32(11):2166-70; discussion 2170.

CHAPTER 39

# Aortic Dissection

## INTRODUCTION

- Occurs in elderly, after 5th decade, incidence 5–30 per million
- Early mortality—very high
- Hyperacute—less than 24 hours
- Acute—1 to 14 days
- Subacute—15 to 90 days
- Chronic—more than 90 days
- Association—Old age, hypertension, Marfan syndrome, Ehler-Danlos syndrome

## CLINICAL PRESENTATION

*Classic symptoms:* Severe tearing or ripping chest or back pain, It may be associated with shock, paraplegia, or pericardial effusion

*Classification*

| ***Classification*** | ***Stanford*** | ***Debakey (Mnemonic as BAD)*** |
|---|---|---|
| | Type A – Ascending Aorta | Ascending aorta + thoracic (Both) |
| | Type B – Descending Aorta | Ascending aorta (ascending) |
| | | Descending aorta +/abdominal aorta (descending) |

*Investigations and the findings*

| | |
|---|---|
| ECG | • May show Left Ventricular Hypertrophy<br>• May show ST-elevation in inferior leads |
| X-ray Chest | • Widening of aortic shadow<br>• Pleural effusion may be seen |
| Trans thoracic Echocardiography | • Pericardial effusion<br>• Aortic regurgitations<br>• Dissecting Flap may be seen |
| Transesophageal Echocardiography | If CT is unavailable or contraindicated |
| CT Aortogram | Classic dissection can be confirmed, and the extent of dissection can be made out |
| Aortogram | Gold standard – being replaced by CT scan nowadays |
| D-dimer | A D-dimer value less than 500 mcg/L may help exclude the diagnosis among those who present with symptoms |

*Aortic dissection detection risk score (ADD-RS):* Score based on the presence of High-risk predisposing conditions, Characteristic pain symptoms, and clinical findings. (maximum score 3). The use of a negative D dimer in combination with a low ADD-RS (0 to 1) has good specificity to rule out aortic dissection

## MEDICAL MANAGEMENT

- *For both types:* Control of pain and medications to reduce the velocity of left ventricular shear stress
- Administer intravenous *beta-blockers* (e.g., Esmolol or labetalol) to control heart rate and blood pressure; target systolic BP <120 mm Hg.
- Provide analgesia to alleviate pain and reduce catecholamine release.

### Multidisciplinary Team Involvement

Multidisciplinary team comprising of cardiologists, vascular surgeons, intensivists, and radiologists for comprehensive care and decision-making regarding ICU management goals, timing of intervention, and technique.

## Specific Management Based on Type

- *Type A dissection*:
  - *Surgical intervention*:
    - Urgent surgical repair is indicated to prevent complications such as rupture or cardiac tamponade.
    - Options include aortic replacement with grafts and reimplantation of coronary arteries if necessary.
- *Type B dissection*:
  - *Medical management*:
    - Continue beta-blocker therapy; consider adding calcium channel blockers if needed.
    - Monitor closely for complications such as organ malperfusion, uncontrolled pain, or impending rupture.
    - If complications develop, consider *Thoracic endovascular aortic repair (TEVAR)* or surgical intervention.

## Follow-up and Long-term Management

- *Post-intervention care:*
  - Regular imaging surveillance (CT/MRI) to monitor aortic dimensions and detect any changes.
  - Manage cardiovascular risk factors aggressively (e.g., hypertension, hyperlipidemia).
  - Educate patients about symptoms that require immediate medical attention.

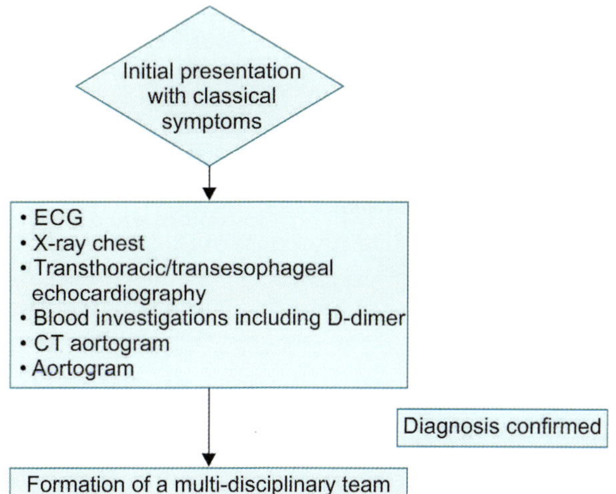


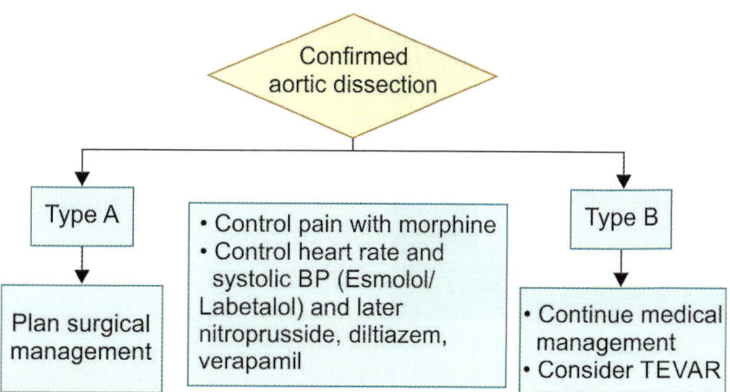


## CONCLUSION

This algorithm emphasizes the importance of rapid assessment, appropriate imaging, classification of the syndrome, and tailored management strategies based on the type of dissection. Early intervention in Type A dissections is critical due to their high mortality risk, while Type B dissections may be managed conservatively unless complications arise. Continuous monitoring and follow-up are essential for improving patient outcomes in AAS management.

## SUGGESTED READING


1. Braverman AC. Acute aortic dissection: Clinician update. Circulation. 2010;122(2):184-8.
2. Carrel T, Sundt TM, Kodolitsch YV, Czerny M. Acute Aortic dissection. Lancet. 2023 4;401(10378):773-88.
3. Flower L, Arrowsmith JE, Bewley J, Cook S, Cooper G, Flower J, Greco R, Sadeque S, Madhivathanan PR. Management of acute aortic dissection in critical care. J Intensive Care Soc. 2023;24(4):409-18.
4. Levy D, Sharma S, Grigorova Y, et al. Aortic Dissection. [Updated 2024 Oct 6]. In: StatPearls [Internet]. Treasure Island (FL): StatPearls Publishing; 2025. Available from: https://www.ncbi.nlm.nih.gov/books/NBK441963/ Accessed on 11/11/2024.

CHAPTER

# 40 Acute Cardiogenic Pulmonary Edema

## INTRODUCTION

Cardiogenic pulmonary edema (CPE) is the accumulation of fluid in the pulmonary interstitium and alveolar spaces due to elevated cardiac filling pressures and, thus, elevated pulmonary venous pressure.

## ETIOLOGY OF CARDIOGENIC PULMONARY EDEMA

- Systolic heart failure (Heart failure with reduced ejection fraction)
- Diastolic heart failure (Heart failure with preserved ejection fraction)
- Heart failure due to left-sided valvular abnormalities
- Heart failure due to arrhythmias

## CLINICAL MANIFESTATIONS AND DIAGNOSTIC ALGORITHM

- Clinically classified into—Warm versus cold and Dry versus wet
- Cold and wet clinical profile—Associated with cardiogenic shock and carries a higher risk of mortality
- Pathophysiology of cardiogenic pulmonary edema

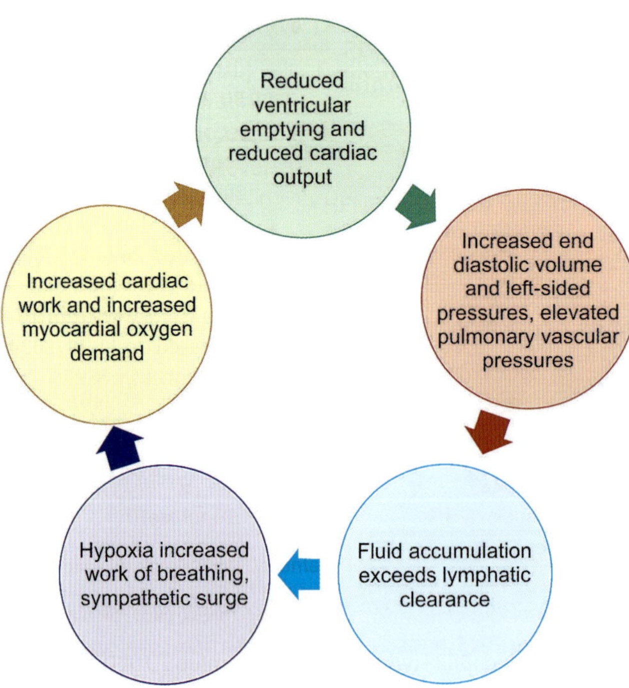

## SIGNS AND SYMPTOMS

- Breathlessness and cough
- Pink frothy sputum is a common symptom
- As hypoxemia worsens, neurologic symptoms such as confusion, anxiety, and disorientation may set in.

## CLINICAL EXAMINATION

Anxious patient with tachypnoea, tachycardia, hypoxia, and elevated jugular venous pulsations. Auscultation of the lungs generally reveals coarse crepitations, but wheezes may also be present.

Hypertension is common, but hypotension due to cardiogenic shock can also occur.

Hypoperfusion is characterized by oliguria, cold extremities, mottling, and altered mental status.

## INVESTIGATIONS

- ECG
- Chest X-ray
- Point of care lung ultrasonography
- Arterial blood gas (ABG)
- Cardiac biomarkers, Brain natriuretic peptide (BNP)
- Bedside echocardiogram

Point of care lung ultrasonography examination reveals B-profile, also known as lung comets. The number of B-lines correlates with extravascular lung water.

Echocardiography is useful to evaluate LV systolic and diastolic function.

Echocardiography also gives clues regarding any valvular abnormality and wall-motion abnormalities that suggest acute myocardial infarction.

## MANAGEMENT

Oxygen is recommended only in cases of hypoxia with a saturation of <90%.

In case of respiratory distress and hypoxia despite oxygen therapy or respiratory acidosis, a trial of non-invasive ventilation (NIV) is warranted.

For Type 1 respiratory failure, CPAP is the initial therapy

Bilevel NIV is preferred for patients with respiratory acidosis.

Patients who fail NIV should be intubated for invasive mechanical ventilation.

### Diuretic Therapy

Patients with pulmonary edema are usually volume overloaded. Intravenous loop diuretics like furosemide form the cornerstone of managing such cases in the absence of cardiogenic shock or profound hypotension.

In patients with volume overload refractory to diuretics or those with oligoanuria, ultrafiltration may be considered.

For patients with sympathetic overactivity and hypertension, a vasodilator like nitroglycerin may be administered as an addition to diuretic therapy. For individuals with elevated diastolic blood pressure, afterload reduction with agents like nitroprusside may be considered.

### Management of Arrhythmias

Atrial fibrillation (AF) is the most common arrhythmia associated with cardiogenic pulmonary edema. The urgency of AF management depends upon whether it is associated with significant hemodynamic instability and whether or not it is believed to be the precipitant of HF decompensation.

AF management starts with rate control and sos cardioversion. Anticoagulation before cardioversion is mandatory for patients with AF for >48 hours or when the duration is unknown.

Rate control can be achieved with beta-blockers. In patients with contraindications to beta-blocker digoxin, calcium channel blockers, such as diltiazem and amiodarone, may be considered.

### Management of Hypotensive Patients

In patients with reduced ejection fraction, inotrope agents such as dobutamine and milrinone may be considered if there is evidence of hypoperfusion (e.g., cool extremities, narrow pulse pressure, low urine output, confusion) and evidence of adequate preload. In case of persistent hypotension, a vasopressor (i.e., norepinephrine) may be added. Dopamine use has now been discouraged due to the increased risk of arrhythmias.

Patients with preserved ejection fraction presenting with hypotension and evidence of adequate preload require a vasopressor and should not receive inotropic therapy. Assessment of the intravascular volume status is critical in such patients to determine the need for diuresis and/or hydration.

For selected patients with acute severe hemodynamic compromise despite adequate pharmacologic therapy, mechanical support (e.g., intra-aortic balloon pump (IABP), extracorporeal circulatory membrane oxygenator (ECMO), or extracorporeal ventricular assist devices) may be considered as a bridge to recovery or transplant.

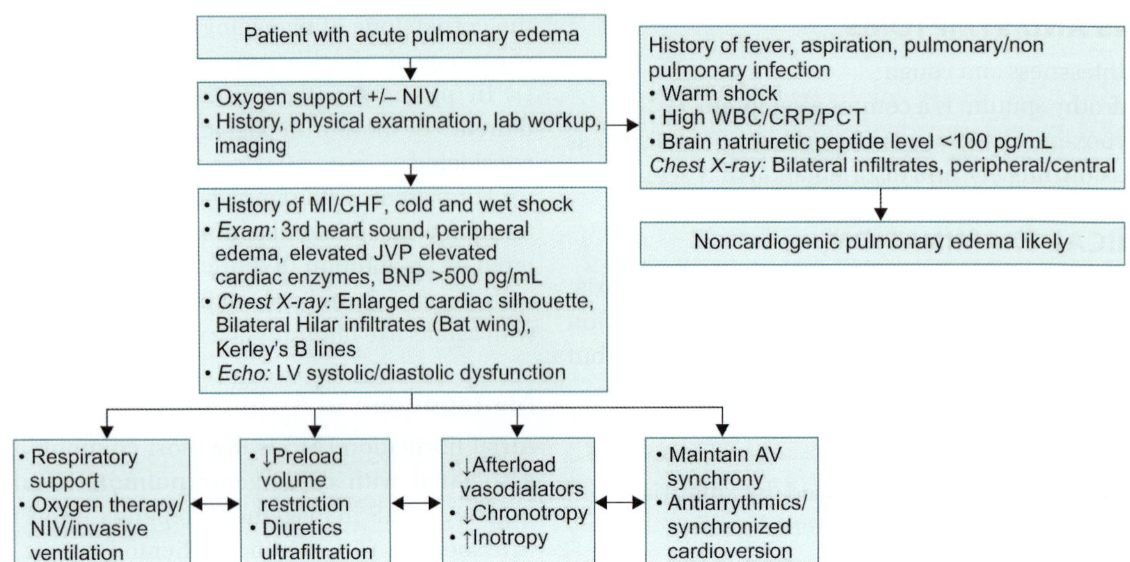


## SUGGESTED READING

1. Dobbe L, Rahman R, Elmassry M, Paz P, Nugent K. Cardiogenic Pulmonary Edema. Am J Med Sci. 2019;358(6): 389-97.
2. Iqbal MA, Gupta M. Cardiogenic Pulmonary Edema. [Updated 2023 Apr 7]. In: StatPearls [Internet]. Treasure Island (FL): StatPearls Publishing; 2024. Available from: https://www.ncbi.nlm.nih.gov/books/NBK544260/ Last accessed on 12//10/2024
3. Zanza C, Saglietti F, Tesauro M, Longhitano Y, Savioli G, Balzanelli MG, et al. Cardiogenic Pulmonary Edema in Emergency Medicine. Adv Respir Med. 2023;91(5):445-63.

# PART 3

# CNS

***Editors:*** Swagata Tripathy, Pratheema Ramachandran

***Associate Editors:*** Lakshmi Kanth Charan S, Sivakumar MN, Ajithkumar BR, Robert James Premkumar, Mahender Prasad, Kalavathy Swarna, Suresh Kumar Sundaramurthy, Kabilan Nallathambi, Dona Saha, Swapnabharati Moharana, Suma R Ahmad, Jyotirmaya Prakash Pati, Devi Prasad Mohapatra, Nivedita J Bodra

CHAPTER 41

# Ischemic Stroke

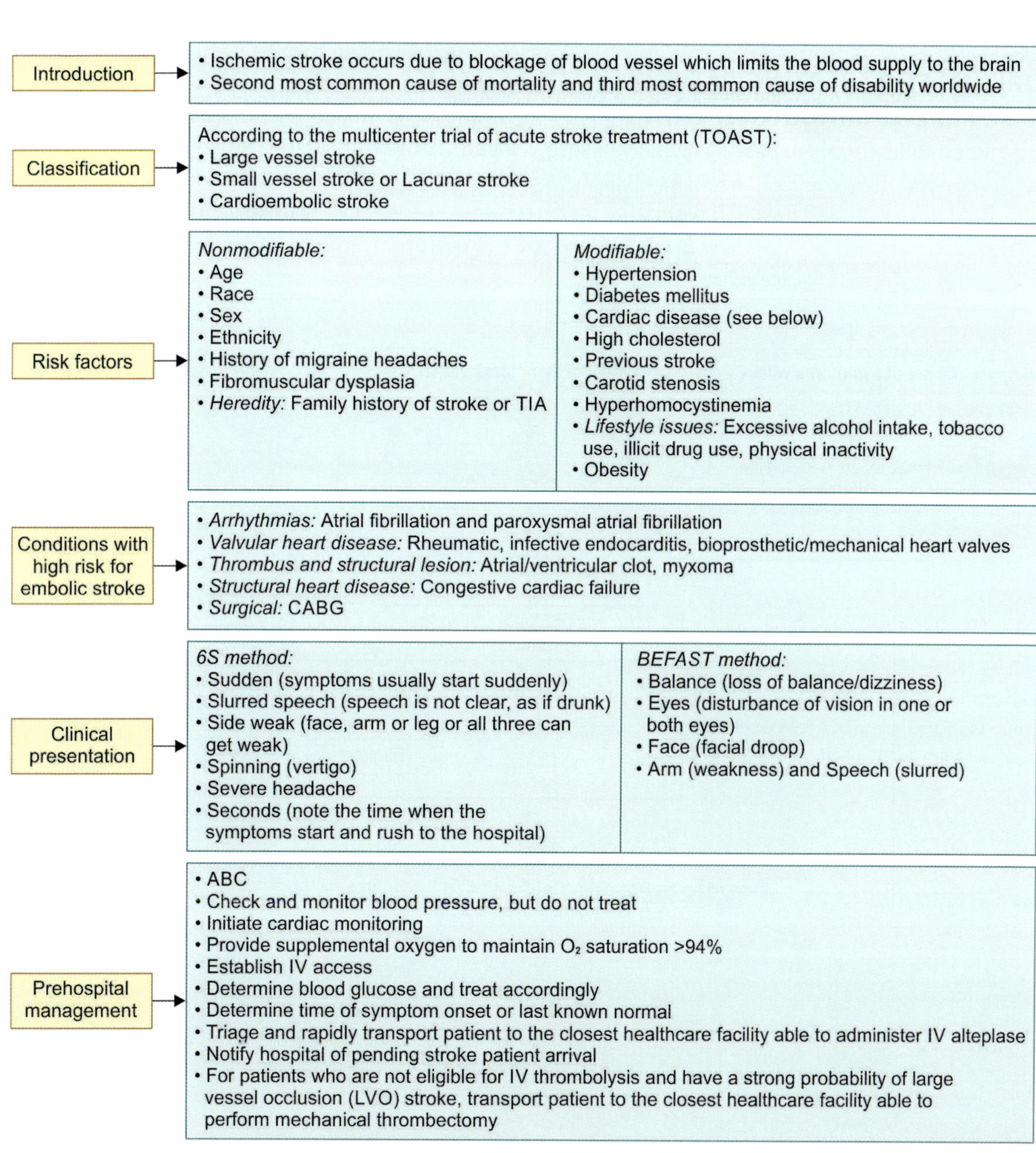

|  |  |
|---|---|
| Introduction | • Ischemic stroke occurs due to blockage of blood vessel which limits the blood supply to the brain<br>• Second most common cause of mortality and third most common cause of disability worldwide |
| Classification | According to the multicenter trial of acute stroke treatment (TOAST):<br>• Large vessel stroke<br>• Small vessel stroke or Lacunar stroke<br>• Cardioembolic stroke |
| Risk factors | *Nonmodifiable:*<br>• Age<br>• Race<br>• Sex<br>• Ethnicity<br>• History of migraine headaches<br>• Fibromuscular dysplasia<br>• *Heredity:* Family history of stroke or TIA<br><br>*Modifiable:*<br>• Hypertension<br>• Diabetes mellitus<br>• Cardiac disease (see below)<br>• High cholesterol<br>• Previous stroke<br>• Carotid stenosis<br>• Hyperhomocystinemia<br>• *Lifestyle issues:* Excessive alcohol intake, tobacco use, illicit drug use, physical inactivity<br>• Obesity |
| Conditions with high risk for embolic stroke | • *Arrhythmias:* Atrial fibrillation and paroxysmal atrial fibrillation<br>• *Valvular heart disease:* Rheumatic, infective endocarditis, bioprosthetic/mechanical heart valves<br>• *Thrombus and structural lesion:* Atrial/ventricular clot, myxoma<br>• *Structural heart disease:* Congestive cardiac failure<br>• *Surgical:* CABG |
| Clinical presentation | *6S method:*<br>• Sudden (symptoms usually start suddenly)<br>• Slurred speech (speech is not clear, as if drunk)<br>• Side weak (face, arm or leg or all three can get weak)<br>• Spinning (vertigo)<br>• Severe headache<br>• Seconds (note the time when the symptoms start and rush to the hospital)<br><br>*BEFAST method:*<br>• Balance (loss of balance/dizziness)<br>• Eyes (disturbance of vision in one or both eyes)<br>• Face (facial droop)<br>• Arm (weakness) and Speech (slurred) |
| Prehospital management | • ABC<br>• Check and monitor blood pressure, but do not treat<br>• Initiate cardiac monitoring<br>• Provide supplemental oxygen to maintain $O_2$ saturation >94%<br>• Establish IV access<br>• Determine blood glucose and treat accordingly<br>• Determine time of symptom onset or last known normal<br>• Triage and rapidly transport patient to the closest healthcare facility able to administer IV alteplase<br>• Notify hospital of pending stroke patient arrival<br>• For patients who are not eligible for IV thrombolysis and have a strong probability of large vessel occlusion (LVO) stroke, transport patient to the closest healthcare facility able to perform mechanical thrombectomy |

*Contd...*

*Contd...*

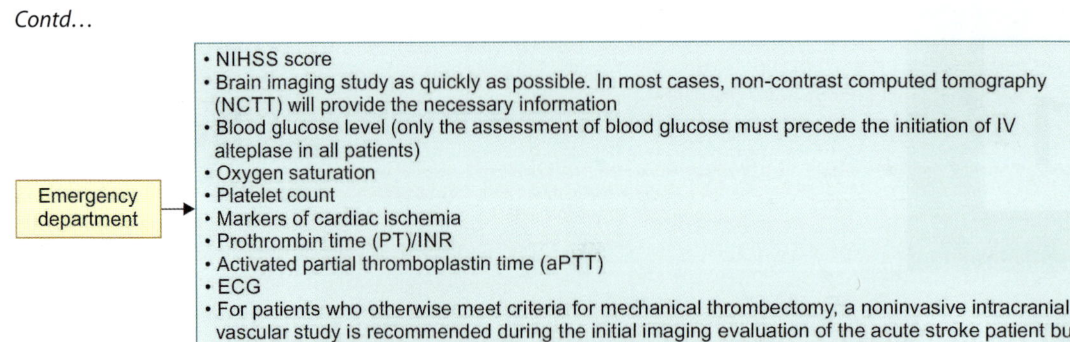


## ALGORITHM FOR TREATING PATIENTS WITH ACUTE ISCHEMIC STROKE WITH DIFFERENT IMAGING OPTIONS[1]

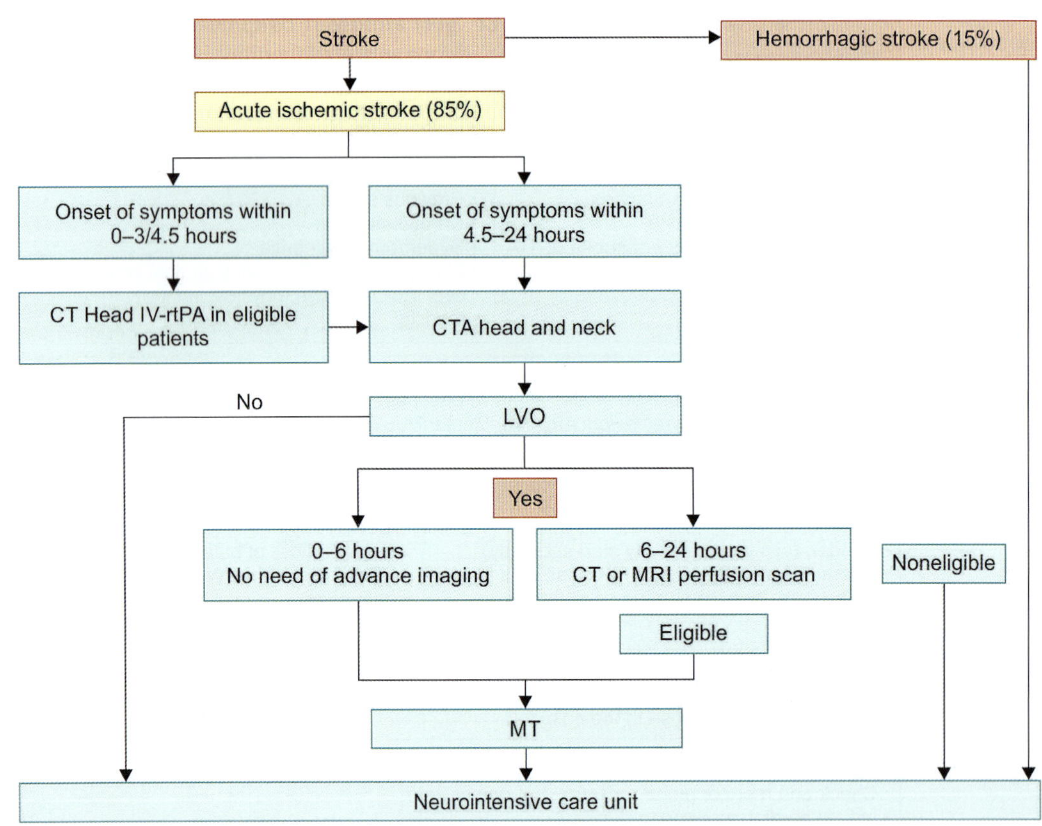

## INCLUSION AND EXCLUSION CRITERIA FOR THROMBOLYSIS

*Inclusion criteria:*
- Stroke onset-to-needle time <3 to 4.5 hours
- No evidence of ICH on CT/MRI
- A measurable deficit on examination, as assessed by NIHSS

*Exclusion criteria:*
- *Absolute*
  - History of stroke or serious head trauma within the prior 3 months
  - Prior history of intracranial hemorrhage
  - Major surgery within 14 days
  - Persistent SBP > 185 mm Hg or DBP > 110 mm Hg
  - Platelets < 100,000
  - INR > 1.7 if on warfarin—elevated PTT if on heparin
- *Relative* (depends on availability of advanced imaging techniques, stroke severity, and examiner and patient preferences)
  - Pregnancy
  - Genitourinary or gastrointestinal bleeding within the previous 21 days
  - Arterial puncture or lumbar puncture within 7 days
  - Improving stroke symptoms
  - Seizure at stroke onset
  - Serum glucose <50 or >400 mg/L
  - NIHSS score <4 or >22

## NIH STROKE SEVERITY SCALE (NIHSS)

| *Item* | *Title* | *Responses and scores* |
|---|---|---|
| 1a. | Level of consciousness | 0—alert<br>1—drowsy<br>2—obtunded<br>3 coma/unresponsive |
| 1b. | Orientation questions (2) | 0—answers both correctly<br>1—answers ono correctly<br>2—answers neither correctly |
| 1c. | Response to commands (2) | 0— performs both tasks correctly<br>1—performs one task correctly<br>2—performs neither |
| 2. | Gaze | 0—normal horizontal movements<br>1—partial gaze palsy<br>2 complete gaze palsy |
| 3. | Visual fields | 0—no visual field defect<br>1—partial hemianopia<br>2—complete hemianopia<br>3—bilateral hemianopia |

*Contd...*

*Contd...*

| *Item* | *Title* | *Responses and scores* |
|---|---|---|
| 4. | Facial movement | 0—normal<br>1—minor facial weakness<br>2—partial facial weakness<br>3—complete unilateral palsy |
| 5. | Motor function (arm)<br>a. Left<br>b. Right | 0—no drift<br>1—drift before 10 seconds<br>2—falls before 10 seconds<br>3—no effort against gravity<br>4—no movement |
| 6. | Motor function (leg)<br>a. Left<br>b. Right | 0—no drift<br>1—drift before 5 seconds<br>2—falls before 5 seconds<br>3—no effort against gravity<br>4—no movement |
| 7. | Limb ataxia | 0—no ataxia<br>1—ataxia in 1 limb<br>2—ataxia in 2 limbs |
| 8. | Sensory | 0—no sensory loss<br>1—mild sensory loss<br>2—severe sensory loss |
| 9. | Language | 0—normal<br>1—mild aphasia<br>2—severe aphasia<br>3—mule or global aphasia |
| 10. | Articulation | 0—normal<br>1—mild dysarthria<br>2—severe dysarthria |
| 11. | Extinction or inattention | 0—absent<br>1—mild toss (1 sensory modality lost)<br>2—severe loss (2 modalities lost) |

*Source:* Adapted from Lyden et al.


*Evaluate for mechanical thrombectomy (<24 hours)*
- Evaluation for IV alteplase and evaluation for mechanical thrombectomy happens simultaneously
- Within 6 hours:
  - Pre stroke mRS score 0–1
  - Causative occlusion of the ICA or proximal MCA (M1)
  - Age ≥18 years
  - NIHSS score of ≥6
  - ASPECTS of ≥6
- Within 6-24 hours
  - Causative occlusion of the ICA or M1
  - Meets eligibility criteria for DAWN or DEFUSE3 trials

*Indications for IV thrombolysis (Class I Recommendations)*
- If within 3 hours of onset and:
  - ≥ 18 years of age
  - Severe stroke (NIHSS score of ≥6)
  - Mild but disabling stroke

*Contd...*

*Contd...*

- If 3-4.5 hours from onset,
  - 18-80 years of age, and
  - Without a history of both diabetes mellitus and prior stroke
  - NIHSS score ≤ 25
  - Not taking any OACs
  - Without imaging evidence of ischemic injury involving more than one third of the MCA territory
- If BP can be lowered safely and maintained < 185/110 mm Hg

## TREATMENT OPTIONS FOR ARTERIAL HYPERTENSION IN ACUTE ISCHEMIC STROKE ELIGIBLE FOR THROMBOLYSIS

| ***Class IIb*** | ***LOE-CEO*** |
|---|---|
| Patient otherwise eligible for acute reperfusion therapy except that BP is >185/110 mm Hg | |
| Labetalol 10-20 mg IV over 1-2 min. may repeat 1 time; or | |
| Nicardipine 5 mg/h IV, titrate up by 2-5 mg/h every 5-15 min, maximum 15 mg/h; when desired BP reached, adjust to maintain proper BP limits; of | |
| Clevidipine 1-2 mg/h IV. Titrate by doubling the dose every 2-5 min until desired BP reached: maximum 21 mg/h | |
| Other agents (e.g., hydralazine, enalaprilat) may also be considered | |
| If BP is not maintained ≤185/110 mm Hg. Do not administer alteplase | |
| Management of BP during and after alteplase or other acute reperfusion therapy to maintain BP ≤180/105 mm Hg | |
| Monitor BP every 15 min for 2 h from the start of alteplase therapy, then every 30 min for 6 h and then every hour for 16 h | |
| If systolic BP >180-230 mm Hg or diastolic BP >105-120 mm Hg | |
| Labetalol 10 mg IV followed by continuous IV infusion 2-8 mg/min; or | |
| Nicardipine 5 mg/h IV titrate up to desired effect by 2.5 mg/h every 5-15 min. maximum 15 mg/h; or | |
| Clevidipine 1-2 mg/h IV titrate by doubling the dose every 2-5 min until desired BP reached: maximum 21 mg/h | |
| If BP not controlled or diastolic BP >140 mm Hg, consider IV sodium nitroprusside | |

## THROMBOLYSIS PROCESS

- Infuse 0.9 mg/kg (maximum dose 90 mg) over 60 min, with 10% of the dose given as a bolus over 1 min.
- Admit the patient to an intensive care or stroke unit for monitoring.
- If the patient develops severe headache, acute hypertension, nausea, or vomiting or has a worsening neurological examination, discontinue the infusion (if IV alteplase is being administered) and obtain emergency head CT scan.
- Measure BP and perform neurological assessments every 15 min during and after IV alteplase infusion for 2 h, then every 30 min for 6 h, then hourly until 24 h after IV alteplase treatment.
- Increase the frequency of BP measurements if SBP is >180 mm Hg or if DBP is >105 mm Hg; administer antihypertensive medications to maintain BP at or below these levels.
- Delay placement of nasogastric tubes, indwelling bladder catheters, or intra-arterial pressure catheters if the patient can be safely managed without them.
- Obtain a follow-up CT or MRI scan at 24 h after IV alteplase before starting anticoagulants or antiplatelet agents.

## INTRAVENOUS THROMBOLYSIS (IVT) DECISION MAKING ALGORITHM

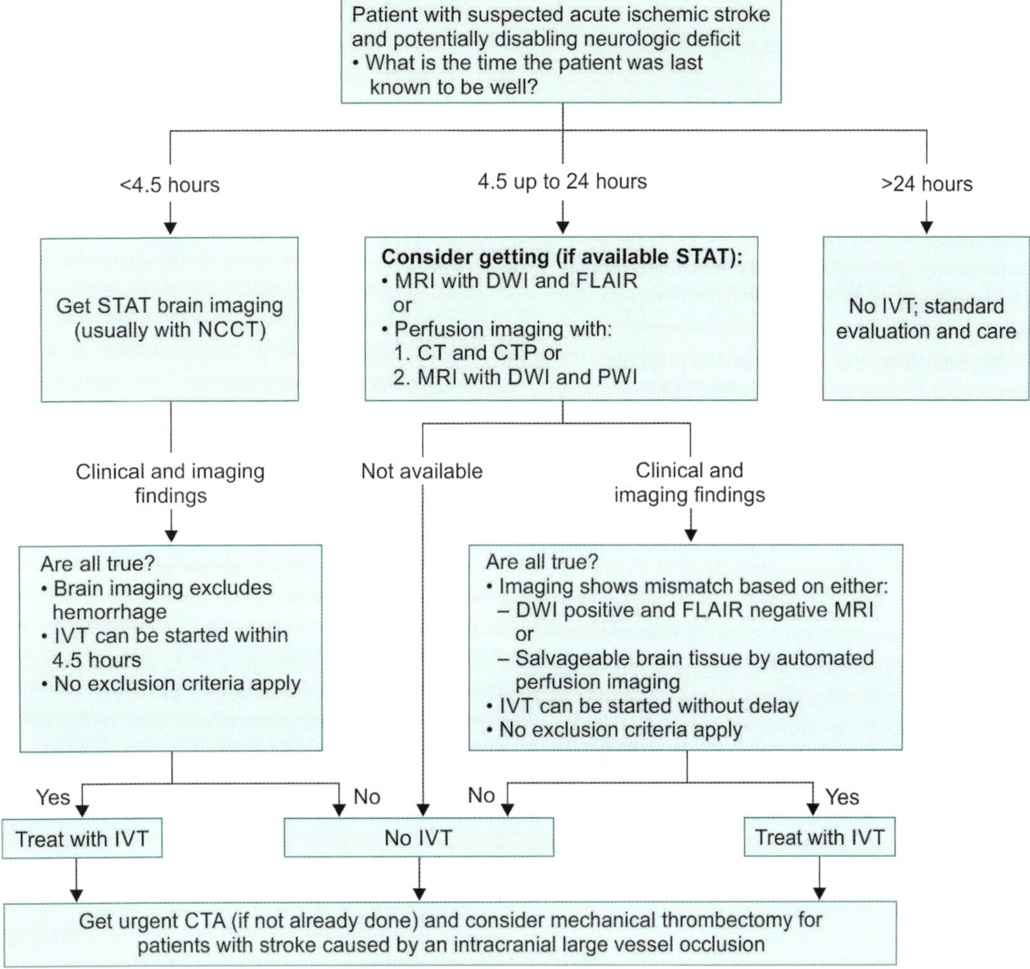

## MECHANICAL THROMBECTOMY (MT) DECISION MAKING ALGORITHM

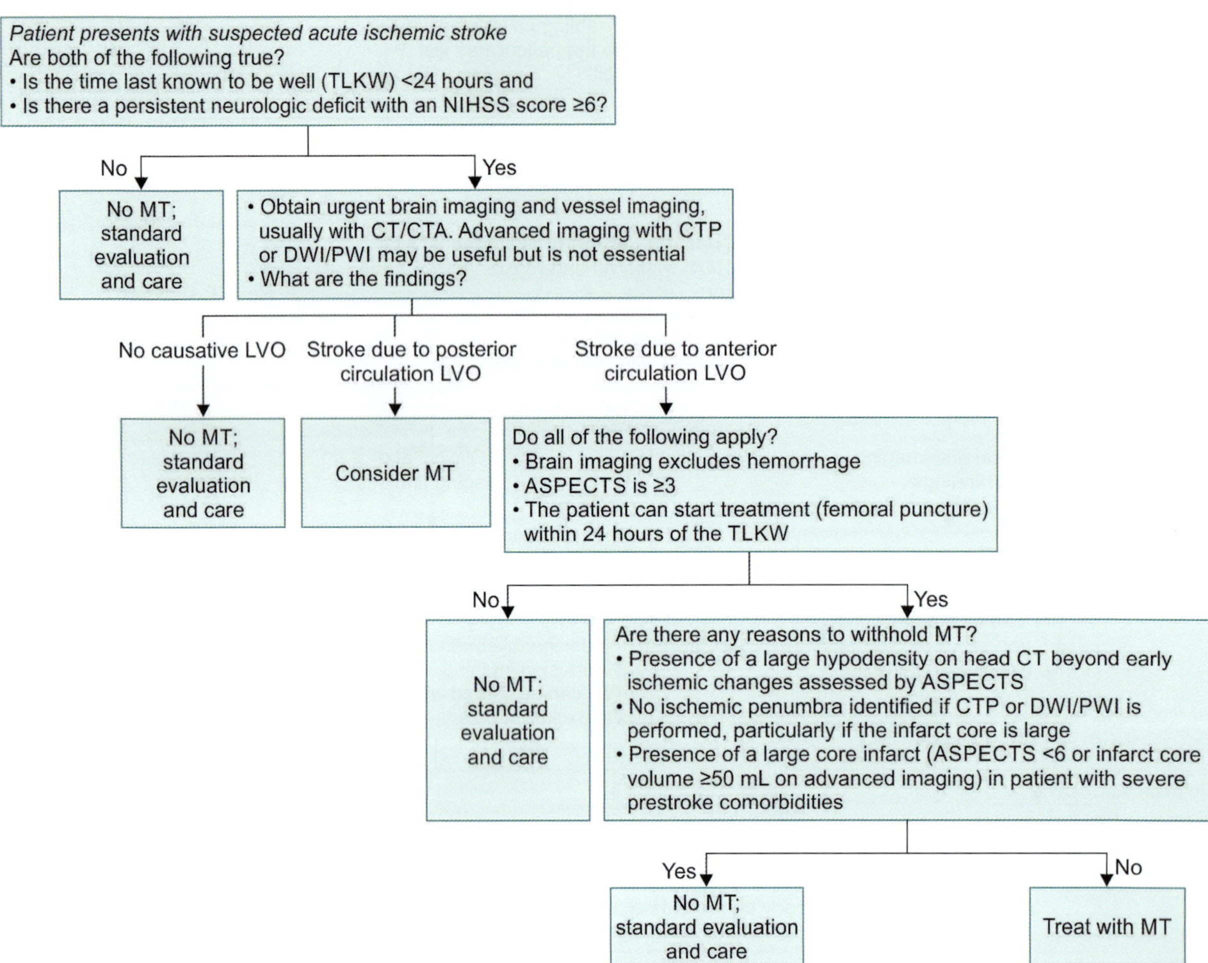


## MANAGEMENT OF SYMPTOMATIC INTRACRANIAL HEMORRHAGE POST-THROMBOLYSIS

- Stop alteplase infusion
- CBC, PT (INR), aPTT, fibrinogen level, and type and crossmatch
- Emergent nonenhanced head CT
- Cryoprecipitate (includes factor VIII): 10 U infused over 10-30 min (onset in 1 h, peaks in 12 h); administer additional dose for fibrinogen level of <150 mg/dL
- Tranexamic acid 1000 mg IV infused over 10 min OR ϵ-aminocaproic acid 4-5 g over 1 h, followed by 1 g IV until bleeding is controlled (peak onset in 3 h)
- Potential for benefit in all patients, but particularly when blood products are contraindicated or declined by patient/family or if cryoprecipitate is not available in a timely manner
- Hematology and neurosurgery consultations
- Supportive therapy, including BP management, ICP, CPP, MAP, temperature, and glucose control

## SUSPECTED STROKE ALGORITHM—AHA: GOALS FOR MANAGEMENT OF STROKE[2]

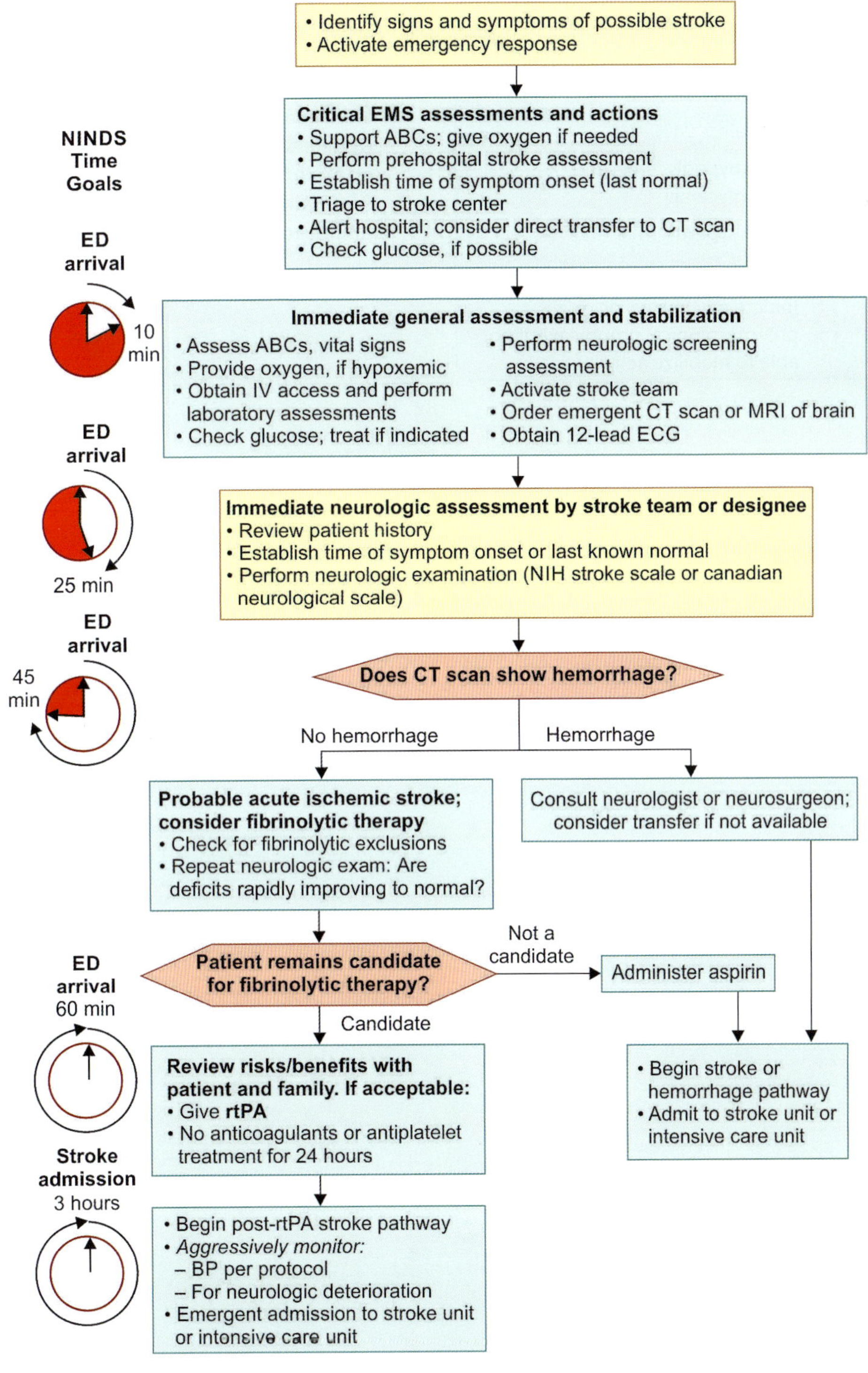

## ANTIPLATELET AND OTHER SUPPORTIVE TREATMENT

| | |
|---|---|
| Antiplatelet | Aspirin within 24-48 hours |
| Anticoagulants | No role for urgent anticoagulation |
| Admission to stroke unit | Improves outcome |
| Oxygenation | Maintain > 94% |
| Glucose | Avoid hypoglycemia and hyperglycemia |
| Temperature | Avoid hyperthermia |
| Nutrition | Initiate early |
| DVT prophylaxis | Initiate mechanical or pharmacological prophylaxis if not able to mobilize actively |

## REFERENCES

1. Patel P, Yavagal D, Khandelwal P. Hyperacute Management of Ischemic Strokes: JACC Focus Seminar. J Am Coll Cardiol. 2020;75(15):1844-56.
2. Powers WJ, Rabinstein AA, Ackerson T, Adeoye OM, Bambakidis NC, Becker K, et al. Guidelines for the Early Management of Patients With Acute Ischemic Stroke: 2019 Update to the 2018 Guidelines for the Early Management of Acute Ischemic Stroke: A Guideline for Healthcare Professionals From the American Heart Association/American Stroke Association. Stroke. 2019;50:e344-418.

CHAPTER 42

# Hemorrhagic Stroke

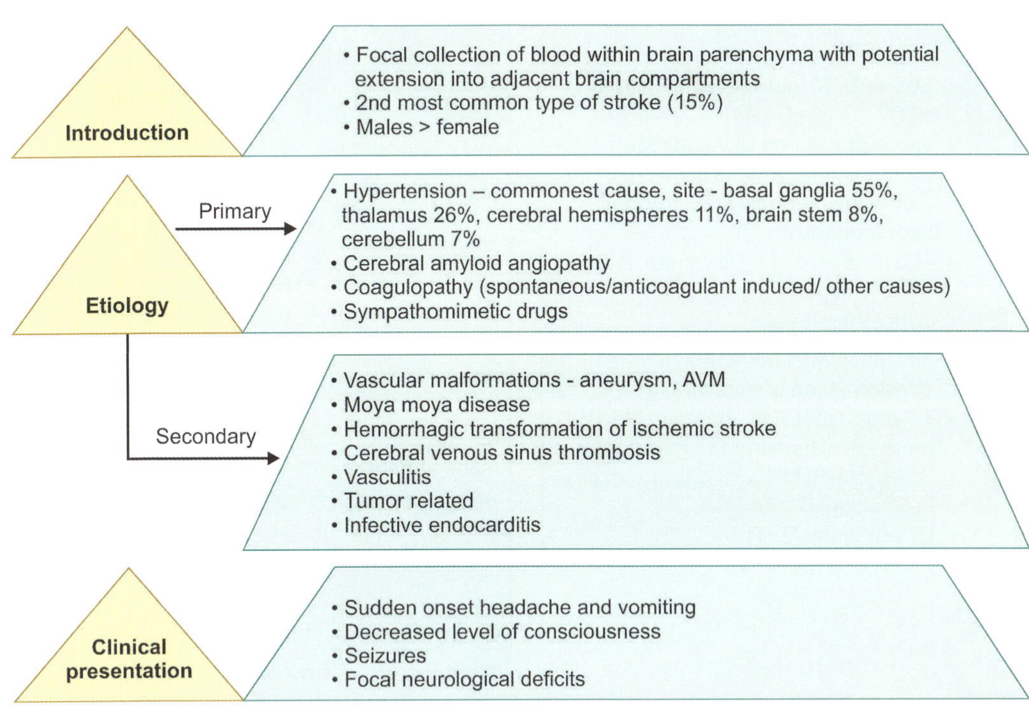

## APPROACH AND DIAGNOSIS

| | |
|---|---|
| History | • Comorbidities (DM/HT/CLD/CKD)<br>• Medications (antiplatelets, anticoagulants, oral contraceptives)<br>• Substance abuse |
| Examination | • Focused neurological assessment<br>• NIHSS score (to quantify the stroke severity)<br>• GCS |
| Non-contrast CT brain | • Distinguishes hemorrhagic and ischemic stroke<br>• Assess ICH volume (> 50-60 mL - poor prognosis) |
| Laboratory tests | • CBC, RFT, LFT, glucose, ESR, PT, INR, aPTT<br>• Specific tests if on DOAC (direct thrombin time, Anti-Xa activity)<br>• Cardiac markers (elevated troponin - poor prognosis)<br>• ECG (evidence of hypertension/MI)<br>• Urine toxicology (for cocaine, sympathomimetics) |
| Evaluation for cause of ICH | • MRI (neoplasm, hemorrhagic transformation of ischemic stroke)<br>• CT angio (spot sign - ongoing bleed, more risk of hematoma expansion)<br>• DSA (isolated IVH with no abnormality in CT angio)<br>• CT venogram (CVT) |

## GENERAL MANAGEMENT

| | |
|---|---|
| ABC | Intubate if GCS ≤8, ICP is high |
| BP control | To decrease hematoma expansion (ATTACH2/INTERACT 2/AHA 2022 recommendation)<br>I. Avoid variability – careful titration for smooth, sustained BP control, sudden lowering not recommended<br>II. Timely control – initiate BP lowering therapies in ≤ 2 hours of ICH onset and reach target in ≤1 hour<br>III. Target BP – goal SBP: 140 (130 – 150) mm Hg, avoid SBP < 130 mm Hg in patients presenting with SBP > 150 mm Hg<br>V. Drugs – IV nicardipine, nimodipine or labetalol infusions |
| Seizure management | • Confirmed seizure - AED to decrease mortality and brain injury<br>• Suspicion of seizure - continuous EEG for > 24 hours<br>• No evidence of seizure - prophylaxis not recommended<br>• Long-term antiepileptics - cortical bleed, volume > 10 mL, age < 65 years, early onset seizure (<7 days of ICH) |
| ICP management | If elevated, tiered approach |
| DVT prophylaxis | • Mechanical thromboprophylaxis on diagnosis of ICH<br>• Pharmacological prophylaxis after 24-48 hours of ICH onset |
| Glycemic control | 140 – 180 mg/dL |
| Temperature management | Avoid hyperthermia |

## REVERSAL OF ANTICOAGULANTS AND ANTIPLATELETS

1. Discontinue immediately
2. For patients on aspirin

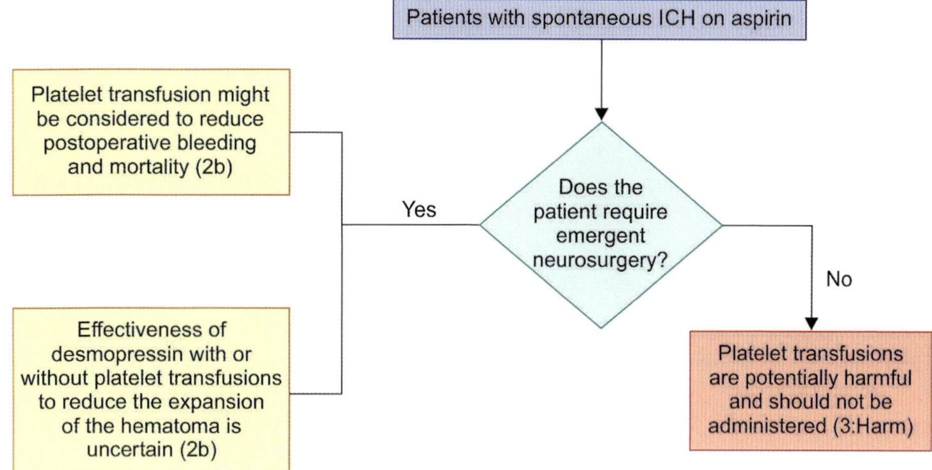


3. For patients on anticoagulants

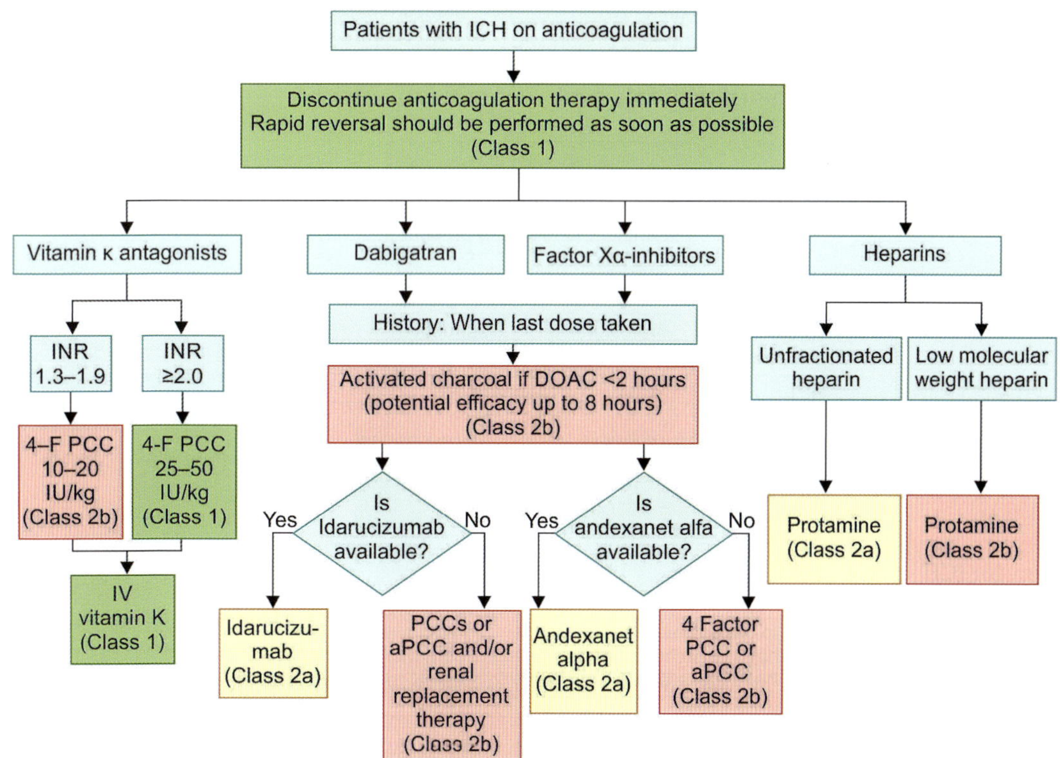

## SURGICAL MANAGEMENT

1. Minimally invasive surgical evacuation (MIS) of ICH

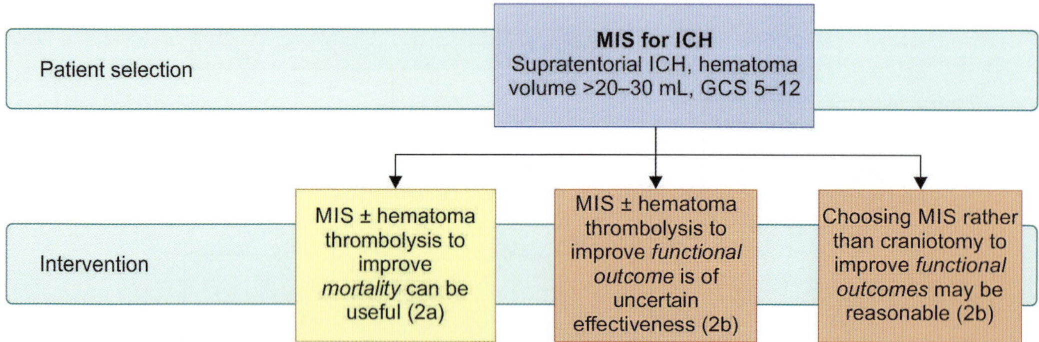


2. Craniotomy for supratentorial hemorrhage

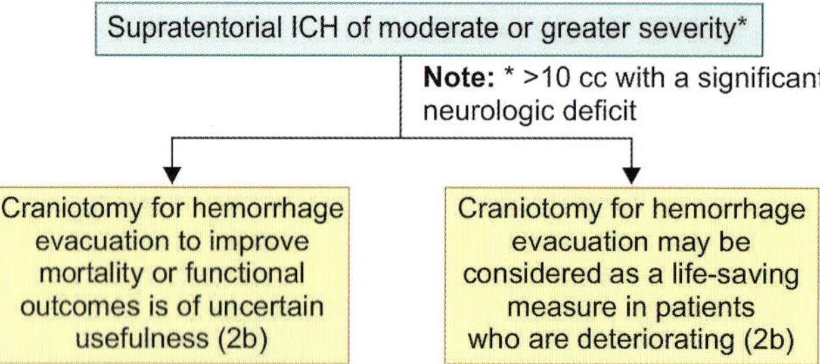


3. Craniotomy for posterior fossa hemorrhage

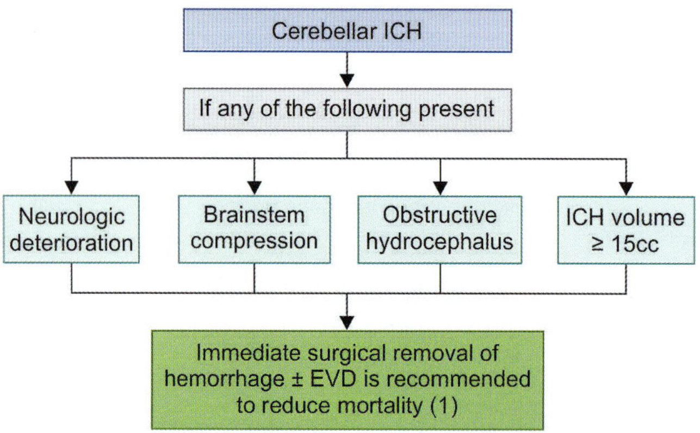


4. Craniectomy for ICH

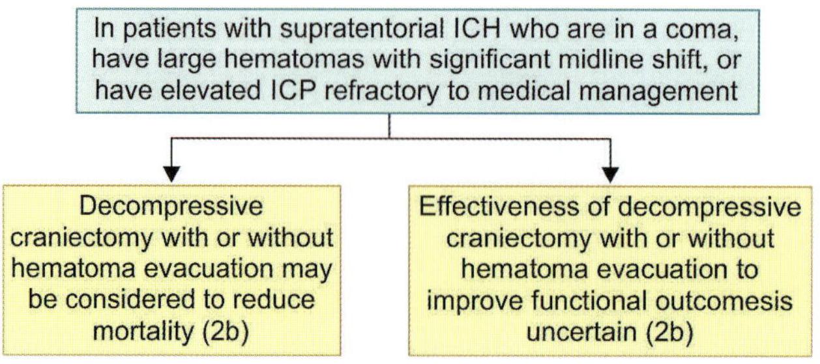

5. Minimally invasive surgical evacuation of intraventricular hemorrhage

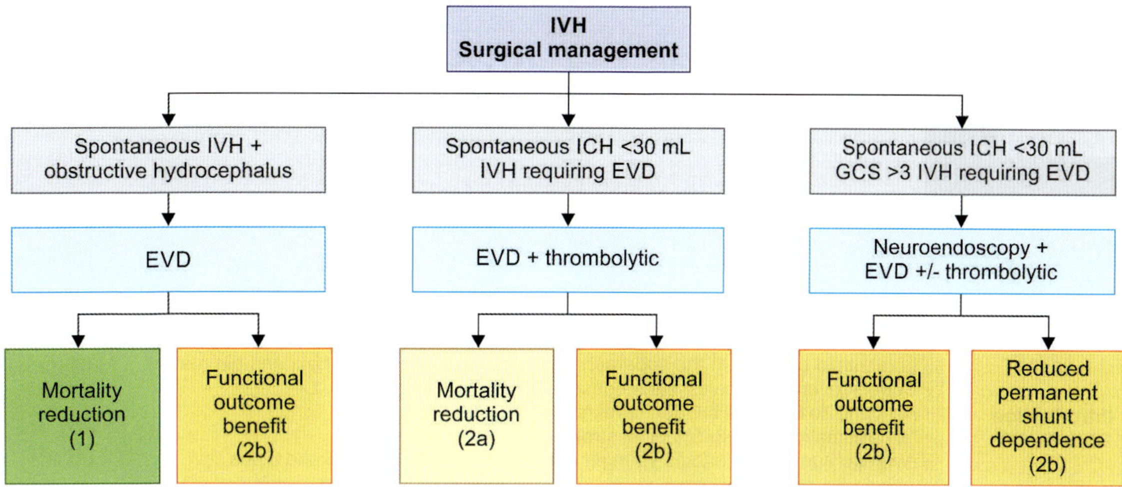


## PROGNOSIS (ICH SCORE)

| ***Component*** | ***Score*** | ***Points*** |
|---|---|---|
| GCS score | 3–4 | 2 |
| | 5–12 | |
| | 13–15 | 0 |
| ICH volume (mL) | >30 | ↑ |
| | <30 | 0 |
| IVH | Present | 1 |
| | Absent | 0 |
| Infratentorial ICH | Yes | 1 |
| | No | 0 |
| Age (years) | >80 | 1 |
| | <80 | 0 |
| *Total points* | *30-day mortality (%)* | |
| 5+ | 100 | |
| 4 | 97 | |
| 3 | 72 | |
| 2 | 26 | |
| 1 | 13 | |
| 0 | 0 | |

## SUGGESTED READING

1. Greenberg SM, Ziai WC, Cordonnier C, Dowlatshahi D, Francis B, Goldstein JN, et al.: 2022 Guideline for the management of patients with spontaneous intracerebral hemorrhage: a guideline from the American Heart Association/American Stroke Association. Stroke. 2022;53:e282-361.

CHAPTER

# 43 Subarachnoid Hemorrhage

**Introduction**

- Intracranial bleeding in the subarachnoid space (between arachnoid and pia mater)
- Sudden event with multisystem consequences
- Accounts to 8% of all sudden cardiac deaths
- Nontraumatic SAH ~3–5% of all strokes
- Average age of ~50, affects younger patients more than other stroke types

**Risk factors**

| Modifiable | Nonmodifiable |
|---|---|
| • Cigarette smoking<br>• Alcoholism<br>• Arterial hypertension | • Female (Postmenopausal—Estrogen deficiency)<br>• Age >50 years<br>• Personal/family history of SAH (or) other aneurysm<br>• Genetic diseases (autosomal dominant polycystic kidney disease, Ehlers-Danlos syndrome, sickle cell disease, Marfan syndrome, and fibromuscular dysplasia) |

**Clinical presentations**

- Thunderclap headache (severe headache that reaches maximal pain in <1 minute, characterized as worst headache of life)—hallmark symptom
- Meningismus (photophobia, nuchal rigidity, neck pain).
- Elevated ICP: Emesis, reduced consciousness
- Brief loss of consciousness
- Focal neurological signs: limb weakness, gait disturbance, visual disturbance
- Seizures (<24 hours – Poor outcome)
- Neurogenic pulmonary edema, ECG – QT prolongation, ST elevation changes
- Sudden death

**Ottawa subarachnoid hemorrhage (SAH) rule**

**For headache evaluation**

- For alert patients > 15 years of age with new onset severe nontraumatic headache reaching maximum intensity within 1 hour. Patients require additional investigation for SAH if they meet any of the following criteria

↓

- Age ≥40 years
- Neck pain or stiffness
- Witnessed loss of consciousness
- Onset during exertion
- Thunderclap headache (instantly peaking pain)
- Limited neck flexion on examination

## CAUSES

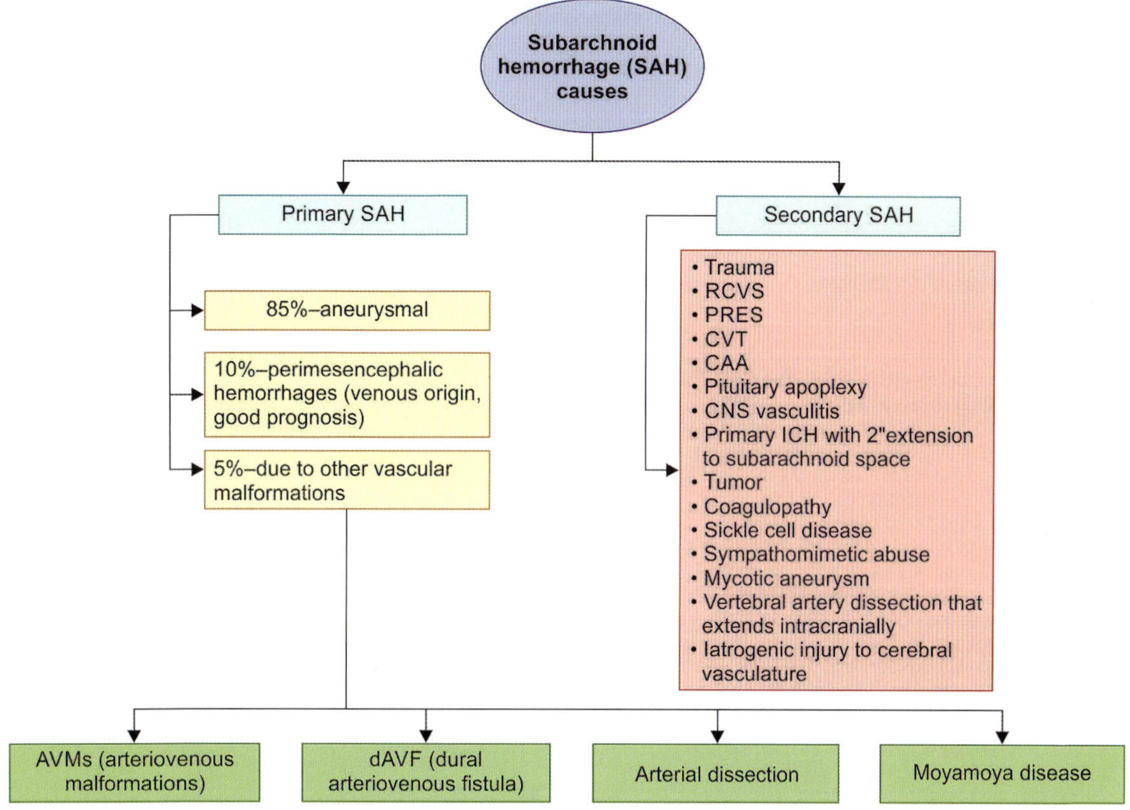


(CAA: cerebral amyloid angiopathy; CVT: cerebral venous sinus thrombosis; PRES: posterior reversible encephalopathy syndrome; RCVS: reversible cerebral vasoconstriction syndrome)

## INVESTIGATIONS

| ***Investigation modalities*** | |
|---|---|
| Plain CT | Diagnosis, Distribution, ICH, Hydrocephalus, Edema |
| CT angio | Highly sensitive and specific (~95%) for aneurysm detection. Detects aneurysm <5 mm but may miss very small aneurysms |
| DSA | Gold standard for diagnosis of aneurysm, can proceed to coiling if needed |
| MRI + MRA | Sensitivity ~100% in subacute phase, for patients who present late and have a negative CT scan. Detect underlying pathology (AV malformations, infections, malignancy, or inflammatory disorders) but doesn't pick small aneurysms |
| Lumbar puncture | Xanthochromia, diagnostic in patients with negative noncontrast head CT scan with have high suspicion for SAH |

## MANAGEMENT

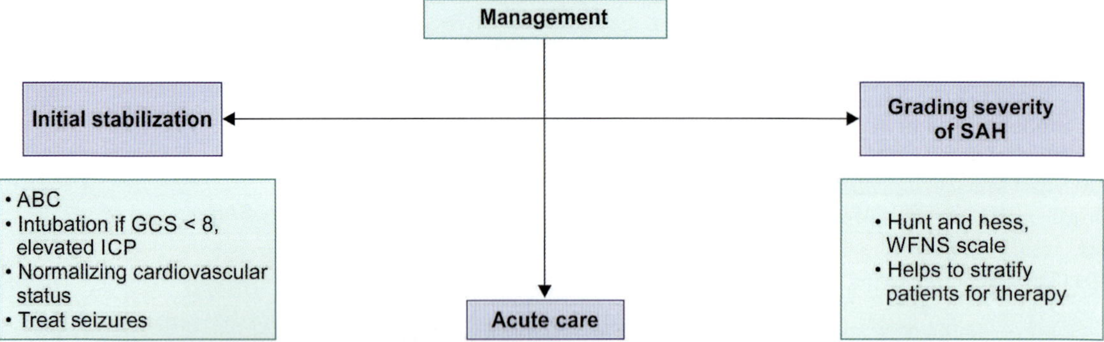


- Routine monitoring–GCS, ECG, BP, $SpO_2$, Na, fluid balance
- Anticoagulation reversal if any
- BP control–SBP <160 (American Heart Association) or MAP <110 mm (Neurocritical Care Society) IV Nicardipine, IV Nimodipine, IV Labetalol can be used. Avoid hypotension
- Seizure prophylaxis for 7 days, Mechanical DVT prophylaxis
- Pain control and maintain euvolemia
- ICP control if indicated-tiered approach
- Promptly securing the aneurysm (either via surgical clipping or endovascular coiling) reduces the risk of rebleeding This should be achieved as soon as possible, usually not later than 72 hours
- The ISAT and BRAT trials demonstrated that endovascular coiling generally yields superior outcomes compared to neurosurgery, choice will depend on the aneurysm's configuration, size, anatomy, presence of a neck, and location
- Coiling is typically favored, except for following situations
  - Aneurysms with an associated hematoma that requires surgical drainage
  - Aneurysms with a broad neck that is not amenable to coiling
  - Associated cerebral edema that may benefit from leaving a craniectomy flap off, to accommodate swelling

## COILING VERSUS CLIPPING

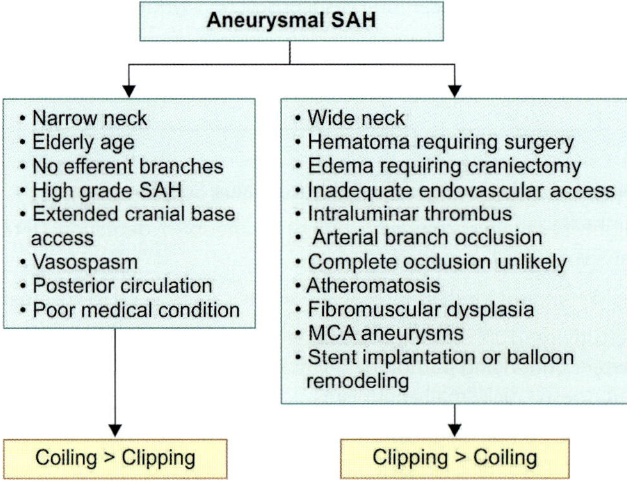

## COMPLICATIONS

**Re-bleeding**

- Risk highest early on
- Deterioration is often rapid and dramatic
- Risk factors – Longer time to aneurysmal treatment, poor neurological status at admission, large aneurysm size, high BP, presence of ICH
- Mortality 70%

**Hydrocephalus (20–30%)**

- Early (Minutes to Hours) – Due to obstruction, very common, may need EVD
- Late (2 weeks or later) – Due to dysfunction of arachnoid granulations in reabsorbing CSF, may need EVD / VP shunt

**Delayed cerebral ischemia**

- Vasospasm leading to ischemia and infarction
- May occur around 3–14 days, peak ~7–10 days
- Deterioration is often gradual and somewhat subtle
- Serial TCD or CT angio to diagnose
- Prevention - nimodipine 60 mg q4hrs for 21 days, maintain euvolemia

**Seizures**

- *Risk factors:* Thick SAH clot, delayed infarction, MCA aneurysm
- *Treatment:* AED Levetiracetam preferred, phenytoin avoided

**Cardiopulmonary**

- Takotsubo cardiomyopathy
- Cardiogenic/Neurogenic pulmonary edema
- Subendocardial ischemia
- QTc prolongation

**Metabolic**

- Hypoglycemia, hypercapnia uremia
- Hyponatremia due to SIADII/CSW

## APPROACH TO DELAYED CEREBRAL ISCHEMIA

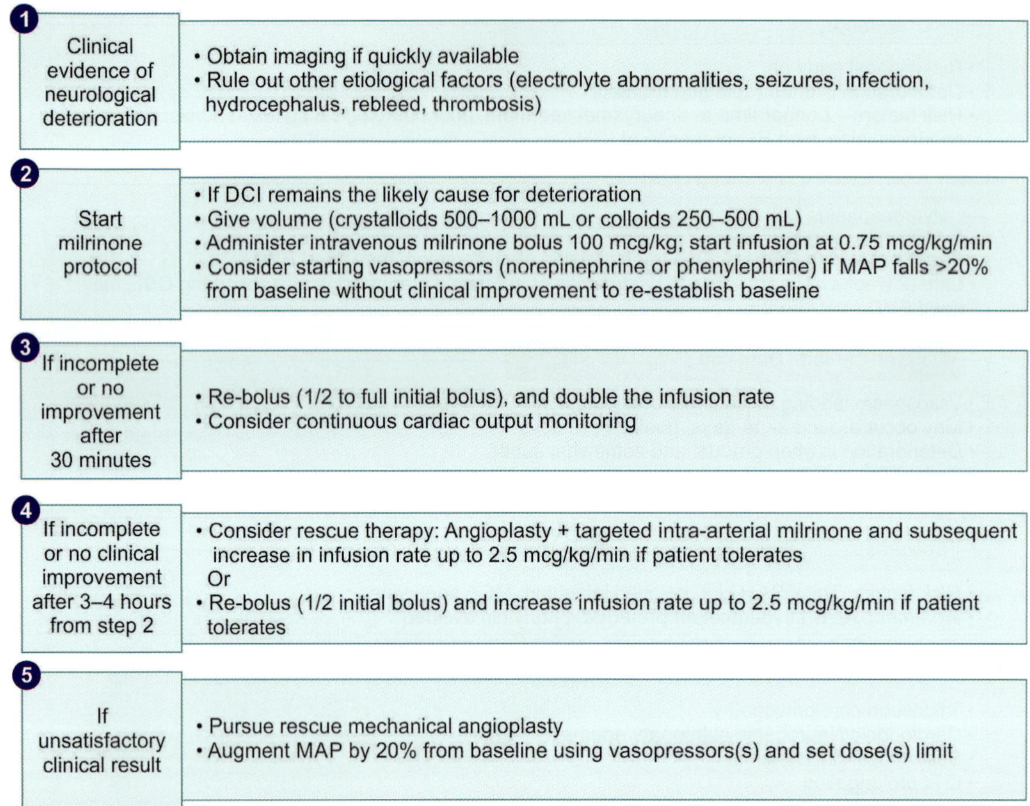


*Source:* Farkas J. (2022). Subarachnoid Hemorrhage (SAH). [online] Available from emcrit.org/ibcc/sah [Last accessed February, 2025].

## MANAGEMENT OF DELAYED CEREBRAL ISCHEMIA

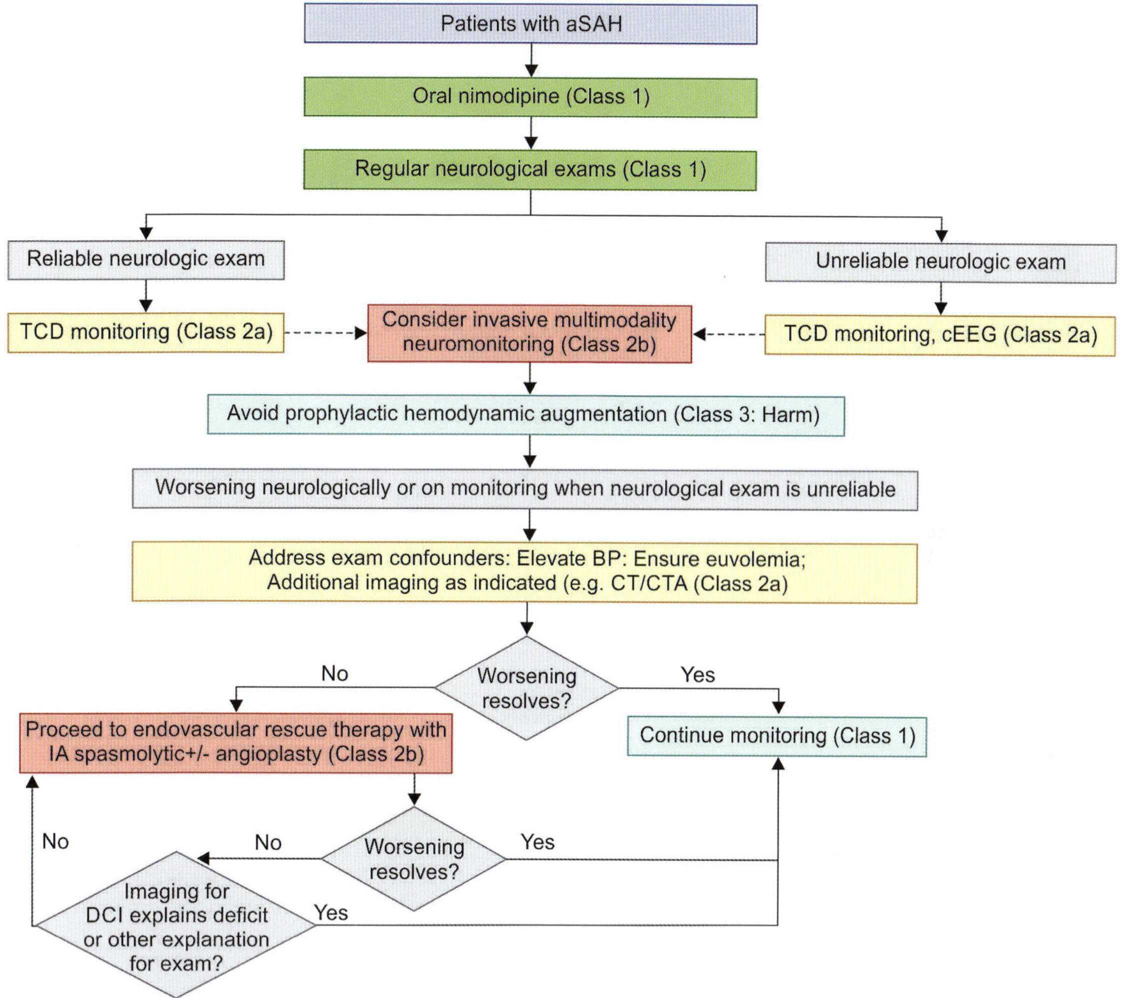


*Source:* Hoh BL, Ko NU, Amin-Hanjani S, Chou SH-Y, Cruz-Flores S, Dangayach NS, et al. 2023 Guideline for the Management of Patients With Aneurysmal Subarachnoid Hemorrhage: a guideline from the American Heart Association/American Stroke Association. Stroke. 2023;54:e31470.

## SAH CARE CONTINUUM

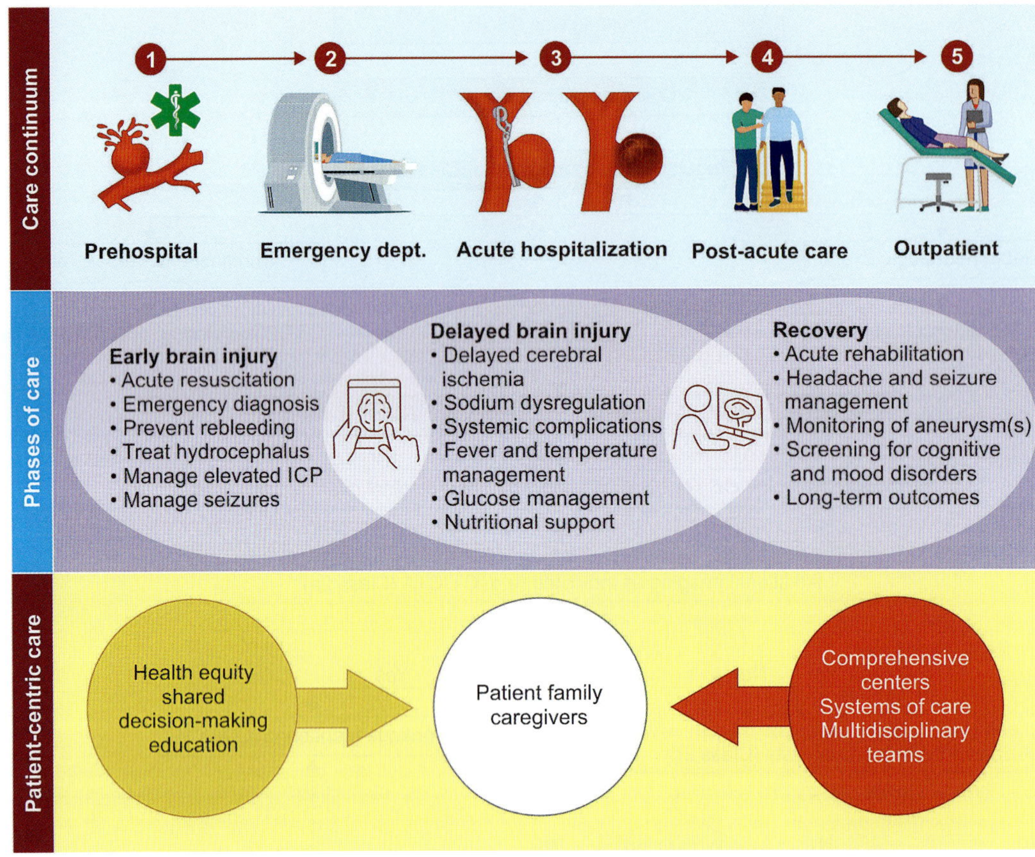


*Source:* Hoh BL, Ko NU, Amin-Hanjani S, Chou SH-Y, Cruz-Flores S, Dangayach NS, et al. 2023 Guideline for the Management of Patients With Aneurysmal Subarachnoid Hemorrhage: a guideline from the American Heart Association/American Stroke Association. Stroke. 2023;54:e31470.

## SUGGESTED READING

1. Farkas J. (2022). Subarachnoid Hemorrhage (SAH). [online] Available from emcrit.org/ibcc/sah [Last accessed February, 2025].
2. Hoh BL, Ko NU, Amin-Hanjani S, Chou SH-Y, Cruz-Flores S, Dangayach NS, et al. 2023 Guideline for the Management of Patients With Aneurysmal Subarachnoid Hemorrhage: a guideline from the American Heart Association/American Stroke Association. Stroke. 2023;54:e31470.

CHAPTER 44

# Management of Severe and Nonsevere Traumatic Brain Injury

| | |
|---|---|
| Airway | • Inspect for foreign bodies, identify facial, mandibular, and/or tracheal/laryngeal fractures<br>• Suction airway to clear accumulated blood or secretions<br>• If GCS 8 or < 8, Consider intubation<br>• If cervical spine tenderness or tenderness during neck movements, apply cervical collar<br>• Manual in line stabilization if intubation is considered for cervical collar patients |
| Breathing and circulation | • Expose neck and chest<br>• Visual inspection and palpation to know chest wall injuries or uneven expansion of chest wall or signs of pneumothorax/hemothorax<br>• Auscultate and confirm b/l equal air entry<br>• Supplementary $O_2$<br>• Assess level of consciousness, skin perfusion, and pulse<br>• Definitive bleeding control is essential, along with appropriate replacement of intravascular volume |
| Disability | • Check pupil size<br>• Check GCS<br>• Decide on airway securing (rule out Hypoglycemia, alcohol, narcotics, and other drugs) |
| Exposure | • Completely undress the patient<br>• Inspection<br>• Assess hypothermia and measures to prevent it |
| Adjuncts | Pulse ox, ventilator/capnography, ABG, urinary cat, Ryles tube, eFAST, X-ray |

## SECTION 1—INITIAL EVALUATION OF TRAUMATIC BRAIN INJURY—AS PER ATLS GUIDELINES

### Primary Survey

*Secondary Survey*

| *Head-to-toe examination once primary survey is over and patient is adequately resuscitated* | |
|---|---|
| History (AMPLE) | • Allergies and ADT<br>• Medications<br>• Past history and pregnancy status<br>• Last meal<br>• Events leading up to injury |
| *Physical examination* | |
| • Head<br>• Cervical spine | • Lacerations<br>• Contusions<br>• Fractures |
| Adjuncts | CT/MRI |

## SECTION 2 : CLASSIFICATION OF TBI

| | | | |
|---|---|---|---|
| Severity | • Mild<br>• Moderate<br>• Severe | | • GCS Score 13–15<br>• GCS Score 9–12<br>• GCS Score 3–8 |
| Morphology | Skull fractures | Vault | Linear vs. stellate<br>Depressed/nondepressed |
| | | Basilar | • With/without CSF leak<br>• With/without seventh nerve palsy |
| | Intracranial lesions | Focal | • Epidural<br>• Subdural<br>• Intracerebral |
| | | Diffuse | • Concussion<br>• Multiple contusions<br>• Hypoxic/ischemic injury<br>• Axonal injury |

## SECTION 3: PATHOPHYSIOLOGY OF ICP/CCP/AUTOREGULATION OF CBF

| *Concept* | *Description* |
|---|---|
| Monro–Kellie Doctrine | • The doctrine states that the total volume of the intracranial contents must remain constant because the cranium is a rigid container.<br>• Initial buffering by venous blood and CSF occurs.<br>• Exceeding normal intracranial volume raises ICP. |
| Cerebral Blood Flow (CBF) | Severe head trauma can drastically reduce CBF initially. Although CBF usually increases over the next few days, it can remain below normal for comatose patients, potentially leading to cerebral ischemia. |
| Intracranial Pressure (ICP) | • ICP is the pressure inside the skull exerted by brain tissue, cerebrospinal fluid (CSF), and blood.<br>• Elevated ICP can reduce cerebral perfusion, worsening ischemia.<br>• Normal resting ICP is around 10 mm Hg. Pressures greater than 22 mm Hg, especially if sustained, are linked with poor outcomes. |
| Cerebral Perfusion Pressure (CPP) | • CPP, calculated as MAP - ICP, is vital for maintaining adequate CBF (60–80 mm Hg)<br>• Severe TBI can disrupt autoregulation, impairing the brain's compensation for changes in CPP and potentially leading to ischemia or brain swelling. |
| Cerebral Autoregulation 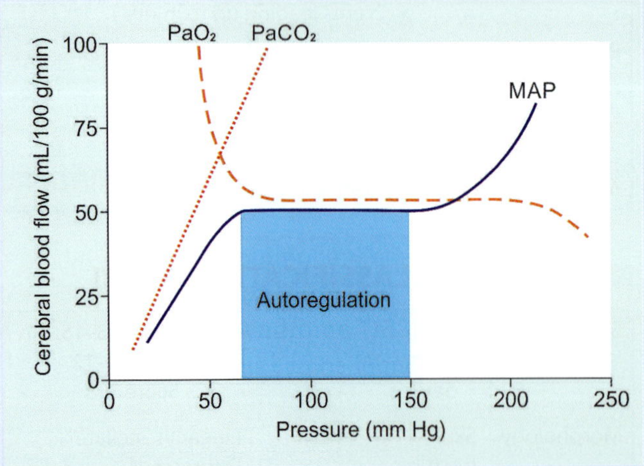 | • Mean Arterial Pressure (MAP) of 50 to 150 mm Hg is autoregulated to maintain constant CBF (pressure autoregulation).<br>• Severe Traumatic Brain Injury (TBI) can disrupt pressure autoregulation, impairing the brain's ability to compensate for CPP changes.<br>• Low MAP can lead to ischemia and infarction.<br>• High MAP can cause marked brain swelling with elevated ICP. |
| Chemical Regulation of Cerebral Blood Vessels | • Cerebral vessels regulate diameter in response to $PaO_2$ and $PaCO_2$ changes.<br>• Hypotension, hypoxia, hypercapnia, or iatrogenic hypocapnia can induce secondary injury by affecting CBF. |

## TBI MANAGEMENT GUIDELINES

| *Tier* | *Intervention* | *Subcategories* | *Key points* |
|---|---|---|---|
| TIER ZERO: Basic Interventions for All TBI Patients | 1. Positioning | - | • Elevate head of bed to 30 degrees.<br>• Maintain head in a neutral position to avoid jugular vein constriction. |
| | 2. Serum Sodium | - | Maintain serum sodium at 140 mEq/L with isotonic intravenous fluids (no dextrose). |
| | 3. Temperature | - | • Maintain normothermia.<br>• Administer acetaminophen 650 mg PO/PT every 4 hours if temperature exceeds 37°C.<br>• Consider a cooling blanket if unable to maintain normothermia. |
| TIER ONE Interventions for Patients with GCS ≤ 8 | 1. General Goals | - | Ensure all physiologic goals from Tier Zero are met. |
| | 2. Airway and Breathing | • Intubation<br>• Ventilation | • Intubate patients with GCS ≤ 8 if needed to protect the airway.<br>• Maintain $PaCO_2$ at 35-40 mm Hg.<br>• Consider obtaining arterial blood gas to correlate with end-tidal $CO_2$ ($EtCO_2$).<br>• Maintain $PaO_2$ at 80-120 mm Hg. |
| | 3. Systemic Perfusion | • Arterial Line<br>• Fluid Management<br>• Blood Pressure<br>• Volume Resuscitation | • Insert an arterial line leveled at the phlebostatic axis.<br>• Maintain euvolemia with a fluid balance positive by 500-1000 mL in the first 24 hours.<br>• Maintain MAP ≥ 65 mm Hg.<br>• Maintain SBP at 100-160 mm Hg.<br>• Ensure adequate volume resuscitation.<br>• Maintain hemoglobin ≥ 8 g/dL during the acute resuscitation phase.<br>• Consider advanced hemodynamic monitoring.<br>• Consider norepinephrine at 0.05 mcg/kg/min to maintain MAP ≥ 65 mm Hg. |
| | 4. Cerebral Perfusion | • Intracranial Pressure (ICP) Monitoring<br>• Cerebral Perfusion Pressure (CPP)<br>• Management of Sustained ICP ≥ 22 mm Hg | • Monitor ICP in all salvageable patients with severe TBI (GCS 3-8 after resuscitation) and an abnormal CT scan within 24 hours.<br>• Prefer using an ICP monitor with external ventricular drainage (EVD) over an ICP monitor alone.<br>• Maintain CPP ≥ 60 mm Hg if ICP monitoring is available.<br>• If CPP is < 60 mm Hg, ensure adequate volume resuscitation, consider advanced hemodynamic monitoring, consider norepinephrine at 0.05 mcg/kg/min.<br>• If ICP remains ≥ 22 mm Hg for 10 minutes and EVD is clamped, open EVD at 0 mm Hg for 15 minutes.<br>• If EVD is opened more than 3 times within 90 minutes, leave EVD open at 0 mm Hg continuously and notify neurosurgery.<br>• Consider osmolar therapy and short-term hyperventilation ($PaCO_2$ 30-34 mm Hg) to acutely reduce ICP. |
| | 5. Osmolar Therapy | | • First line therapy: 3% sodium chloride 500 mL IV bolus over 15 min x 1 if serum sodium < 160 mmol/L.<br>• Alternate therapy: Mannitol 0.25-1.0 gm/kg (nearest 12.5g) IV push x 1 if serum sodium < 160 and/or serum osmolality < 320 mOsm/L. |

*Contd...*

*Contd…*

| Tier | Intervention | Subcategories | Key points |
|---|---|---|---|
| | | - | • Measure serum sodium every 4 hours (and serum osmolality every 4 hours if using mannitol).<br>• Notify intensivist if serum sodium changes by 2 mEq/L within 4 hours from previous measurement.<br>• Hold hypertonic saline therapy for serum sodium ≥ 160 mEq/L.<br>• Hold mannitol therapy for serum sodium ≥ 160 mEq/L and/or serum osmolality ≥ 320 mOsm/L. |
| | 6. Protect the Brain | - | • Provide judicious analgesia and sedation to control pain and agitation.<br>• Fentanyl: 25-500 mcg/h IV infusion titrate to CPOT < 2 or ICP < 22.<br>• Propofol: 10-50 mcg/kg/min IV infusion titrate to ICP < 22.<br>• Obtain spot EEG monitoring within 24 hours of admission to rule out non-convulsive status epilepticus in patient GCS 10 or less.<br>• Levetiracetam x 7 days (discontinue after 7 days if no seizure activity):<br>– Age < 75 years: 1,000 mg IV/PO q12 hours x 7 days.<br>– Age ≥ 75 years OR CrCl < 50 mL/min: 500 mg IV/PO q12 hours x 7 days.<br>– ESRD: 500 mg IV/PO QHS x 7 days. |
| | 7. Avoid | - | • Hypotension (SBP < 100 mm Hg) or CPP < 60 mm Hg.<br>• Hypoxemia ($SpO_2$ < 92%).<br>• Hypercarbia ($PaCO_2$ > 40 mm Hg).<br>• Hyponatremia (Serum Sodium < 136 mmol/L).<br>• Hypoglycemia or Hyperglycemia (serum glucose < 70 mg/dL or > 180 mg/dL).<br>• Hypovolemia.<br>• Fever (temperature > 37°C).<br>• Anemia (maintain hemoglobin ≥ 8 g/dL) in the first seven days. |
| TIER TWO Interventions for Persistent ICP > 22 mm Hg | 1. Ensure All Tier One Goals Are Met | - | Review and confirm that all physiologic goals from Tier One are achieved and maintained. |
| | 2. Repeat Osmolar Therapy | - | • If serum sodium is less than 160 mmol/L, recommend 23.4% sodium chloride, 30 mL IV syringe over 15 minutes.<br>• If volume resuscitation is needed, use 3% sodium chloride, 500 mL IV bolus.<br>• Continue to check serum sodium every 4 hours. |
| | 3. Consider head CT scan | - | Obtain a head CT scan to rule out a space-occupying lesion. |
| | 4. Continuous EEG Monitoring | - | Initiate continuous EEG monitoring to rule out non-convulsive status epilepticus, if not already in place. |
| | 5. Sedative and Analgesic Therapy | - | Consider bolusing and then increasing sedative and analgesic therapy to manage agitation and pain more effectively. |

*Contd…*

*Contd...*

| Tier | Intervention | Subcategories | Key points |
|---|---|---|---|
| | 6. Paralysis | - | • Ensure a Richmond Agitation-Sedation Scale (RASS) score of -5 before initiating paralytic agents.<br>• Start rocuronium with a 50 mg IV push loading dose, followed by 8 mcg/kg/h continuous infusion. Adjust the dose according to Train of Four (TOF) monitoring to achieve a TOF ratio of 1/4. |
| | 7. Hypothermia | - | Early (within 2.5 hours), short-term (48 hours post-injury) prophylactic hypothermia is not recommended to improve outcomes in patients with diffuse injury. |
| | 8. Mild Hyperventilation | - | Begin mild hyperventilation with a goal $PaCO_2$ of 35-40 mm Hg. |
| TIER THREE Interventions for Persistent ICP > 22 mm Hg Despite Tier Two Interventions | 1. Maximize Medical Therapy with Hypertonic Saline | - | Ensure medical therapy with hypertonic saline is maximized (e.g., serum sodium 160 mEq/L). |
| | 2. Revised ICP Threshold | - | Consider a revised ICP threshold of 25 mm Hg with strict adherence to maintaining CPP > 60 mm Hg. |
| | 3. Continuous EEG | - | Initiate continuous EEG monitoring if not already present. |
| | 4. Surgical Decompression | - | • Note that craniectomy solely for ICP management does not improve long-term neurological outcomes.<br>• Consider decompressive craniectomy or craniotomy in patients with a surgical lesion. |
| | 5. Barbiturate Coma | - | • If not a surgical candidate and refractory to all other interventions, consider a pentobarbital coma.<br>• Hemodynamic stability is essential before and during pentobarbital therapy. |

## SECTION 5 : TARGETS OF THERAPY IN TBI

| | |
|---|---|
| Decompressive craniectomy | 1. NEW–Secondary DC performed for early (72 hrs) refractory ICP elevation is not recommended to improve mortality and favorable outcomes<br>2. NEW–Secondary DC performed for late (10 days) refractory ICP elevation is recommended to improve mortality and favorable outcomes. |
| Prophylactic hypothermia | No outcome benefit |
| Hyperosmolar therapy | • No outcome benefit proven as yet but none the less useful in lowering ICP<br>• Mannitol - 0.25 g/kg to 1 g/kg body weight. |
| CSF Drainage | Continuous drainage of CSF may be considered to lower ICP burden more effectively than intermittent use. |
| Ventilation therapies | Hyperventilation is recommended as a temporizing measure for the reduction of elevated ICP. |
| Anesthetics, analgesics and Sedatives | High-dose barbiturate administration is recommended to control elevated ICP refractory to maximum standard medical and surgical treatment.(2B) |
| Nutrition | • Feeding patients to attain basal caloric replacement at least by the 5th day and at most by the 7th day post-injury is recommended to decrease mortality.(2A)<br>• Transgastric jejunal feeding is recommended to reduce the incidence of ventilator-associated pneumonia.(3A) |

*Contd...*

*Contd...*

| | |
|---|---|
| Infection prophylaxis | Early tracheostomy is recommended to reduce mechanical ventilation day bhut not mortality (Level 2A) |
| Thromboprophylaxis | In addition to compression stockings, pharmacologic prophylaxis may be considered if the brain injury is stable and the benefit is considered to outweigh the risk of increased intracranial hemorrhage. |
| Seizure prophylaxis | Phenytoin is recommended to decrease the incidence of early PTS (within 7 days of injury) |
| ICP Monitoring | Management of severe TBI patients using information from ICP monitoring is recommended to reduce in-hospital and 2-week post-injury mortality. (level 2b) |
| CPP Monitoring | Management of severe TBI patients using guidelines-based recommendations for CPP monitoring is recommended to decrease 2-week mortality. |
| Advanced cerebral monitoring | Jugular bulb monitoring of arteriovenous oxygen content difference (AVDO2), as a source of information for management decisions, may be considered to reduce mortality and improve outcomes at 3 and 6 months post-injury.(3) |
| Blood pressure thresholds | Maintaining SBP at ≥100 mm Hg for patients 50 to 69 years old or at ≥110 mm Hg or above for patients 15 to 49 or over 70 years old may be considered to decrease mortality and improve outcomes.(3) |
| Intracranial pressure thresholds | Treating ICP above 22 mm Hg is recommended because values above this level are associated with increased mortality. (3) |
| CPP Thresholds | The recommended target cerebral perfusion pressure (CPP) value for survival and favorable outcomes is between 60 and 70 mm Hg.(2b) |
| Advanced cerebral monitoring thresholds | Jugular venous saturation of <50% may be a threshold to avoid in order to reduce mortality and improve outcomes. |

## SUGGESTED READING

1. American College of Surgeons Committee on Trauma. Advanced Trauma Life Support : Student Course Manual. Tenth. Chicago, Illinois, United States: American College of Surgeons; 2018.
2. Birrer K, Helmick E, Schuemann K, Hunter J, Wisniewski P, Semon G, et al.(2019). Severe Traumatic Brain Injury Management Evidence Based Medicine Guideline. [online] Available from https://www.surgicalcriticalcare.net/Guidelines/Traumatic%20Brain%20Injury%202023.pdf [Last accessed February, 2025].
3. Hawryluk, GWJ, Rubiano AM, Totten AM, O'Reilly C, Ullman JS, Bratton SL, et al. Guidelines for the Management of Severe Traumatic Brain Injury: 2020 Update of the Decompressive Craniectomy Recommendations. Neurosurgery. 2020;87(3):427-34.

CHAPTER 45

# Traumatic Spinal Cord Injury

## INTRODUCTION

The global incidence of traumatic spinal injury is approximately 10.5 cases per 100,000 persons. The severity of the damage and extent of neurological impairment will determine the prognosis. Timely intervention can mitigate more harm and consequences. A primary survey leading to appropriate action, followed by secondary survey and stabilization of the patient, choosing between conservative or surgical management, monitoring the patient's status over time, and providing long-term care are all part of managing patients with traumatic spinal cord injury (TSCI).

## PATHOPHYSIOLOGY AND MECHANISM OF INJURY

Sequential order of events is categorized into two phases:

1. Primary injury results from compression of the spinal cord by pressure from bony fragments, blood products, soft tissue, and/or foreign objects.
2. After the onset of the first insult, there is a release of cytokines, free radicals and vasoactive proteins leading to oxidative damage.

## CLINICAL PRESENTATION

- Complete injury (AIS - American Spinal Injury Association Impairment Scale, grade A)
    - No motor or sensory function below neurological level of injury, and no sacral sparing.
    - In the acute setting, reflexes are absent (including bulbocavernosus) and male patients may have priapism.
    - Urinary retention and bladder distension
    - Patients with cervical or high thoracic complete cord injuries—variable sympathetic dysfunction including hypotension and bradycardia
- Incomplete injury (AIS, grades B through D) preserves voluntary anal contraction, has nonzero perineal sensory scores and often preserved bulbocavernosus reflex
    - Various degrees of motor function and sensation caudal to the level of injury.
    - Central cord syndrome:
        - Hyperextension injury which is exacerbated by preexisting cervical spondylosis and/or central canal stenosis
        - Disproportionally greater motor impairment in the upper (especially distal upper) versus lower extremities, often with bladder dysfunction and variable degree of caudal sensory loss.
- Anterior cord syndrome:
    - Direct mechanical injury to the anterior cord from disc/bone fragment retropulsion, often with flexion as the causative mechanism.
    - Corticospinal tracts, spinothalamic tracts, and descending autonomic tracts affected with preservation of the posterior column.
    - Complete motor paralysis and loss of pain and temperature, and preservation of tactile position and vibration.
- Lateral hemisection or hemicord syndrome or Brown-Sequard injuries:
    - Unilateral damage to the dorsal column, corticospinal tract, and spinothalamic tract
    - Ipsilateral weakness, loss of vibration and proprioception, and contralateral loss of pain and temperature sensation beginning approximately two spinal levels below the injured level.
    - Contralateral sensation loss is due to the decussation of spinothalamic fibers that occurs approximately two spinal levels above the level of injury since these fibers have yet to decussate and are thus preserved.
    - Common causes of this syndrome include ballistic and penetrating injuries.

## SPINAL SHOCK

- Spinal shock is "an acute state of diminished spinal function characterized by loss of all sensorimotor functions caudal to the site of injury."
- Transient condition which can mislead initial neurological examination.
- Continual and ongoing assessment is vital to determine the true extent of SCI.
- Physiologic reflex depression of spinal cord function rather than anatomic.
- Characterized by loss of reflexes, flaccid paralysis, and decreased blood pressure.
- Course is measured by the return of spinal reflexes usually starting with the bulbocavernosus reflex (as early as 1 hour after injury), followed by the anal cutaneous reflex, and subsequently the plantar reflex.

## CAVEATS

- Permanent areflexia with or without replacement by pathological reflexes is more likely due to mechanical spinal cord injury.
- Differentiate spinal shock and neurogenic shock. Spinal shock occurs from spinal cord damage, while neurogenic shock is due to injury at cervical and high thoracic vertebral levels, causing sympathetic dysfunctions such as hypotension and bradycardia.

## EVALUATION

As per advanced trauma and life support (ATLS) guidelines, prioritize airway, breathing, and circulation "A, B, C's".

Place the patients in spinal precautions on a backboard, secured with tape or blocks, and placed in a rigid cervical collar (typically a Miami J collar or Aspen collar).

Arms secured at the patient's side with spider straps.

### Spinal Precautions

Spinal precautions should be implemented in all patients who have sustained an acute traumatic injury until a spinal fracture is ruled out. Precautions include:

- Limiting flexion, extension, rotation, and twisting of the spine to avoid exacerbating an injury to the spinal cord.
- Cervical collars for suspected cervical-level spinal fractures.
- Use of cervical collars can elevate intracranial pressure (ICP) or lead to skin breakdown, and increase the risk of aspiration in elderly persons. Rule out cervical-level spinal injuries as early as possible to allow for safe removal of the cervical collar.
- For injuries below T8 skeletal level, hip should not be allowed to actively or passively flex beyond 90° to avoid kyphotic stress on the lumbar spine. Instead, a unilateral, isometric examination should be completed to ensure extension of the contralateral hip to stabilize the pelvis.

### In the Trauma Bay

Assume spinal cord injury in polytrauma patients, until appropriate diagnostic testing is performed.

Reassess ABC

Maintain MAP between 85 and 90 mmHg, keeping in mind other injuries and bleeding.

Common *neurological signs and symptoms* associated with ATSCI:

In one or more limbs:

- Paralysis
- Sensory loss
- Reflex loss
- Hypoesthesia
- Hyperesthesia
- Bowel and bladder dysfunction
- Autonomic dysreflexia

*Neurological levels:* Use the International Standards for Neurological Classification of Spinal Cord Injury (ISNCSCI) to classify the level of spinal cord injury. The ISNCSCI system assesses motor function in eight segments (C5-T1) and assigns a score based on the level of motor function preserved.

### Spinal Cord Injury Severity Classification

The ISNCSCI, commonly referred to as the ASIA Exam, consists of a:

- Myotomal-based motor examination;
- Dermatomal-based sensory examination, and
- An anorectal examination.

Upon completion of these three components, an injury grade and level are assigned. This designation can be used for rehabilitation.

**ASIA Impairment Scale (AIS).**

| Grade | Type of injury | Description of injury |
|---|---|---|
| A | Complete | No sensory or motor function is preserved in sacral segments S4-S5. no sacral sparing |
| B | Sensory Incomplete | • Sensory but not motor function is preserved below the neurological level and includes sacral segments S4-S5 AND<br>• No motor function is preserved more than three levels below the motor level on either side of the body |
| C | Motor Incomplete | Motor function is preserved below the neurological level<br>AND<br>More than half of the key muscle functions below the neurological level of injury have a muscle grade of less than 3 (Grades 0-2) |
| D | Motor Incomplete | Motor function is preserved below the neurological level<br>AND<br>At least half (half or more) of the key muscle functions below the neurological level of injury have a muscle grade ≥ 3 |
| E | Normal | If sensation and motor function are graded as normal in all segments<br>AND<br>the patient had prior SCI-related deficits<br>Individuals without a spinal cord injury do not receive an AIS Grade. |

Information in the above table is adapted from the 2011 version of International Standards for Neurological Classification of Spinal Cord Injury

## IMAGING

A trauma series computed tomography (CT) of brain, cervical spine, chest, abdomen, and pelvis.

Plain radiographs to characterize orthopedic injuries to the extremities.

MRI of the relevant section to assess the severity of the injury.

If an injury pattern is suspicious for head/neck vascular injury, a CT head and neck angiogram.

### Resuscitation and Supportive Care

- *Fluid management:* Prevent hypovolemia, hypotension, and shock.
- *Cardiovascular support*: Monitor and manage blood pressure (MAP above 85–90 mm Hg), heart rate, and cardiac rhythm.
- *Respiratory support:*
  - Supplemental oxygen to maintain oxygen saturation levels.
  - High cervical cord injury often requires ventilatory support and continued mechanical ventilation with tracheostomy.
  - Vaccination against influenza and pneumococcus for all patients with respiratory impairment due to SCI is recommended
  - Aggressive daily chest physiotherapy
  - Pain management
- *Nutritional support:* Adequate nutrition and hydration
- *Steroid therapy:* No recommendation for methylprednisolone as a routine in SCI.
- *Alternative approaches:* To reduce inflammation and edema in acute SCI,:
  - Minocycline, for its anti-inflammatory properties
  - N-acetylcysteine (NAC), to reduce oxidative stress
  - Hyperbaric oxygen therapy, to improve tissue oxygenation and reduce inflammation.

## SURGICAL MANAGEMENT

Aims to stabilize the spine, decompress the spinal cord, and promote optimal healing.

### Indications for Surgical Therapy in ATSCI

- *Severe trauma:* Including fractures, dislocations, or instability in the spine.
- *Spinal cord compression:* Compressive lesions, such as herniated disks or bone fragments that cause pressure on the spinal cord.
- *Spinal instability:* Unstable spines that are at risk of further injury or collapse.
- *Progressive neurologic deficit:* Worsening neurologic symptoms, such as weakness, numbness, or paralysis.
- *Unstable fracture:* Unstable fractures that require stabilization to prevent further injury.

Some of the most common surgical therapies used for ATSCI:

- Decompressive surgery
- Spinal fusion
- Laminectomy
- Anterior cervical discectomy and fusion (ACDF)
- Surgical stabilization

### Early Rehabilitation

- Passive range of motion exercises to prevent contractures and maintain joint mobility and maintain muscle strength and tone.
- Early mobilization
- Multidisciplinary team management
- Homecare for services, such as physical therapy, occupational therapy, and speech therapy, as needed.
- *Follow-up care:* With the healthcare team to monitor progress and address any concerns.

### Common Complications of ATSCI

- Spinal shock
- Hypotension
- Hypoxia
- Respiratory failure
- Pneumonia
- Pneumothorax
- Rhabdomyolysis
- Sepsis
- Deep vein thrombosis (DVT)
- Organ failure
- Infections
- Skeletal complications
- Neurological complications
- Pressure ulcers
- Nutritional complications and malnutrition
- Psychological complications
- Rehabilitation challenges

### Late Complications

Occur weeks, months, or even years after ATSCI.

Early recognition and provide timely and effective management minimize their impact on the patient's quality of life and outcome. Some of the complications are:

- Chronic pain
- Respiratory complications
- Cardiometabolic syndrome
- Thermoregulation disorders
- Endocrine disorders
- Gastrointestinal complications
- Spinal cord compression
- Herniated disks
- Spasticity
- Pressure ulcers
- Osteoporosis
- Heterotopic ossification
- Neurogenic bladder
- Neurogenic bowel
- Painful spasticity
- Anxiety and depression
- Sleep disturbances
- Musculoskeletal complications
- Autonomic dysreflexia
- Syringomyelia

It is essential for individuals with SCI to receive regular medical care and rehabilitation to prevent or manage these late complications. Early detection and intervention can help improve outcomes and quality of life for individuals with SCI.

## REGULAR FOLLOW-UP CARE

To monitor for late complications and address early any concerns or issues that arise.

- *Preventive measures:* To reduce the risk of developing late complications, such as practicing good skin care, maintaining a healthy diet, and engaging in regular exercise.
- *Patient education:* Educate patients on their specific condition and provide them with resources to manage their condition effectively.
- *Multidisciplinary care:* Including physical therapists, occupational therapists, speech therapists, psychologists, and other specialists.

By addressing these late complications of acute traumatic SCI through a multidisciplinary approach, healthcare providers can improve patient outcomes, reduce morbidity, and enhance quality of life for individuals with SCI.

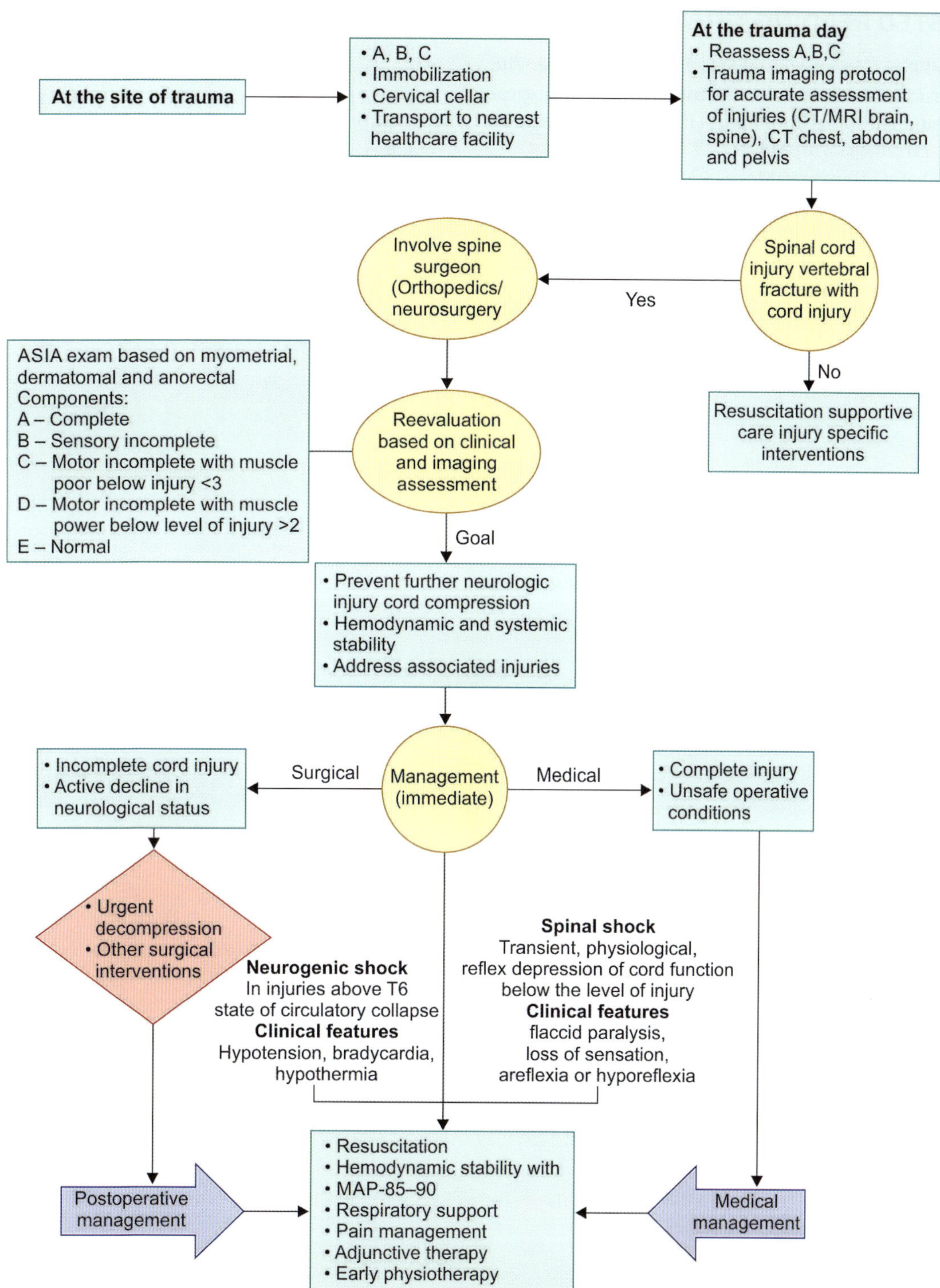

At the site of trauma
• A, B, C
• Immobilization
• Cervical cellar
• Transport to nearest healthcare facility
At the trauma day
• Reassess A,B,C
• Trauma imaging protocol for accurate assessment of injuries (CT/MRI brain, spine), CT chest, abdomen and pelvis
Spinal cord injury vertebral fracture with cord injury
Yes
Involve spine surgeon (Orthopedics/ neurosurgery
No
Resuscitation supportive care injury specific interventions
ASIA exam based on myometrial, dermatomal and anorectal Components:
A – Complete
B – Sensory incomplete
C – Motor incomplete with muscle poor below injury <3
D – Motor incomplete with muscle power below level of injury >2
E – Normal
Reevaluation based on clinical and imaging assessment
Goal
• Prevent further neurologic injury cord compression
• Hemodynamic and systemic stability
• Address associated injuries
Management (immediate)
Surgical
Medical
• Incomplete cord injury
• Active decline in neurological status
• Complete injury
• Unsafe operative conditions
• Urgent decompression
• Other surgical interventions
Neurogenic shock
In injuries above T6 state of circulatory collapse
Clinical features
Hypotension, bradycardia, hypothermia
Spinal shock
Transient, physiological, reflex depression of cord function below the level of injury
Clinical features
flaccid paralysis, loss of sensation, areflexia or hyporeflexia
Postoperative management
• Resuscitation
• Hemodynamic stability with
• MAP-85–90
• Respiratory support
• Pain management
• Adjunctive therapy
• Early physiotherapy
Medical management

## SUGGESTED READING

1. ASIA and ISCoS International Standards Committee. The 2019 revision of the International Standards for Neurological Classification of Spinal Cord Injury (ISNCSCI)-What's new? Spinal Cord. 2019;57(10):815-7.
2. Crozier-Shaw G, Denton H, Morris S. Management strategies in acute traumatic spinal cord injury: a narrative review. Neuroimmunol Neuroinflammation. 2020;7:335-44.
3. Roberts TT, Leonard GR, Cepela DJ. Classifications in brief: American spinal injury association (ASIA) impairment scale. 2017:475(5):1499-504.
4. Sandean D. Management of acute spinal cord injury: a summary of the evidence pertaining to the acute management, operative and non-operative management. World journal of orthopedics. 2020;11(12):573.
5. Schuld C, Wiese J, Franz S, Putz C, Stierle I, Smoor I, et al. Effect of formal training in scaling, scoring and classification of the international standards for neurological classification of spinal cord injury. Spinal Cord. 2013;51(4):282-8.
6. Wang TY, Park C, Zhang H, Rahimpour S, Murphy KR, Goodwin CR, et al. Management of Acute Traumatic Spinal Cord Injury: A Review of the Literature. Front Surg. 2021;8:698736.

# CHAPTER 46 Acute Flaccid Paresis

## INTRODUCTION

Acute flaccid paresis (AFP) is a complex condition that is characterized by the sudden onset of weakness or paralysis in one or more limbs, often accompanied by a distinctive pattern of neurophysiological changes.

## COMMON CLASSIFICATIONS OF AFP IN ADULTS

### Etiological Classification

#### Autoimmune

*Guillain-Barré syndrome (GBS):* This is the most common cause of acute flaccid paralysis in adults, accounting for approximately 70% of cases. GBS is an autoimmune disorder leading to inflammation and damage to nerve fibers.

- *Acute motor axonal neuropathy (AMAN):* This is a subtype of GBS characterized by rapid onset of weakness, often with a predominance of motor symptoms. AMAN is caused by an autoimmune response to gangliosides, which are complex lipids found on the surface of nerve cells.
- *Acute inflammatory demyelinating polyneuropathy (AIDP):* This is another subtype of GBS characterized by a slower onset of weakness and a more prominent sensory component. AIDP is also caused by an autoimmune response to the myelin sheath, which surrounds and protects nerve fibers.
- *Chronic inflammatory demyelinating polyneuropathy (CIDP):* While typically presenting in adults over the age of 50, CIDP can also occur in younger adults. It is characterized by progressive weakness, sensory loss, and demyelination of nerve fibers.
- *Acute flaccid paralysis of childhood (AFPC):* This condition is characterized by sudden onset of weakness or paralysis in children, often accompanied by fever and respiratory symptoms. AFPC is thought to be caused by an autoimmune response to a viral or bacterial infection.

*Other causes:* Other potential causes of AFP in adults include:

- *Infectious diseases* such as West Nile virus, tick-borne relapsing fever, herpes simplex virus, and human immunodeficiency virus (HIV) can cause AFP. Bacterial infections such as Lyme disease, meningitis, and sepsis can also cause AFP.
- *Trauma or injury* to the spinal cord or peripheral nerves
- *Tumors or neoplasms* affecting the nervous system
- *Vitamin deficiencies or toxicity* (e.g., thiamine deficiency)
- *Neurodegenerative disorders* such as amyloidosis or multiple sclerosis

## CLASSIFICATION BASED ON MYELIN SHEATH INTEGRITY

*AFP with demyelination (e.g., Guillain-Barré syndrome and Miller Fisher syndrome):*

- *Primary pathology is the destruction of the myelin sheath, leading to a loss of nerve function.*
- *Typical clinical presentation:* Weakness, usually starting in the legs, followed by ascending paralysis, and often accompanied by sensory symptoms.
- *Electrophysiological features:* Abnormalities on electromyography (EMG) and NCSs, such as prolonged distal latency, slowed conduction velocity, and decreased compound muscle action potential (CMAP) amplitude.
- *Imaging studies:* Magnetic resonance imaging (MRI) may show white matter lesions or diffuse signal changes in the spinal cord, brainstem, and peripheral nerves.

- *Laboratory findings:* Elevated cerebrospinal fluid (CSF) protein and abnormal CSF electrophoresis.
- *Treatment:* Plasmapheresis or intravenous immunoglobulin (IVIG) therapy is typically used to manage the autoimmune response.

*AFP without demyelination (e.g., direct peripheral nerve damage):*

- The primary pathology is damage to the nerve fibers themselves, rather than demyelination.
- *Common causes of AFP in adults without demyelination:*
  - *Traumatic spinal cord injury:* Direct trauma to the spinal cord
  - *Infections:* Meningitis, encephalitis, and sepsis can cause AFP.
  - *Neoplastic processes:* Spinal cord tumors, metastases, and lymphoma
- *Clinical presentation:* Weakness, often starting in the limbs or face, with variable distribution and progression.
- *Electrophysiological features:* Abnormalities on EMG and NCS may include reduced or absent CMAP amplitude, prolonged distal latency, and slowed conduction velocity.
- *Imaging studies:* MRI may show focal or diffuse lesions in specific nerve roots or peripheral nerves, but these findings are not always present.
- *Laboratory findings:* Normal or slightly elevated CSF protein levels; no abnormal CSF electrophoresis.
- *Treatment:* Management is often focused on supportive care, such as physical therapy, pain management, and rehabilitation.

*Key differences between the two conditions:*

- Demyelination is a hallmark feature of Guillain-Barré syndrome and related conditions, whereas direct nerve damage is more characteristic of other conditions that cause AFP in adults.
- The clinical presentation of demyelinating diseases often includes a more gradual onset of weakness, ascending paralysis, and sensory symptoms, whereas direct nerve damage may present with more rapid onset of weakness or other symptoms.
- Electrophysiological features and laboratory findings are distinct between the two conditions.
- Keep in mind that some cases may not fit neatly into one category or the other, and a thorough diagnostic evaluation is necessary to determine the underlying cause of AFP in adults.

## PATHOPHYSIOLOGICAL MECHANISMS

The pathophysiology of AFP is complex and involves multiple factors. A thorough understanding of these mechanisms is essential for developing effective treatment strategies for this condition.

- *Immune-mediated inflammation:* AFP is often associated with acute inflammation in the peripheral nervous system, which can be triggered by a variety of factors, including viral infections, autoimmune disorders, and environmental toxins.
- *Demyelination:* In some cases, AFP may be associated with demyelination of peripheral nerves, which can lead to the disruption of normal nerve conduction and the development of symptoms.
- *Neurotransmitter imbalance:* Infections can disrupt the normal balance of neurotransmitters in the brain and spinal cord, leading to changes in pain perception and muscle tone.
- *Neuroinflammation:* Infections can trigger an inflammatory response in the central nervous system (CNS), leading to damage to nerve fibers and axons.
- *Axonal degeneration:* Inflammation and damage to nerve fibers which can be mediated by immune-mediated inflammation, compression, or ischemia. can lead to axonal degeneration, resulting in muscle weakness and paralysis.
- *Disruption of neural circuits:* Infections can disrupt normal neural circuits in the brain and spinal cord, leading to changes in motor function and sensation.
- *Neuropraxia:* Neuropraxia is a type of nerve damage that occurs when the nerve is compressed or stretched, leading to the disruption of normal nerve function.
- *Ganglionitis:* Ganglionitis is a type of inflammation that occurs in the ganglia (nerve cell clusters) of peripheral nerves, which can lead to damage to the axons and the development of symptoms.
- *Microvasculitis:* Microvasculitis is a type of inflammation that occurs in the small blood vessels of the peripheral nervous system, which can lead to damage to the nerves and the development of symptoms.

## ALGORITHM SUMMARY

The algorithm for managing AFP in adults involves:

- Initial assessment to determine the patient's presentation and symptoms.
- Diagnostic considerations to determine the underlying cause of the patient's symptoms.

- Treatment with supportive care, immunotherapy (if indicated), and physical therapy.
- Follow-up and monitoring to assess the patient's progress and adjust treatment as necessary.
- By following this algorithm, healthcare providers can help manage AFP in adults effectively and improve patient outcomes.

### Initial Assessment and Diagnostics

The diagnosis of AFP in adults typically involves a combination of thorough history, clinical evaluation, laboratory tests, imaging studies and other ancillary tests.

### History

Perform a thorough medical history, of symptoms, including the onset, duration, and progression of the illness, and identify potential triggers, including:

- Recent travel or exposure to affected areas
- Recent respiratory or gastrointestinal symptoms
- History of immunosuppression or chronic medical conditions
- Trauma (e.g., spinal cord injury and nerve compression)
- Infections (e.g., meningitis, encephalitis, and sepsis)
- Neoplastic processes (e.g., spinal cord tumors, and metastases)
- Autoimmune disorders (e.g., lupus and rheumatoid arthritis)

### Clinical Features

The clinical features associated with AFP include sudden onset of weakness or paralysis in one or more limbs, but can also be bilateral or asymmetric, often accompanied by pain, numbness, or tingling.

Arrive at a diagnosis through thorough history taking, physical examination and appropriate laboratory tests.

Assess the patient's level of consciousness, muscle strength, reflexes, and sensory function.

*Onset:* AFP typically develops within hours to days after the onset of infection.

*Progressive weakness:* Muscle weakness or paralysis progresses over time, often affecting multiple limbs.

*Flaccid weakness:* The affected muscles are weak and flaccid, with no muscle spasticity or rigidity.

*Loss of reflexes:* Reflexes are often absent or diminished due to damage to the peripheral nervous system.

*Pain:* Many patients with AFP experience significant pain, which can be severe and debilitating.

*Physical Examination:* Perform a thorough neurological examination to assess:

1. *Muscle strength and tone:* Using the Medical Research Council (MRC) scale to assess muscle power (0-5).
2. *Reflexes:* Assess deep tendon reflexes, including the biceps, triceps, patellar, and Achilles reflexes.
3. *Sensation:* Assess sensory function, including pain, temperature, and light touch.
4. *Cranial nerves:* Assess cranial nerves I-XII for any signs of weakness or dysfunction.

## DIAGNOSIS AND CLASSIFICATION

Based on the initial evaluation, classify the patient as having:

- AFP without a clear cause
- AFP with suspected underlying etiology (e.g., myasthenia gravis, WNV infection, and Guillain-Barré syndrome)
- Perform additional testing as needed to confirm the diagnosis

## LABORATORY TESTING

The diagnosis of AFP in adults is based on a combination of clinical features, electrophysiological studies, and neuroimaging findings.

- Complete blood count (CBC) with differential to evaluate for any signs of infection or inflammation.
- Electrolyte panel to evaluate for any electrolyte imbalances that may be contributing to the patient's symptoms.
- Serum creatine phosphokinase (CPK) to evaluate for any signs of muscle damage or necrosis.
- Blood urea nitrogen (BUN) and creatinine
- Liver function tests (LFTs)
- Blood cultures
- Rapid strep test (if there is a history of streptococcal pharyngitis)
- Mononucleosis (Epstein-Barr virus) titer
- Lyme disease serology (if there is a history of tick exposure)
- West Nile virus (WNV) IgM and IgG antibodies (if there is a history of recent travel or exposure to mosquitoes)
- West Nile virus (WNV)(if suspected WNV infection)

- Cytomegalovirus (CMV) serology (if there is a history of immunosuppression or organ transplantation)
- Perform a lumbar puncture (if suspected central nervous system infection or meningitis)
- Consider ordering additional tests based on the patient's symptoms and clinical presentation.
- Acetylcholine receptor antibody (AChRAb) titers (if suspected myasthenia gravis)

## IMAGING STUDIES

Magnetic resonance imaging of the spine and brain to evaluate for compressive lesions or inflammatory lesions.

*Neuroimaging findings:* The neuroimaging findings associated with AFP include swelling or enhancement of affected nerves on MRI, as well as evidence of nerve damage or compression on computed tomography (CT) scans.

*Electrophysiological studies:* Perform EMG and NCSs to evaluate the severity of demyelination and axonal damage. The electrophysiological changes associated with AFP include prolonged latency and decreased amplitude of CMAPs, as well as reduced sensory nerve action potentials (SNAPs).

*Histopathological changes:* The histopathological changes associated with AFP include inflammation, axonal damage, and demyelination in affected nerves.

Based on the results of the laboratory tests and imaging studies, consider the following possible causes of AFP in adults:

### Infections

- Streptococcal pharyngitis
- Lyme disease
- West Nile virus
- Cytomegalovirus
- Herpes simplex virus
- *Autoimmune disorders:*
    - *Guillain-Barré Syndrome (GBS):* A post-infectious autoimmune disorder that can cause rapid onset of weakness and paralysis. A common cause of AFP in adults, characterized by rapid progression of weakness, sensory deficits, and autonomic dysfunction.
    - *Miller Fisher Syndrome (MFS):* A variant of GBS that is characterized by ataxia, areflexia, and ophthalmoplegia.
    - Chronic inflammatory demyelinating polyneuropathy
    - *Multiple sclerosis (MS):* A chronic autoimmune disease characterized by demyelination in the central nervous system
- *Porphyria:* A group of genetic disorders that can cause acute weakness and neuropathy.
- Neoplastic disorders:
    - Primary tumors of the brain or spinal cord
    - Metastatic cancer
- *Other causes:* Such as stroke, spinal cord injury (traumatic or non-traumatic), or polyneuropathy.

## CLASSIFICATION ACCORDING TO SITE OF INVOLVEMENT

### Myelopathies

- Compressive myelopathy
- Transverse myelitis, brainstem encephalitis
- Necrotizing myelopathy
- *Infection:* Poliomyelitis, enterovirus, and flavivirus

### Neuropathies

- *Primary:*
    - Guillain barre syndrome variants
    - Acute inflammatory demyelinating polyneuropathy
    - Acute motor axonal neuropathy
    - Acute motor and sensory axonal neuropathy
    - Miller fisher syndrome
- *Secondary:*
    - Diabetes, uremia, porphyria
    - Infection—Lyme disease, diphtheria, HIV, and hepatitis C
    - Drugs/toxins—alcohol, organophosphates, heavy metals
    - Autoimmune—vasculitic neuropathy with or without connective tissue disorder
    - Malignant paraneoplasia
    - Other—critical illness polyneuropathy

### Neuromuscular Junction Transmission Disorder

- Myasthenia graves
- Lambert Eaton myasthenic syndrome
- Botulism
- Venom:snake, sea urchin

### Myopathies

Acute inflammatory myopathies.

### Others

- Conversion disorder/factitious disorder
- Brainstem infarction (locked-in syndrome)

## TREATMENT AND MANAGEMENT

Based on the results of the evaluation, it provides appropriate treatment and management for the underlying cause of AFP.

Consider the following treatment options.

### Specific Treatment

Based on the underlying cause of AFP, provide targeted therapy:

- Antimicrobial agents for infections (e.g., antibiotics, antivirals)
- Anti-inflammatory agents—immunosuppressive therapy for patients with suspected immune-mediated inflammation.
- Radiation therapy or chemotherapy for neoplastic processes
- Corticosteroids for autoimmune disorders
- Consider the following therapies based on the underlying etiology:
- *Myasthenia gravis:* Cholinesterase inhibitors, immunosuppressive therapy, and plasmapheresis
- *WNV infection:* Supportive care, antiviral therapy (if indicated), and plasma exchange
- *Guillain-Barré syndrome:* Plasmapheresis, IVIG, and corticosteroids
- *Immunotherapy:* Consider immunotherapy for patients with suspected GBS or MFS:
    - *Immunomodulatory therapy:* Consider immunomodulatory therapy to reduce the immune response and promote recovery
    - *Intravenous immunoglobulin:* Administer IVIG at a dose of 2–4 g/kg of body weight per day for 3–5 days.
    - *Plasmapheresis:* Perform plasmapheresis sessions to remove pathogenic antibodies from the bloodstream that are contributing to the autoimmune response.
    - *Consider administering corticosteroids to reduce inflammation:* Methylprednisolone: Administer 1 g IV every 6 hours for 3–5 days.

### General Management

Provide supportive care, as needed including:

- Monitor vital signs and neurological function regularly
- Provide supportive care to maintain stability and promote recovery.
- Collaborate with specialists to develop a comprehensive rehabilitation plan.
- Close monitoring of respiratory function
- *Respiratory support:* Monitor vital signs and provide respiratory support Providing oxygen therapy and mechanical ventilation if necessary

*Treatment of underlying medical conditions:*

- Pain management with analgesics anti-inflammatory medications and muscle relaxants. Patients with AFP often require aggressive pain management strategies to manage their symptoms.
- *Nutritional support:* Ensuring adequate nutrition and hydration.
- *Physical therapy:* Physical therapy is important for maintaining muscle strength and function during the recovery period. It helps maintain muscle strength and prevent contractures and promote muscle recovery. It is Performed daily to prevent contractures.
- *Occupational therapy:* Assist with daily activities and provide strategies for adaptation. Collaborate with physical medicine and rehabilitation specialists to develop a comprehensive rehabilitation plan

## FOLLOW-UP EVALUATION

To assess the patient's response to treatment and to monitor for any signs of complications or worsening of symptoms and adjust treatment as necessary.

*Serial Neurological Examinations:* Perform serial neurological examinations to assess for any changes in muscle strength, sensation, or reflexes.

Consider ordering repeat laboratory tests and imaging studies as needed to monitor the patient's response to treatment.

*Imaging studies:* Repeat imaging studies as necessary to monitor the progression of demyelination and for any changes in the spinal cord or surrounding tissues.

### Complications Monitoring

Monitor for potential complications, including:

- *Respiratory failure:* Close monitoring of vital signs, oxygen saturation, and respiratory function; consider mechanical ventilation if necessary

- *Pneumonia:* Perform chest imaging studies and treat with antibiotics if necessary
- *Deep vein thrombosis (DVT) or pulmonary embolism (PE):* Perform Doppler ultrasound studies and treat with anticoagulation therapy if necessary
- *Autonomic dysfunction:* Monitor for signs of autonomic instability, such as changes in heart rate, blood pressure, or temperature; consider treatment with anticholinergics or beta blockers if necessary.

### Follow-up and Rehabilitation

Arrange for follow-up appointments with a neurologist or primary care physician to monitor the patient's progress and adjust therapy as needed

Provide rehabilitation services, including:

- Physical therapy to improve range of motion and strength, to improve motor function and prevent long-term disability.
- Occupational therapy to improve functional ability and daily living skills
- Speech therapy to improve communication skills.

## KEY TAKEAWAYS

Acute flaccid paresis in adults with demyelination is a neurological emergency that requires prompt diagnosis and management.

A comprehensive diagnostic approach includes clinical evaluation, lumbar puncture, MRI, electrophysiological studies, and blood tests.

Management involves supportive care, immunomodulatory therapy, corticosteroids, rehabilitation, and monitoring.

Differential diagnosis includes GBS, MS, spinal cord injury, and infectious diseases.

By following this approach, healthcare providers can effectively diagnose and manage AFP in adults with demyelination, reducing the risk of long-term disability and improving outcomes.

## SUGGESTED READING


1. Antoine JC, Mosnier JF, Absi L, Convers P, Honnorat J, Michel D. Carcinoma associated paraneoplastic peripheral neuropathies in patients with and without anti-onconeural antibodies. J Neurol Neurosurg Psychiatry. 1999;67:7-14.
2. D'Ercole M, Cipriani L, Picciotto D, Bianzina S, Russo E, Viazzi F, wt al. Hyperkalemia-induced acute flaccid paralysis: a case report. G Ital Nefrol. 2021;38(2):2021-vol2.
3. Hughes RA, Wijdicks EF, Barohn R, Benson E, Cornblath DR, Hahn AF, et al. Practice parameter: Immunotherapy for Guillain-Barré syndrome: Report of the Quality Standards Subcommittee of the American Academy of Neurology. Neurology. 2003;61:736-40.
4. Lim R, Sathasivam S, Larner AJ. An acute evolving flaccid quadriparesis in an elderly woman. PLoS Med. 2008; 5(8):e180.
5. Lim R, Sathasivam S, Larner AJ. An acute evolving flaccid quadriparesis in an elderly woman. PLoS Med. 2008;5(8): e180.
6. Van der Meche FGA, Van Doorn PA, Meulstee J, Jennekens FGI; GBS-consensus group of the Dutch Neuromuscular Research Support Centre. Diagnostic and classification criteria for the Guillain-Barré syndrome. Eur Neurol. 2001; 45:133-9.
7. Walter E. Case Reports in Neurocritical Care/Thematic Poster Session/Monday, May 22/09:00 AM-04:15 PM. Washington: Washington Convention Center, Area I, Hall C (Lower Level).

CHAPTER 47

# Acute Inflammatory Demyelinating Polyneuropathy

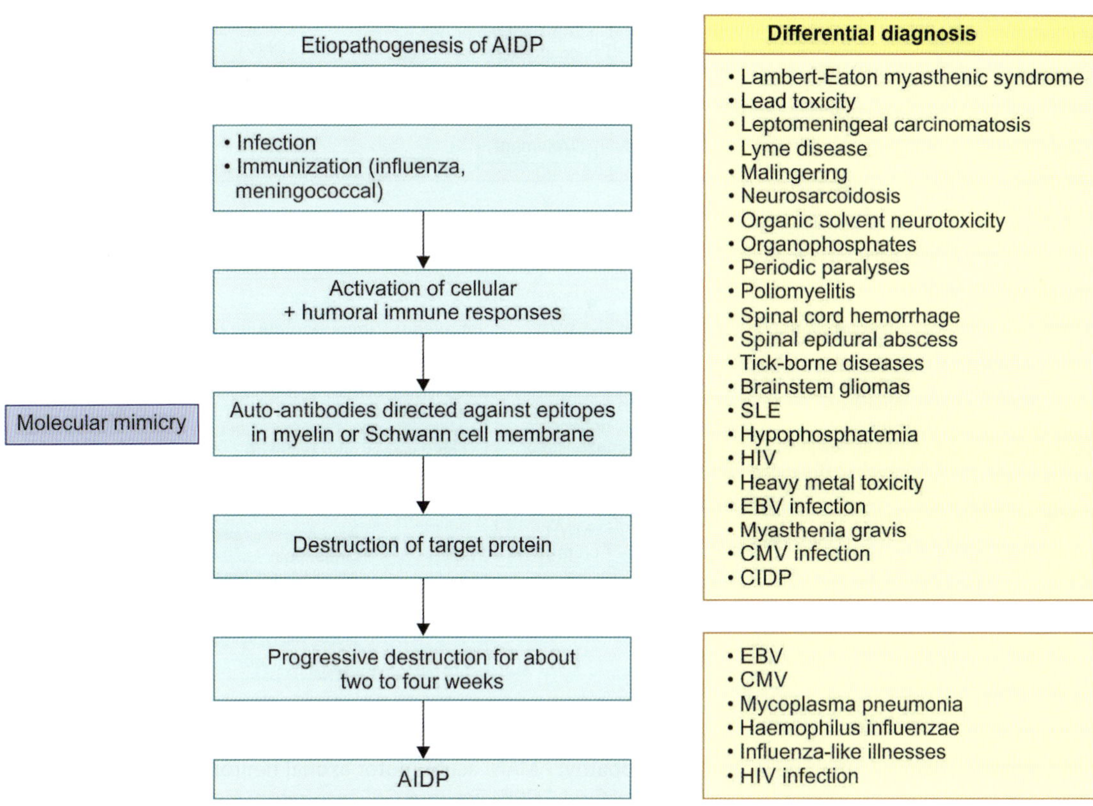

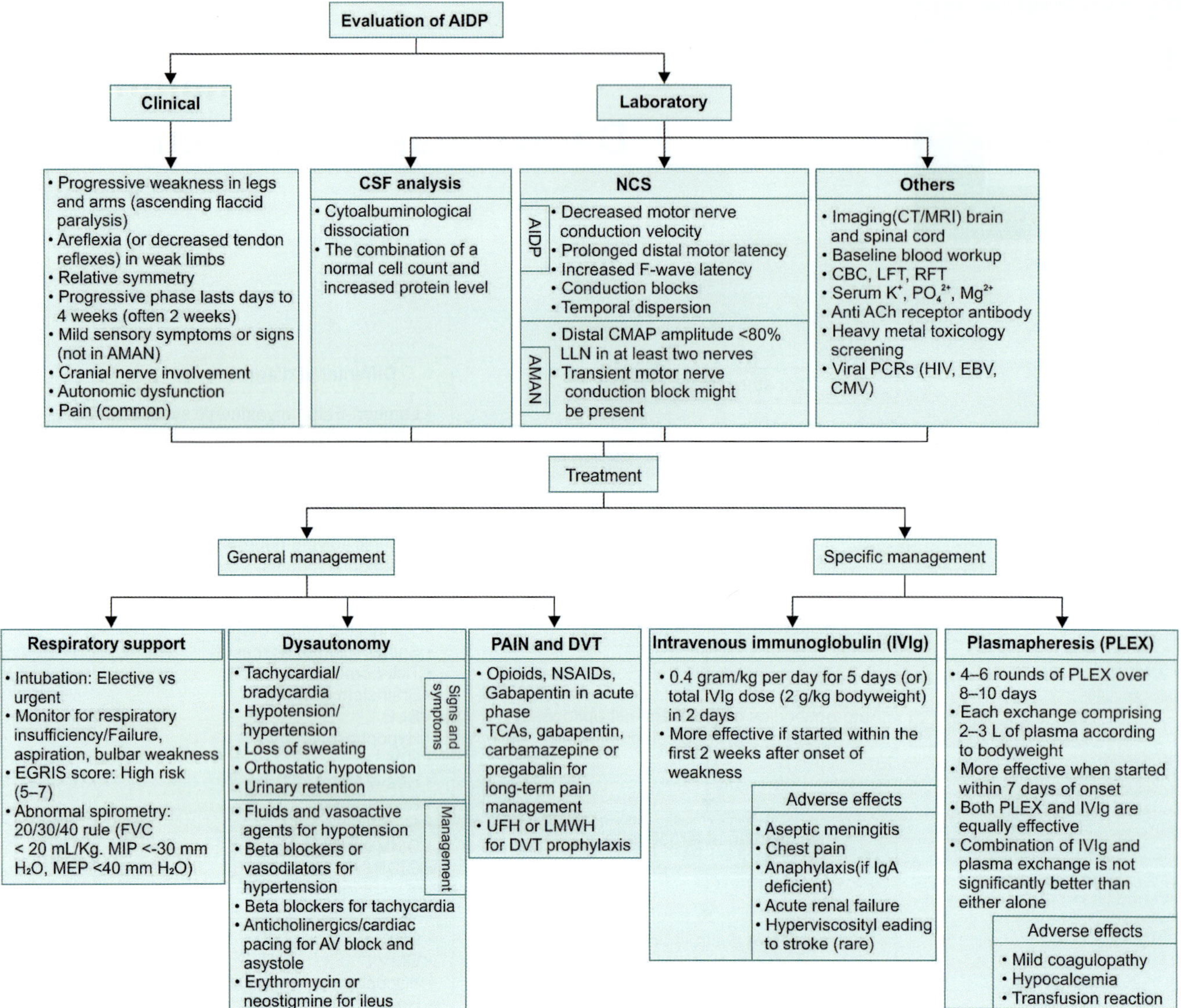


(AIDP: acute inflammatory demyelinating polyradiculoneuropathy; AMAN: acute motor axonal neuropathy; CMAP: compound muscle action potential; LLN: lower limit of normal; CSF: cerebrospinal fluid; EGRIS: Erasmus GBS respiratory insufficiency score; FVC: forced vital capacity; MIP: maximum inspiratory pressure; MEP: maximum expiratory pressure)

## SUGGESTED READING

1. Rao G. (2024). Critical Care in Guillain-Barré Syndrome. J Neuroanaesthesiol Crit Care. 2024;11:77-85.
2. Shang P, Feng J, Wu W, Zhang HL. Intensive Care and Treatment of Severe Guillain-Barré Syndrome. Front Pharmacol. 2021;12:608130.
3. Tan CY, Sekiguchi Y, Goh KJ, Kuwabara S, Shahrizaila N. A model to predict the probability of acute inflammatory demyelinating polyneuropathy. Clin Neurophysiol. 2020;131(1):63-9.

CHAPTER 48

# Myasthenia Gravis

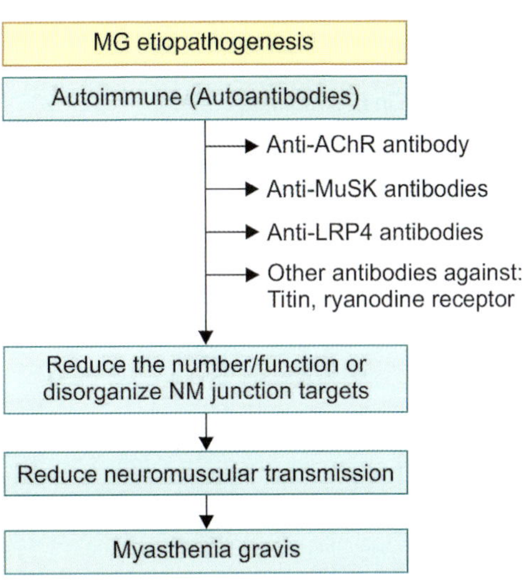


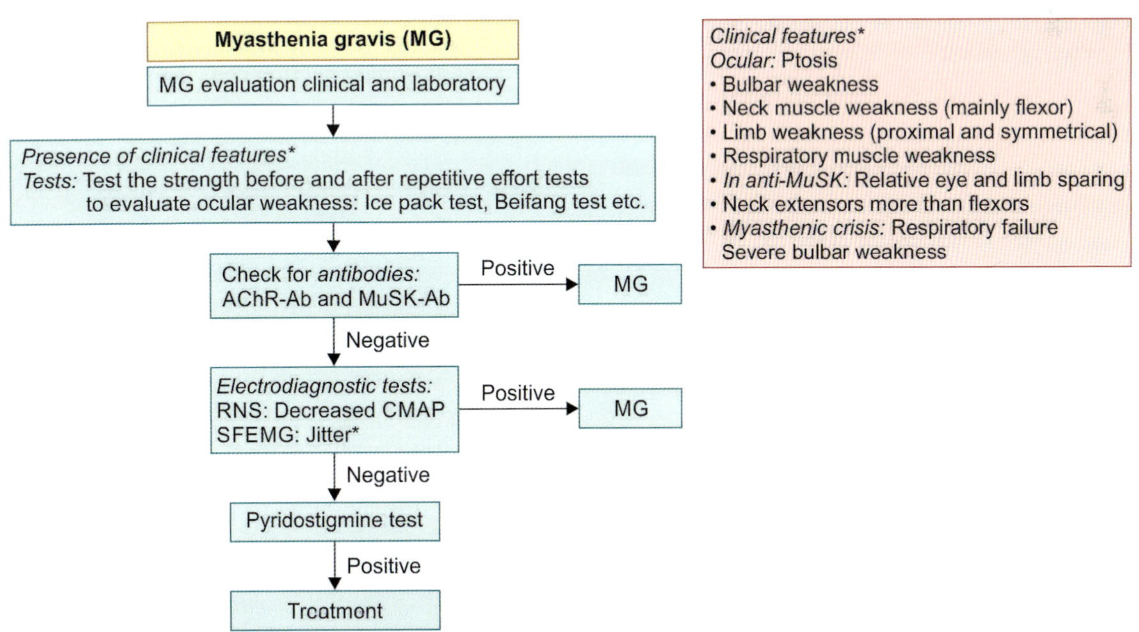

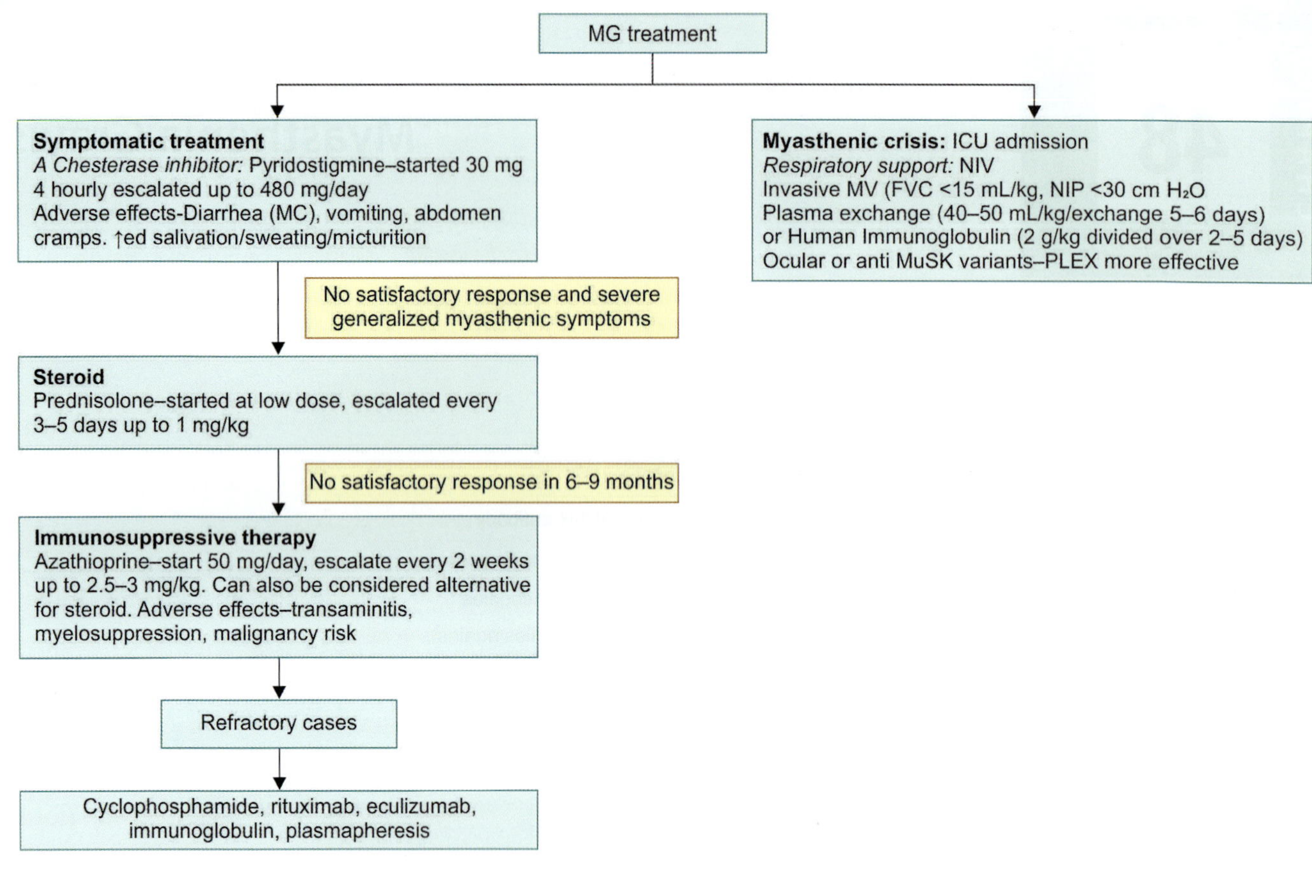


## SUGGESTED READING

1. Estephan EP, Baima JPS, Zambon AA. Myasthenia gravis in clinical practice. Arq Neuropsiquiatr. 2022;80(5 Suppl 1): 257-65.
2. Narayanaswami P, Sanders DB, Wolfe G, Benatar M, Cea G, Evoli A, et al. International Consensus Guidance for Management of Myasthenia Gravis: 2020 Update. Neurology. 2021;96(3):114-22.

CHAPTER 49

# Status Epilepticus and Super-refractory Status Epilepticus

## DEFINITIONS

*Status epilepticus (SE):* In 2015, the International League Against Epilepsy defined status epilepticus as "a condition resulting either from the failure of the mechanisms responsible for seizure termination or from the initiation of mechanisms which lead to abnormally prolonged seizures".[1] In this guideline two time points are mentioned in SE, as t1 and t2; t1 represents the duration beyond which seizures are likely to be prolonged, while t2 represents the time beyond which seizures can result in long-term consequences. For tonic-clonic seizures, t1 is set at 5 minutes, and t2 is set at 30 minutes. However, for focal SE or absence status, these specific time points either differ or remain unknown.

If a delay in SE treatment persists beyond five minutes, or if SE is undertreated, progression to refractory status epilepticus (RSE) and super-refractory status epilepticus (SRSE) may occur.[1] Therefore, SE is a critical condition that requires prompt treatment to minimize long-term consequences from continuous seizure activity.

*Refractory status epilepticus (RSE):* SE that persists despite treatment with benzodiazepine and at least two appropriately dosed parenteral antiepileptic drugs (AEDs).

*Super refractory status epilepticus (SRSE):* SE persisting at least 24 hours after the onset of continuous anesthetic medications (i.e., midazolam, propofol, pentobarbital, and ketamine) or during the weaning of these medications.[2] Delayed treatment of SRSE can lead to neuronal injury, irreversible damage to vulnerable regions in the hippocampus, thalamus, and neocortex, and in some cases, brain tissue hypoxia and increased intracranial pressure.[3]

The American Epilepsy Society has proposed an integrated treatment algorithm for the management of convulsive status epilepticus (CSE).[4] Immediate pharmacological management to terminate the seizure (both clinical and electro-graphical) and stabilization of the patient, along with diagnostic workup to search for the underlying cause, should start simultaneously.

## IMMEDIATE MANAGEMENT AND STABILIZATION

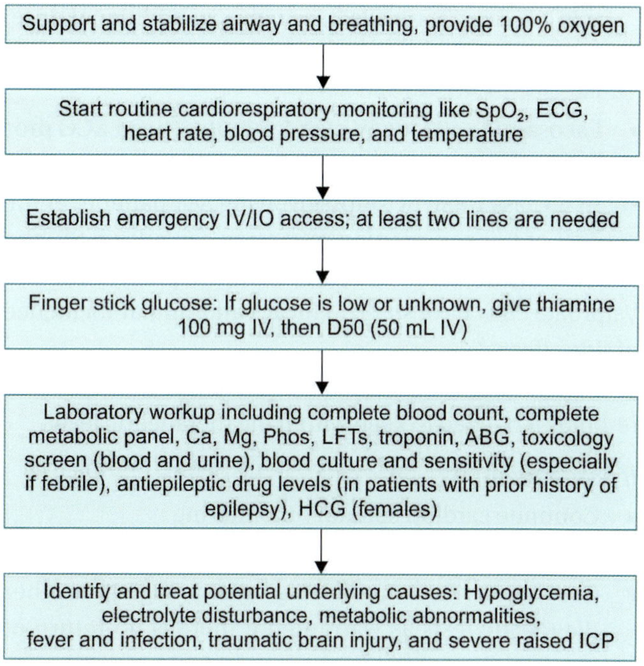

Support and stabilize airway and breathing, provide 100% oxygen

↓

Start routine cardiorespiratory monitoring like $SpO_2$, ECG, heart rate, blood pressure, and temperature

↓

Establish emergency IV/IO access; at least two lines are needed

↓

Finger stick glucose: If glucose is low or unknown, give thiamine 100 mg IV, then D50 (50 mL IV)

↓

Laboratory workup including complete blood count, complete metabolic panel, Ca, Mg, Phos, LFTs, troponin, ABG, toxicology screen (blood and urine), blood culture and sensitivity (especially if febrile), antiepileptic drug levels (in patients with prior history of epilepsy), HCG (females)

↓

Identify and treat potential underlying causes: Hypoglycemia, electrolyte disturbance, metabolic abnormalities, fever and infection, traumatic brain injury, and severe raised ICP

## ANTICONVULSANT THERAPY

Simultaneous with the above steps, give the first dose of benzodiazepine in the initial 5–10 minutes *(Seizure ongoing for 5 minutes or recurrent episodes of seizures without regaining consciousness in between: Diagnosed SE).*

## First Line

- Lorazepam 4 mg IV (push over 2 minutes)
- If seizure is not controlled within 5 minutes, repeat 4 mg IV × 1
- If no IV access: Diazepam 20 mg rectally (use IV solution if rectal form is unavailable)
- Midazolam 10 mg intranasal/buccal/IM (use IV solutions if a rectal form is unavailable).

*If seizure persists (10–30 minutes)*

## Second Line

Choose from the following (may be used in combination):

- Valproic acid 40 mg/kg IV (max rate 6 mg/kg/min)
- Levetiracetam 20 mg/kg IV (max rate 100 mg/min)
- Phenobarbital 20 mg/kg IV (max rate 50–75 mg/min)
- Fosphenytoin 20 mg PE/kg IV (max rate 150 mg PE/min) or Phenytoin 20 mg/kg IV (max rate 25–50 mg/min). If there is no effect, can give an additional dose: Fosphenytoin 10 mg PE/kg IV or Phenytoin 10 mg/kg IV
- Lacosamide 400 mg IV over 5 minutes (need ECG pre/post)

In a Class I ESETT study involving 384 patients in the context of benzodiazepine refractory convulsive SE, the anticonvulsant drugs Levetiracetam, Fosphenytoin, and Valproate each have similar efficacy and similar incidence of side effects.[5]

At this time, check anticonvulsant levels post-load and re-bolus if needed to keep within the therapeutic level.

*If seizure stops:*

- Continue cardiorespiratory monitoring
- Complete neurological assessment
- Continuous EEG monitoring, neuroimaging or other diagnostic tests as warranted if there is no return of responsiveness after 1–2 hours of seizure cessation.

*Seizure persists (30–60 minutes)*

*(The persistence of either clinical or electrographic seizures despite the administration of appropriate doses of an initial benzodiazepine and suitable second-line antiepileptic drugs (AEDs) irrespective of the time: Diagnosed RSE)*

## Third Line

Choose from the following (may be used in combination):

| Drugs | Dose | Side effects |
|---|---|---|
| Midazolam (most suitable when BP is unstable) | 0.2 mg/kg, followed by 0.05–2 mg/kg/h | Respiratory depression, hypotension |
| Propofol | 1–2 mg/kg, followed by 30–200 µg/kg/min | Propofol infusion syndrome, peripheral accumulation, respiratory depression, hypotension, pancreatitis |
| Barbiturates (thiopental/pentobarbital) | 2–7 mg/kg (thiopental) or 5–15 mg/kg (pentobarbital) followed by 0.5–5 mg/kg/h | Respiratory depression, hypotension, ileus, cardiac depression, and immune suppression |

There are currently no randomized controlled trials to provide guidance on the selection of anesthetic drugs for the treatment of RSE. As such, which anesthetic third-line treatment for RSE offers superior outcomes, minimizes adverse effects, and is most effective in halting seizures in the ICU currently remains unclear.[6]

## ENDPOINT AND DURATION OF ANESTHETIC INFUSION

- Continuous EEG monitoring is mandatory
- Titrate infusions to stop seizures or induce burst suppression (currently, no evidence to guide the best depth/duration of suppression).
- There are no data to support the superiority of electrographic seizure control or burst suppression. However, treatment for EEG suppression was associated with lower occurrence of breakthrough seizures.[7]
- Once seizure-free for >24–48 hours, start slow taper of 3rd line medications over 24 hours while maintaining high therapeutic levels of AEDs to avoid recurrent seizures.
- Continue EEG monitoring is recommended until seizure-free and the patient is off third-line medications for >24 hours to monitor for recurrence of nonconvulsive seizures or NCSE.

## ADDITIONAL INTENSIVE CARE MANAGEMENT OF RSE

- At this point, intubate the patient for airway protection
- Treat respiratory failure, neurocardiogenic pulmonary edema, and infection
- Avoid prolonged neuromuscular blocking agent infusion
- Use IV fluids and pressors appropriately to support BP (anesthetic doses required to treat refractory SE are much higher than doses used for routine sedation).
- Prolonged seizures can lead to complications such as rhabdomyolysis, hyperkalemia, hyperphosphatemia, hypocalcemia, and precipitate acute kidney injury: have a high index of suspicion.
- Monitor side effects of different anesthetic drugs with specific laboratory parameters such as creatinine kinase, acid/base balance, serum lactate, and lipid profile
- Continue the workup to determine the underlying cause of SE. Neuroimaging - brain MRI (preferred) or head CT. Lumbar puncture - evaluate for infection, inflammatory, and autoimmune causes.

### Promising Treatment for RSE

| *Promising drug* | *Mechanism of action* | *Dose* |
|---|---|---|
| Ketamine | • Non-competitive NMDA receptor antagonist<br>• Reduction in glutaminergic neuronal transmission and excitotoxicity<br>• Neuroprotective | 0.5–3 mg/kg followed by 0.1–5 mg/kg/h |
| Volatile anesthetic | • Inhibition of seizure activity via inhibition of NMDA. Excitotoxicity and activation of GABA receptors<br>• Ultra short-acting | • Not established/end-tidal concentrations<br>• 0.8–2% titrated to EEG |
| Perampanel | AMPA receptor antagonist | • Variable loading dose<br>• Maintenance: 2–12 mg/day |
| Topiramate | • Block voltage-gated sodium channels, increase GABA activity, antagonize AMPA glutamate receptors, weak carbonic anhydrase inhibitor | • Variable loading dose<br>• Maintenance: 300–1,600 mg/d in divided doses |
| Clobazam | GABA A agonist | • 20 mg/d in two divided doses (range 10–60 mg/day) |

## MANAGEMENT STRATEGIES FOR SPECIAL SUBGROUPS OF RSE

### Nonconvulsive Status Epilepticus (NCSE)

| *Diagnostic criteria* | *Management* | *Evidence* |
|---|---|---|
| *The Salzburg consensus criteria*[8]<br>EEG evidence of rhythmic epileptiform discharges at a frequency >2.5 Hz,<br>Or<br>Rhythmic EEG discharges at a frequency ≤2.5 Hz accompanied by spatiotemporal evolution<br>Plus<br>Subtle clinical changes correlating with EEG alterations,<br>Or<br>EEG and clinical improvement after intravenous AED therapy | • Currently, there is little high-quality evidence to guide the best management practices or advice on how aggressively to pursue treatment<br>• Treat as convulsive RSE as described before<br>• Newer AEDs, including levetiracetam and lacosamide, are safe and effective in the treatment of NCSE<br>• Explore trial of non-sedative intravenous second-line AEDs before resorting to anesthetic induction in NCSE, e.g., IV lacosamide | • A Study showed a 30-minute delay in therapy initiation in NCSE was linked to elevated morbidity and mortality[9]<br>• A Prospective study showed early initiation of treatment leads to good control of NCSE[10] |

*Contd...*

*Contd...*

| ***Diagnostic criteria*** | ***Management*** | ***Evidence*** |
|---|---|---|
| Plus<br>Continuous presence of EEG changes indicative of NCSE for a minimum duration of 10 minutes or 20% of any 60-minute EEG recording | • IV Mega dose phenobarbitone could be a viable and advantageous treatment choice for refractory NCSE. (PB dose >10 mg/kg/day)<br>• The prognosis depends heavily on the etiology; therefore, when contemplating the use of anesthetic drugs for third-line therapy in refractory NCSE, it is imperative to assess risk versus benefits | |

*New onset refractory status epilepticus (NORSE) and Febrile infection-related epilepsy syndrome (FIRSE):*

| ***Definition*** | ***Management*** | ***Evidence*** |
|---|---|---|
| • NORSE is characterized by the sudden onset of uncontrollable seizures, referred to as RSE, without any identifiable acute or active structural, toxic, or metabolic cause in a patient without epilepsy or other neurological disorder known to precipitate seizure[11]<br>• FIRES is regarded as a subset of NORSE and is characterized by the presence of a preceding febrile infection occurring between 2 weeks and 24 hours before the onset of RSE with or without fever at the onset of SE[12] | • Should be managed in a tertiary neurological center with multidisciplinary involvement<br>• Initial treatment of SE and RSE starts with benzodiazepine, AEDs, and anesthetic drugs in the initial 48 hours in a stepwise approach<br>• Acute diagnostic workup during initial 48-72 hours<br>– MRI brain with contrast<br>– *Serum and CSF:* Infection and rheumatological panel, autoimmune and paraneoplastic antibodies, CSF cytokines, or inborn errors of metabolism panel<br>– Malignant screening of chest, abdomen, pelvis, ovaries, and testicles and whole-body PET scan<br>– Genetic testing<br>• Initiate first-line immune therapies:<br>– IV Methylprednisolone: 20–30 mg/kg/day (max 1 g/day) for 3–5 days<br>or<br>– IV immunoglobulin: 2 g/kg in divided doses over 2–5 days<br>or<br>– Therapeutic plasma exchange within the first 72 hours of onset<br>• Initiate ketogenic diet<br>• Initiate second-line immune therapies within one week after ruling out infectious etiology or if there is an insufficient response to first-line immune treatment.<br>– If antibody-mediated or strong suspicion (Autoimmune encephalitis), IV Rituximab<br>– If cryptogenic,<br>*IL-1R antagonist:* IV Anakinra or<br>*IL-6 antagonists:* IV Tocilizumab | In 2022, the International NORSE Consensus Group presented recommendations for managing NORSE, including FIRES[13] |

## SUPER REFRACTORY STATUS EPILEPTICUS (SRSE)

SE persisting at least 24 hours after the onset of continuous anesthetic medications (i.e., midazolam, propofol, pentobarbital, and ketamine) or during the weaning of these medications

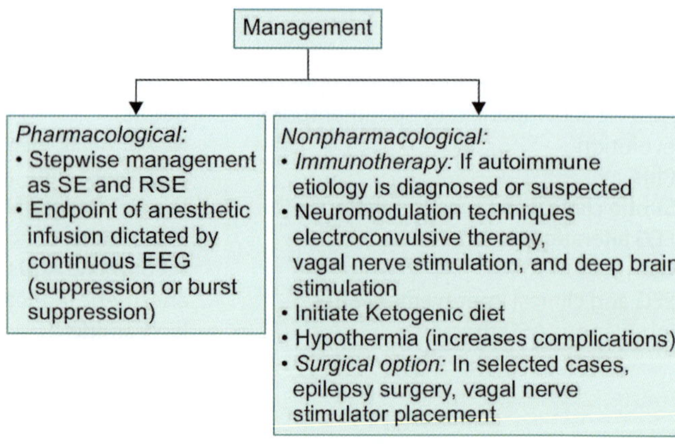

## REFERENCES


1. Trinka E, Cock H, Hesdorffer D, Rossetti AO, Scheffer IE, Shinnar S, et al. A definition and classification of status epilepticus: Report of the ILAE Task Force on Classification of Status Epilepticus. Epilepsia. 2015;56:1515-23.
2. Brophy GM, Bell R, Claassen J, Alldredge B, Bleck TP, Glauser T, et al. Guidelines for the Evaluation and Management of Status Epilepticus. Neurocrit Care. 2012;17:3-23.
3. Vespa PM, Miller C, McArthur D, Eliseo M, Etchepare M, Hirt D, et al. Nonconvulsive electrographic seizures after traumatic brain injury result in a delayed, prolonged increase in intracranial pressure and metabolic crisis. Crit Care Med. 2007;35:2830-36.
4. Glauser T, Shinnar S, Gloss D, Alldredge B, Arya R, Bainbridge J, et al. Evidence-based guideline: treatment of convulsive status epilepticus in children and adults: report of the Guideline Committee of the American Epilepsy Society. Epilepsy Curr. 2016;16:48-61.
5. Kapur J, Elm J, Chamberlain JM, Barsan W, Cloyd J, Lowenstein D, et al. Randomized trial of three anticonvulsant medications for status epilepticus. N Engl J Med. 2019;381:2103-13.
6. Minicucci F, Ferlisi M, Brigo F, Mecarelli O, Meletti S, Aguglia U, et al. Management of status epilepticus in adults: position paper of the Italian League against Epilepsy. Epilepsy Behav. 2020;102:106675.
7. Claassen J, Hirsch L, Emerson RG, Mayer SA. Treatment of Refractory Status Epilepticus with Pentobarbital, Propofol, or Midazolam: A Systematic Review. Epilepsia. 2002;43:146-53.
8. Trinka E, Leitinger M. Which EEG patterns in coma are nonconvulsive status epilepticus? Epilepsy Behav. 2015;49:203-22.
9. Cheng JY. Latency to treatment of status epilepticus is associated with mortality and functional status. J Neurol Sci. 2016;370:290-5.
10. Gutiérrez-Viedma Á, Parejo-Carbonell B, Cuadrado ML, Serrano-García I, Abarrategui B, et al. The relevance of timing in nonconvulsive status epilepticus: a series of 38 cases. Epilepsy Behav. 2018;82:11-6.
11. Hirsch LJ, Gaspard N, van Baalen A, Nabbout R, Demeret S, Loddenkemper T, et al. Proposed consensus definitions for new-onset refractory status epilepticus (NORSE), febrile infection-related epilepsy syndrome (FIRES), and related conditions. Epilepsia. 2018;59:739-44.
12. Gaspard N, Hirsch LJ, Sculier C, Loddenkemper T, van Baale A, Lancrenon J, et al. New-onset refractory status epilepticus (NORSE) and febrile infection-related epilepsy syndrome (FIRES): State of the art and perspectives. Epilepsia. 2018;59:745-52.
13. Wickstrom R, Taraschenko O, Dilena R, Payne ET, Specchio N, Nabbout R, et al. International consensus recommendations for the management of New Onset Refractory Status Epilepticus (NORSE) incl. Febrile Infection-Related Epilepsy Syndrome (FIRES): statements and supporting evidence. Epilepsia. 2022;63:2840-64.

# CHAPTER 50 Delirium in Intensive Care Unit

## INTRODUCTION AND DEFINITION

Delirium is a syndrome of acute onset characterized by a change in mental state with confusion, inattention, disorganized thinking and an altered level of consciousness.

It is a nonspecific but generally reversible manifestation of an acute illness.[1]

According to the Diagnostic and Statistical Manual of Mental Disorders DSM -5, delirium is defined as inattention (reduced ability to focus, sustain or shift attention) that develops over a short period with the additional feature of disturbance in cognition.[2]

It is an independent predictor of mortality, prolonged ICU and hospital stay, increased cost of care and long-term cognitive impairment.[3]

Delirium commonly occurs in elderly patients who are critically ill, but the incidence in mechanically ventilated patients in ICU remains as high as 80%.[4]

## PATHOPHYSIOLOGY

- Pathophysiology of delirium is poorly understood.
- There is an increased risk of delirium with the use of GABA agonists and anticholinergics.
- Recent theories show the role of imbalance in neurotransmitters like GABA, acetylcholine and dopamine in the development of delirium.

## TYPES OF DELIRIUM

There are three subtypes of delirium according to the psychomotor behavior of the patients.[5,6]

| *Types of delirium* | *symptoms manifested* |
|---|---|
| 1. Hypoactive delirium (24.5–43.5%) | Decreased responsiveness, lethargic, withdrawn attitude, drowsiness, apathy, confusion, slowed motor function |
| 2. Hyperactive delirium (1.6–23%) | Agitation, restlessness, emotional lability, paranoid |
| 3. Mixed delirium (52.5%). Most common type | Fluctuation of features of both types |

- Hypoactive delirium has the worst prognosis among all types.[7]
- Hypoactive delirium is often diagnosed late and not given immediate attention as the patients remain calm despite having delirium.

## ASSESSMENT OF DELIRIUM

- Early diagnosis or assessment is imperative to prevent long-term complications.
- Routine assessments will increase the rate of early detection of delirium, and risk factors can be minimized.
- Routine assessments are recommended at least once per shift per the pain, agitation, and delirium guidelines.[8]

The confusion assessment method (CAM-ICU) is the most used screening tool for assessment of delirium in clinical settings

### CAM-ICU Delirium Assessment

Involves two step assessment:[9]

1. *Step one:* Evaluate the level of consciousness/arousal by using Richmond Agitation sedation scale (RASS) **(Table 1)**.
2. *Step two:* Assess patients (moderately sedated, RASS score –3 or more alert) for four characteristics of delirium, i.e., acute onset of altered mental status, inattention and altered level of consciousness or disorganized thinking. Three out of four features diagnose delirium **(Fig. 1)**.

## ETIOLOGY OF DELIRIUM

The potential causes broadly include:

- Infectious (sepsis, pneumonia, meningitis/encephalitis, urinary tract infection)
- Alcohol/substance intoxication or withdrawal
- Medications side effects
- Trauma
- Neurologic disorder (dementia, Parkinson's disease, cerebrovascular accident, traumatic brain injury and nerve degenerative disease)
- Toxins and heavy metal ingestion
- Endocrinopathies (hypo/hyperparathyroidism, hypo/hyperthyroidism)
- Seizures
- Acute vascular (stroke, hemorrhage)
- Vitamin deficiencies (Wernicke's encephalopathy, vitamin $B_{12}$ deficiency)
- Metabolic and electrolyte disturbances (hyponatremia, hypocalcemia, hypo/hyperglycemia)
- Hypoxia
- Autoimmune (CNS vasculitis, neuropsychiatric lupus)
- Neoplastic (primary tumor, paraneoplastic syndrome)

**TABLE 1:** Richmond agitation sedation scale (RASS).

| | |
|---|---|
| +4 | Overtly combative, violent, immediate danger to staff |
| +3 | Pulls or removes tubes or catheters; aggressive |
| +2 | Frequent nonpurposeful movement, fights ventilator |
| +1 | Anxious, apprehensive but not aggressive |
| 0 | Alert and calm |
| –1 | Drowsy, awakens to voice (eye opening/eye contact) >10 sec |
| –2 | Light sedation, briefly awakens to voice (eye opening/eye contact) <10 sec |
| –3 | Moderate sedation, movement or eye opening to voice. But no eye contact |
| –4 | Deep sedation, no response to voice, but movement or eye opening to physical stimulation |
| –5 | Unarousable, no response to voice or physical stimulation |

## RISK FACTORS FOR DELIRIUM

- Predisposing and precipitating risk factors
- Important to identify the precipitating risk factors so that they can be minimized or avoided.[10]

*Predisposing factors:*

- Advanced age
- Male gender
- Pre-existing cognitive dysfunction

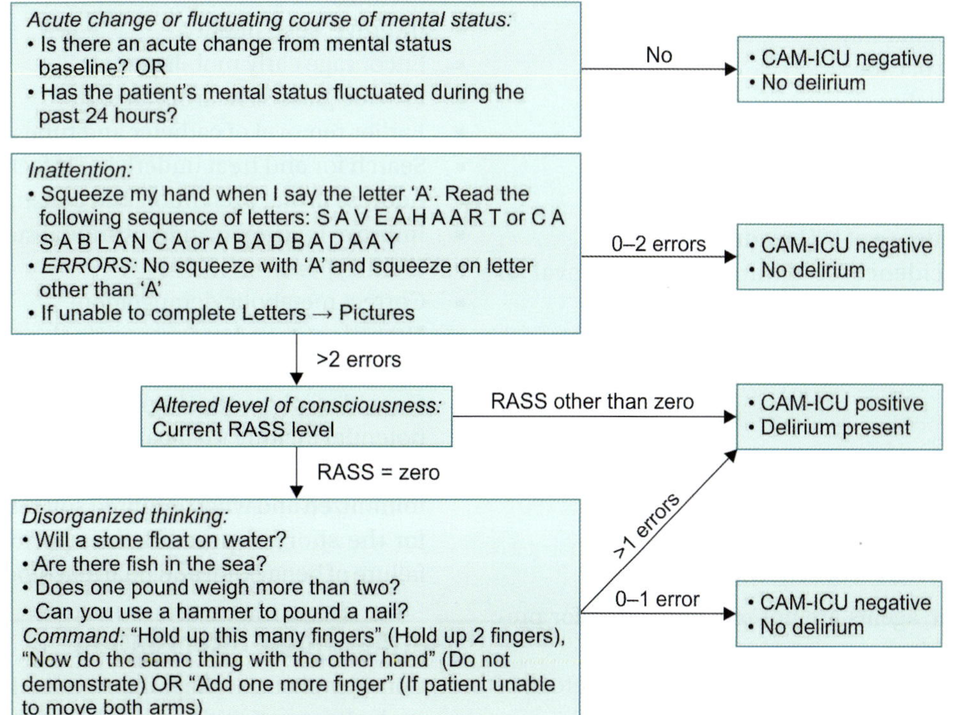


**Fig. 1:** Confusion assessment method for the Intensive Care Unit (CAM-ICU) for the diagnosis of delirium.

- Frailty
- Multiple comorbid condition
- Coexisting medical disease (uremia, lung disease, cardiac, and hepatic disease)
- Surgery (orthopedic and cardiac)
- Trauma

*Precipitating factors:*

- *Nonpharmacologic:*
  - Poor pain control
  - Hypoxia
  - Infection
  - Metabolic disturbances
  - Prolonged mechanical ventilation
  - Immobility (physical restraints, catheters)
  - Chronic sleep disturbances
  - Urinary retention or fecal impaction
  - Reduced sensory inputs (blindness, deafness)
- *Pharmacologic factors:*
  - Deep sedation
  - Benzodiazepines
  - Opioids
  - Anticholinergics
  - Corticosteroids
  - Antipsychotics
  - Anticonvulsants

*Complications of delirium:*[11]

- Prolonged hospital stay
- Increased cost of care
- Increased mortality
- Risk of long-term cognitive impairment
- Prolonged ICU stays
- Longer duration of mechanical ventilation
- Increased incidence of ICU readmission
- Increased incidence of unintentional removal of catheter and tubes

## MANAGEMENT OF DELIRIUM

*It includes:*

- Prevention
- Nonpharmacologic intervention
- Pharmacologic intervention

## PREVENTION OF DELIRIUM

- Pharmacologic agents are not recommended for prevention of delirium.
- Avoid or minimize the precipitating risk factors of delirium
- Consider analgesia first before sedation.
- Maintain minimal to moderate sedation as it allows earlier mobilization and also allows earlier detection of delirium.[12]
- Dexmedetomidine is recommended over benzodiazepines (midazolam) in mechanically ventilated patients as it decreases duration and incidence of delirium.[13,14]
- Follow ABCDEF bundle checklist.[8]

### ABCDEF Bundle Checklist

- *A:* Assess and manage pain
- *B:* Both spontaneous awakening trial (SAT) and spontaneous breathing trial (SBT)
- *C:* Choice of sedation and analgesia
- *D:* Delirium assessment and management
- *E:* Early mobilization and exercise
- *F:* Family engagement and empowerment

### Nonpharmacologic Intervention

- Cognitive behavior therapy (frequent patient orientation and occupational therapy)
- Show some familiar objects to the patient.
- Encourage communication with family members.
- Environmental intervention (noise reduction, exposure to natural bright light, darkened lighting in the evening.
- Improve sleep quality
- Encourage early mobilization
- Provide glasses, hearing aids
- Earlier removal of catheter and tubes
- Search for and treat underlying infection
- Address urinary retention and constipation problem
- Improve hydration and nutritional status
- Treat hypoxia
- Correct metabolic derangement
- Neurologic and neurosurgical causes should be treated.
- Consider pharmacologic etiologies and eliminate potential inciting medications.
- Restraints-use of physical restraints should be minimized and when required soft restraints to be used for the shortest possible time period and only after failure of behavioral and pharmacologic intervention.[15]

### Pharmacologic Intervention

- Consider pharmacologic intervention if delirium persists even after treating the possible causes or if treating the underlying etiology is not feasible.

- According to pain, agitation and delirium guidelines, not a single drug is effective in all type of delirium.
- Atypical antipsychotic (olanzapine, risperidone, quetiapine) may reduce the duration of delirium.[16]
- Haloperidol is used for treating agitation in the dose of 2–5 mg intravenously
- Caution should be taken while using atypical antipsychotic and haloperidol in patients with QT prolongation or used with other QT interval prolonging medications.
- The patients treated with antipsychotics should have a baseline and daily electrocardiogram.
- Short acting benzodiazepine (midazolam) is useful in patients with alcohol withdrawal.
- Dexmedetomidine is the drug of choice in patients with delirium requiring continuous intravenous infusion of a sedative agent.
- Nonbenzodiazepines (propofol, dexmedetomidine) should be preferred over benzodiazepine (midazolam) as sedative agent for better clinical outcomes in mechanically ventilated patients like reduced duration and incidence of delirium, shortened mechanical ventilation duration, reduced hospital and ICU stay.

## CONCLUSION

Delirium is a very frequent yet serious event in clinical settings. It is associated with higher mortality rate, increased cost of care and a risk of permanent cognitive dysfunction. Delirium is a clinical diagnosis and require a multidisciplinary approach to identify the cause. Perform daily CAM-ICU assessment and follow delirium protocol. identify and minimize the precipitating risk factors. Consider minimal to moderate sedation and use nonbenzodiazepines as sedative agent if possible. Consider analgesia first before starting sedation.

## REFERENCES


1. Reade MC, Finfer S. Sedation and delirium in the intensive care unit. N Engl J Med. 2014;370:444-54.
2. American psychiatric association. Diagnostic and statistical manual of mental disorders: DSM-5. USA: American psychiatric association; 2013.
3. Stollings JL, Kotfis K, Chanques G, Pun BT, Pandharipande PP, Ely EW. Delirium in critical illness: clinical manifestations, outcomes, and management. Intensive Care Med. 2021;47: 1089-103.
4. Ely EW, Inouye SK, Bernard GR, Gordon S, Francis J, May L, et al. Delirium in mechanically ventilated patients: validity and reliability of the confusion assessment method for the intensive care unit (CAM-ICU). JAMA. 2001;286: 2703-10.
5. Cascella M, Fiore M, Leone S, Carbone D, Di Napoli R. Current controversies and future perspectives on treatment of intensive care unit delirium in adults. World J Crit Care Med. 2019;8:18-27.
6. Collet MO, Caballero J, Sonneville R, Bozza FA, Nydahl P, Schandl A, et al; AID-ICU cohort study co-authors. Prevalence and risk factors related to haloperidol use for delirium in adult intensive care patients: the multinational AID-ICU inception cohort study. Intensive Care Med. 2018;44:1081-9.
7. Robinson TN, Raeburn CD, Tran ZV, Brenner LA, Moss M. Motor subtypes of postoperative delirium in older adults. Arch Surg. 2011;146:295-300.
8. Barr J, Fraser GL, Puntillo K, Ely EW, Gélinas C, Dasta JF, et al; American College of Critical Care Medicine. Clinical practice guidelines for the management of pain, agitation, and delirium in adult patients in the intensive care unit. Crit Care Med. 2013;41:263-306.
9. Gusmao-Flores D, Salluh JI, Chalhub RA, Quarantini LC. The confusion assessment method for the intensive care unit (CAM-ICU) and intensive care delirium screening checklist (ICDSC) for the diagnosis of delirium: a systematic review and meta-analysis of clinical studies. Crit Care. 2012;16:R115.
10. Hayhurst CJ, Pandharipande PP, Hughes CG. Intensive Care Unit Delirium: A Review of Diagnosis, Prevention, and Treatment. Anesthesiology. 2016;125:1229-41.
11. Goldberg TE, Chen C, Wang Y, Jung E, Swanson A, Ing C, et al. Association of Delirium With Long-term Cognitive Decline: A Meta-analysis. JAMA Neurol. 2020;77:1373-81.
12. Hughes CG, McGrane S, Pandharipande PP. Sedation in the intensive care setting. Clin Pharmacol. 2012;4:53-63.
13. Fraser GL, Devlin JW, Worby CP, Alhazzani W, Barr J, Dasta JF, et al. Benzodiazepine versus nonbenzodiazepine-based sedation for mechanically ventilated, critically ill adults: a systematic review and meta-analysis of randomized trials. Crit Care Med. 2013;41(9 Suppl 1):S30-8.
14. Riker RR, Shehabi Y, Bokesch PM, Ceraso D, Wisemandle W, Koura F, et al; SEDCOM (Safety and Efficacy of Dexmedetomidine Compared With Midazolam) Study Group. Dexmedetomidine vs midazolam for sedation of critically ill patients: a randomized trial. JAMA. 2009;301:489-99.
15. Mitchell DA, Panchisin T, Seckel MA. Reducing Use of Restraints in Intensive Care Units: A Quality Improvement Project. Crit Care Nurse. 2018;38:e8-e16.
16. Sadlonova M, Duque L, Smith D, Madva EN, Amonoo HL, Vogelsang J, et al. Pharmacologic treatment of delirium symptoms: A systematic review. Gen Hosp Psychiatry. 2022;79:60-75.

CHAPTER 51

# Community-acquired Meningitis

## INTRODUCTION

Community acquired meningitis is caused by infection of the meninges and subarachnoid space. Infection can be viral, bacterial, fungi, or protozoal **(Table 1)**. It can be associated with encephalitis, an infection of the brain parenchyma. Acute meningitis is considered a medical emergency, and if treatment is not instituted, the disease is fatal. The initial approach begins with a strong clinical suspicion and proper investigation **(Flowchart 1)**. The classical triad of fever, neck stiffness, and altered mental status are not present in all cases. Therefore, a thorough neurological and systemic examination should be done to rule out the associated complications **(Table 2 and 3)**. First, a blood culture should be sent in all cases before the institution of antibiotics, followed by other investigations **(Table 4)**. Proper choice of intravenous antimicrobial therapy with a prior dose of dexamethasone and antiviral should be administered immediately. Viral meningitis is more common, but bacterial meningitis is more serious.

## CSF FLUID EXAMINATION—SALIENT POINTS OF IMPORTANCE (TABLE 5)

- Confirms the diagnosis of bacterial meningitis, but treatment should not be delayed for this purpose.
- CSF examination after empirical antibiotics does not necessarily decrease the diagnostic sensitivity. Therefore, empirical antibiotics should not be delayed for lumbar puncture
- Forgo Lumbar puncture in the following conditions: Altered mental status/GCS, Immunocompromised patient, known CNS disease, New-onset CNS disease, New-onset seizure, Papilledema, focal neurological deficit

**TABLE 1:** Etiology of community-acquired meningitis.

| *Types* | *Etiology* | *Prevalence* |
|---|---|---|
| Acute bacterial meningitis | *Streptococcus pneumoniae* | Most common |
| | *Neisseria meningitidis* | Most common in 11–17-year age group |
| | Group B *Streptococcus* | In Infants <2 months of age |
| | *Haemophilus influenzae* type B | Was the most common cause before the vaccination program |
| | *Listeria monocytogenes* | Elderly, immunocompromised, Patients with chronic illnesses such as alcoholic, diabetic, or with malignancy |
| Acute viral meningitis | • Cytomegalovirus<br>• Others—Enterovirus, Herpes Simplex Virus (HSV) type 2, Varicella Zoster virus, West Nile virus<br>• HSV type1—encephalitis is more common<br>• Others—HIV, mumps | Immunocompromised Host (e.g., HIV or organ transplant patients) |
| Acute fungal meningitis | Cryptococcal | Immunocompromised Host |
| Tubercular meningitis | Mycobacterial | Immunocompromised Host |

In these cases, a CT Scan should be done.

- DVT prophylaxis is to be withheld accordingly.
- Gram Stain is positive in 50–60 % of cases

## CT Findings in Meningitis

- Noncontrast CT *usually normal.*
- Contrast CT scan—occasionally leptomeningeal enhancement, sulcal and cisternal effacement
- *Other findings:* Otitis media, sinusitis, mastoiditis, abscess formation, subarachnoid hemorrhage, and hydrocephalus
- CTA/CTV (arteriography/venography): If there is a focal neurological deficit in a comatose patient.

**Flowchart 1:** Initial approach.

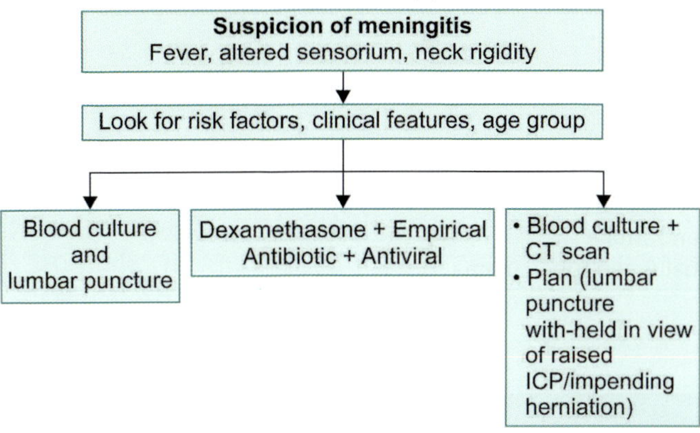


## MRI Findings in Meningitis

- 50% contrast-enhanced MRIs may be *normal.*
- MRI—not be waited to establish a diagnosis, may be helpful in some situations—comatose patient with a high index of suspicion
- T1 Sequence—purulent exudates in superficial sulci and basal cistern may be isointense with brain parenchyma
- FLAIR hyperintensity—CSF a "dirty" appearance-nonspecific
- Diffusion restriction due to purulent exudates—more specific for infection

**TABLE 2:** Clinical features.

| | |
|---|---|
| History of clinical complaints | Acute onset of fever, headache, neck stiffness, meningism, altered consciousness, irritability, photophobia, retrobulbar pain, seizures (children and 25% of cases), vertigo, nausea and vomiting |
| Antecedent History (in preceding days or hours) | • Trauma<br>• Upper respiratory tract infection<br>• Ear infection<br>• Travel history—suggestive of viral meningitis<br>• History of exposure |
| Neurological Signs | • Nuchal rigidity, stiffness, Positive Kernig's sign<br>• Convulsions (present because of raised ICP, cerebral abscess, cerebritis, septic venous thrombosis)<br>• Focal neurological signs, papilledema |
| Systemic Signs | • Ear and sinus examination<br>• Skin rashes (Meningococcal disease)<br>• Sepsis<br>• ARDS<br>• DIC |
| Complications | • Acute ischemic stroke—the possibility of underlying endocarditis to be ruled out<br>• Cerebral venous thrombosis<br>• Intracerebral hemorrhage<br>• Progression of infection: Cerebritis, brain abscess, subdural empyema.<br>• Hydrocephalus:<br>– Communicating hydrocephalus: In most cases- due to impaired CSF reabsorption<br>– Noncommunicating hydrocephalus: due to a diffuse brain edema or space-occupying lesion<br>• Ventriculitis<br>• Cranial nerve palsies (especially hearing loss) |

(ARDS: acute respiratory distress syndrome, DIC: disseminated intravascular coagulopathy; ICP: intracranial pressure)

**TABLE 3:** Diagnostic dilemma.

| *Feature of meningitis* | *Clinical pearls* |
|---|---|
| The classical triad of fever, neck stiffness and altered mental status may be absent | Present in < 50% of cases |
| Viral meningitis | • Less severe systemic features<br>• It may be associated with generalized malaise<br>• Self-limiting usually lasts 7 to 10 days<br>• Presence of focal neurological deficit: Indicative of meningoencephalitis |
| Immuno-compromised, elderly, or infant patient | Nonspecific features such as low-grade fever or mild behavioral change |
| Tubercular Meningitis | Risk factors:<br>• Immunocompromised, HIV, diabetes mellitus, recent use of steroids<br>Clinical features:<br>• Varied clinical features<br>• Non-specific prodromal features<br>– Cranial nerve palsies<br>– Vasculitis and stroke<br>– Hydrocephalus and tuberculoma |

**TABLE 4:** Investigations.

| *S. No.* | *Investigations* |
|---|---|
| 1. | Immediate paired blood cultures |
| 2. | • Lumbar Puncture / CSF fluid examination<br>• Cytology, biochemistry, Gram's stain, culture |
| 3. | Neuroimaging:<br>• CT Scan Brain<br>• MRI Brain with or without MRV<br>• CTA/CTV (arteriography/venography) |
| 4. | Throat swab for culture and sensitivity |
| 5. | Complete Blood Count, Renal Function Test, Liver Function Test, and Coagulation tests like PT, INR, and Blood glucose |
| 6. | EEG if seizures are ongoing |
| 7. | Diagnostic PCR studies, if available |
| 8. | Chest Radiograph |
| 9. | Blood Gas Analysis |
| 10. | Other relevant tests as per systemic examination findings<br>HIV screening |

(CSF: cerebrospinal fluid; CT: commuted tomography; EEG: electroencephalogram; MRI: magnetic resonance imaging; PCR: polymerase chain reaction)

- Abnormalities in the basal cisterns, prepontine cisterns, and Sylvian fissures suggestive of tuberculosis, fungal meningitis, or sarcoidosis
- MRI Brain with MRV if diagnosis is indeterminant—to rule out encephalitis, septic emboli, stroke

## DIFFERENTIAL DIAGNOSIS OF COMMUNITY-ACQUIRED MENINGITIS

- Subarachnoid hemorrhage—history of severe headache and CT findings
- Migraine—Headache pattern and aura
- Encephalitis—presence of focal neurological symptoms, altered consciousness, seizures more frequently suggestive of brain parenchyma
- Tumor—Absence of fever **(Tables 6 to 8)**

*Empirical antivirals:* IV Acyclovir 10 mg/kg 8th Hourly for 14 days

## DEFINITIVE ANTIBIOTICS

- Isolates susceptible to third-generation cephalosporins (MIC <1.0 μg/mL): ceftriaxone (2 g IV every 12 hours) or cefotaxime (2 g IV every 4 to 6 hours).
- Isolates with reduced sensitivity to third-generation cephalosporins (MIC ≥1.0 μg/mL): vancomycin should be added
- If a patient is not responding to an initial regimen—we would add a fluoroquinolone (moxifloxacin or levofloxacin)
- If fluoroquinolone is unavailable or should be avoided, rifampin can be used if the organism is susceptible. Total duration of antimicrobial therapy: 10 to 14 days.

**TABLE 5:** CSF findings in meningitis.

| | ***Normal*** | ***Pyogenic/bacterial*** | ***Viral*** | ***Tubercular/fungal*** |
|---|---|---|---|---|
| Appearance | Clear | Turbid/purulent | Clear/turbid | Fibrin web/Cobweb (TB) |
| Opening pressure | 90–180 mm Hg | Increased | Normal or moderate increased | Increased<br>If obstruction to CSF flow in TB meningitis then decreased |
| WBC count | <5/mm$^3$, Mononuclear | 200–10000/mm$^3$<br>PMN Predominantly | <500/mm$^3$<br>Lymphocytes mainly | 100–500<br>Lymphocytes/ Mixed |
| Protein (mg/dL) | 15–45 | 100–500 | Normal to a mild increase | 50–300 |
| CSF: Blood glucose ratio | 0.6 | Normal or ≤0.6 | Usually, normal | <0.4 |
| CSF lactate | <3.5 mmol/L | >3.5 mmol/L | <3.5 mmol/L | >3.5 mmol/L |

**TABLE 6:** Management of meningitis.

| | |
|---|---|
| 1. | Resuscitation and stabilization of airway, breathing and circulation |
| 2. | General ICU care |
| 3. | Steroid administration:<br>• Dexamethasone IV 15 to 20 minutes before the first antibiotic dose<br>• 0.4 mg/kg IV BD for 2 days<br>• 0.15 mg/kg QID for 4 days<br>• Dexamethasone should be continued if culture grows *S. pneumoniae* or *H. influenzae* |
| 4. | • Empirical therapy-antibiotics and antiviral<br>• Should be started immediately |
| 5. | Anticonvulsants |
| 6. | Cerebral protection strategies for raised intracranial pressure |
| 7. | • Management of other complications<br>• Fever prevention with antipyretics<br>• If SIADH – appropriate treatment |
| 8. | Definitive Therapy-Subsequently adjust antibiotics based on LP results |

**TABLE 7:** Empirical antibiotic for bacterial meningitis.

| *Indication* | *Antibiotic* | *Dose* |
|---|---|---|
| <60 years | • Ceftriaxone<br>• Cefotaxime<br>• *Vancomycin<br>• **Rifampicin | • 2 g IV 12th hourly<br>• 2 g IV 6th hourly<br>• 15-20 mg/kg IV 12th hourly<br>• 600 mg 12th hourly IV/oral |
| >60 years or impaired cell immunity (diabetes/alcohol misuse) | • Ceftriaxone<br>• Cefotaxime<br>• AND Ampicillin or Amoxicillin[#] | • 2 g IV 12th hourly<br>• 2 g IV 6th hourly<br>• 2g IV 4th hourly |

*And ** Drug-resistant *Streptococcus pneumoniae*-where prevalence of penicillin-resistant pneumococcal meningitis is high or travel history to such place within last 6 months
**Not commonly used for this indication in high mycobacterium prevalent areas due to the risk of development of resistance to rifampicin
[#]Ampicillin is useful for Listeria infection

**TABLE 8:** Alternative empirical antibiotic therapy (in case of allergy to third-generation cephalosporins or penicillin).

| *Patient profile* | *Antibiotic* | *Dose* |
|---|---|---|
| <60 years | Chloramphenicol | 25 mg/kg 6 hourly |
| >60 years or impaired cell immunity | Chloramphenicol<br>AND<br>Co-trimoxazole 10–20 mg/kg (of the trimethoprim component) | 25 mg/kg 6 hourly<br><br>In four divided daily doses |

Local hospital sensitivity and resistance patterns to be checked

## TUBERCULAR MENINGITIS

### Diagnosis

- Ideally, a minimum 3 serial lumbar punctures increase the sensitivity of mycobacterial culture.
- CSF ADA ranges from 8.6–28 IU/L- mean of 13.58 IU/L.
- Use of PCR increases sensitivity
- *Newer modalities:* Xpert/RIF can provide information about resistance pattern
- HIV with TB-multidrug-resistant TB risk is high. The resistance pattern should be determined
- CSF culture takes 6 weeks

### Treatment of Tubercular Meningitis

- *Antitubercular Drugs:* 2 months of intensive phase
    - Isoniazid oral/IV 300 mg daily
    - Rifampicin oral/IV 450 mg (<50 kg) and 600 mg (≥ 50 kg)
    - Pyrazinamide oral 1.5 g (<50 kg) and 2 g (≥ 50 kg)
    - Ethambutol oral 15 mg/kg OR Streptomycin
    - Fluroquinolones-Moxifloxacin/levofloxacin-alternative
    - AND continuation phase of 7 to 10 months of Isoniazid and Rifampicin
- *Steroids:* Dexamethasone and tapered over 4-6 weeks

### Treatment of Cryptococcal Meningitis

Amphotericin B 0.7 to 1 mg/kg /day AND flucytosine 100 mg/kg/day

OR

Liposomal amphotericin B 3 to 4 mg/kg/day AND flucytosine 100 mg/kg/day

## SUGGESTED READING

1. Taledano M, Davies NWS. Meningitis and encephalomyelitis. In: Bersten AD, Handy JM (Eds). OH'S Intensive Care Manual, eighth edition. Philadelphia: Elsevier; 2019. pp. 681-91.
2. Tunkel AR, Hartman BJ, KaplanSL, Kaufman BA, Roos KL, Scheld WM, et al. Practice Guidelines for the Management of Bacterial Meningitis. Clin Infect Dis. 2004;39(9):1267-84.

CHAPTER

# 52 Nosocomial Meningitis

## INTRODUCTION

Nosocomial meningitis is considered acquired when meningitis occurs at least 48 hours after hospital admission. It has high mortality, and the diagnosis is challenging. The presence of associated ventriculitis increases mortality. The management is also difficult due to the presence of drug-resistant strains of microbes. The etiology and risk factors of Nosocomial meningitis are described in **Boxes 1 and 2**, respectively.

## DIAGNOSIS

### Clinical Features

- New onset fever with or without deterioration of mental status
- In the absence of another definite source of infection
- In the context of recent head trauma or neurosurgery
- It should always raise suspicion of CNS infection and prompt CSF analysis.
- It may be difficult to detect in the backdrop of the antecedent pathology causing altered sensorium and ongoing sedation
- Overdiagnosis of meningitis—due to meningeal reactions to cerebral hemorrhage or TBI

**BOX 1:** Etiology of nosocomial meningitis.

| *Systemic nosocomial pathogens* | |
|---|---|
| 1. | Main etiological agents: Cutaneous Gram-positive bacteria-*Staphylococcus* species-coagulase-negative *Staphylococci*, *Staphylococcus aureus*, epidermidis and *Cutibacterium acnes*, *P. acnes* |
| 2. | • Gram-negative infections are increasing (prevalence 52% in few reports)<br>• *Escherichia coli*, *Pseudomonas* spp., *Klebsiella* and *Acinetobacter* spp. |

**BOX 2:** Risk factors for nosocomial meningitis.

1. Invasive devices: Internal ventricular catheters/ventriculoperitoneal shunts (VP), external ventricular drains (EVD), external lumbar catheters
2. Lumbar puncture (LP)
3. Tumor neurosurgery/craniotomy
4. Moderate or severe head trauma
5. Basilar Skull Fracture
6. Subarachnoid hemorrhage
7. Metastatic infection in patients with bacteremia—rare

### Investigations

- *Nonspecific Cerebrospinal Fluid (CSF) findings*:
  - Raised CSF white blood count (WBC), low CSF glucose
  - Culture is negative in 11–30% of cases (because of prior antibiotic therapy)
  - Altered nonspecific biochemistry (because of intracerebral hemorrhage and/or inflammation)
  - Elevated CSF lactate is better than CSF WBC in differentiating bacterial meningitis from aseptic meningitis
  - Elevated serum procalcitonin may be useful (poor quality of evidence)
  - β-D-glucan and galactomannan in CSF for fungal meningitis detection
- Contrast-enhanced—magnetic resonance imaging and diffusion-weighted imaging
- Ultrasound or computed tomography of the abdomen
  - For VP shunt with abdominal pain
  - Recommended to detect CSF loculations at the shunt terminal end

### Treatment

- *Steroids:* Dexamethasone is not routinely used for management of inflammation or elevated intracranial pressure in patients with nosocomial meningitis.

- *Antimicrobial therapy:*
  - *Empirical choice:* This condition is associated with different pathogenetic mechanisms and different spectrum of microorganisms. Therefore, the choice of empirical antimicrobial therapy will vary according to the condition.
  - *Route:*
    - *Intravenous:* CSF penetration of the antibiotics varies.
    - *Empiric:*
      - Usual empiric therapy: Vancomycin and an anti-pseudomonal beta-lactam (such as cefepime, ceftazidime, or meropenem)
      - Vancomycin trough concentration to be maintained at 15–20 µg/mL
      - In case of anaphylaxis to beta-lactam antimicrobials, aztreonam or ciprofloxacin
      - For a highly antimicrobial-resistant organism, colonized or infected elsewhere, adjusting the empiric regimen is to be done accordingly

      *Definite:* This is described in **Table 1**.

Intraventricular/Intrathecally Antimicrobial therapy through LP/EVD:

- Combined IV and intraventricular antimicrobial agents improve CSF antimicrobial concentration without side effects
- Should be considered in refractory infection, which responds poorly to systemic antibiotics
- Ventricular drain should be clamped for 15–60 minutes after instillation into the CSF through it to allow time for equilibrium
- Dosage and frequency are to be adjusted based on CSF antimicrobial concentration (sent 24 hours after administration of first dose) of at least 10-20 times the MIC of the etiological organism, ventricular size, and daily drain output **(Tables 2 and 3)**.
- However—efficacy and safety are not well established and not recommended in pediatric shunts
- Commonly used—Polymyxin B, colistimethate sodium, gentamicin, vancomycin
- Not to be given intraventricularly—penicillins and cephalosporins-risk of neurotoxicity and seizures
- *Other therapeutic measures:*
  - Complete removal of an infected CSF shunt and replacement with an external ventricular drain
  - Removal of an infected CSF drain is recommended.

**TABLE 1:** Choice of definitive antimicrobial therapy.

| *Pathogen* | *Antibiotic recommended* |
|---|---|
| Methicillin-susceptible *S. aureus* | Nafcillin or oxacillin |
| Methicillin-resistant *S. aureus* | Vancomycin<br>If the vancomycin minimal inhibitory concentration (MIC) is ≥1 µg/mL/beta-lactam agents cannot be used: Linezolid, daptomycin, or trimethoprim-sulfamethoxazole<br>For any patient with intracranial or spinal hardware such as a CSF shunt or drain: Rifampin, if sensitive may be combined with other agents |
| Coagulase-negative staphylococci | Vancomycin |
| Propionibacterium acnes | Penicillin G |
| Gram-negative bacilli | Third-generation cephalosporins- ceftriaxone or cefotaxime |
| Extended-spectrum beta-lactamase-producing gram-negative bacilli | Meropenem |
| *Acinetobacter* species | Meropenem<br>Carbapenem resistance: Colistimethate sodium or polymyxin B |
| *Candida* species | Liposomal amphotericin B<br>5-flucytosine is often added |
| *Aspergillus* or *Exserohilum* species | Voriconazole |

**TABLE 2:** Frequency of intraventricular antimicrobial therapy as per drain output.

| *Drain output* | *Frequency* |
|---|---|
| >100 mL/day | Once daily dosing |
| 50–100 mL/day | Every other day |
| <50 mL/day | Every third day |

**TABLE 3:** Dose of intraventricular antimicrobial therapy.

| *Antibiotic* | *Dose* |
|---|---|
| Vancomycin | • *15–20 mg/kg IV 12th hourly:* Enlarged ventricles<br>• *10 mg/kg IV 12th hourly:* Normal-sized ventricles<br>• *5 mg/kg IV 12th hourly:* Slit ventricles |
| Meropenem | 2 g IV 6th hourly |

### Prophylaxis

- *Antibiotic-impregnated EVD:*
  - Effective and safe in lowering the risk, especially against gram-positive organisms
  - Currently impregnated with clindamycin/rifampicin or minocycline/rifampicin or sliver
- Neurosurgery, including procedures to place CSF shunts or other hardware: Perioperative antimicrobial prophylaxis is recommended
- Basilar skull fracture and cerebrospinal fluid leak:
  - No role of prophylactic antimicrobials
  - Patients with a basilar skull fracture and a prolonged CSF leak (> seven days): repair of the leak is advised
  - Any patient with a CSF leak—should receive pneumococcal vaccination

## SUGGESTED READING

1. Tunkel AR, Hasbun R, Bhimraj A, Byers K, Kaplan SL, Scheld WM, et al. 2017 Infectious Diseases Society of America's Clinical Practice Guidelines for Healthcare-Associated Ventriculitis and Meningitis. Clin Infect Dis. 2017;64(6):e34-e65.
2. Valdoleiros SR, Torrão C, Freitas LS, Mano D, Gonçalves C, Teixeira C. Nosocomial meningitis in intensive care: a 10-year retrospective study and literature review. Acute Crit Care. 2022;37(1):61-70.

CHAPTER 53

# Neurogenic Shock

## INTRODUCTION

Traumatic spinal cord injury can present with shock in <20% of cases when the lesion is above the T6 level due to loss of sympathetic autonomic control.

The classical triad of neurogenic shock:

- Hypotension
- Bradycardia
- Autonomic dysreflexia

| *Neurogenic shock* | *Spinal shock* |
|---|---|
| • Hemodynamic phenomenon (distributive shock)<br>• Caused by a sudden loss of sympathetic outflow below the level of injury<br>• It can last up to 6 weeks | • Neurological phenomenon<br>• Results in immediate loss of motor power, reflexes and sensation below the level of injury<br>• Can last hours to weeks, depending on severity and level of injury<br>*Phases:*<br>1. Areflexia/hyporeflexia (first 24 hours)<br>2. Return of some reflexes (1–3 days)<br>3. Early autonomic hyperreflexia (4 days–1 month)<br>4. Spasticity (1–12 months) |

## PATHOPHYSIOLOGY

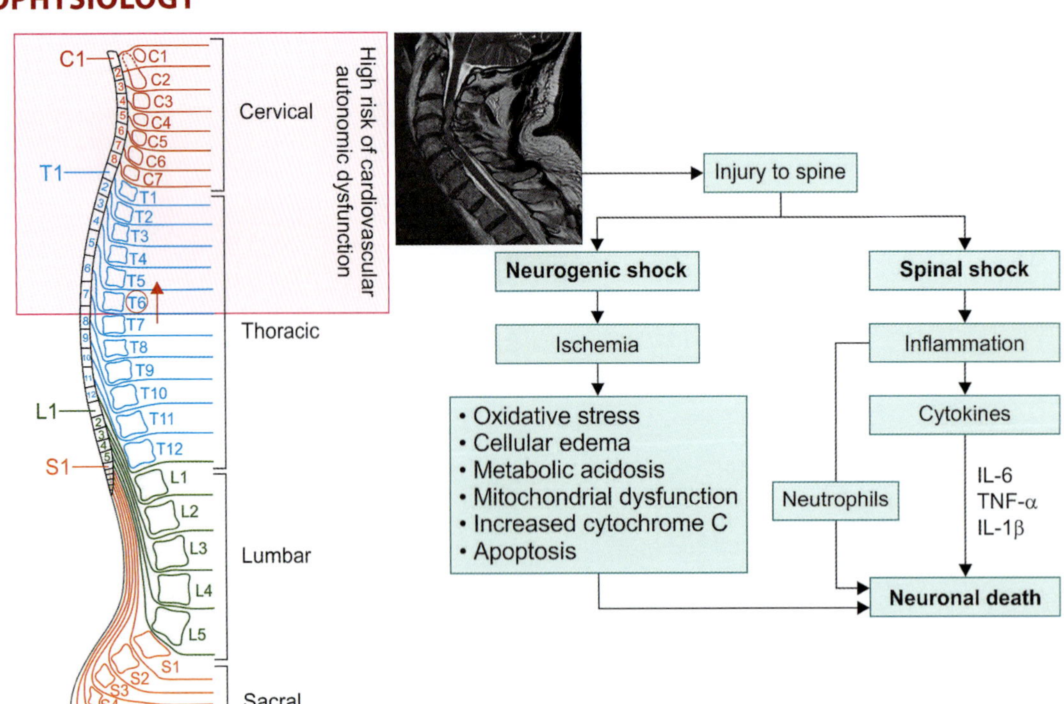

## MANAGEMENT

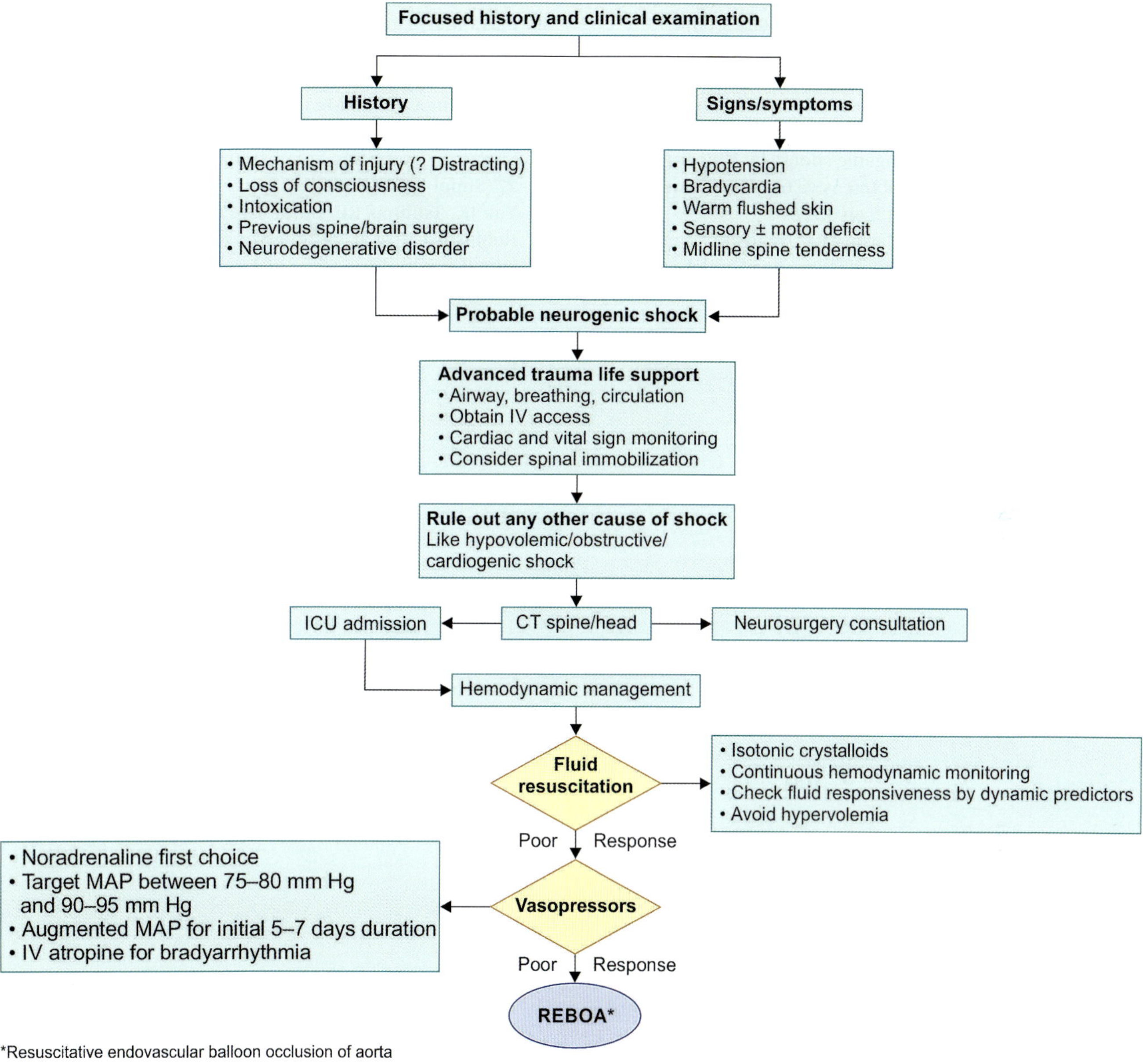


*Resuscitative endovascular balloon occlusion of aorta

## ANCILLARY MEASURES

- There is no definitive role of neuroprotection, especially corticosteroids
- Decubitus ulcer prevention
- Management of gastroparesis
- Prophylaxis for deep vein thrombosis (pharmacologic/mechanical)
- Prevention of spasticity and contracture by early employment of physical rehabilitation
- Infection prevention measures
- Psychological support

## SUGGESTED READING


1. American College of Surgeons; Committee on Trauma (2018). "Spine and spinal cord trauma". ATLS®—Advanced Trauma Life Support: Student Course Manual (Tenth ed.). Chicago: American College of Surgeons; pp. 129-46.
2. Coleman WP, Benzel D, Cahill DW, Ducker T, Geisler F, Green B, et al. A critical appraisal of the reporting of the National Acute Spinal Cord Injury Studies (II and III) of methylprednisolone in acute spinal cord injury. J Spinal Disord. 2000;13(03):185-99.
3. Fox AD. Spinal shock Assessment & treatment of spinal cord injuries & neurogenic shock. JEMS. 2014;39:64-7

4. Furlan JC, Fehlings MG. Cardiovascular complications after acute spinal cord injury: pathophysiology, diagnosis, and management. Neurosurg Focus. 2008;25(05):E13.
5. Go Steven. Spine Trauma (Chapter 258). In: Tintinalli JE, Stapczynski J, Ma O, Yearly DM, Meckler GD, Cline DM (Eds.) Tintinalli's Emergency Medicine. Philadelphia: McGraw-Hill Education; 2016. pp. 1696-714.
6. Jordan JR, Witt JP. Neurogenic shock. In: Vincent JL, Hall J.B (Eds). Encyclopedia of Intensive Care Medicine. Berlin, Heidelberg: Springer; 2012. pp. 1527-8.
7. Kwon BK, Tetreault LA, Martin AR, Arnold PM, Marco RAW, Newcombe VFJ, et al. A clinical Practice Guideline for the Management of Patients With Acute Spinal Cord Injury: Recommendation on Hemodynamic Management. Global Spine J. 20124;14(3_suppl):187S-211S.
8. Parra MW, Ordoñez CA, Mejia D, Caicedo Y, Lobato JM, Castro OJ, et al. Damage control approach to refractory neurogenic shock: a new proposal to a well-established algorithm. Colomb Med (Cali). 2021;52(2):e4164800.
9. Stein DM, Knight WA. Emergency Neurological Life Support: Traumatic Spine Injury. Neurocrit Care. 2017; 27 (Suppl 1):170-80.
10. Yue JK, Tsolinas RE, Burke JF, Deng H, Upadhyayula PS, Robinson CK, et al. Vasopressor support in managing acute spinal cord injury: Current knowledge. J Neurosurg Sci. 2019;63(3):308-17.

CHAPTER 54

# New-onset Weakness in the Intensive Care Unit

**Flowchart 1:** Algorithm for initial assessment of new onset nontraumatic weakness in the ICU (Modified).[1]

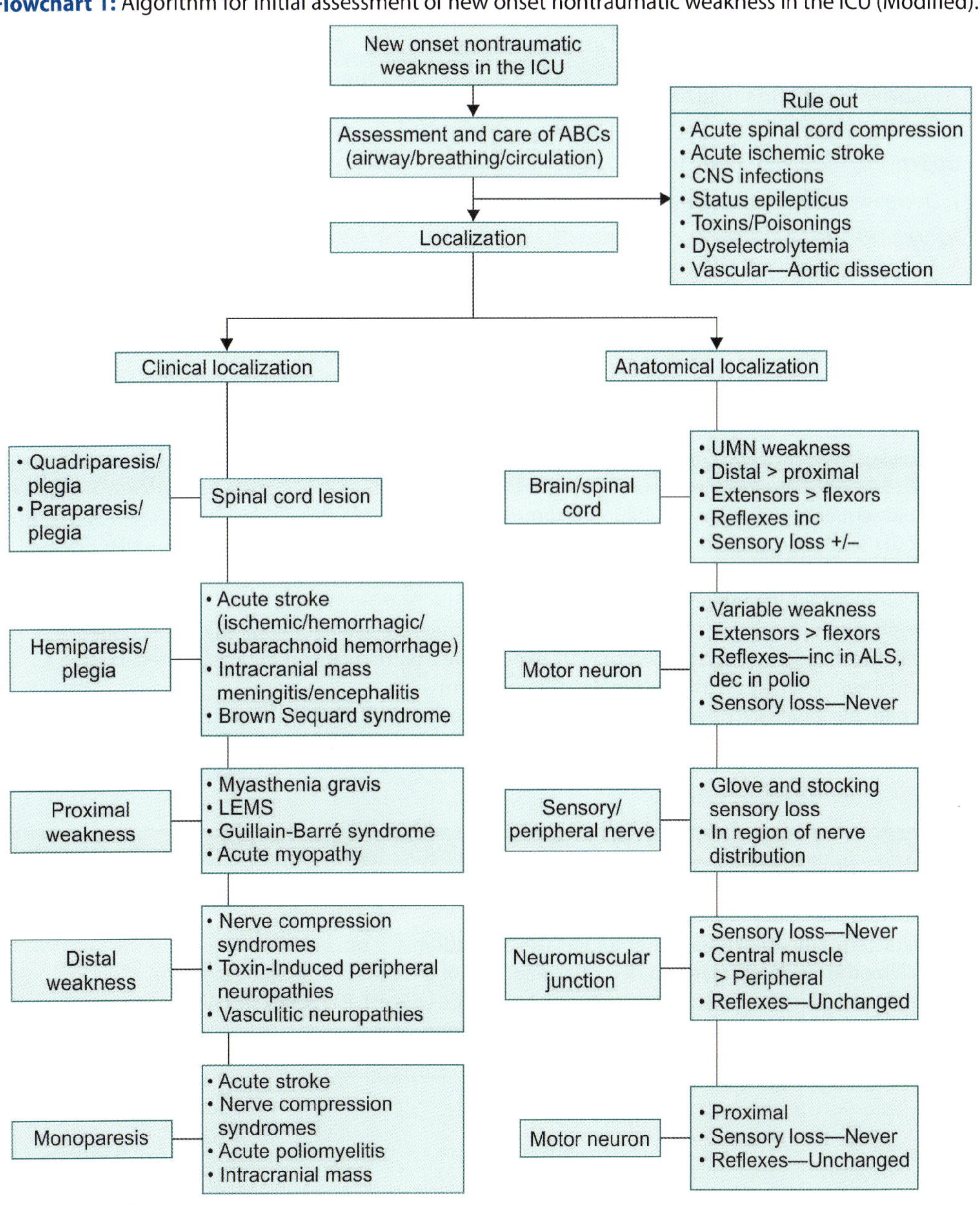

**BOX 1: Indications of intubation in acute nontraumatic weakness.[2]**

*General*

- Increasing generalized muscle weakness
- Dysphagia
- Dysphonia
- Dyspnea on exertion and at rest

*Subjective*

- Rapid Shallow Breathing
- Tachycardia
- Weak cough
- Interrupted speech
- Use of accessory muscles
- Abdominal paradoxical breathing
- Orthopnea
- Weakness of trapezius and neck muscles: Inability to lift head
- Inability to perform single breath count (less than 20)
- Cough after swallowing

*Objective*

- Decreased level of consciousness
- Hypoxemia
- Vital capacity < 1 L or 20 mL/kg, or 50% decrease in VC in a day
- Maximum Inspiratory Pressure > –30 $cmH_2O$
- Maximum Expiratory pressure < 40 $cmH_2O$
- Hypercarbia

**BOX 2: Special considerations for intubation.[2]**

- Rapid sequence induction/intubation recommended
- Avoid use of succinylcholine if there is evidence of underlying progressive neuromuscular disease (Guillain-Barré syndrome, chronic muscular weakness, or prolonged immobility). Consider Rocuronium as alternative
- Consider non-invasive ventilation as a temporizing measure in a neurologically stable patient, while the diagnosis is established or with a known neuromuscular condition expected to have a rapid resolution (e.g. myasthenia gravis exacerbation)
- Prepare Atropine/Glycopyrrolate, fluids, and vasopressors (risk of autonomic instability)

**BOX 3: Acute weakness checklist for the first hour.[2]**

- Assess and manage Airway, Breathing, and Circulation
- Rule out emergency etiologies
- Characterize the weakness by neurological examination
- Localize the lesion to create a differential diagnosis of the causes of weakness
- *Initial Labs:* Glucose, electrolytes, Ca, Mg, $pO_4$, BUN/Cr, LFTs, PT, PTT, CBC, and ABG
- *Special Labs:* TFTs, CPK or CK, ESR, parathyroid hormone, GGT
- Relevant MRI and CT imaging

**TABLE 1:** Management options for common etiologies of new-onset weakness in the ICU.

| | |
|---|---|
| *Intracranial* | |
| Intracranial mass | • Steroids for peri tumoral vasogenic edema<br>• Tier approach for raised ICP<br>• Surgical evacuation and excision of lesion SOS |
| Acute ischemic stroke | • Stroke Protocol<br>• Thrombolysis/thrombectomy |
| Metabolic/hypertensive encephalopathy | • IV anti-hypertensive agents<br>• Invasive BP monitoring |
| *Spinal cord lesions* | |
| Transverse myelitis | • IV Methylprednisolone<br>• IVIG<br>• Plasma exchange |
| Guillain-Barré syndrome | • Plasma exchange<br>• IVIG |
| Myasthenia gravis/LEMS | • Mechanical ventilation when indicated<br>• Plasmapheresis/IVIG<br>• High dose steroids<br>• Immunosuppressants<br>• Withdraw anticholinesterase medications<br>• Consider 3,4-diaminopyridine for LEMS |
| Vasculitic neuropathy | Combination therapy with steroids and cyclophosphamide |
| Nerve compression syndromes | • Treat and remove precipitants<br>• Decompressive surgery |
| Botulism | • *Adults/Children > 1 year:* Equine serum heptavalent<br>• *Infants < 1 year:* Human derived botulism immunoglobulin<br>• Penicillin G (or metronidazole) for wound care |
| *Muscle* | |
| Dermatomyositis | • Corticosteroids<br>• Immunosuppressive or cytotoxic steroid sparing agents<br>• IVIG in refractory cases |
| Dyselectrolytemia | • Correct dyselectrolytemia<br>• Fluid therapy<br>• Diuretics<br>• Addressing the cause of dyselectrolytemia |
| *Miscellaneous* | |
| Envenomation | • Care of ABCs<br>• Specific anti-venom |
| Locked in syndrome | Follow acute Stroke Protocol |
| *Supportive care* | |
| • Spinal cord infarction<br>• Brown-Sequard syndrome<br>• Amyotrophic lateral sclerosis | |

## REFERENCES

1. Jangra K, Bhagat H, Takkar A. Acute Nontraumatic Muscle Weakness. J Neuroanaesthesiol Crit Care. 2019;6(3):236-56.
2. Caulfield AF, Flower O, Pineda JA, Uddin S. Emergency Neurological Life Support: Acute Non-traumatic Weakness. Neurocrit Care. 2017;27(S1):29-50.

CHAPTER 55

# Cerebral Venous Thrombosis

## INTRODUCTION

Cerebral venous thrombosis is the presence of a blood clot in the dural venous sinuses, cerebral veins, or both.

| | | |
|---|---|---|
| *Site* | • Transverse sinus (25–60%)<br>• Sup sagittal sinus (25–45%)<br>• Straight sinus (15–18%)<br>• Cortical veins (15–17%)<br>• Sigmoid sinus (5–15%)<br>• Deep venous system (10%)<br>• Internal jugular vein (10%)<br>• Multiple sinuses (18–50%) | |
| *Symptoms* | • Headache<br>• Nausea<br>• Eye signs—visual disturbances or vision loss, papilledema, diplopia<br>• Increased ICP<br>• Seizures<br>• Focal neurological deficit | |
| *Diagnosis* | CT scan | Look for cord sign (rare finding), dense triangle, empty triangle sign (10–20%) |
| | Four vessel angiography | Partial or complete lack of filling of veins or sinuses. The gold standard for the diagnosis of CVT |
| | MRI | Dilated and tortuous cortical vein with a corkscrew appearance |
| | Others | • Method of choice for diagnosis and follow-up for CVT<br>Benefit—noninvasive, better visualization of thrombus, sensitive to blood flow.<br>– CSF examination<br>– EEG—abnormal in 75%<br>– Isotropic brain scanning with $^{99}$TC<br>– Coagulation studies—increase platelet adhesiveness and aggregability and decrease fibrinolytic activity |

*Contd...*

*Contd…*

| *Treatment* | Symptomatic treatment | • Anticonvulsants<br>• Antibiotics<br>• To decrease ICP:<br>– Head end elevation<br>– Hyperventilation to maintain $PaCO_2$ of 30–35 mm Hg<br>– IV mannitol—1–1.5 g/kg<br>– Acetazolamide- 500 mg bd<br>– Sedation<br>– Lumbar puncture CSF drainage<br>– Peritoneal shunting<br>– Barbiturate induced coma<br>– Craniotomy |
|---|---|---|
| | Antithrombotic treatment* | • *Anticoagulant of choice*—low molecular weight heparin (LMWH) for the acute phase as per body weight; subcutaneous, therapeutic dose<br>• Dose-adjusted IV Heparin can be given to maintain an APPT (2 times normal)<br>• Followed by warfarin (Vitamin K agonist) with a target INR of 2.5 (Range 2–3)<br>• Warfarin may be continued for 3–12 months to prevent recurrences |

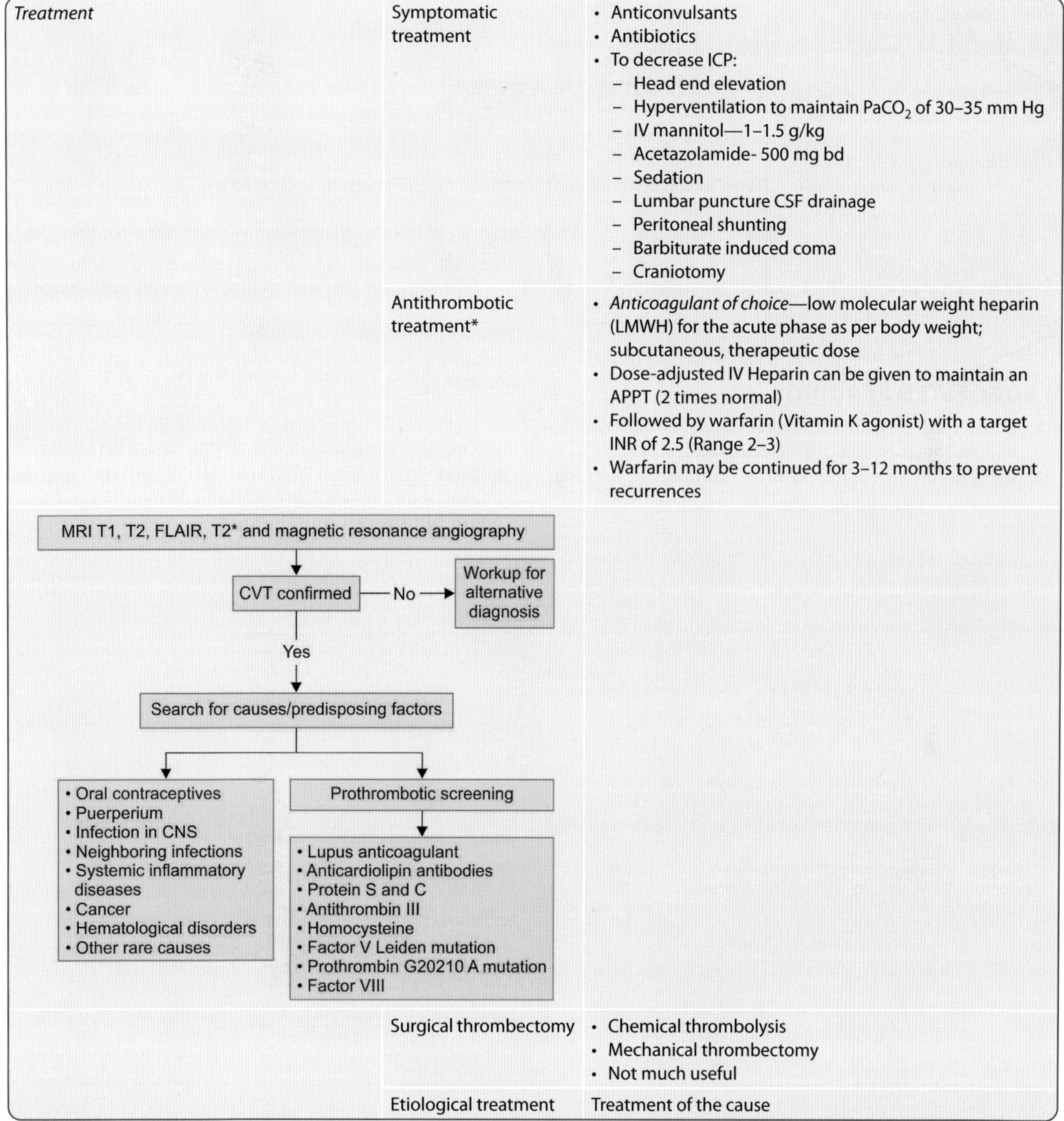


| | | |
|---|---|---|
| | Surgical thrombectomy | • Chemical thrombolysis<br>• Mechanical thrombectomy<br>• Not much useful |
| | Etiological treatment | Treatment of the cause |

*Contd…*

*Contd...*

| *Poor prognostic features* | • Rate of evolution of thrombus<br>• Coma<br>• Age of patient<br>• Presence of focal symptom<br>• Presence of hemorrhagic infarct<br>• Empty delta sign on CT scan |
|---|---|
| *Special mentions:*<br>• *CVT in pregnancy:* Anticoagulant (LMWH) should be continued throughout the pregnancy and followed by warfarin with a target INR 2.0-3.0 to be continued till 6 weeks postdelivery.<br>• *CVT in pediatric:* Initial treatment involves parenteral anticoagulation, which is typically followed by low molecular weight heparin (LMWH), vitamin K antagonists (VKAs), or rivaroxaban for a minimum of 6 weeks | |
| *The presence of isolated subarachnoid hemorrhage, hemorrhagic venous infarction, and intracerebral hemorrhage are *not contraindications for anticoagulant treatment in CVT.* | |

## SUGGESTED READING


1. Bousser MG, Ferro JM. Cerebral venous thrombosis: An update. Lancet Neurol. 2007;6(2):162-70.
2. Bousser MG. Cerebral venous thrombosis: nothing, heparin, or local thrombolysis? Stroke. 1999;30(3):481-3.
3. Saposnik G, Bushnell C, Coutinho JM, Field TS, Furie KL, Galadanci N, et al. Diagnosis and management of cerebral venous thrombosis: a Scientific Statement from the American Heart Association. Stroke. 2024;55(3):e77-90.
4. Silvis SM, De Sousa DA, Ferro JM, Coutinho JM. Cerebral venous thrombosis. Nat Rev Neurol. 2017;13(9):555-65.

# PART 4

# GASTROENTEROLOGY/HEPATOLOGY

***Editors:*** Shrikanth Srinivasan, Lalita Gouri Mitra

***Associate Editors:*** Krishna Murari Dhaker, Anuradha Pandey, Nitin Saluja, Priyankar Datta, Sunil Kumar Karhana, Nitin Jain, Vishal Khandelwal, Rishikant Birla, Raghvendra Kumar Giri, Ankit Sharma, Rajathadri Hosur Ravikumar

CHAPTER **56**

# Massive Upper Gastrointestinal Bleed

## DEFINITION

GI bleed is proximal to the ligament of Treitz.

## CAUSES

- Peptic ulcer disease
- Gastric ulcers
- Duodenal ulcers
- Gastric erosions and gastritis
- Esophageal and/or gastric varices

*Contd...*

- Stress ulcers
- Mallory-Weiss tear
- Esophagitis and esophageal ulcers
- Vascular abnormalities—angiodysplasia, Dieulafoy lesions, and telangiectasia
- Portal hypertensive gastropathy
- Neoplasms
- Hemobilia—bleeding into bile duct
- Hemosuccus—bleeding into pancreatic duct
- Aortoenteric fistula

## INITIAL EVALUATION

| History | Past medical history | *History* | *Possible abnormality* |
|---|---|---|---|
| | | • *H. pylori* infection<br>• NSAID use<br>• Antithrombotic use<br>• Smoking | Peptic ulcer disease |
| | | • History of liver disease<br>• Alcohol | Varices or PHG |
| | | • Kidney disease<br>• AS<br>• Hereditary hemorrhagic telangiectasia | Gastrointestinal angiodysplasia |
| | | • Abdominal aortic aneurysm<br>• Aortic graft | Aortoenteric fistula |
| | | • Smoking<br>• Alcohol<br>• *H. pylori* infection | Malignancy |
| | | • Gastroenteric anastomosis | Marginal ulcer |

*Contd...*

*Contd...*

| | | | |
|---|---|---|---|
| | Medication history | *Drugs* | *Remark* |
| | | • NSAIDs intake | |
| | | • Pill esophagitis<br>– Antibiotics<br>– NSAIDs<br>– Bisphosphonates<br>– Chemo drugs | |
| | | • Anticoagulants | |
| | | • SSRI<br>• Calcium channel blockers<br>• Aldosterone antagonists | Associated with GI bleed. |
| | | • Bismuth<br>• Charcoal<br>• Licorice<br>• Iron | Can turn the stool color black and give false sense of GI bleed. |
| Physical examination | • Tachycardia: Hypotension may be a late finding<br>• Hemodynamic Assessment (Refer table below)<br>• Stool color<br>• Abdominal pain/rebound tenderness/guarding | | |
| Laboratory data | • CBC<br>• KFT<br>• LFT<br>• Coagulation studies | | |
| • Nasogastric lavage | | | |

(AS: aortic stenosis; PHG: portal hypertensive gastropathy)

## Assessment of Hemodynamic Stability

| ***Category*** | ***Whole blood volume loss*** | ***Hemodynamics*** |
|---|---|---|
| Mild | <15% | Resting tachycardia |
| Moderate | >15% and <40% | Orthostatic hypotension |
| Severe | At least 40% | Supine hypotension |

## MANAGEMENT

*Resuscitation:*
- Assessment airway status
- Supplemental oxygen, may require intubation for airway protection
- Establish two large bore IV lines (16 gauge or larger)
- Record vitals
- Obtain blood for routine investigations including CBC and coagulation profile
- Treat hypotension initially with rapid, bolus infusions of isotonic crystalloid. Vasopressors support if required

↓

*Blood transfusion:*
- For severe, ongoing bleeding, immediately transfuse blood products in 1:1:1 ratio of PRBCs, plasma, and platelets, as for trauma patients
- Give plasma for coagulopathy or after transfusing four units of RBCs
- Give platelets for thrombocytopenia (platelets <50,000) or platelet dysfunction (e.g., chronic aspirin therapy) or after transfusing four units of RBCs
- Avoid over-transfusion with possible upper GI bleeding

↓

*Factors propagating bleeding:*
- Discontinue antiplatelets and anticoagulants if any
- Correction of coagulopathy
- Correction of thrombocytopenia

↓

*Pharmacotherapy:*
- *PPI infusion*: Inj. Pantoprazole 80 mg IV stat followed by 8 mg/h infusion
- Give somatostatin 250 mg/h infusion or an analog (e.g., octreotide, terlipressin)
- IV antibiotic
- *Prokinetics*: For better visualization during endoscopy. Erythromycin 250 mg IV stat or metoclopramide 5–10 mg IV stat
- Tranexamic acid: No added benefits in UGI bleed patient

↓

*Consultations:*
- Gastroenterology
- Surgeon
- Interventional radiology
- Hematology
- Transfusion medicine

↓

*Specific treatment:*
- *Upper GI endoscopy:* Diagnostic/therapeutic
- *Balloon tamponade:* Sengstaken-Blakemore tube, Minnesota tube

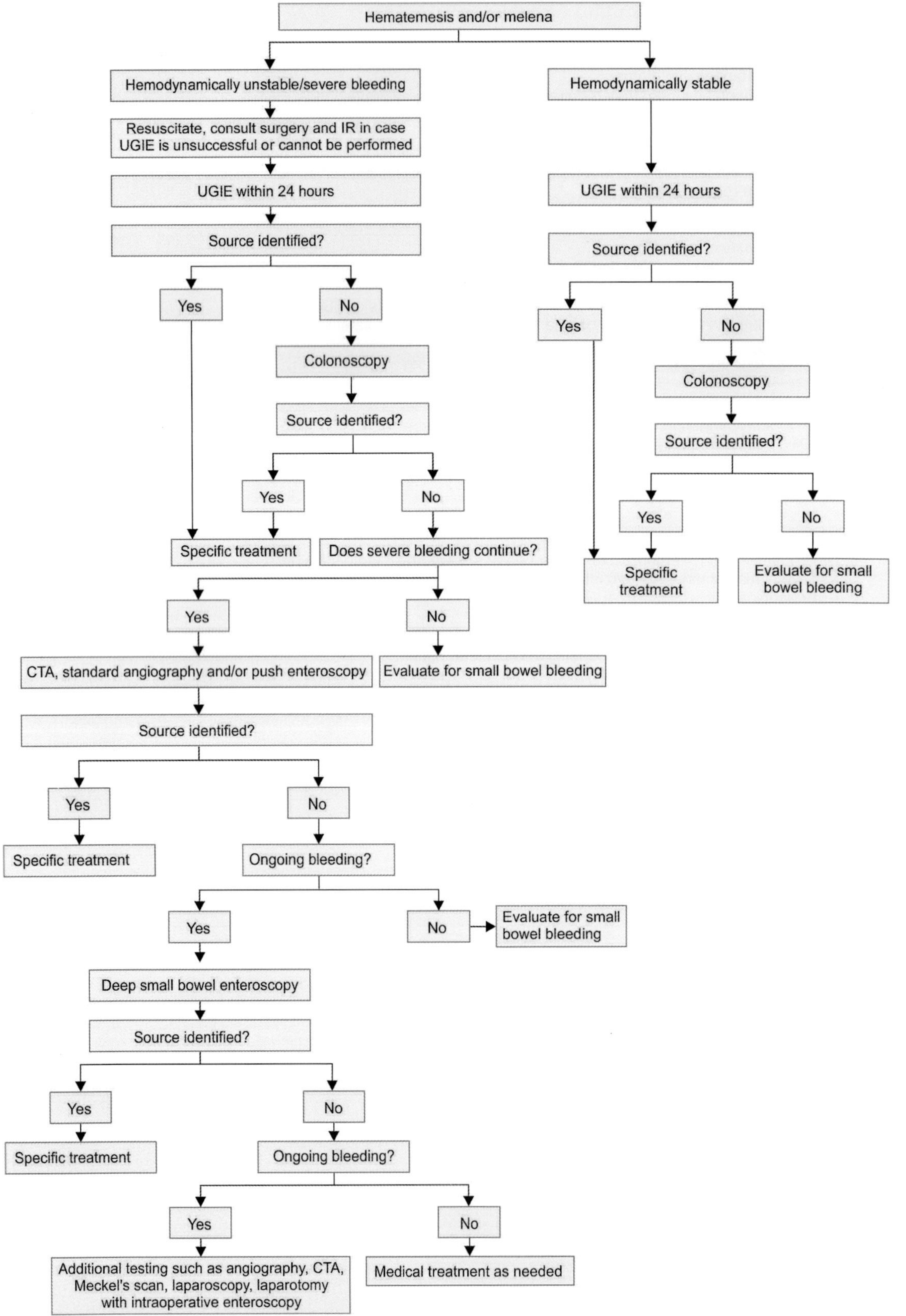


(CT: computed tomographic; CTA: computed tomographic angiography; GI: gastrointestinal; IR: interventional radiology; MR: magnetic resonance; UGIE: upper GI endoscopy)

## UGI ENDOSCOPY FINDINGS

| Diagnosis | UGI endoscopic findings |
|---|---|
| Duodenal and/or gastric Ulcer | • Ulcer with smooth, regular, rounded edges; ulcer base often filled with exudate. Examination of the ulcer may reveal:<br>– Active bleeding or oozing<br>– Nonbleeding visible vessel<br>– Adherent clot<br>– Flat pigmented spot<br>– Clean ulcer base |
| Esophagitis | • Erythema, mucosal breaks/erosions, exudative lesions, superficial or deep ulcers, stenosis, and scarring<br>• *Peptic esophagitis*: The ulcerations are usually irregularly shaped or linear, multiple, and distal; may be accompanied by Barrett's esophagus.<br>• *Pill-induced*: Ulcerations are usually singular and deep, occurring at points of stasis (especially near the carina), with sparing of the distal esophagus.<br>• Infectious esophagitis—different findings in HSV, CMV, Candida, and HIV |
| Gastritis/gastropathy<br>Duodenitis/duodenopathy | • Erythematous mucosa<br>• Superficial erosions<br>• Nodularity<br>• Diffuse oozing |
| Esophagogastric varices | • Vascular structures that protrude into the esophageal and/or gastric lumen<br>• Findings associated with an increased risk of hemorrhage:<br>– Longitudinal red streaks on the varices (red wale marks).<br>– Cherry-colored spots that are flat and overlie varices.<br>– Raised, discrete red spots (hematocystic spots)<br>• Esophageal varices:<br>– F1: Small, straight varices<br>– F2: Enlarged, tortuous varices that occupy less than one-third of the lumen<br>– F3: Large, coil shaped varices that occupy more than one-third of the lumen<br>• *Gastric varices*:<br>– GOV1: Gastroesophageal varices along the lesser curvature of the stomach<br>– GOV2: Gastroesophageal varices along the greater curvature of the stomach<br>– IGV1: Isolated gastric varices in the fundus<br>– IGV2: Isolated gastric varices at other loci in the stomach |
| Ectopic varices | Vascular structures that protrude into areas of the gastrointestinal tract lumen other than the esophagus or stomach (e.g., small bowel, and rectum) |
| Portal hypertensive gastropathy | • Mosaic-like pattern that gives the gastric mucosa a "snakeskin" appearance<br>• Mucosal changes are usually most evident in the fundus and body; in more severe cases, oozing, bleeding, subepithelial hemorrhages, and increased vascularity similar to angiomas are evident, often involving the gastric fundus, gastric body, and antrum |
| Angiodysplasia | Small (5–10 mm), flat, cherry-red lesions, often with a fern-like pattern of arborizing, and ectatic blood vessels radiating from a central vessel |
| Dieulafoy's lesion | • Usually located in the proximal stomach (within 6 cm of the esophagogastric junction) along the lesser curvature (although can be found anywhere in the GI tract)<br>• May have active arterial spurting from the mucosa without an associated ulcer or mass<br>• If the bleeding has stopped, there may be a raised nipple or visible vessel without an associated ulcer<br>• Endoscopic ultrasound may help confirm the diagnosis |
| Gastric antral vascular ectasia (GAVE) | • Longitudinal rows of flat, reddish stripes radiating from the pylorus into the antrum that resemble the stripes on a watermelon |
| Blue rubber bleb nevus syndrome (Bean syndrome) | • Blue or purple nodules, round or multilobular; may occur anywhere in the gastrointestinal tract |

*Contd…*

*Contd…*

| *Diagnosis* | *UGI endoscopic findings* |
|---|---|
| Mallory-Weiss syndrome | • Tear in the esophagogastric junction<br>• Usually singular and longitudinal, but may be multiple<br>• Visualization may require retroflexion of the gastroscope in the cardia of the stomach<br>• The tear may be covered by an adherent clot |
| Foreign body ingestion | • Visualization of the foreign body endoscopically (plain radiographs of the neck, chest, and abdomen may reveal a radiopaque foreign body or signs of perforation) |
| Marginal ulcers | • Ulceration/friable mucosa at an anastomotic site |
| Cameron lesions | • Linear ulcers or erosions on the mucosal folds of a hiatal hernia at the diaphragmatic impression |
| Aortoenteric fistula | • Enteroscope or side viewing duodenoscope may reveal a graft, an ulcer or erosion at the site of an adherent clot, or an extrinsic pulsatile mass in the distal duodenum or esophagus |
| Upper GI tumors | • Ulcerated mass in esophagus, stomach, or duodenum.<br>• In gastric malignancies, the folds surrounding the ulcer crater may be nodular, clubbed, fused, or stop short of the ulcer margin; the margins may be overhanging, irregular, or thickened. Bleeding lymphoma may appear as an ulcerated mass or polypoid lesion or as a gastric ulcer |
| Hemobilia | • Blood or clot emanating from ampulla (a side-viewing duodenoscope may be required to visualize ampulla)<br>• If a clot has formed in the bile duct, bleeding may not be appreciated until the clot is removed ERCP may reveal a filling defect in the bile duct |
| Hemosuccus pancreaticus | • Blood or clot emanating from the ampulla (a side-viewing duodenoscope may be required to visualize the ampulla)<br>• Cross-sectional imaging or angiography is often required to confirm the diagnosis |

## DECISION FOR RBC TRANSFUSION

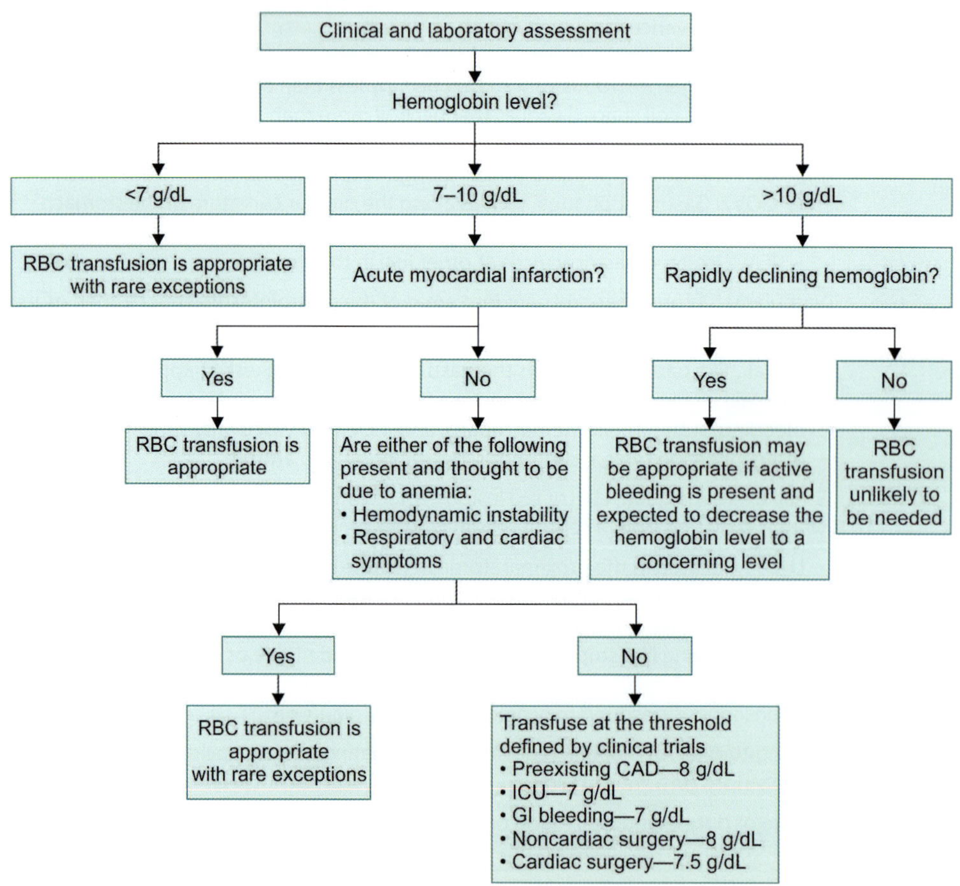


(CAD: coronary artery disease; ICU: intensive care unit; RBC: red blood cell)

## RISK STRATIFICATION

Factors associated with rebleeding:

- Hemodynamic instability (systolic blood pressure < 100 mm Hg, heart rate > 100 beats/min)
- Hemoglobin < 10 g/L
- Active bleeding at the time of endoscopy
- Large ulcer size (>1–3 cm in various studies)
- Ulcer location (posterior duodenal bulb or high lesser gastric curvature)

## RISK SCORES

### Glasgow-Blatchford Score

| *Variable* | *Score* | *Variable* | *Score* |
|---|---|---|---|
| *Blood urea (mmol/L)* | | *Systolic BP (mm Hg)* | |
| 6.5–7.9 | 2 | 100–109 | 1 |
| 8–9.9 | 3 | 90–99 | 2 |
| 10–25 | 4 | <90 | 3 |
| >25 | 6 | *Other markers* | |
| *Hb for men (g/L)* | | Pulse ≥ 100 | 1 |
| 120–129 | 1 | Presentation with melena | 1 |
| 100–119 | 3 | Presentation with syncope | 2 |
| <100 | 6 | Hepatic disease | 2 |
| *Hb for women* | | Cardiac failure | 2 |
| 100–119 | 1 | | |
| <100 | 6 | | |
| Score > 6—intervention required (blood transfusion or endoscopic) | | | |

### Rockall Score

| *Rockall Scoring System* | | | | |
|---|---|---|---|---|
| Variables | Score = 0 | Score = 1 | Score = 2 | Score = 3 |
| Age (Years) | <60 | 60–79 | >80 | |
| Comorbidity | | | Congestive heart failure, ischemic heart disease | Renal failure, liver disease, metastatic disease |
| Shock | No shock | Pulse > 100 bpm | SBP < 100 mm Hg | |
| Source of bleeding | Mallory-Weiss tear | All other diagnosis, e.g., esophagitis, gastritis, peptic ulcer disease, variceal bleed | Malignancy | |
| Stigmata of recent bleeding | None | | Adherent clot or spurting vessel | |
| Score < 5—Risk of recurrent bleeding < 14.1%; risk of death < 5.3%<br>Score > 5—Risk of recurrent bleeding > 24.1%; risk of death > 10.8%<br>(SBP: systolic blood pressure) | | | | |

## MANAGEMENT: VARICEAL VERSUS NONVARICEAL BLEED

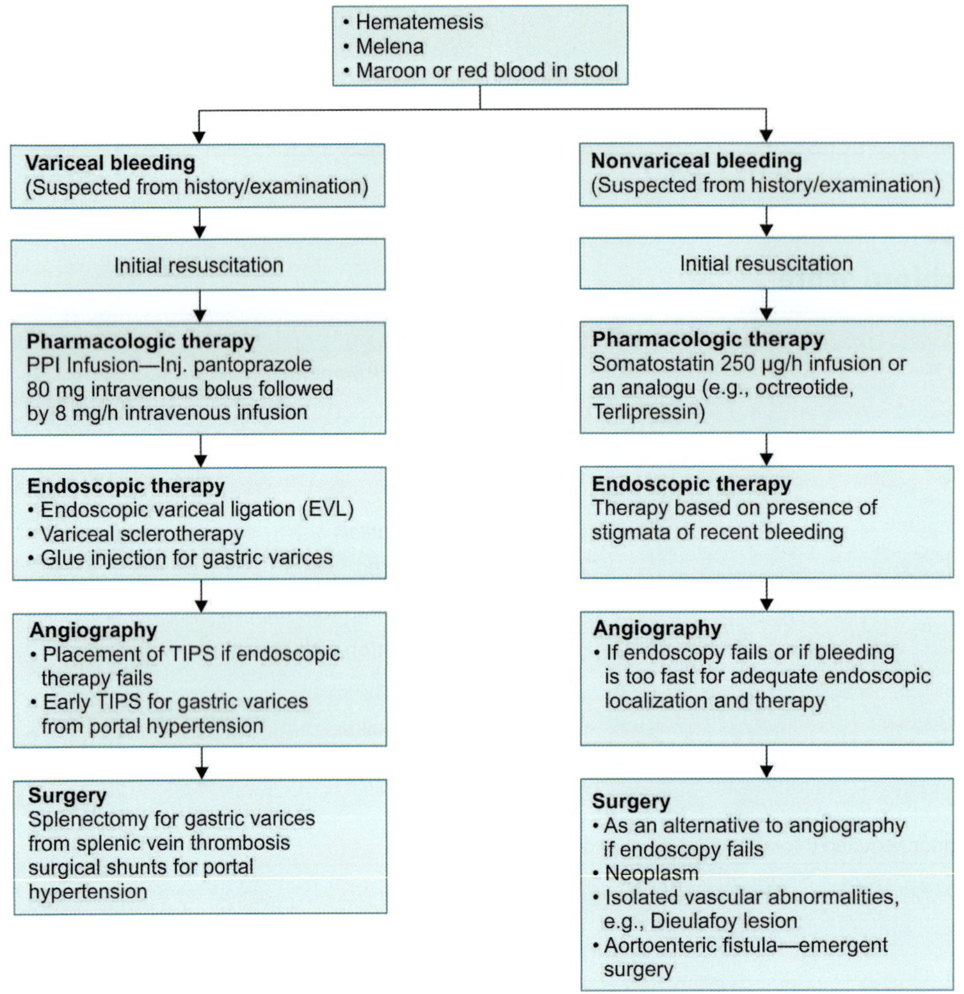


(TIPS: transjugular intrahepatic portosystemic shunt)

## MANAGEMENT OF PEPTIC ULCERS

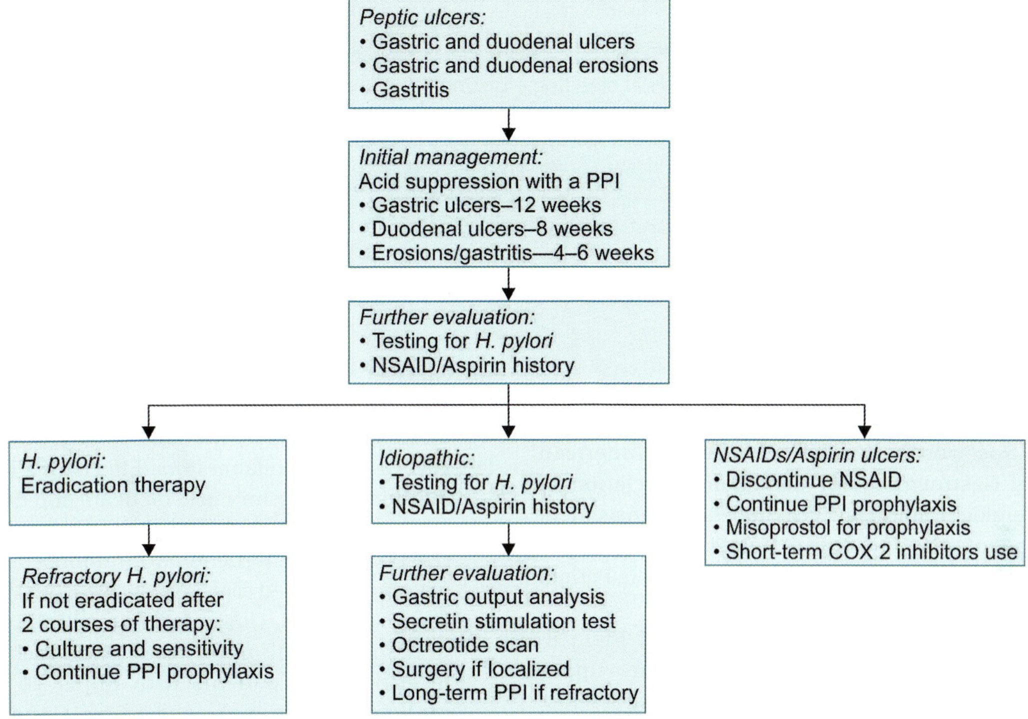


### Balloon Tamponade

- *Indications:*
  - Temporary control of variceal bleeding (gastric esophageal or both)
  - Access to endoscopic or radiologic therapy not immediately available, to stabilize patient for transport
- *Equipment:*
  - Tube:
    - Sengstaken-Blakemore tube
    - Minnesota tube
    - Linton-Nachlas tube
  - Tube clamps
  - Surgical scissors
  - Topical anesthetics
  - Tube connectors
  - Syringes
  - Traction system
- Technique
- Patient needs to be intubated and sedated
- Insert lubricated tube through mouth and confirm the position radiographically
- Fill gastric lumen with air (typically 450-500 mL), clamp air inlet
- If esophageal inflation is required, inflate esophageal balloon to 30-45 mm Hg pressure
- Traction can be applied if bleeding persists
- Deflate balloons every 5–6 hours for 5 minutes to reduce the risk of pressure necrosis

## ENDOSCOPIC PREDICTORS OF RECURRENT PEPTIC ULCER HEMORRHAGE

| *Endoscopic stigmata of recent hemorrhage* | *Prevalence (%)* | *Risk of rebleeding on medical management (%)* |
|---|---|---|
| Active arterial bleeding (Forrest Ia) | 12 (Arterial bleeding + oozing) | 55 (Arterial bleeding + oozing) |
| Oozing without visible vessel (Forrest Ib) | | |
| Nonbleeding visible vessel (Forrest IIa) | 8 | 43 |
| Adherent clot (Forrest IIb) | 8 | 22 |
| Flat spot (Forrest IIc) | 16 | 10 |
| Clean ulcer base (Forrest III) | 55 | 5 |

## SUGGESTED READING


1. Abraham NS, Barkun AN, Sauer BG, Douketis J, Laine L, Noseworthy PA, Telford JJ, et al. American College of Gastroenterology-Canadian Association of Gastroenterology Clinical Practice Guideline: Management of Anticoagulants and Antiplatelets During Acute Gastrointestinal Bleeding and the Periendoscopic Period. Am J Gastroenterol. 2022;117:542.
2. Adão D, Gois AF, Pacheco RL, Pimentel CF, Riera R. Erythromycin prior to endoscopy for acute upper gastrointestinal haemorrhage. Cochrane Database Syst Rev. 2023;2:CD013176.
3. Barkun AN, Almadi M, Kuipers EJ, Laine L, Sung J, Tse F, et al. Management of Nonvariceal Upper Gastrointestinal Bleeding: Guideline Recommendations From the International Consensus Group. Ann Intern Med. 2019;171:805.
4. Blatchford O, Murray WR, Blatchford M. A risk score to predict need for treatment for upper-gastrointestinal haemorrhage. Lancet. 2000;356:1318.
5. Carson JL, Guyatt G, Heddle NM, Grossman BJ, Cohn CS, Fung MK, et al. Clinical Practice Guidelines From the AABB: Red Blood Cell Transfusion Thresholds and Storage. JAMA. 2016;316:2025.
6. Cooper GS, Chak A, Connors AF Jr, Harper DL, Rosenthal GE. The effectiveness of early endoscopy for upper gastrointestinal hemorrhage: a community-based analysis. Med Care. 1998;36:462.
7. de Franchis R, Bosch J, Garcia-Tsao G, Reiberger T, Ripoll C; Baveno VII Faculty. Baveno VII-Renewing consensus in portal hypertension. J Hepatol. 2022;76:959.
8. Gralnek IM, Ching JY, Maza I, Wu JC, Rainer TH, Israelit S, et al. Capsule endoscopy in acute upper gastrointestinal hemorrhage: a prospective cohort study. Endoscopy. 2013;45:12.
9. Gralnek IM, Stanley AJ, Morris AJ, Camus M, Lau J, Lanas A, et al. Endoscopic diagnosis and management of nonvariceal upper gastrointestinal hemorrhage (NVUGIH): European Society of Gastrointestinal Endoscopy (ESGE) Guideline - Update 2021. Endoscopy. 2021;53:300.
10. Guo CLT, Wong SH, Lau LHS, Lui RNS, Mak JWY, Tang RSY, et al. Timing of endoscopy for acute upper gastrointestinal bleeding: a territory-wide cohort study. Gut. 2022;71:1544.
11. HALT-IT Trial Collaborators. Effects of a high-dose 24-h infusion of tranexamic acid on death and thromboembolic events in patients with acute gastrointestinal bleeding (HALT-IT): an international randomised, double-blind, placebo-controlled trial. Lancet. 2020;395:1927.
12. Hayat U, Lee PJ, Ullah H, Sarvepalli S, Lopez R, Vargo JJ. Association of prophylactic endotracheal intubation in critically ill patients with upper GI bleeding and cardiopulmonary unplanned events. Gastrointest Endosc. 2017;86:500.
13. Jung DH, Huh CW, Kim NJ, Kim BW. Optimal endoscopy timing in patients with acute variceal bleeding: A systematic review and meta-analysis. Sci Rep. 2020;10:4046.
14. Jutabha R, Jensen DM. Management of upper gastrointestinal bleeding in the patient with chronic liver disease. Med Clin North Am. 1996;80:1035.
15. Kaplan DE, Ripoll C, Thiele M, Fortune BE, Simonetto DA, Garcia-Tsao G, et al. AASLD Practice Guidance on risk stratification and management of portal hypertension and varices in cirrhosis. Hepatology. 2024;79:1180.
16. Karakonstantis S, Tzagkarakis E, Kalemaki D, Lydakis C, Paspatis G. Nasogastric aspiration/lavage in patients with gastrointestinal bleeding: A review of the evidence. Expert Rev Gastroenterol Hepatol. 2018;12:63.
17. Laine L, Barkun AN, Saltzman JR, Martel M, Leontiadis GI. ACG Clinical Guideline: Upper Gastrointestinal and Ulcer Bleeding. Am J Gastroenterol. 2021;116:899.
18. Laine L, Jensen DM. Management of patients with ulcer bleeding. Am J Gastroenterol. 2012;107:345.
19. Laine L, Laursen SB, Zakko L, Dalton HR, Ngu JH, Schultz M, et al. Severity and Outcomes of Upper Gastrointestinal Bleeding With Bloody Vs. Coffee-Grounds Hematemesis. Am J Gastroenterol. 2018;113:358.
20. Lau JYW, Yu Y, Tang RSY, Chan HCH, Yip HC, Chan SM, et al. Timing of Endoscopy for Acute Upper Gastrointestinal Bleeding. N Engl J Med. 2020;382:1299.
21. Laursen SB, Oakland K, Laine L, Bieber V, Marmo R, Redondo-Cerezo E, et al. ABC score: a new risk score that

accurately predicts mortality in acute upper and lower gastrointestinal bleeding: an international multicentre study. Gut. 2021;70:707.

22. Odutayo A, Desborough MJ, Trivella M, Stanley AJ, Dorée C, Collins GS, et al. Restrictive versus liberal blood transfusion for gastrointestinal bleeding: a systematic review and meta-analysis of randomised controlled trials. Lancet Gastroenterol Hepatol. 2017;2:354.
23. O'Donoghue ML, Murphy SA, Sabatine MS. The Safety and Efficacy of Aspirin Discontinuation on a Background of a P2Y12 Inhibitor in Patients After Percutaneous Coronary Intervention: A Systematic Review and Meta-Analysis. Circulation. 2020;142:538.
24. Pallin DJ, Saltzman JR. Is nasogastric tube lavage in patients with acute upper GI bleeding indicated or antiquated? Gastrointest Endosc. 2011;74:981.
25. Rockey DC, Ahn C, de Melo SW Jr. Randomized pragmatic trial of nasogastric tube placement in patients with upper gastrointestinal tract bleeding. J Investig Med. 2017;65:759.
26. Stanley AJ, Laine L, Dalton HR, Ngu JH, Schultz M, Abazi R, et al. Comparison of risk scoring systems for patients presenting with upper gastrointestinal bleeding: international multicentre prospective study. BMJ. 2017;356:i6432.
27. Villanueva C, Colomo A, Bosch A, Concepción M, Hernandez-Gea V, Aracil C, et al. Transfusion strategies for acute upper gastrointestinal bleeding. N Engl J Med. 2013;368:11.
28. Vimonsuntirungsri T, Thungsuk R, Nopjaroonsri P, Faknak N, Pittayanon R. The Efficacy of Metoclopramide for Gastric Visualization by Endoscopy in Patients With Active Upper Gastrointestinal Bleeding: Double-Blind Randomized Controlled Trial. Am J Gastroenterol. 2024;119:846.
29. Zakko L, Rustagi T, Douglas M, Laine L. No Benefit From Platelet Transfusion for Gastrointestinal Bleeding in Patients Taking Antiplatelet Agents. Clin Gastroenterol Hepatol. 2017;15:46.

CHAPTER 57

# Acute Severe Pancreatitis

## DEFINITION

Acute pancreatitis diagnosis requires at least two of the following features:

1. Characteristic abdominal pain
2. Biochemical evidence of pancreatitis (SERM AMYLASE/LIPASE > 3 TIMES)
3. Radiologic evidence of pancreatitis

Severe acute pancreatitis (SAP) is defined as persistent organ failure including respiratory, cardiovascular or renal. It is associated with pancreatic and extra pancreatic complications and high mortality as high as 85%.[1]

## CLINICAL FEATURES

1. Fever, tachycardia, abdominal pain, jaundice
2. Uncommon findings in severe necrotizing pancreatitis include Cullen's sign, grey turner sign, erythematous skin nodules

*Clinical course:* Develops in two phases

1. 1-2 weeks - Pro inflammatory response results in SIRS (Severe Inflammatory Response Syndrome).
2. More than 2 weeks - transitions from pro to anti-inflammatory response. During this duration, the patient is at higher risk of translocation of intestinal flora due to intestinal barrier failure.[1]

Diagnosis of acute severe pancreatitis is established with classification, Revised Atlanta[2] classification and determinant bases classification of acute pancreatitis (WES guidelines 2019).[3]

## SEVERITY GRADING

| ***Revised Atlanta classification (RAC) 2012*** | ***Determinant-based classification (DBC)*** |
|---|---|
| *Mild acute pancreatitis* | |
| No organ failure | *Mild AP* |
| No local or systemic complications | No organ failure or no peripancreatic necrosis |
| *Moderated severe AP* | *Moderate AP* |
| Transient organ failure (<48 hour) | Transient organ failure AND/OR |
| Local/systemic complications without persistent organ failure | Sterile per/pancreatic necrosis |
| *Severe AP* | *Severe AP* |
| Persistent single or multiple organ failure >48 hour | Persistent organ failure or |
| | Infected peri pancreatic necrosis |
| | *Critical AP* |
| | Persistent organ failure and infected peripancreatic necrosis |

## DIAGNOSIS

### Laboratory Parameters

1. Raised serum amylase and lipase by three times upper limit.
2. CRP >150 mg/L on day 3 can be used as a prognostic factor for severe pancreatitis.
3. Hematocrit >44% represents an independent risk factor for pancreatic necrosis.
4. Urea >20 mg/dL—independent risk factor for mortality.
5. Procalcitonin is the most sensitive lab test for detection of pancreatic infection and low serum values indicate negative predictors of infected necrosis.

## IMAGING

1. USG Abdomen should be performed on admission to rule out etiology of acute pancreatitis mainly biliary pancreatitis.

2. *CT scan*: Patient with severe pancreatitis needs to be assessed with contrast enhanced CT or MRI, optimal timing is 72–96 hours after onset of symptoms.[4]

If CTSI > 3, follow-up CT scan is advised 7–10 days from initial scan, additional scans are recommended if clinical condition deteriorates or if invasive intervention are planned.

## CT SEVERITY INDEX (MODIFIED BALTHAZAR)[4]

| *CT grade* | *Grade score* | *Definitions* |
|---|---|---|
| A | 0 | Normal pancreas |
| B | 1 | Pancreatic enlargement |
| C | 2 | Pancreatic inflammation and or peri-pancreatic fat |
| D | 3 | Single peripancreatic fluid collection |
| E | 4 | >2 or more fluid collections or retroperitoneal air |
| *% of Necrosis* | *Necrosis score* | *Definition* |
| None | 0 | Uniform pancreatic enhancement |
| Less than 30% | 2 | Nonenhancement of regions of gland equivalent in size of pancreatic head |
| 30-50% | 4 | Nonenhancement of 30–50% of the gland |
| More than 50% | 6 | Nonenhancement of >50% of the gland |
| CT Severity index | Morbidity | Mortality |
| 0–1 | 0 | 0 |
| 2–3 | 8% | 3% |
| 4–6 | 35% | 6% |
| 7–10 | 92% | 17% |

1. Endoscopic ultrasound (EUS)—assessment of choledocholithiasis, helps in categorizing patients who require ERCP.[5]
2. MRCP may replace ERCP in diagnostic evaluation, should be considered to screen for common bile duct stones and to screen for occult common bile ducts in patients with unknown etiology.

## RISK ASSESSMENT

1. **BISAP SCORE—**BED SIDE INDEX OF SEVERITY OF ACUTE PANCREATITIS—most accurate and applicable for prediction severity, death, and organ dysfunction
2. Ranson criteria 3 or more score within 48 hours of onset
3. 9 or more on APACHE 2 criteria

| ***BISAP score—one point for each of the following criteria*** | |
|---|---|
| Blood urea nitrogen >25 mg/dL | |
| Impaired mental status | |
| Systemic inflammatory response syndrome is present | |
| Age >60 years | |
| BISAP Score <2 | 0–0.5% Mortality |
| BISAP Score =2 | 2% Mortality |
| BISAP Score >3 | 5–20% Mortality |

## MANAGEMENT OF SEVERE ACUTE PANCREATITIS

### Medical Management[6]

- Routine prophylactic antibiotics are not recommended but always recommended for severe pancreatitis.[7]
- Serum procalcitonin is useful in predicting risk of development of severe pancreatitis.
- Patient should be shifted to ICU if organ dysfunction occurs/ SIRS response present.
- Early fluid resuscitation is indicated to maintain organ perfusion guided by hemodynamic assessment.
- Enteral nutrition is recommended to prevent gut failure , both gastric route and jejunal feed can be delivered safely. If enteral is not tolerated, partial TPN can be used for support.
- Adequate pain management including NSAIDS, epidural analgesia, patient-controlled analgesia.
- Monitor intra-abdominal pressure.
- Appropriate antibiotics penetrating necrosis should be used. Broad spectrum antibiotics should include gram positive and gram-negative microorganism.
- Routine antifungal is not recommended , although candida species are common in patients and indicate high risk of mortality.
- Fine needle-guided aspiration for gram stain and culture may help in confirmation of infected pancreatitis and drive antibiotic therapy.

## IMAGE-GUIDED PERCUTANEOUS TREATMENT

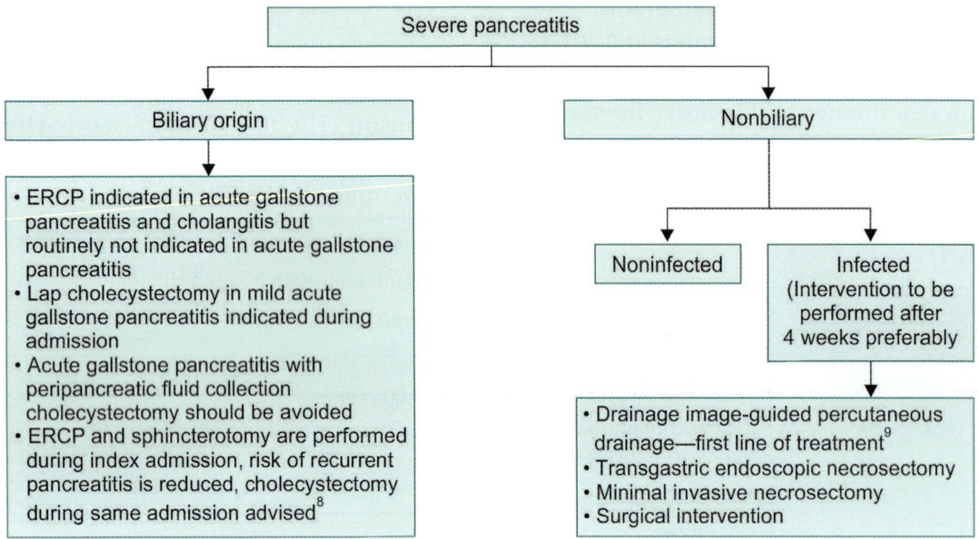


### Surgical Approach

*Indications*

1. Continuum step-up approach after percutaneous/endoscopic procedure with same indication
2. Abdominal compartment syndrome
3. Acute on-going bleeding when endovascular is unsuccessful
4. Bowel fistula extending in peripancreatic collection
5. Bowel ischemia extending intraperipancreatic collection

### Surgical Treatment Modalities[10]

| | |
|---|---|
| Open necrosectomy with open packing | Abdomen is left open and repeated debridement done until no residual necrosis and closed by secondary suturing |
| Open necrosectomy with closed packing | After removal of necrosed tissue, abdomen is closed with external drains |
| Open necrosectomy with continuous post operative lavage | Based on insertion of two or more double lumen catheters, repeated open necrosectomy is performed and drains are used for inflow and outflow of lavage |
| Programmed open necrosectomy | After necrosectomy pancreatic bed is packed with sponges and abdomen is closed |

### Open Abdomen Recommendations

- Avoid open abdomen if other strategies can be used to treat severe Intra-abdominal hypertension
- Avoid open abdomen after necrosectomy unless severe IAH
- Avoid debridement or undertaking early necrosectomy if early open abdomen surgery is undertaken
- Recommends the use of negative pressure peritoneal therapy
- Early fascial and or abdominal definitive closure should be planned after cessation of open abdomen or source control or there is no further need for surgical exploration

## COMPLICATIONS AND MANAGEMENT OF SEVERE ACUTE PANCREATITIS[2]

| ***Complications*** | ***Management*** |
|---|---|
| Acute pancreatic fluid collection and necrosis | Percutaneous drainage or endoscopic transmural drainage |
| Infected pancreatic necrosis | • Early surgical intervention (before 3 week) could result in worse prognosis.<br>• Minimal invasive nonsurgical management including drainage of infected necrotic tissue should be considered when conservative management fails<br>• Surgical necrosectomy should be performed in later stage when demarcation between necrotic and vital tissue occurs, carries high risk of bleeding |

*Contd...*

*Contd...*

| ***Complications*** | ***Management*** |
|---|---|
| Pancreatic walled of necrosis (WON) | • Can be located intrapancreatically or extrapancreatically<br>• Symptomatic WON may require minimum invasive treatment strategies |
| Peri pancreatic collection (PPC) | Symptomatic PPC requires endoscopic, and image guided drainage |
| Pancreatic fistula | • Due to disruption of pancreatic duct, Pancreatic juice may spill over causing ascites, pleural effusion, pseudo cyst, or pancreaticoduodenal fistula<br>• ERCP and MRCP utilized as diagnostic tool, managed with TPN and pancreatic secretary inhibitors octreotide<br>• Medical management fails interventions, and surgical therapy is next option |
| Hemorrhage | Due to gastroduodenitis, bleeding peptic ulcer and enzymatic damage of vessels, rupture of aneurysm. Diagnosis by Angio CT, embolization can be performed, may need definitive surgery if method fails |

## SUMMARY

1. Characterized by persistent organ failure and high mortality
2. USG at admission is advised for diagnosis of etiology, CT is indicated for determination of severity score and in case of clinical deterioration
3. Routine ERCP is not indicated, indicated in case of acute gall stones and cholangitis
4. Infected percutaneous necrosis, percutaneous drainage delays surgical intervention
5. Lap cholecystectomy

## REFERENCES


1. Bruennler T, Langgartner J, Lang S, Wrede CE, Klebl F, Zierhut S, et al. Outcome of patients with acute, necrotizing pancreatitis requiring drainage-does drainage size matter? World J Gastroenterol. 2008;14:725-30.
2. Banks PA, Bollen TL, Dervenis C, Gooszen HG, Johnson CD, Sarr MG, et al. Classification of acute pancreatitis—2012: revision of the Atlanta classification and definitions by international consensus. Gut. 2013;62:102-11.
3. Leppäniemi A, Tolonen M, Tarasconi A, Segovia-Lohse H, Gamberini E, Kirkpatrick AW, et al. 2019 WSES guidelines for the management of severe acute pancreatitis. World J Emerg Surg. 2019;14:27.
4. Balthazar EJ. Acute pancreatitis: assessment of severity with clinical and CT evaluation. Radiology. 2002;223:603-13.
5. Freeman ML, Werner J, van Santvoort HC, Baron TH, Besselink MG, Windsor JA, et al. Interventions for necrotizing pancreatitis: summary of a multidisciplinary consensus conference. Pancreas. 2012;41:1176-94.
6. Wada K, Takada T, Hirata K, Mayumi T, Yoshida M, Yokoe M, et al. Treatment strategy for acute pancreatitis. J Hepatobiliary Pancreat Sci. 2010;17:79-86.
7. Werner J, Feuerbach S, Uhl W, Büchler MW. Management of acute pancreatitis: from surgery to interventional intensive care. Gut. 2005;54:426-36.
8. Fölsch UR, Nitsche R, Lüdtke R, Hilgers RA, Creutzfeldt W. Early ERCP and papillotomy compared with conservative treatment for acute biliary pancreatitis. The German Study Group on Acute Biliary Pancreatitis. N Engl J Med. 1997;336:237-42.
9. Maher MM, Lucey BC, Gervais DA, Mueller PR. Acute pancreatitis: the role of imaging and interventional radiology. Cardiovasc Intervent Radiol. 2004;27:208-25.
10. Doctor N, Agarwal P, Gandhi V. Management of severe acute pancreatitis. Indian J Surg. 2012;74:40-6.

CHAPTER 58

# Dysmotile Gut in Critical Care Settings

## OVERVIEW

Dysmotility of the gastrointestinal (GI) tract is a frequent complication in critically ill patients, characterized by delayed gastric emptying, ileus, and impaired bowel function. This dysfunction can result from a variety of factors, including sepsis, surgery, medications (e.g., opioids), and prolonged mechanical ventilation. Early recognition and management are essential to prevent complications such as aspiration, malnutrition, and bowel ischemia.

## SYMPTOMS OF DYSMOTILE GUT

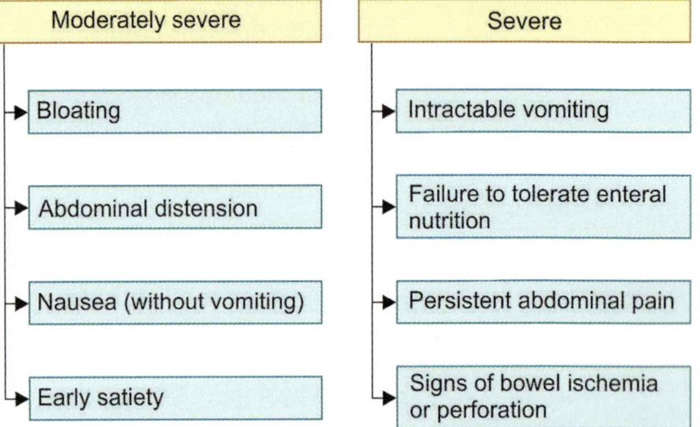


## CLINICAL APPROACH TO DYSMOTILE GUT

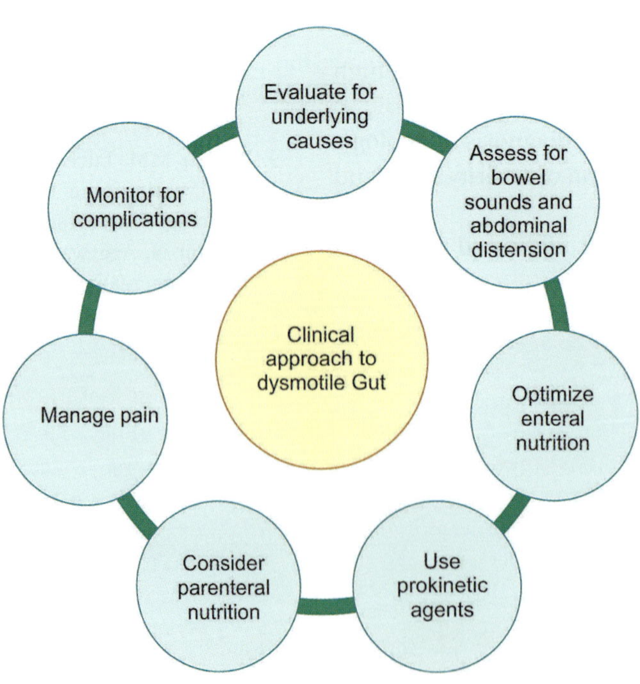

- *Evaluate for underlying causes:* Assess for contributing factors such as medications (e.g., opioids, anticholinergic), electrolyte imbalances (e.g., hypokalemia), or sepsis.
- *Assess for bowel sounds and abdominal distension:* Perform regular physical exams to monitor for changes in bowel sounds and increasing abdominal girth.
- *Optimize enteral nutrition:* Begin with small, continuous feeding rather than bolus feeding to reduce gastric overload. Monitor gastric residual volumes.
- *Use prokinetic agents:* Consider medications like metoclopramide or erythromycin to enhance GI motility. Avoid in cases of suspected bowel obstruction.
- *Consider parenteral nutrition:* If enteral feeding is not tolerated and the patient is at risk of malnutrition, transition to total parenteral nutrition (TPN) while investigating the cause of dysmotility.
- *Manage pain:* Use non-opioid pain management strategies where possible to avoid exacerbating dysmotility.
- *Monitor for complications:* Be vigilant for signs of bowel ischemia, perforation, or aspiration pneumonia. These may necessitate surgical intervention.

## DIAGNOSTIC CRITERIA FOR DYSMOTILITY

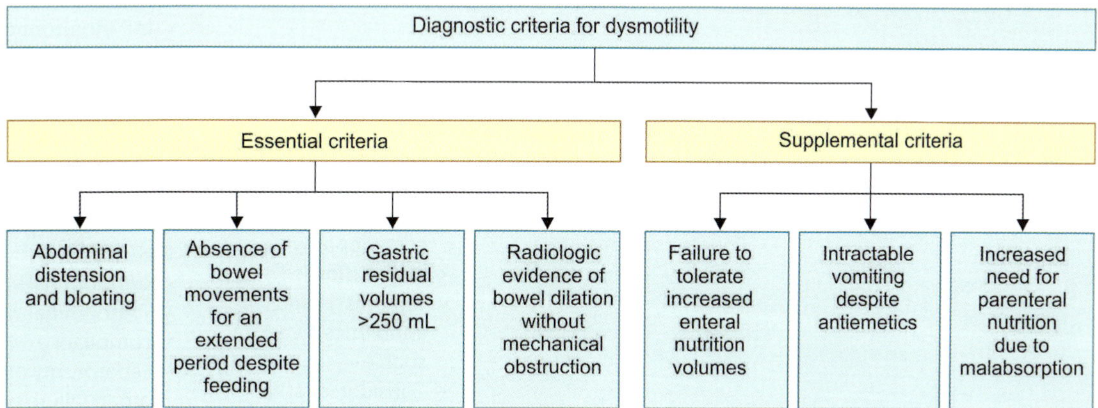


*Algorithm for Management of Dysmotile Gut in Critical Care:*

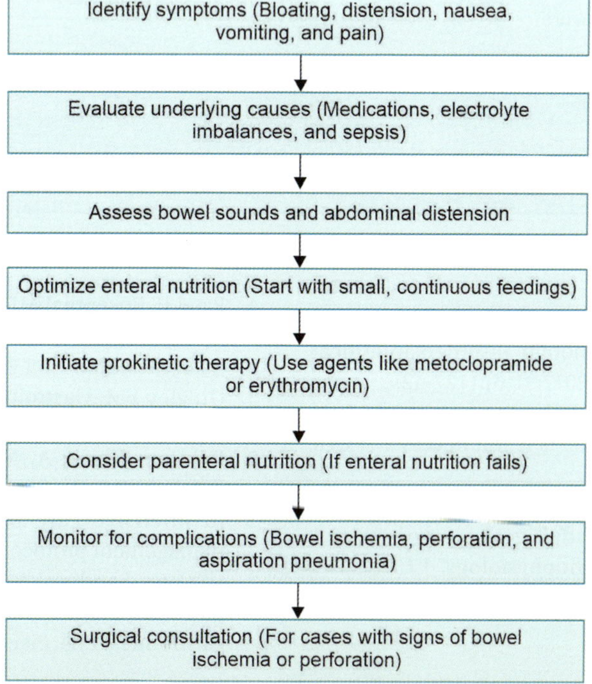

This approach ensures a systematic evaluation and treatment of dysmotile gut in critical care settings, minimizing complications and improving patient outcomes.

Gastrointestinal dysfunction (including dysmotility) management summary

| Nutrition | • *First line:* Oral supplements<br>• *Second line:* Enteral nutrition (EN) and initiate early<br>• *Third line:* Parenteral nutrition: Not before 7 days, or failure of EN | • Estimation of requirements.<br>• *First line:* Indirect calorimetry<br>• *Second line:* Simple weight-based calculation: 20–30 Kcal/kg | • Avoid overfeeding in first 48 hours (*Aim:* <70% of energy requirements)<br>• Aim to reach 80–100% by 7 days.<br>• Aim 1.2– 2.0 gm/ kg per day protein administration | |
|---|---|---|---|---|
| Classification | Gut Dysmotility | Infection | GI bleeding | Disorder of perfusion |
| Preventive measures | • Early enteral nutrition<br>• Consider bowel protocols | Selective digestive decontamination | • Early EN<br>• PPI or H2B for high-risk patients | • Limited fluid resuscitation aiming for euvolemia<br>• IAP monitoring<br>• VTE prophylaxis |
| Management | Gastroparesis<br>• Erythromycin<br>• Metoclopramide<br>• STOP EN only if GRV > 550 mL | Gut derived sepsis<br>• Supportive<br>• Broad-spectrum antibiotics or targeted to culture positivity<br>• Source control | Active bleeding (any cause)<br>• Blood products if active uncontrolled bleeding: Hb <7.0 gm/dL or coagulopathy<br>• PPI infusion<br>• Terlipressin and antibiotics if variceal source<br>• Consider invasive procedures:<br>– Endoscopic<br>– Interventional<br>– Surgical | • Limited fluid resuscitation aiming Euvolemia<br>• IAP monitoring<br>• VTE prophylaxis |
| | Ileus<br>• Conservative Measures | | | IAH/ACS<br>• ↓Abdominal volume<br>• ↑Abdominal wall compliance<br>• Laparotomy only if new organ failure persistent+ Severe IAH |
| | Acute pseudo-obstruction<br>• Conservative measure<br>• Neostigmine<br>• Endoscopic<br>• Decompression | | | Bowel Ischemia<br>• Consider anticoagulation or endovascular intervention<br>• Targeted vasodilator therapy for nonocclusive disease<br>• Transmural ischemia mandates laparotomy |

## SUGGESTED READING


1. Camilleri M. Gastrointestinal motility disorders in critical illness. Clin Gastroenterol Rev. 2017;31(6):1127-42.
2. Chapman MJ, Nguyen NQ. Monitoring gastric residual volumes in critically ill patients: Is it still necessary? Crit Care Med. 2018;46(9):1603-08.
3. Nguyen NQ, Chapman M. Gastrointestinal dysmotility in critically ill patients: Bridging the gap between clinical management and pathophysiology. J Crit Care. 2019;46:75-83.
4. Patel JJ, Rosenthal MD. Clinical implications of dysmotility and management in critical care: A focus on nutrition and outcomes. Nutr Clin Pract. 2020;35(4):591-602.
5. Quigley EM. Gastrointestinal motility and critical illness. World J Gastroenterol. 2017;23(18):3311-3323.
6. Reintam-Blaser A, Malbrain ML, Starkopf J, Fruhwald S, Jakob SM, De Waele J, et al. Gastrointestinal function in intensive care patients: A systematic review and management protocol. Crit Care. 2017;21(1):1-12.
7. Vázquez-Sandoval A, Ghamande S, Surani S. Critically ill patients and gut motility: Are we addressing it? World J Gastrointest Pharmacol Ther. 2017;8(3):174-9.

CHAPTER **59**

# Enteral and Parenteral Nutritional Support in Intensive Care Unit

## INDICATION OF NUTRITIONAL SUPPORT

- Any patient unable to accept adequate oral feed
- At high risk of malnutrition

## NUTRITIONAL RISK ASSESSMENT (USE ANY OF THE FOLLOWING TOOLS)

- *Nutrition risk in critically ill (NUTRIC) score:* Specifically designed for critically ill patients, IL6 optional
- Nutrition risk screening (NRS)-2002
- Malnutrition universal screening tool (MUST)
- Nutritional risk index (NRI)
- *Subjective global assessment:* Weight loss, dietary intake, gastrointestinal (GI) symptoms, functional status, disease severity and comorbidities, muscle, and fat wasting

High nutritional risk patients in ICU:

- Intensive care unit (ICU) stay for >2 days
- Mechanical ventilation
- Sepsis
- Underfed for >5 days
- Severe chronic disease

## CONTRAINDICATIONS TO ENTERAL NUTRITIONAL SUPPORT

- Uncontrolled shock (high vasopressor dose and rising lactate)
- Uncontrolled hypoxemia/acidosis
- Active upper GI bleed
- Bowel ischemia
- High-output intestinal fistula without distal feeding access
- Abdominal compartment syndrome
- Gastric residual volume (GRV) >500 mL/6h

## PRINCIPLES OF NUTRITIONAL SUPPORT (AND TROUBLESHOOTING FEED INTOLERANCE)

- If patient can take orally, encourage—should cover 70% of need by day 7
- If oral intake is not possible, start early enteral nutrition (EN) support (within 48 hours) in critical patients
- If oral/EN contraindicated, start parenteral nutrition (PN) within 3–7 days (or earlier if severely malnourished)
- Consider supplementary PN if EN goal is not achieved by day 7
- Gastric route—standard
- Continuous administration preferred over intermittent bolus—less diarrhea
- No need to routinely measure GRV, measure only if intolerance suspected
- In case of gastric intolerance (GRV >500 mL/6 h)—trial of prokinetics (IV erythromycin +/- metoclopramide) for maximum 72 hours
- Postpyloric feeding—refractory gastric intolerance/high aspiration risk
- Use standard polymeric formula over semielemental/elemental formula

## TIMING OF PARENTERAL NUTRITIONAL SUPPORT

- Early trials showed higher incidence of infective complications with early PN.
- Later trials (with lower calorie target) show no difference in infective complications.
- Start PN early in patients with long-term contraindications to oral/EN.
- Start PN early in severely malnourished patients with short-term contraindications to EN.
- Consider supplemental PN if EN goals are not achieved by day 7.

## DOSE OF NUTRITIONAL SUPPORT

- Resting energy expenditure (REE) is calculated from indirect calorimetry, volumetric capnography, or weigh-based equations (approximately 25–30 kcal/kg/day).
- Avoid overfeeding during acute phase (1st week) of critical illness.
- *Day 1–3:* Do not exceed 70% REE (endogenous energy production).
- *Day 3–7:* Gradually increase to 80–100% of REE.
- *Protein requirement:* 1.2–2 g/kg/day
- Use adjusted body weight for obese individuals.
- Monitor blood glucose, serum electrolytes (K, Mg, and P) during initiation phase.
- *Refeeding hypophosphatemia (phosphate <2 mg/dL of fall by >0.5 mg/dL):* Restrict energy intake for 48 hours)

Algorithm for initiation of nutritional support in hospitalized patients:

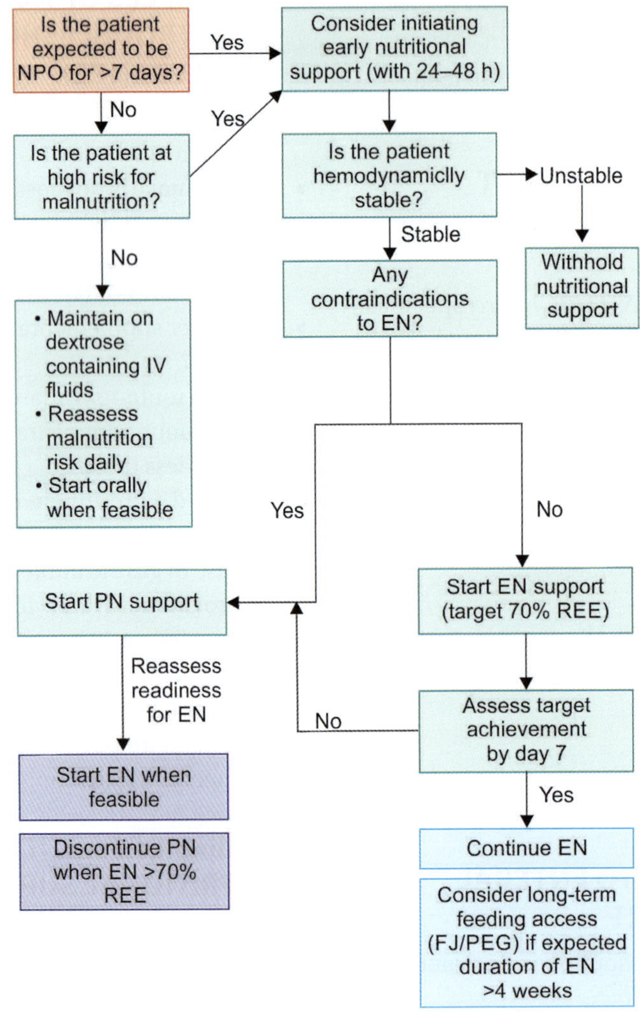

## SUGGESTED READING


1. Compher C, Bingham AL, McCall M, et al. Guidelines for the provision of nutrition support therapy in the adult critically ill patient: The American Society for Parenteral and Enteral Nutrition. JPEN J Parenter Enteral Nutr 2022; 46:12.
2. da Silva JSV, Seres DS, Sabino K, et al. ASPEN Consensus Recommendations for Refeeding Syndrome. Nutr Clin Pract 2020; 35:178.
3. Gudivada KK, Kumar A, Sriram K, et al. Antioxidant micronutrient supplements for adult critically ill patients: A bayesian multiple treatment comparisons meta-analysis. Clin Nutr ESPEN 2022; 47:78.
4. Lee ZY, Lew CCH, Ortiz-Reyes A, et al. Benefits and harm of probiotics and synbiotics in adult critically ill patients. A systematic review and meta-analysis of randomized controlled trials with trial sequential analysis. Clin Nutr 2023; 42:519.
5. McClave SA, Taylor BE, Martindale RG, et al. Guidelines for the Provision and Assessment of Nutrition Support Therapy in the Adult Critically Ill Patient: Society of Critical Care Medicine (SCCM) and American Society for Parenteral and Enteral Nutrition (A.S.P.E.N.). JPEN J Parenter Enteral Nutr 2016; 40:159.
6. Mirtallo JM, Ayers P, Boullata J, et al. ASPEN Lipid Injectable Emulsion Safety Recommendations, Part 1: Background and Adult Considerations. Nutr Clin Pract 2020;35:769.
7. Nakamura K, Kihata A, Naraba H, et al. β-Hydroxy-β-methylbutyrate, Arginine, and Glutamine Complex on Muscle Volume Loss in Critically Ill Patients: A Randomized Control Trial. JPEN J Parenter Enteral Nutr 2020; 44:205.
8. Pradelli L, Mayer K, Klek S, et al. ω-3 Fatty-Acid Enriched Parenteral Nutrition in Hospitalized Patients: Systematic Review With Meta-Analysis and Trial Sequential Analysis. JPEN J Parenter Enteral Nutr 2020; 44:44.
9. Qu J, Xu X, Xu C, et al. The effect of intermittent versus continuous enteral feeding for critically ill patients: a meta-analysis of randomized controlled trials. Front Nutr 2023;10:1214774.
10. Schaller SJ, Scheffenbichler FT, Bein T, et al. Guideline on positioning and early mobilisation in the critically ill by an expert panel. Intensive Care Med 2024; 50:1211.
11. TARGET Investigators, for the ANZICS Clinical Trials Group, Chapman M, Peake SL, et al. Energy-Dense versus Routine Enteral Nutrition in the Critically Ill. N Engl J Med 2018; 379:1823.
12. Viana MV, Becce F, Pantet O, et al. Impact of β-hydroxy-β-methylbutyrate (HMB) on muscle loss and protein metabolism in critically ill patients: A RCT. Clin Nutr 2021; 40:4878.

CHAPTER 60

# Total Parenteral Nutrition

## INTRODUCTION

Feeding nutritionally compromised patients has never been as easy, or as hard, as it is today. We are able to provide nutrients parenterally and enterally to patients who once would have been considered "unfeedable." Today's inpatient population is sicker than patients in the past; the same may be said for patients needing specialized nutrition support. This results in challenges to clinicians caring for these patients. Our goal in writing this chapter is to provide a succinct and easy-to-follow guide for the practicing clinician.

## ABSOLUTE INDICATIONS

*Parenteral nutrition is usually indicated in the following situations:*

- Documented inability to absorb adequate nutrients via the GI tract such as:
    - Massive small-bowel resection/short bowel syndrome
    - Radiation enteritis
    - Severe diarrhea
    - Untreatable steatorrhea/malabsorption (i.e., small bowel disease, i.e., celiac disease)
- Complete bowel obstruction, or intestinal pseudo-obstruction
- Severe catabolism with or without malnutrition when GI tract is not usable within 5–7 days
- Inability to obtain enteral access
- Inability to provide sufficient nutrients/fluids enterally
- Pancreatitis accompanied by abdominal pain with jejunal delivery of nutrients
- Persistent GI hemorrhage
- Acute abdomen/ileus
- Lengthy GI work-up requiring NPO status for several days in a malnourished patient
- High output enterocutaneous fistula (>500 mL) and inability to gain enteral access distal to the fistula site
- Trauma requiring repeat surgical procedures

## RELATIVE INDICATIONS

- Enterocutaneous fistula
- Inflammatory bowel disease not responding to medical therapy
- Hyperemesis gravidarum when nausea and vomiting persist longer than 5–7 days and enteral nutrition is not possible
- Partial small bowel obstruction
- Intensive chemotherapy/severe mucositis
- Major surgery/stress when enteral nutrition not expected to resume within 7–10 days
- Intractable vomiting when jejunal feeding is not possible
- Chylous ascites or chylothorax when low fat/fat-free EN does not adequately decrease output

## CONTRAINDICATIONS FOR PARENTERAL NUTRITION

- Functioning gastrointestinal tract
- Treatment anticipated for <5 days in patients without severe malnutrition
- Inability to obtain venous access
- A prognosis that does not warrant aggressive nutrition support
- When the risks of PN are judged to exceed the potential benefits

## DAILY ENERGY AND SUBSTRATE GUIDELINES FOR ADULT PARENTERAL NUTRITION

| Nutrient | Acute care | Critical care |
|---|---|---|
| Energy | 25–30 total kcals/kg/d | 25 total kcals/kg/d |
| • Refeeding<br>• Obesity (≥130% IBW) | • 15–25 kcal/kg/d<br>• 15–20 kcal/kg/ adjusted weight | • 15–25 kcal/kg/d<br>• 15–20 kcal/kg/d adjusted weight |
| Protein | • 0.8–1.0 g/kg/d maintenance<br>• 1.2–2.0 g/kg/d catabolism | 1.5–2.2 g/kg/d |
| Dextrose | <7 g/kg/d | <5 g/kg/d |
| Lipid | <2.5 g/kg/d | 0.4–0.75 g/kg/d |

## REVIEW OF ACCESS DEVICES FOR TOTAL PARENTERAL NUTRITION

The selection of an appropriate access device is crucial for the successful administration of total parenteral nutrition (TPN). The choice of device depends on the duration of therapy, patient's condition, and clinical requirements. Here is a review of the common access devices used for TPN.

### Central Venous Catheters

*Description:* Central venous catheters (CVCs) are long, flexible tubes inserted into a large central vein, typically in the chest (subclavian vein) or neck (internal jugular vein). They are used for long-term TPN administration. Infuse solutions >900 mOsm/L (central solutions range from ~1,500–2,800 mOsm/L).

- *Types:*
  - *Nontunneled CVCs:* Inserted directly into the central vein. Used for short-term access (usually less than 1–2 weeks)
  - *Tunneled CVCs (e.g., Hickman, Broviac):* Inserted into the central vein and tunneled under the skin to the insertion site; designed for long-term use (weeks to months or more)
  - *Implanted ports (e.g., Port-a-Cath):* A device implanted under the skin with a catheter leading to a central vein. Suitable for long term use and minimizes infection risk.
- *Advantages:*
  - *Long-term use:* Suitable for extended TPN therapy
  - *High-flow rate:* Allows for the infusion of large volumes and high-osmolarity solutions.
  - *Reliable access:* Provides stable and reliable access to the central venous system.
- *Disadvantages:*
  - *Infection risk:* Increased risk of catheter-related infections
  - *Complications:* Potential complications include catheter occlusion, thrombosis, and mechanical issues.

### Peripheral Venous Catheters

*Description:* Inserted into a peripheral vein, usually in the arm. Typically used for short-term or less aggressive TPN therapy.

- *Types:*
  - *Peripheral short-term catheters:* Inserted for a few days to a week
  - *Peripheral midline catheters:* Longer than short-term catheters and can be used for up to 2–4 weeks. Inserted into a vein in the upper arm and can reach veins near the shoulder.
- *Advantages:*
  - *Simplicity:* Easier and quicker to insert compared to central lines
  - *Lower infection risk:* Generally lower risk of infection compared to central lines
- *Disadvantages:*
  - *Short-term use:* Not suitable for long-term TPN due to the risk of vein irritation and phlebitis
  - *Limited flow rates:* Not ideal for high-osmolarity solutions or high-flow rates

## PERIPHERALLY INSERTED CENTRAL CATHETERS

*Description:* Peripherally inserted central catheters (PICCs) are inserted into a peripheral vein in the arm and advanced until the tip resides in a central vein near the heart.

- *Advantages:*
  - *Long-term use:* Suitable for medium to long-term use (weeks to months)

- *Reduced infection risk:* Lower risk of major infections compared to traditional CVCs
- *Versatile:* It can be used for both TPN and other intravenous therapies.

- *Disadvantages:*
  - *Insertion complexity:* Requires skilled insertion and might not be suitable for all patients.
  - *Risk of complications:* Potential complications include thrombosis and catheter occlusion.

### Implanted Ports

*Description:* A device implanted under the skin with a catheter leading to a central vein. The port is accessed through the skin with a special needle.

- *Advantages:*
  - *Long-term use:* Suitable for long-term use with minimal external components
  - *Reduced infection risk:* Lower risk of infection as the port is completely under the skin
  - *Cosmetic:* Less visible and more comfortable for the patient compared to external catheters
- *Disadvantages:*
  - *Surgical placement:* Requires a minor surgical procedure for implantation
  - *Access:* Requires special needles for access, and regular flushing and maintenance are needed

## CHOOSING THE APPROPRIATE ACCESS DEVICE

*Factors to consider:*

- *Duration of therapy:* Short-term versus long-term needs
- *Patient condition:* Any contraindications, risk of infection, or coagulation issues
- *Flow rates and osmolarity:* High-osmolarity solutions may require central venous access.
- *Patient preferences:* Comfort and lifestyle considerations

*Milliosmoles of selected additives:*

- Additive mOsm/Unit
- Sterile Water 0.00

*Dextrose Options (3.4 cal/g)*

- Dextrose 5, 10, 30, 50, 70% ~5 mOsm/g

*Amino acid options (4 cal/g)*

- Amino Acid 8.5, 10, 15% ~10 mOsm/g

*Intravenous fat emulsion (IVFE) options*

- 10% (1.1 cal/mL)
- 20% (2.0 cal/mL) ~0.280 mOsm/mL
- 30% (3.0 cal/mL)

*Micronutrients*

- Calcium gluconate 0.662 mOsm/mEq
- Magnesium sulfate 1 mOsm/mEq
- Multi-trace elements (MTE-5) 0.36 mOsm/mL
- MVI infusion concentrate (MVI-12) 41.1 mOsm/dose
- Potassium acetate 2 mOsm/mEq
- Potassium chloride 2 mOsm/mEq
- Potassium phosphate 2.47 mOsm/mM
- Sodium acetate 2 mOsm/mEq
- Sodium chloride 2 mOsm/mEq
- Sodium phosphate 4.0 mOsm/mM

## PERIPHERAL PARENTERAL NUTRITION "VEIN PROTECTOR"

- Hydrocortisone, 15 mg
- Heparin, 1,500 units
- *Plus:* Transdermal nitroglycerin (NTG) patch, 0.1 mg/hour

## CRITERIA FOR USE OF PERIPHERAL PARENTERAL NUTRITION

- Nutritional needs <1,800 kcals per day
- Patient requires <10–14 days of intravenous nutrition
- Peripheral venous access is available (good peripheral veins)
- Requires only one intravenous line with intravenous fat emulsion (IVFE) administration via piggyback infusion.
- Fluid restriction is not an issue

## ADVANTAGES AND DISADVANTAGES OF THE TOTAL NUTRIENT ADMIXTURE (3-IN-1) SYSTEM

*Advantages:*

- All components aseptically compounded by the pharmacy
- Preparation is more efficient for pharmacy personnel, especially if automated
- Less manipulation of the system during administration
- Less risk of contamination during administration

- Less nursing time needed for one bag/d and no piggyback to administer
- Less supply and equipment expense for only one pump and IV tubing
- More convenient storage, fewer supplies, easier administration in home care settings
- Glucose and venous access tolerance maybe better in some situations
- Possible applications in fluid-restricted patients
- Maybe more cost-effective overall in certain settings

*Disadvantages:*
- Larger particle size of admixed lipid emulsion precludes use of 0.22-micron (bacteria-eliminating) filter and requires larger pore size filter of 1.2 microns.
- Admixed lipid emulsion is less stable, more prone to separation of lipid components.
- Admixtures are more sensitive to destabilization with certain electrolyte concentrations or the addition of iron.
- Difficult to visualize precipitate or particulate material in the opaque admixture.
- Certain medications are incompatible with lipid emulsion portion of admixture.
- Catheter occlusion is more common with daily lipid administration.
- Less attractive in pediatric settings due to pH and compatibility considerations.

## SUGGESTED MONITORING FOR PARENTERAL NUTRITION (IN-PATIENT)

| *Parameter* | *Baseline* | *Initiation* | *Critically ill* | *Stable patients* |
|---|---|---|---|---|
| CBC with differential | Yes | Daily × 3 Day 1 | Weekly | Weekly |
| PT and PTT | Yes | Day 1 | Weekly | Weekly |
| Basic chemistry—Na, K, Cl, $CO_2$, | Yes | Day 1 | Daily | 1–2 times per week |
| BUN, creatinine | Yes | Daily | As needed | Weekly |
| Magnesium, calcium, phosphorus | Yes | As needed | As needed | As needed |
| Serum triglycerides | Yes | Daily | Daily | 1–2 times per week |
| Serum glucose | Yes | Daily | 3 × day until consistently <150 mg/dL | As needed |
| Capillary glucose | Q 6 hours × 48 hours; stop if WNL | Day 1 | | 2–3 times per week<br>As needed |
| Weight | Yes | | Daily | Monthly |
| Intake and output | Yes | | Daily | As needed |
| ALT, AST, ALP, total bilirubin | Yes | | Weekly | |
| Nitrogen balance | As needed | | As needed | |

## COMPLICATIONS OF LONG-TERM PARENTERAL NUTRITION

### Problem 1: Fatty Liver

*Possible causes:*
- *Exact etiology unknown. Theories include:* Overfeeding of dextrose and/or total calories; overfeeding of fat; EFAD; carnitine deficiency, and choline deficiency

*Symptoms:* Elevation of LFTs

*Treatment/prevention:*
- Avoid overfeeding
- Do not exceed recommended dosages of macronutrients (*See* Table below)
- Enteral nutrition as soon as possible (even if trophic)
- Enteric antibiotics if blind loops/bacterial overgrowth possible
- Add Taurine to PN

### Problem 2: Cholestasis

*Possible causes:* Exact etiology unknown. Theories include lack of nutrition in the bowel leading to decreased bile stimulation and impaired bile flow; overfeeding of glucose, lipid, and/or amino acids; toxic tryptophan metabolites, and choline deficiency.

*Symptoms:* Elevated alkaline phosphatase; progressive increase in total bilirubin

*Treatment/prevention:*
- Avoid overfeeding
- Do not exceed recommended dosages of macronutrients (*See* Table below)

- Enteral nutrition as soon as possible
- Enteric antibiotics if blind loops/bacterial overgrowth possible

### Problem 3: Gastrointestinal Atrophy

*Possible causes:* Atrophy of villi in the GI tract due to lack of enteral nutrients

*Symptoms:* Observed in vitro; in vivo only symptom maybe enteric bacteremia and sepsis without clear source.

*Treatment/prevention:* Enteral/oral nutrition concurrent or as soon as possible

## SUMMARY

- Determine if PN is truly indicated.
- Assess the patient (medical/surgical history, review drug/medication profile, anthropometric data, and lab values).
- Determine need for long-term versus short-term <7–10 days IV access.
- Determine estimated kcal, protein, and lipid needs
  - 20–30 kcal/kg
  - Protein 0.8–1.5 gm/kg
    - Higher levels may be needed in severe catabolic states
  - Lipid to provide ≤30% of kcals

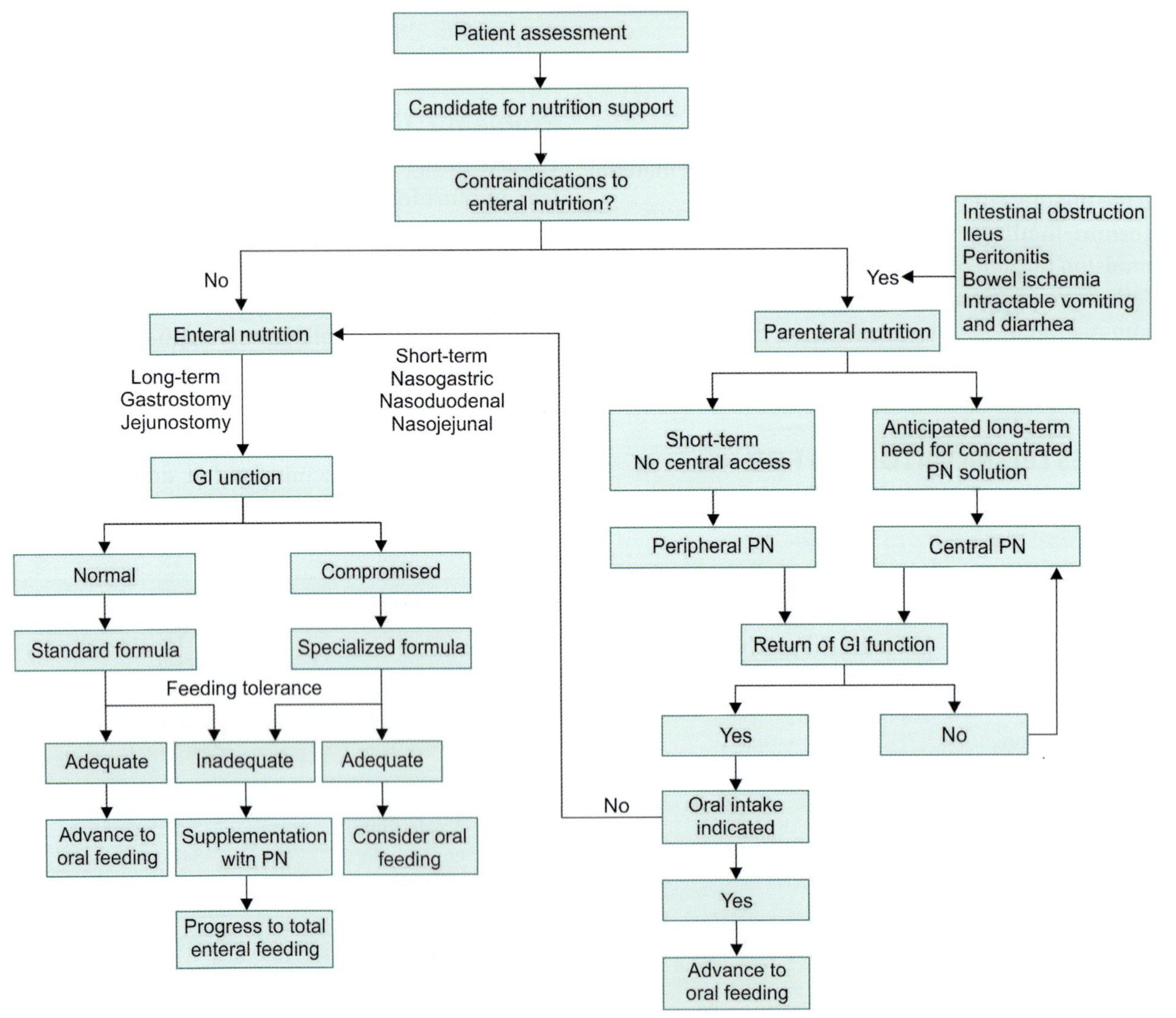

- Determine initial electrolyte, vitamin, and trace element requirements; consider ongoing losses
- Consider any additional additives to PN formulation including insulin and H2-antagonists
- Monitor for:
    - Risk of refeeding syndrome
    - Glucose intolerance
        - If so initiate feeding at a low dextrose level and advance cautiously as lab values are stable. If not, then attempt to advance to goal within the first 24–48 hours.
- Initiate trophic feedings or convert patient to PO or enteral feeding when feasible.

## SUGGESTED READING


1. Braunschweig CL, Levy P, Sheean PM, Wang X. Enteral compared with parenteral nutrition: A meta-analysis. Am J Clin Nutr. 2001;74(4):534-42.
2. Cerra FB, Benitez MR, Blackburn GL, Irwin RS, Jeejeebhoy K, Katz DP, et al. Applied nutrition in ICU patients. A consensus statement of the American College of Chest Physicians. Chest. 1997;111(3):769-77.
3. Frankenfield D. Energy and macro substrate requirements. In: Gottschlich MM (Ed). The Science and Practice of Nutrition Support: A Case-based Core Curriculum. Dubuque, IA: Kendall/Hunt Publishing Co.; 2001. p. 36.
4. Grimm H, Tibell A, Norrlind B, Blecher C, Wilker S, Schwemmle K. Immunoregulation by parenteral lipids: Impact of the n-3 to n-6 fatty acid ratio. JPEN J Parent Enteral Nutr. 1994;18(5):417-21.
5. Haber LM, Hawkins EP, Seilheimer DK, Saleem A. Fat overload syndrome. An autopsy study with evaluation of the coagulopathy. Am J Clin Pathol. 1988;90(2):223-7.
6. Heyland DK, Dhaliwal R, Drover JW, Gramlich L, Dodek P. Canadian clinical practice guidelines for nutrition support in mechanically ventilated, critically ill adult patients. JPEN J Parent Enteral Nutr. 2003;27(5):355-73.
7. Infusion Nurses Society. Infusion Nursing Standards of Practice. J Infus Nurs. 2006;29(1 Suppl):S1-92.
8. Khawaja HT, Williams JD, Weaver PC. Transdermal glyceryl trinitrate to allow peripheral total parenteral nutrition: a double-blind placebo controlled feasibility study. J Royal Soc Med. 1991;84(2):69-72.
9. Krenitsky J. Adjusted body weight, pro: evidence to support the use of adjusted body weight in calculating calorie requirements. Nutr Clin Pract. 2005;20(4):468-73.
10. Lipman TO. The chicken soup paradigm. J Parenter Enteral Nutr. 2003;27:93-9.
11. Mirtallo JM. Introduction to Parenteral Nutrition. In: Gottschlich MM, Ed. The Science and Practice of Nutrition Support: A Case-Based Core Curriculum. Dubuque, IA: Kendall/Hunt Publishing Co.; 2001. p. 217.
12. O'Grady NP, Alexander M, Dellinger EP, Gerberding JL, Heard SO, Maki DG, et al. Guidelines for the prevention of intravascular catheter-related infections. MMWR Recomm Rep. 2002;51(RR-10):1-29.
13. Roongpisuthipong C, Puchaiwatananon O, Songchitsomboon S, Kanjanapanjapol S. Hydrocortisone, heparin, and peripheral intravenous infusion. Nutrition. 1994;10(3):211-3.
14. Safe Practices for Parenteral Nutrition Formulations. National Advisory Group on Standards and Practice Guidelines for Parenteral Nutrition. JPEN J Parent Enteral Nutr. 1998;22(2):49-66.
15. Tighe MJ, Wong C, Martin IG, McMahon MJ. Do heparin, hydrocortisone, and glyceryl trinitrate influence thrombophlebitis during full intravenous nutrition via a peripheral vein? JPEN J Parent Enteral Nutr. 1995;19(6):507-9.
16. Tokars JI, Cookson ST, McArthur MA, Boyer CL, McGeer AJ, Jarvis WR. Prospective evaluation of risk factors for bloodstream infection in patients receiving home infusion therapy. Ann Inter Med. 1999;131(5):340-7.
17. Veterans Affairs Total Parenteral Nutrition Cooperative Study Group. Perioperative total parenteral nutrition in surgical patients. N Engl J Med. 1991;325(8):525-32.
18. Von Allmen D, Fisher JF. Metabolic Complications. In: Fischer JF (Ed). Total Parenteral Nutrition. 2nd edition. Boston, MA: Little Brown Company; 1991.

CHAPTER 61

# Fulminant Hepatic Failure

## DEFINITION

Fulminant hepatic failure (FHF) or acute liver failure (ALF) is a life-threatening condition that occurs in patients with no preexisting liver disease and is characterized by liver injury, coagulopathy [international normalized ratio (INR) >1.5], and hepatic encephalopathy.

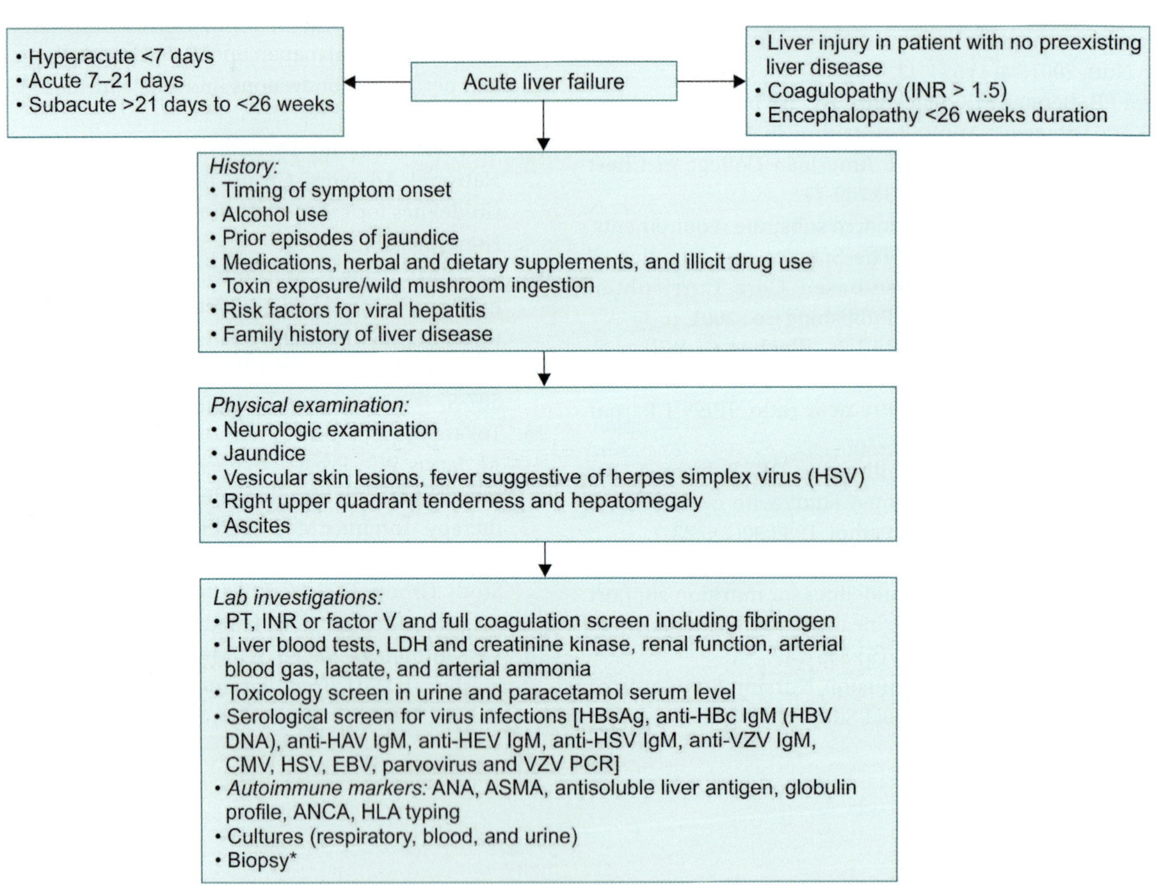


* Through transjugular approach to rule out underlying chronic liver disease, malignancies or alcohol-induced liver disease, and Wilson disease.

## SYMPTOMS

| |
|---|
| Fatigue/malaise/lethargy |
| Anorexia, nausea and/or vomiting |
| Right upper quadrant pain |
| Jaundice |
| Pruritus |
| Abdominal distension from ascites |

## NEUROLOGIC EXAMINATION

Hepatic encephalopathy (HE)

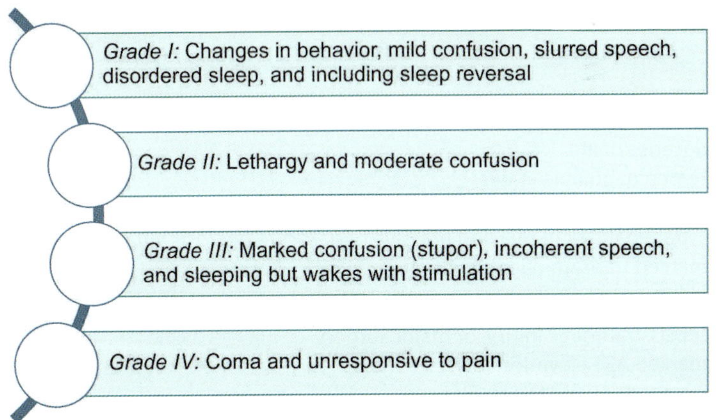


| *Etiology* | *Clinical features* | *Treatment* |
|---|---|---|
| Acetaminophen toxicity | • Rapid progression with hypoglycemia, lactic acidosis, and renal failure<br>• Very high aminotransferase levels (>3,500 international units/L), low bilirubin, and high INR | • *IV NAC:* 150 mg/kg loading dose, then 50 mg/kg IV over 4 hours, then 100 mg/kg IV over 16 hours as a continuous infusion<br>• *Oral NAC:* 140 mg/kg loading dose, then 70 mg/kg every 4 hours |
| Idiosyncratic drug-induced liver injury | Not necessarily dose-dependent, and latency period is highly variable Antimicrobials followed by complementary and alternative medications are the most common culprits | Discontinue offending agent Consider NAC for early coma Corticosteroids for those with hypersensitivity or autoimmune features |
| Viral hepatitis | • Hepatitis A, B, and E virus infections are the most common causes.<br>• Laboratory-marked transaminase elevation<br>• Viral prodrome with symptoms of acute gastroenteritis | • *HSV:* Acyclovir<br>• *CMV:* Ganciclovir<br>• *Hep B:* Entecavir/tenofovir |
| Pregnancy-related | Hemolysis, elevated liver enzymes, and low platelet (HELLP) syndrome and acute fatty liver of pregnancy (AFLP) | Delivery of fetus |
| Autoimmune hepatitis | • Marked transaminase elevation, accompanied by elevated antinuclear antibody, antismooth muscle actin antibody, and elevated IgG levels.<br>• Characteristic findings on liver biopsy include centrilobular hemorrhagic necrosis and confluent necrosis | *Methylprednisolone:* 60 mg/day IV |

*Contd...*

*Contd...*

| *Etiology* | *Clinical features* | *Treatment* |
|---|---|---|
| Wilson disease | • Transaminase elevation and normal or very low alkaline phosphatase<br>• Coombs-negative hemolytic anemia with features of acute intravascular hemolysis and rapid progression to renal failure<br>• Alkaline phosphatase (international units/L) to total bilirubin (mg/dL) ratio <4, rapidly progressive renal failure, and low uric acid levels | • Continuous hemofiltration<br>• Plasma exchange |
| Mushroom poisoning | Mostly associated with ingestion of Amanita species with marked transaminase elevation. Patient presents with severe gastroenteritis symptoms 6–12 hours after ingestion | • *Charcoal:* Via NGT every 4 hours alternating with silymarin<br>• *Penicillin G:* 1 g/kg/day IV and NAC (dosing as for acetaminophen overdose)<br>• *Silymarin:* 300 mg PO/NGT every 12 hours |
| Budd–Chiari syndrome | • Most commonly affects women in their fourth to fifth decades of life.<br>• Hypercoagulable states<br>• Obstruction of hepatic venous outflow tract causes severe intrahepatic ischemia and massive hepatocyte necrosis with marked transaminase elevation | • Heparin as initial therapy in the absence of contraindications to anticoagulation<br>• TIPS is the preferred intervention in those who fail anticoagulation |
| Ischemic liver injury | • Often occurs in the setting of congestive heart failure, sepsis, traumatic injury, or major surgery<br>• marked AST elevation (25–250 times)<br>• Elevated serum LDH levels<br>• Bilirubin and INR often worsen despite improvement in transaminase levels | Restoration of hemodynamic |
| Malignant infiltration | • Lymphoma, leukemia, breast cancer, and colon cancer are the most common causes<br>• Patients often present with abdominal pain, jaundice, hepatic encephalopathy, and hepatomegaly | |

Differentiation of ALF versus acute on chronic liver failure (ACLF).

| | *ALF* | *ACLF* |
|---|---|---|
| Chronic liver disease | Absent | Present signs of portal hypertension |
| Precipitating factors (by frequency) | Drug-induced liver injury, viral hepatitis, and autoimmune hepatitis | Infection, alcohol, and GI bleeding |
| Clinical signs | Liver injury, INR.1.5, and HE | Coagulopathy, elevated bilirubin, shock, and multiorgan dysfunction |
| Liver biopsy | Necrosis and collapse | Fibrosis |
| CNS | • Increased intracranial pressure<br>• Use CRRT early for HE | HE responds to lactulose/rifaximin |
| Infection | Late (>5 days) | Early (<5 day) |
| Renal failure | Hypoperfusion and ATN | HRS-AKI |
| Liver transplantation | KCC, MELD Status 1A listing | MELD, No priority in MELD system |

## MANAGEMENT

### General Management

| |
|---|
| *Hemodynamic:* Volume resuscitation with crystalloids avoids volume overload, and persistent hypotension requires vasopressor agents (norepinephrine is the vasopressor of choice) |
| *Ventilation:* Standard sedation and lung protective ventilator techniques should be utilized |
| *Nutrition:* Enteral or parenteral nutrition, consider stopping PPI when enteral feeding has been established |
| *Metabolic:*<br>• Hypoglycemia needs to be corrected avoiding hyperglycemia<br>• Hyponatremia should be corrected to maintain concentrations 140–150 mmol/L |
| *Blood product:* The routine use of fresh frozen plasma and other coagulation factors is not recommended<br>Hemoglobin target for transfusion is 7 g/dL |
| Prophylactic antibiotics, nonabsorbable antibiotics, and antifungal is not recommended (may be considered in the setting of clinical deterioration of the patient) |
| • Encephalopathy grades 1 and 2 monitored in ICU, and grade 3 or 4 encephalopathy, intubation should be undertaken<br>• In patients with ALF and grade 2 or higher encephalopathy, we suggest early CRRT for management of hyperammonemia |
| In acute kidney injury, CRRT is preferred over intermittent hemodialysis |
| Mannitol or hypertonic saline should be administered for surges of ICP with consideration for short-term hyperventilation |
| There is no conclusive evidence to recommend for or against the use of lactulose or rifaximin for the treatment of encephalopathy in patients with ALF |

Specific management according to etiology.

### Liver Transplant Criteria

Patients with ALF, potential for deterioration, and who may be candidates for liver transplant, should be transferred to specialist units before the onset of HE to facilitate assessment.

| ***King's College criteria*** | |
|---|---|
| ***Acetaminophen overdose*** | ***Nonacetaminophen overdose*** |
| Arterial pH <7.3<br>Or<br>*All of the following:*<br>1. PT >100 seconds (INR >6.5)<br>2. Creatinine level >3.4 mg/dL<br>3. Grade 3/4 encephalopathy | PT >100 seconds (INR > 6.5)<br>Or<br>*Any 3 of the following:*<br>1. NANB/drug/halothane etiology<br>2. Time from jaundice to encephalopathy >7 days<br>3. Age 40 years<br>4. PT >50 sec (INR >3.5)<br>5. Bilirubin level > 17.4 mg/dL |

| ***MELD score*** |
|---|
| 3.78 [Ln serum bilirubin (mg/dL)] + 11.2 [Ln INR] + 9.57 [Ln serum creatinine (mg/dL)] + 6.43 |
| Utilized to prioritize transplant recipients |
| *In hospitalized patients, the 3 month mortality is:*<br>• *40 or more:* 100% mortality<br>• *30–39:* 83% mortality<br>• *20–29:* 76% mortality<br>• *10–19:* 27% mortality<br>• *<10:* 4% mortality |

## SUGGESTED READING


1. European Association for the Study of the Liver; Clinical practice guidelines panel; Wendon, J; Panel members; Cordoba J, Dhawan A, Larsen FS, Manns M, Samuel D, Simpson KJ, et al; EASL Governing Board representative; Bernardi M. EASL Clinical Practical Guidelines on the management of acute (fulminant) liver failure. J Hepatol. 2017;66(1):1047-81.
2. Lee WM, Stravitz RT, Larson AM. Introduction to the revised American Association for the Study of Liver Diseases position paper on acute liver failure 2011. Hepatology. 2012;55(3):965-7.
3. Nanchal R, Subramanian R, Karvellas CJ, Hollenberg SM, Peppard WJ, Singbartl K, et al. Guidelines for the management of adult acute and acute-on-chronic liver failure in the ICU: Neurology, peri-transplant medicine, infectious disease, and gastroenterology considerations. Crit Care Med. 2020;48(3):657-76.
4. Shingina A, Mukhtar N, Wakim-Fleming J, Alqahtani S, Wong RJ, Limketkai BN, et al. Acute liver failure guidelines. Am J Gastroenterol. 2023;118(7):1128-53.

CHAPTER 62

# Enteral Nutrition

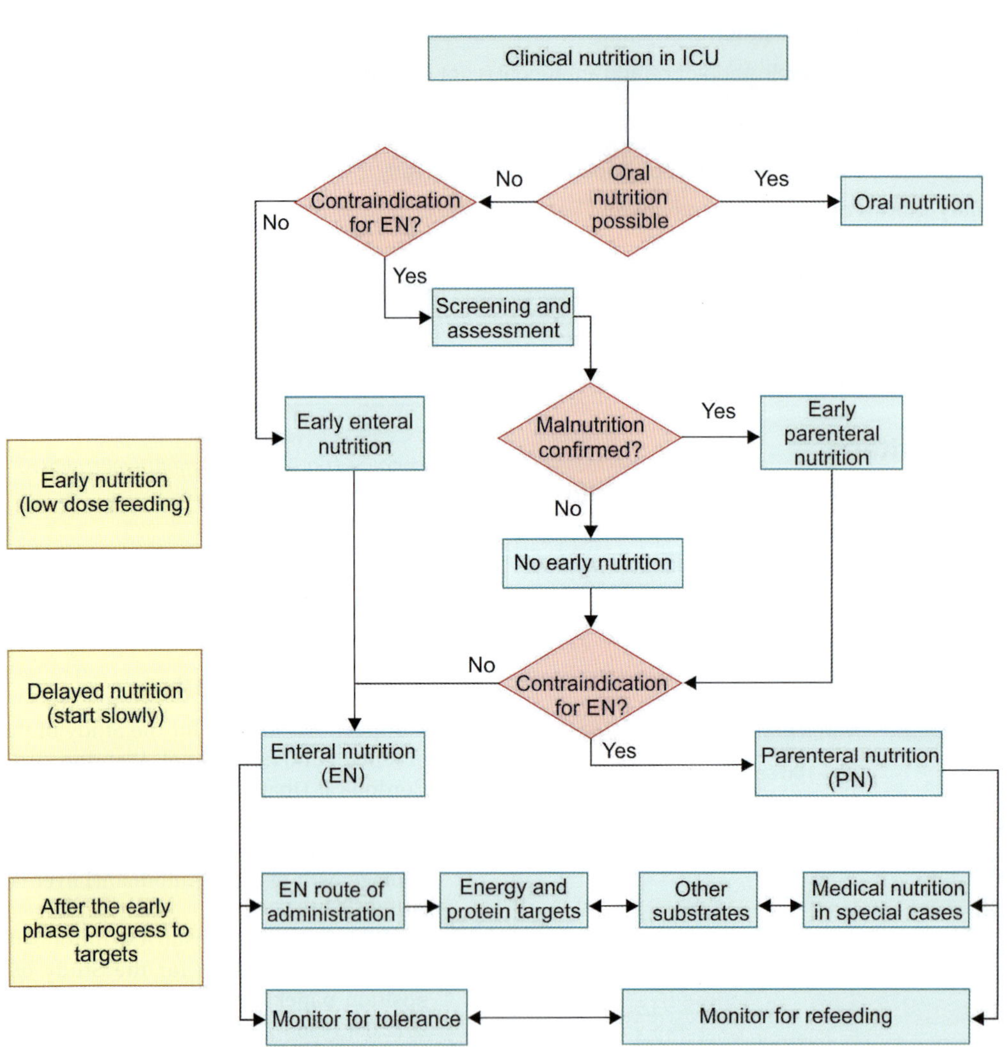

Early medical nutrition (EN/PN)

**Early enteral nutrition**

If oral intake is not possible, early EN (within 48 hours) in critically ill adult patients should be performed/initiated rather than delaying EN (114, 8, 100%)

If oral intake is not possible, early EN (within 48 hours) shall be performed/initiated in critically ill adult patients rather than early PN (R5, A, 100%)

Early EN should be performed
- in patients receiving extracorporeal membrane oxygenation (ecmo)
- in patients with traumatic brain injury
- in patients with stroke (ischemic or hemorrhagic)
- in patients with spinal cord injury
- in patients with severe acute pancreatitis
- in patients after gastrointestinal surgery
- in patients after abdominal aortic surgery
- in patients with abdominal trauma when the continuity of the GI tract is confirmed/restored
- in patients receiving neuromuscular blocking agents
- in patients managed in prone position
- in patients with open abdomen
- regardless of the presence of bowel sounds unless bowel ischemia or obstruction is suspected
- in patients with diarrhea (R40, B, 96%)

**Early parenteral nutrition**

Early and progressive PN can be provided instead of no nutrition in case of contraindications for EN in severely malnourished patients. (R7, 0, 95%)

In patients who do not tolerate full dose EN during the first week in the ICU, the safety and benefits of initiating PN should be weighed on a case-by-case basis. (R20, GPP, 96)

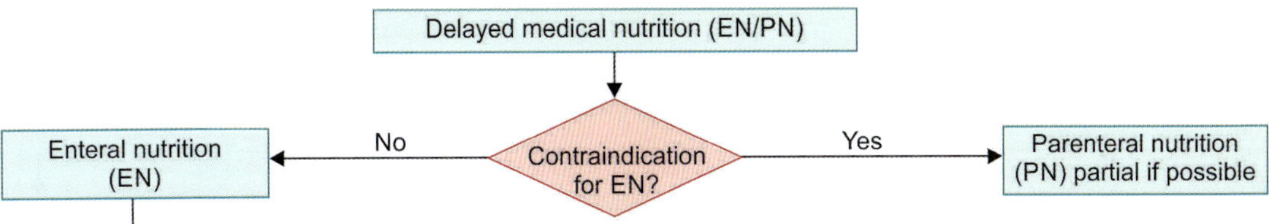


EN should be delayed
- if shock is uncontrolled and hemodynamic and tissue perfusion goals are not reached, whereas low dose EN can be started as soon as shock is controlled with fluids and vasopressors/inotropes, while remaining vigilant for signs of bowel ischemia;
- in case of uncontrolled life-threatening hypoxemia, hypercapnia or acidosis, whereas EN can be started in patients with stable hypoxemia, and compensated or permissive hypercapnia and acidosis;
- in patients suffering from active upper gastrointestinal bleeding, whereas EN can be started when the bleeding has stopped and no signs of re-bleeding are observed;
- in patients with overt bowel ischemia;
- in patients with high-output intestinal fistula if reliable feeding access distal to the fistula is not achievable;
- in patients with abdominal compartment syndrome; and
- if gastric aspirate volume is above 500 mL/6 h. (R38, B, 100%)

Low dose EN should be administered
- in patients receiving therapeutic hypothermia and increasing the dose after rewarming
- in patients with intra-abdominal hypertension without abdominal compartment syndrome, whereas temporary reduction or discontinuation of EN should be considered when intra-abdominal pressure values further increase under EN; and
- in patients with acute liver failure when acute, immediately life-threatening metabolic derangements are controlled with or without liver support strategies, independent on grade of encephalopathy. (R39, B, 96%)

In case of contraindications to oral and EN, PN should be implemented within three to seven days. (R6, B, 89%)

PN should not be started until all reasonable strategies to improve EN tolerance have been attempted. (R21, updated, GPP,100%)

**EN route of administration**

In patients deemed to be at high risk for aspiration, postpyloric, mainly jejunal feeding can be performed. (R12, GPP, 95%)

Continuous rather than bolus EN should be used. (R9, B,95%)

Gastric access should be used as standard approach to initiate EN. (R10, GPP, 100%)

In patients with gastric feeding in-tolerance not solved with prokinetic agents, postpyloric feeding should be used. (R11, B, 100%)

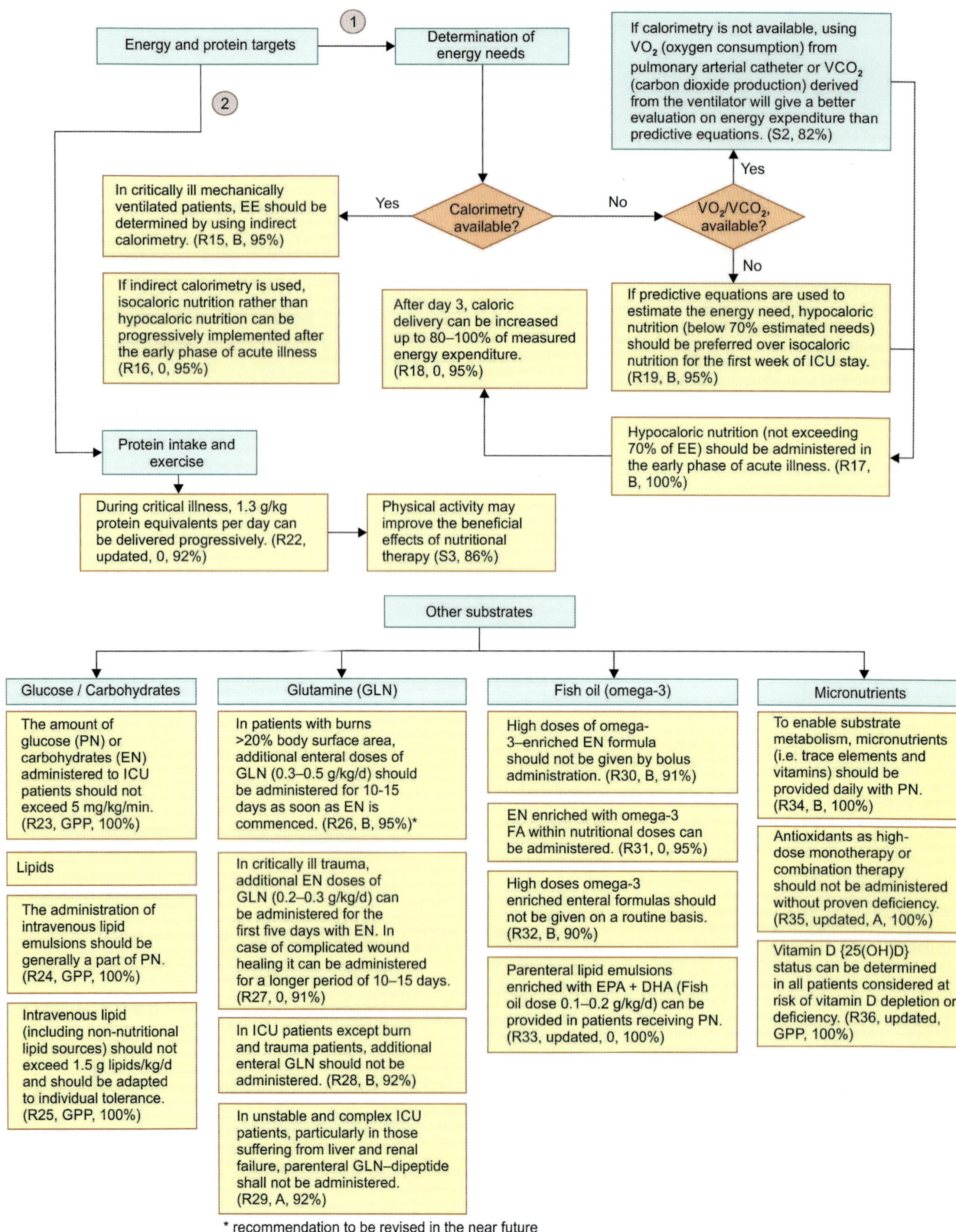


* recommendation to be revised in the near future

## Medical nutrition in special cases

### The non-intubated patient

In non-intubated patients not reaching the energy target with an oral diet, oral nutritional supplements should be considered first and then EN. (R41, GPP, 96%)

In non-intubated patients with dysphagia, texture-adapted food can be considered. If swallowing is proven unsafe, EN should be administered. (R42, GPP, 94%

In non-intubated patients with dysphagia and a very high aspiration risk, postpyloric EN or, if not possible, temporary PN during swallowing training with removed nasoenteral tube can be performed. (R43, GPP, 92%)

### The surgical patient

In patients after abdominal or esophageal surgery, early EN can be preferred over delayed EN. (R45, 0, 96%)

In critically ill patients with surgical complications after abdominal or esophageal surgery and unable to eat orally, EN (rather than PN) should be preferred unless discontinuity or obstruction of GI tract, or abdominal compartment syndrome is present. (R46, GPP, 96%)

In the case of an unrepaired anastomotic leak, internal or external fistula, a feeding access distal to the defect should be aimed for to administer EN. (R47, GPP, 96%)

In the case of an unrepaired anastomotic leak, internal or external fistula, or if distal feeding access is not achieved, EN should be withheld and PN may be commenced. (R48, GPP, 100%)

In case of high output stoma or fistula, the appropriateness of chyme reinfusion or enteroclysis should be evaluated and performed if adequate. (R49, GPP, 100%)

### The trauma patient

Trauma patients should preferentially receive early EN instead early PN. (R50, B, 96%)

#### The septic patient

Early and progressive EN should be used in septic patients after hemodynamic stabilization. If contraindicated, EN should be replaced or supplemented by progressive PN. (R44, GPP, 94%)

### The obese patient

An iso-caloric high protein diet can be administered to obese patients, preferentially guided by indirect calorimetry measurements and urinary nitrogen losses. (R51, 0, 89%)

In obese patients, energy intake should be guided by indirect calorimetry. Protein delivery should be guided by urinary nitrogen losses or lean body mass determination (using computerized tomography or other tools). If indirect calorimetry is not available, energy intake can be based on "adjusted body weigh". If urinary nitrogen losses or lean body mass determination are not available, protein intake can be 1.3 g/kg "adjusted body weight"/d. (R52, GPP, 89%)

## Monitoring of medical nutrition

### Monitor for tolerance, overfeeding and underfeeding

#### Glucose and insulin

Blood glucose should be measured initially (after ICU admission or after artificial nutrition initiation) and at least every four hours, for the first two days in general. (R53, GPP, 93%)

Insulin shall be administered, when glucose levels exceed 10 mmol/L (R54, A, 93%)

#### EN feeding intolerance

In critically ill patients with gastric feeding intolerance, intravenous erythromycin should be used as a first line prokinetic therapy. (R13, B, 100%)

Alternatively, intravenous metoclopramide or a combination of metoclopramide and erythromycin can be used as a prokinetic therapy. (R14, 0, 100%)

### Monitor for refeeding

#### Electrolytes

Electrolytes (potassium, magnesium, phosphate) should be measured at least once daily for the first week. (R55, A, 93%)

#### Refeeding hypophosphatemia

In patients with refeeding hypophosphatemia (<0.65 mmol/L or a drop of >0.16 mmol/L), electrolytes should be measured 2-3 times a days and supplemented if needed. (R56, GPP, 92%)

In patients with refeeding hypophosphatemia energy supply should be restricted for 48 h and then gradually increased. (R57, B, 100%)

## SUGGESTED READING


1. Arabi YM, Preiser JC. A critical view on primary and secondary outcome measures in nutrition trials. Intensive Care Med. 2017;43:1875-7.
2. Bendavid I, Singer P, Theilla M, Themessl-Huber M, Sulz I, Mouhieddine M, et al. Nutrition Day ICU: A 7 year worldwide prevalence study of nutrition practice in intensive care. Clin Nutr. 2017;36:1122-9.
3. Bischoff SC, Singer P, Koller M, Barazzoni R, Cederholm T, van Gossum A. Standard operating procedures for ESPEN guidelines and consensus papers. Clin Nutr. 2015;34:1043-51.
4. Bordeje ML, Montejo JC, Mateu ML, Solera M, Acosta JA, Juan M, et al. Intraabdominal pressure as a marker of enteral nutrition intolerance in critically ill patients. The PIANE study. Nutrients. 2019;11:2616.
5. Cederholm T, Bosaeus I, Barazzoni R, Bauer J, Van Gossum A, Klek S, et al. Diagnostic criteria for malnutrition e an ESPEN consensus statement. Clin Nutr. 2015;34:335-40.
6. Cederholm T, Jensen GL, Correia M, Gonzalez MC, Fukushima R, Higashiguchi T, et al. GLIM criteria for the diagnosis of malnutrition: a consensus report from the global clinical nutrition community. Clin Nutr. 2019;38(1):1-9.
7. Compher C, Bingham AL, McCall M, Patel J, Rice TW, Braunschweig C, et al. Guidelines for the provision of nutrition support therapy in the adult critically ill patient: the American Society for Parenteral and Enteral Nutrition. J Parenter Enter Nutr. 2022;46:12-41.
8. Elke G, van Zanten ARH, Lemieux M, McCall M, Jeejeebhoy KN, Kott M, et al. Enteral versus parenteral nutrition in critically ill patients: an updated systematic review and meta-analysis of randomized controlled trials. Crit Care. 2016;20:117.
9. Ellia M. The 'MUST'report. Nutritional screening for adults: a multidisciplinary responsibility. Redditch: BAPEN; 2003.
10. Jenkins B, Calder PC, Marino LV. A systematic review of the definitions and prevalence of feeding intolerance in critically ill adults. Clin Nutr ESPEN. 2022;49:92-102.
11. Kondrup J. Nutritional risk screening (NRS 2002): A new method based on an analysis of controlled clinical trials. Clin Nutr. 2003;22:321-36.
12. Murthy TA, Plummer MP, Tan E, Chapman MJ, Chapple LAS. Higher versus lower enteral calorie delivery and gastrointestinal dysfunction in critical illness: a systematic review and meta-analysis. Clin Nutr. 2022;41:2185-94.
13. Pardo E, Lescot T, Preiser JC, Massanet P, Pons A, Jaber S, et al. Association between early nutrition support and 28-day mortality in critically ill patients: the FRANS prospective nutrition cohort study. Crit Care. 2023;27:7.
14. Patel JJ, Rosenthal MD, Heyland DK. Intermittent versus continuous feeding in critically ill adults. Curr Opin Clin Nutr Metab Care. 2018;21:116-20.
15. Reignier J, Boisrame-Helms J, Brisard L, Lascarrou JB, Ait Hssain A, Anguel N, et al. Enteral versus parenteral early nutrition in ventilated adults with shock: a randomised, controlled, multicentre, open-label, parallel-group study (NUTRIREA-2). Lancet (London, England). 2018;391: 133-43.
16. Reignier J, Plantefeve G, Mira JP, Argaud L, Asfar P, Aissaoui N, et al. Low versus standard calorie and protein feeding in ventilated adults with shock: a randomised, controlled, multicentre, open-label, parallel-group trial (NUTRIREA-3). Lancet Respir Med. 2023;11:602-12.
17. Reintam Blaser A, Padar M, M€andul M, Elke G, Engel C, Fischer K, et al. Development of the Gastrointestinal Dysfunction Score (GIDS) for critically ill patients e a prospective multicenter observational study (iSOFA study). Clin Nutr 2021;40:4932-40.
18. Reintam Blaser A, Starkopf J, Alhazzani W, Berger MM, Casaer MP, Deane AM, et al. Early enteral nutrition in critically ill patients: ESICM clinical practice guidelines. Intensive Care Med. 2017;43:380-98.
19. Singer P, Blaser AR, Berger MM, Alhazzani W, Calder PC, Casaer MP, et al. ESPEN guideline on clinical nutrition in the intensive care unit. Clin Nutr. 2019;38:48-79.
20. Taylor BE, McClave SA, Martindale RG, Warren MM, Johnson DR, Braunschweig C, et al. Guidelines for the provision and assessment of nutrition support therapy in the adult critically ill patient. Crit Care Med 2016;44: 390-438.
21. Wischmeyer PE. Tailoring nutrition therapy to illness and recovery. Crit Care. 2017;21:316.

CHAPTER

# 63 Decompensated Cirrhosis Management

## CHRONIC LIVER DISEASE OVERVIEW

- *Definition:* Progressive deterioration of liver functions (synthesis of clotting factors, proteins, detoxification, and excretion) for >6 months.
- *Pathophysiology:* Continuous inflammation, destruction, and regeneration of liver parenchyma leading to fibrosis and cirrhosis.

## DECOMPENSATION

*Definition:* Acute deterioration in liver function in a patient with cirrhosis, characterized by:

- Jaundice
- Ascites
- Hepatic encephalopathy
- Hepatorenal syndrome
- Variceal hemorrhage

## INITIAL PATIENT ASSESSMENT

The ABC approach for initial patient assessment is as follows:

- *Airway:*
  - Compromise may occur with severe hepatic encephalopathy (Grade 3 or 4) or large-volume hematemesis.
  - Early intubation and mechanical ventilation may be necessary.
- *Breathing:*
  - Assess for pneumonia, pulmonary edema, hepatic hydrothorax, and splinting of the diaphragm due to ascites.
  - Consider portopulmonary hypertension and hepatopulmonary syndrome.
  - Stabilize as appropriate (oxygen supplementation, intubation, mechanical ventilation, paracentesis, and thoracocentesis).
- *Circulation:*
  - Monitor for hypotension and tachycardia (*causes:* sepsis, hypovolemia, over-diuresis, and GI bleeding).
  - Fluid resuscitation hypovolemic/shocked patients with IV crystalloid or human albumin solution, aiming for MAP >80 mm Hg.
  - Assess hydration status carefully due to intravascular depletion despite peripheral overload.
- *Disability:* Document Glasgow Coma Scale score, encephalopathy grade **(Table 1)**, alcohol withdrawal signs, temperature, and blood glucose levels.
- *Exposure:*
  - Abdominal exam to assess for ascites, tenderness (SBP), and perform a rectal exam for bleeding.
  - Check for signs of infection (cellulitis and septic arthritis) and conduct a neurological exam to rule out other causes of altered mental status.
  - Identify signs of chronic liver disease (muscle atrophy, spider naevi, palmar erythema, caput medusae, and gynecomastia).

**TABLE 1:** Hepatic encephalopathy.

| *Grade of encephalopathy* | *Symptoms/signs* |
|---|---|
| Grade 1 | Trivial lack of awareness, euphoria or anxiety, shortened attention span, and impaired performance of addition or subtraction |
| Grade 2 | Lethargy or apathy, minimal disorientation for time or place, subtle personality change, inappropriate behavior, and asterixis |
| Grade 3 | Somnolence to semistupor, but responsive to verbal stimuli, confusion, and gross disorientation |
| Grade 4 | Coma |

**TABLE 2:** Workup of newly diagnosed decompensated CLD.

| *Etiology* | *Investigations* |
|---|---|
| Viral hepatitis | Serology and PCR |
| Hemochromatosis | Serum iron, ferritin, liver biopsy, and genetic testing |
| Wilson disease | Urine copper, serum ceruloplasmin, liver biopsy, and genetic testing |
| Autoimmune hepatitis | ANA, ASMA, and LKM-1 |
| Alpha 1 antitrypsin deficiency | Decreased alpha one antitrypsin level |
| Primary biliary cirrhosis | Alkaline phosphatase and antimitochondrial antibody |
| Budd–Chiari syndrome | CBC, clotting profile, and imaging studies |
| Alcoholic liver disease | Elevated AST >ALT and history of alcohol intake |
| NAFLD | ALT > AST and ultrasonography |

## INVESTIGATIONS

- *Routine investigations:* Complete blood count (CBC), kidney function test (KFT), liver function test (LFT), and coagulation profile.
- Specific investigation are given in **Table 2**.
- *Radiologic Investigations:* Abdominal ultrasound, Triple phase CT scan, fibro scan, hepatic wedge pressure, endoscopy, EEG, TIPS, and Doppler scan.

## SPECIFIC MANAGEMENT OF DECOMPENSATED CIRRHOSIS

- *Infection:*
  - Common infections include SBP, UTI, pneumonia, and cellulitis (typically Gram-negative bacteria like *E. coli* and gram-positive cocci)[1]
  - Diagnostic ascitic tap for all patients with ascites
  - *Source identification:* Blood culture, chest X-ray/HRCT, fluid analysis, and culture
  - *SBP diagnosis:* Ascitic fluid PMN count >250/mm$^3$ or positive fluid culture[2]
  - Broad-spectrum antibiotics, rationalized by source, antimicrobial, and antimicrobial resistance detection
  - Albumin administration
- *Ascites:*
  - Low albumin content, difference between serum and ascites albumin concentration (SAAG) >1.1g/dL
  - *Salt restriction:* No added salt diet and diuretics for mild/moderate ascites
  - *Diuretics:* Spironolactone and furosemide titrated based on response and renal function
  - *Large volume paracentesis:* For tense ascites, with albumin replacement to prevent hepatorenal syndrome (100 mL 20% albumin for every 2.5 L drained).[3]
  - TIPS
- *Gastrointestinal bleeding:*
  - IV access, fluid resuscitation, and blood product transfusion
  - Coagulopathy, thrombocytopenia correction (FFP, platelets, and cryoprecipitate)
  - Restrictive blood transfusion strategy (target Hb 8.0 g/L)[4]
  - Terlipressin and IV antibiotics for variceal bleeding[5,6]
  - Early endoscopy within 12 hours (variceal band ligation preferred)[7]
  - Endoscopic injection of *N*-butyl-2-cyanoacrylate (glue) for gastric varices
  - Balloon tamponade if bleeding persists
  - Transjugular intrahepatic portosystemic shunt should be considered if hemostasis cannot be achieved endoscopically or the patient rebleeds
  - Nonselective beta-blocker (such as carvedilol 6.25–12.5 mg daily) in addition to variceal band ligation for secondary prophylaxis of variceal bleeds following discharge[5]
- *Hepatic encephalopathy:*
  - Diagnosis based on history and exam, ruling out other causes like SDH and cerebrovascular accident (NCCT Head)
  - Grading of hepatic encephaopathy[8]
  - Correct underlying causes (Infection, constipation, electrolyte disturbances, and TIPS)
  - *Lactulose:* Titrate to achieve 2–3 soft stools/day
  - *Rifaximin:* Added if no response to lactulose
- *Alcohol-related hepatitis:*
  - Syndrome of rapid onset jaundice, liver failure, systemic inflammation, associated with prolonged heavy alcohol consumption
  - *Prognostic score:* Poor prognosis (*Maddrey's discriminant function >32) may be helped by steroids administration
  - *Treatment:* Long-term abstinence, corticosteroids,[9] NAC, and SAMe.

**BOX 1:** Diagnostic criteria for HRS.

- Diagnosis of cirrhosis and ascites
- Diagnosis of AKI
- No response after two consecutive days of diuretics withdrawal and plasma volume expansion with albumin 1 gm/kg body weight
- Absence of shock
- No current and recent nephrotoxic drugs
- No macroscopic sign of parenchymal kidney injury
  - Absence of Proteinuria (>500 mg/day)
  - Absence of microhematuria >50 RBCs/HPF
  - Normal findings in renal ultrasound

- *Hepatopulmonary Syndrome (HPS):*
- *Triad:* Liver dysfunction, intrapulmonary vasodilation, and arterial oxygenation defects
- *Symptoms:* Platypnea (shortness of breath worsening when upright) and orthodeoxia (hypoxia that worsens in the upright position and improves when lying flat)
- Diagnosis: Bubble echocardiography
- *Treatment:* Both portopulmonary hypertension and HPS show improvement following liver transplantation.[10]
- *AKI in Cirrhosis*[11]
  - Begin treatment by correcting hypovolemia with intravenous fluids
  - Administer human albumin solution at a dose of 1 g/kg for 2 days.
    - Use 5% albumin if the patient is hypovolemic.
    - Use 20% albumin if the patient is euvolemic.
    - Avoid 0.9% NS and 5% dextrose

    Stop diuretics, nephrotoxins, and vasodilators to prevent further renal damage.

    Investigate and rule out other intrinsic causes of renal dysfunction.

    If hepatorenal syndrome **(Box 1)** is suspected, add terlipressin at a dose of 0.5–1 mg four times per day.
  - Titrate the dose up to a maximum of 12 mg/day if needed.
  - Administer 20–40 g of albumin per day in combination with terlipressin.

## REFERENCES

1. Bunchorntavakul C, Chamroonkul N, Chavalitdhamrong D. Bacterial infections in cirrhosis: A critical review and practical guidance. World J Hepatol. 2016;8(6):307-21.
2. Rimola A, García-Tsao G, Navasa M, Piddock LJ, Planas R, Bernard B, et al. Diagnosis, treatment, and prophylaxis of spontaneous bacterial peritonitis: A consensus document. International Ascites Club. J Hepatol. 2000;32(1):142-53.
3. Runyon BA; AASLD Practice Guidelines Committee. Management of adult patients with ascites due to cirrhosis: An update. Hepatology. 2009;49(6):2087-107.
4. Villanueva C, Colomo A, Bosch A, Concepción M, Hernandez-Gea V, Aracil C, et al. Transfusion strategies for acute upper gastrointestinal bleeding. N Engl J Med. 2013;368(1):11-21. Erratum in: N Engl J Med. 2013;368(24): 2341.
5. Tripathi D, Stanley AJ, Hayes PC, Patch D, Millson C, Mehrzad H, et al; Clinical Services and Standards Committee of the British Society of Gastroenterology. U.K. guidelines on the management of variceal haemorrhage in cirrhotic patients. Gut. 201;64(11):1680-704.
6. Chavez-Tapia NC, Barrientos-Gutierrez T, Tellez-Avila FI, Soares-Weiser K, Mendez-Sanchez N, Gluud C, et al. Meta-analysis: antibiotic prophylaxis for cirrhotic patients with upper gastrointestinal bleeding - An updated Cochrane review. Aliment Pharmacol Ther. 2011;34(5):509:18.
7. National Institute for Health and Care Excellence. Acute upper gastrointestinal bleeding in over 163: management. NICE clinical guideline No 141. Available from https://www.nice.org.uk/guidance/cg141 [Last accessed February, 2025].
8. Leise MD, Poterucha JJ, Kamath PS, Kim WR. Management of hepatic encephalopathy in the hospital. Mayo Clin Proc. 2014;89(2):241-53.
9. Thursz MR, Richardson P, Allison M, Austin A, Bowers M, Day CP, et al; STOPAH Trial. Prednisolone or pentoxifylline for alcoholic hepatitis. N Engl J Med. 2015;372(17):1619-28.
10. Müller C, Schenk P. Hepatopulmonary syndrome. Wien Klin Wochenschr. 1999;111(9):339-47.
11. Angeli P, Gines P, Wong F, Bernardi M, Boyer TD, Gerbes A, et al; International Club of Ascites. Diagnosis and management of acute kidney injury in patients with cirrhosis: revised consensus recommendations of the International Club of Ascites. Gut. 2015;64(4):531-7.

CHAPTER 64

# Drug-induced Liver Injury

## DEFINITION

An adverse toxic drug reaction resulting in liver injury.

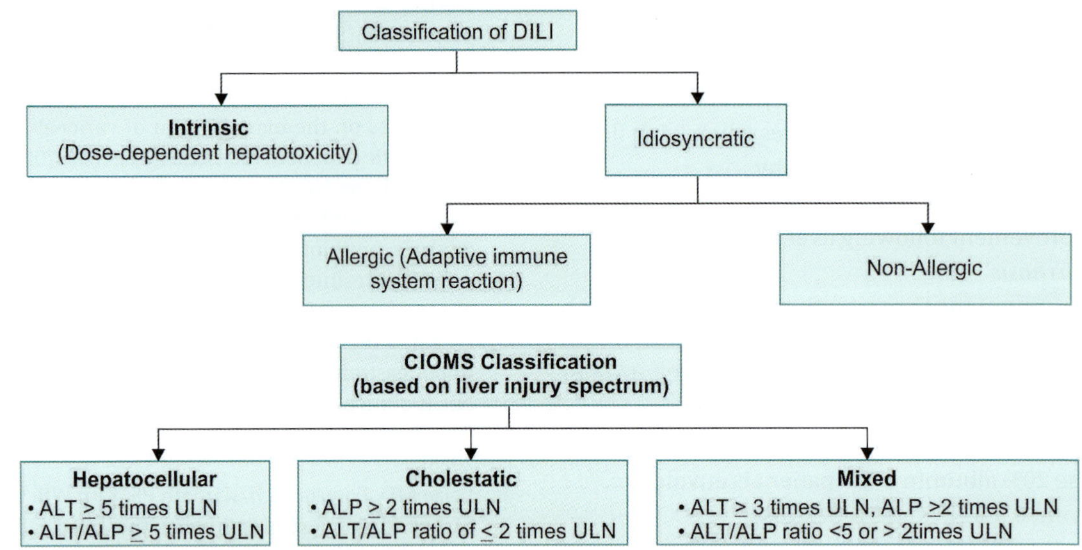


(CIOMS: Council for International Organizations of Medical Sciences; ULN: upper limit of normal)

## CLINICAL SPECTRUM OF DRUG-INDUCED LIVER INJURY

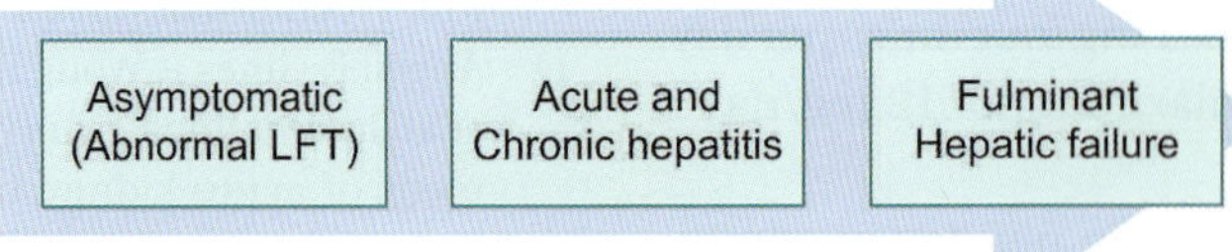

## ALGORITHM FOR CLINICAL DIAGNOSIS OF DILI

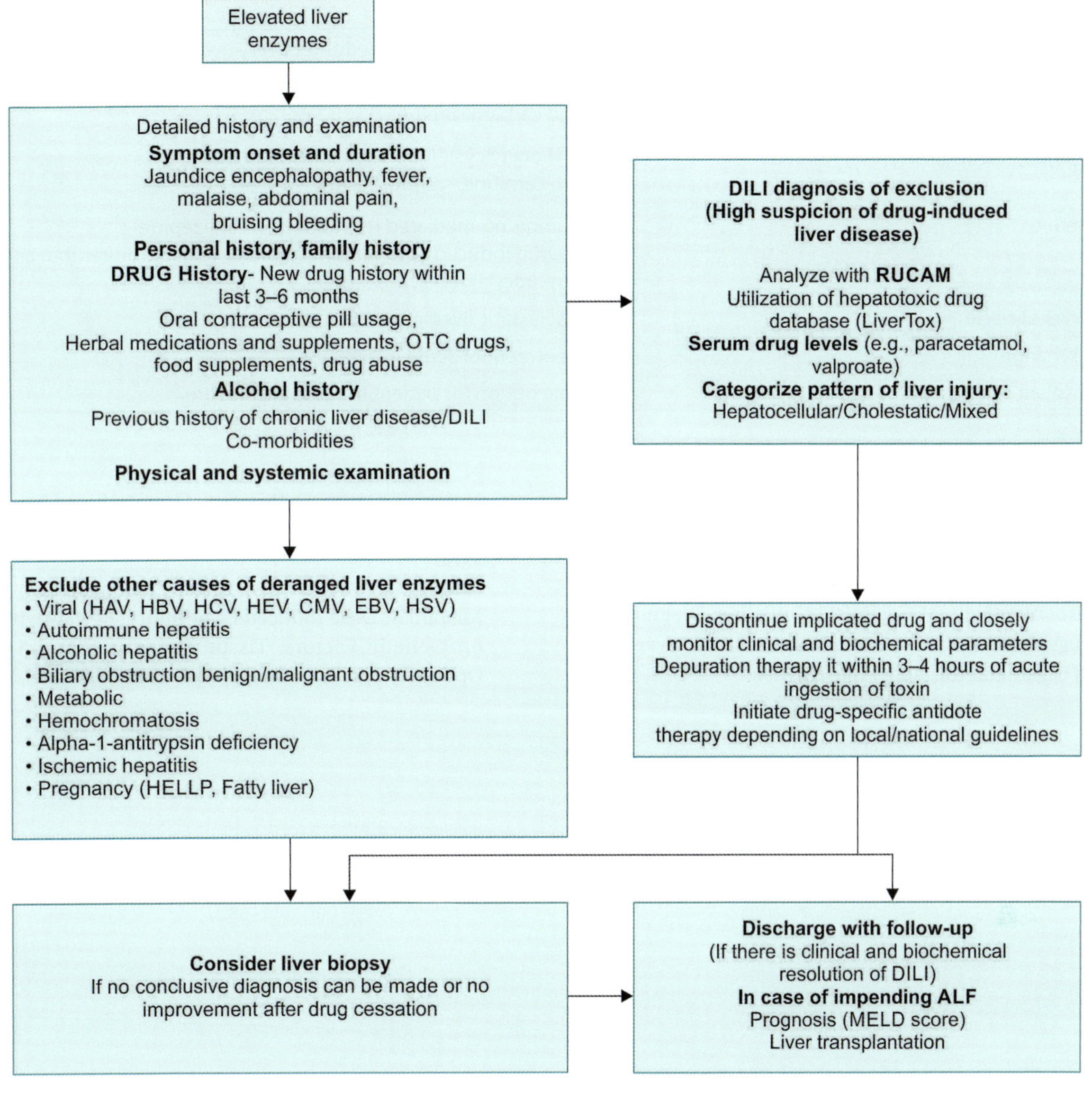

## MANAGEMENT OF DILI

| | |
|---|---|
| Prompt cessation of the implicated drug | Often leads to spontaneous recovery in days to weeks |
| Rapid depuration of the toxic drug (helpful in intrinsic DILI) | Activated charcoal - drug overdoses (e.g., paracetamol, phenobarbital and carbamazepine) |
| Administration of a drug-specific antidote | • N-acetylcysteine (NAC) -paracetamol<br>• L-carnitine –valproic acid |
| Corticosteroids | • Immune-mediated reactions (carbamazepine)<br>• Drug induced autoimmune hepatitis (e.g. nitrofurantoin and minocycline) |
| Ursodeoxycholic acid | Cholestatic liver injury |
| Plasma exchange | Treatment of acute liver failure |
| Liver transplant | Sole option for patient in acute liver failure |

## SUGGESTED READING

1. Chalasani NP, Maddur H, Russo MW, Wong RJ, Reddy KR; Practice Parameters Committee of the American College of Gastroenterology. ACG Clinical Guideline: Diagnosis and Management of Idiosyncratic Drug-Induced Liver Injury. Am J Gastroenterol. 2021;116(5):878-98.
2. Hosack T, Damry D, Biswas S. Drug-induced liver injury: a comprehensive review. Ther Adv Gastroenterol. 2023;16: 1-13.
3. Khoury T, Rmeileh AA, Yosha L, Benson AA, Daher S, Mizrahi M.Drug Induced Liver Injury: Review with a Focus on Genetic Factors, Tissue Diagnosis, and Treatment Options. J Clin Translat Hepatol. 2015;3:99-108.

CHAPTER 65

# Spontaneous Bacterial Peritonitis

## DEFINITION

Spontaneous bacterial peritonitis (SBP) is an infection of ascitic fluid that cannot be attributed to any intra-abdominal, ongoing inflammatory, or surgically correctable condition.

## RISK FACTORS

- Ascitic fluid total protein concentration <1 g/dL
- Prior episode of SBP
- Serum total bilirubin >2.5 mg/dL
- Variceal hemorrhage
- Use of proton pump inhibitors (PPI)
- Use of nonselective beta-blocker (NSBB)
- Ascitic fluid total protein <1.5 g/d: + child Pugh score >9 + plasma creatinine >1.2 mg/dL

## PATHOGENESIS

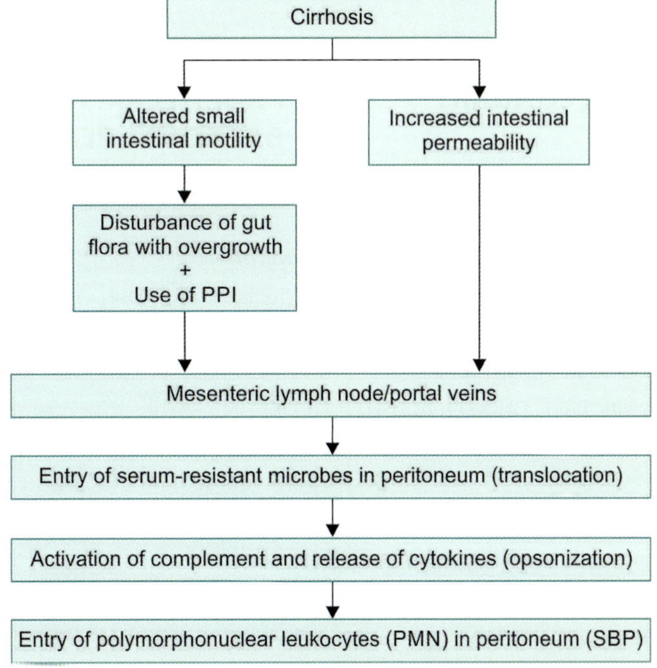

## DIAGNOSIS

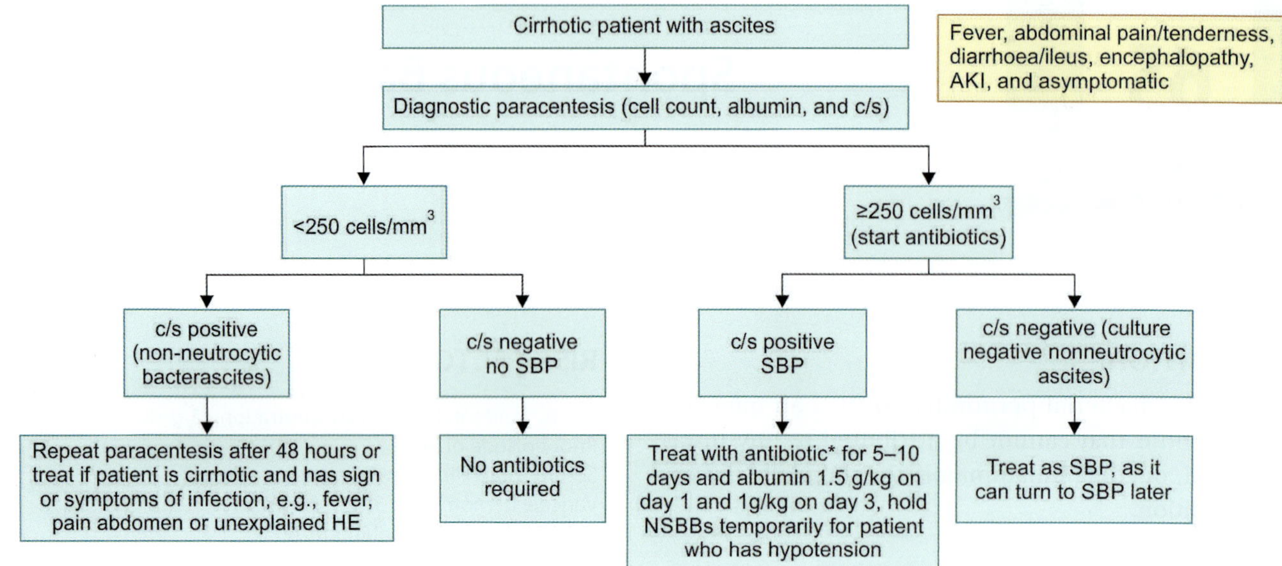


*Most common organism causing SBP are gram-negative bacteria, for example, *E. coli, Klebsiella pneumoniae, and Streptococcus pneumoniae.*

Start with ceftriaxone if chronic liver failure-sequential organ failure assessment (CLIF SOFA) ≤7 (less severe) and with carbapenem if more severe disease or CLIF SOFA score >7.

Routine repeat paracentesis for treatment is not recommended but if patient is not improving and repeats paracentesis shows rising PMN then need to change antibiotic.

(c/s: culture and sensitivity; HE: hepatic encephalopathy; NSBBs: nonselective beta-blockers; SBP: spontaneous bacterial peritonitis)

## SPONTANEOUS VERSUS SECONDARY BACTERIAL PERITONITIS

| ***Spontaneous bacterial peritonitis*** | ***Secondary bacterial peritonitis*** |
|---|---|
| Normally with high serum albumin globulin ratio | Ascitic fluid bilirubin >6.0 |
| Ascitic fluid total protein <1.0 | Ascitic fluid total protein >1.0 |
| Ascitic/serum bilirubin <1 | Ascitic/serum bilirubin >1 |
| Ascitic fluid LDH < serum LDH | Ascitic fluid LDH > serum LDH |
| Ascitic fluid glucose >50 mg/dL | Ascitic fluid glucose <50 mg/dL |
| Monomicrobial | Polymicrobial |
| Medically treated | Surgically treated |

## PROPHYLAXIS FOR SPONTANEOUS BACTERIAL PERITONITIS

Norfloxacin/ciprofloxacin/cotrimoxazole.

| ***Indication*** | ***Duration of antibiotic prophylaxis*** |
|---|---|
| Prior episode of SBP | Indefinite duration |
| Pt with cirrhosis and ascites with total protein <1.5 g/dL and at least one of the following:<br>• Serum creatinine ≥1/2 mg/dL<br>• Blood urea nitrogen ≥25 mg/dL<br>• Serum sodium ≤130 mEq/L<br>• Child–Pugh score ≥9 + bilirubin ≥3 mg/dL | Indefinite duration |
| Acute gastrointestinal bleed | For up to 7 days (ceftriaxone/cefotaxime IV) |

## SUGGESTED READING

1. Aithal GP, Palaniyappan N, China L, Härmälä S, Macken L, Ryan JM, et al. Guidelines on the management of ascites in cirrhosis. Gut. 2021;70(1):9-29.
2. Biggins SW, Angeli P, Garcia-Tsao G, Ginès P, Ling SC, Nadim MK, et al. diagnosis, evaluation, and management of ascites, spontaneous bacterial peritonitis and hepatorenal syndrome: 2021 Practice Guidance by the American Association for the Study of Liver Diseases. Hepatology. 2021;74(2):1014-48.
3. Chang CS, Chen GH, Lien HC, Yeh HZ. Small intestine dysmotility and bacterial overgrowth in cirrhotic patients with spontaneous bacterial peritonitis. Hepatology. 1998; 28:1187.
4. Dunn DL, Barke RA, Knight NB, Humphrey EW, Simmons RL. Role of resident macrophages, peripheral neutrophils, and translymphatic absorption in bacterial clearance from the peritoneal cavity. Infect Immun. 1985; 49(2):257-64.
5. Goel GA, Deshpande A, Lopez R, Hall GS, van Duin D, Carey WD. Increased rate of spontaneous bacterial peritonitis among cirrhotic patients receiving pharmacologic acid suppression. Clin Gastroenterol Hepatol. 2012;10(4): 422-7.
6. Runyon BA, Morrissey RL, Hoefs JC, Wyle FA. Opsonic activity of human ascitic fluid: A potentially important protective mechanism against spontaneous bacterial peritonitis. Hepatology. 1985;5(4):634-7.
7. Würstle S, Hapfelmeier A, Karapetyan S, Studen F, Isaakidou A, Schneider T, et al. Differentiation of spontaneous bacterial peritonitis from secondary peritonitis in patients with liver cirrhosis: Retrospective multicentre study. Diagnostics (Basel). 2023;13(5):994.
8. Yim HJ, Kim TH, Suh SJ, Yim SY, Jung YK, Seo YS, et al. Response-guided therapy with cefotaxime, ceftriaxone, or ciprofloxacin for spontaneous bacterial peritonitis: A randomized trial: A Validation Study of 2021 AASLD Practice Guidance for SBP. Am J Gastroenterol. 2023;118(4): 654-63.

CHAPTER 66

# Diarrhea in Intensive Care Unit

## CLASSIFICATION

Diarrhea is classified based on the duration:

- *Acute diarrhea:* 14 days or fewer in duration
- *Persistent diarrhea:* <14 but fewer than 30 days in duration
- *Chronic diarrhea:* <30 days in duration

## CAUSES OF DIARRHEA IN INTENSIVE CARE UNIT

- *Infective:*
    - Community-acquired gastroenteritis
    - Hospital-acquired infection
    - Antibiotic-associated diarrhea
    - Neutropenic enterocolitis
    - CMV infection
- *Noninfective:*
    - Osmotic diarrhea
    - Lactose intolerance
    - Laxatives/prokinetics
    - Malabsorption
    - Inflammatory bowel disease
    - Macrolides and MMF therapy
    - Pancreatic failure
    - Acute mesenteric ischemia

## COMMON PHYSIOLOGICAL DERANGEMENTS IN PATIENTS WITH DIARRHEA

- Hypovolemia
- Hyperchloremic metabolic acidosis
- Hypokalemia

## APPROACH TO PATIENT WITH DIARRHEA IN INTENSIVE CARE UNIT

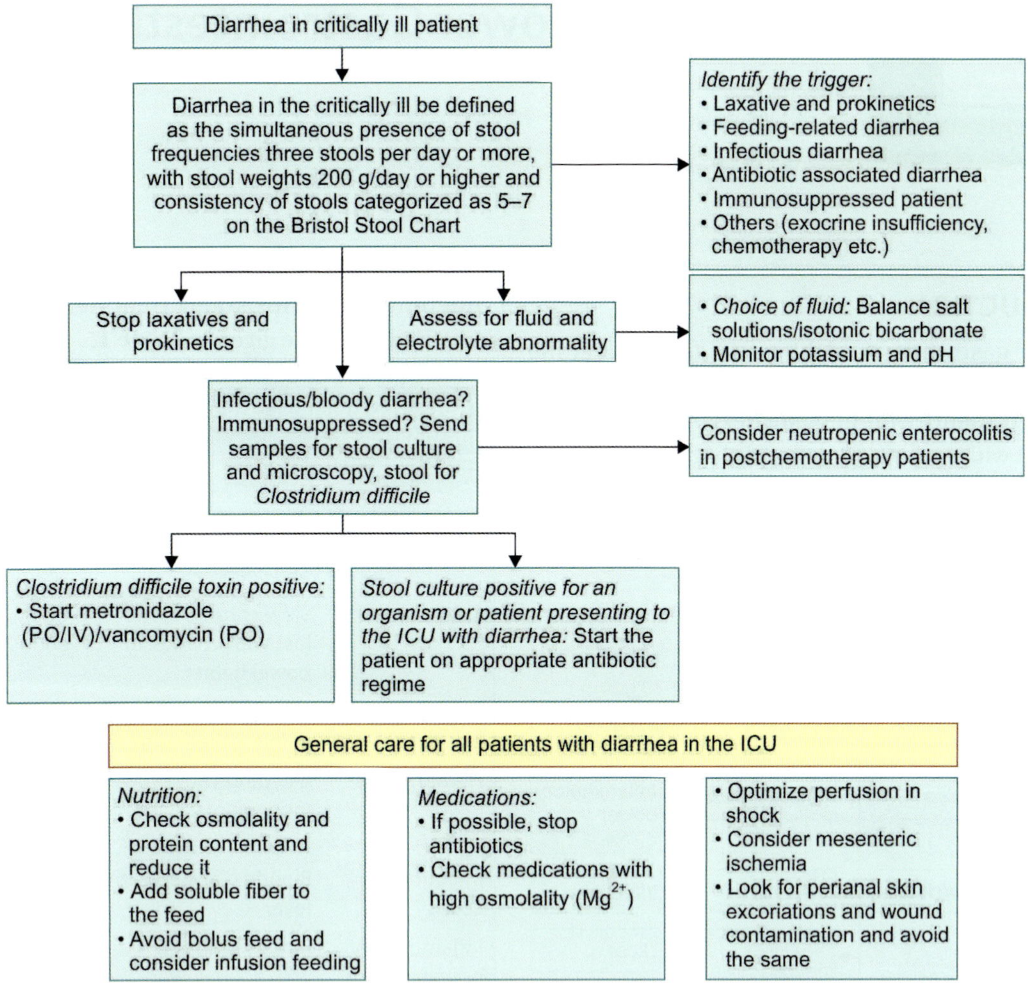


## SUGGESTED READING


1. Gadewar S, Fasano A. Current concepts in the evaluation, diagnosis and management of acute infectious diarrhea. Curr. Opin. Pharmacol. 5, 559-65.
2. Kelly TW, Patrick MR, Hillman KM. Study of diarrhea in critically ill patients. Crit. Care Med. 1983;11:7-9.
3. Montejo JC Enteral nutrition-related gastrointestinal complications in critically ill patients: a multicenter study. The Nutritional and Metabolic Working Group of the Spanish Society of Intensive Care Medicine and Coronary Units. Crit. Care Med. 1999;27:1447-53.
4. Reintam Blaser A, et al. Gastrointestinal function in intensive care patients: terminology, definitions and management. Recommendations of the ESICM Working Group on Abdominal Problems. Intensive Care Med. 38, 384-94.
5. Thibault R, et al. Diarrhoea in the intensive care unit: respective contribution of feeding and antibiotics. Crit. Care 17, R153, 2013. doi: 10.1186/cc12832.
6. Wiesen P, Van Gossum A, Preiser JC. Diarrhoea in the critically ill. Current Opin. Crit. Care 12, 149-154.
7. Zahar JR, et al. Outcome of ICU patients with Clostridium difficile infection. Crit. Care 16, R215.

CHAPTER 67

# Lower Gastrointestinal Bleeding

## INTRODUCTION

Acute lower gastrointestinal bleed is acute bleeding originating from site distal to the ligament of Treitz. Generally, it presents with hematochezia but can sometimes present with melena, for example, right-side colonic bleed.

## ETIOLOGY

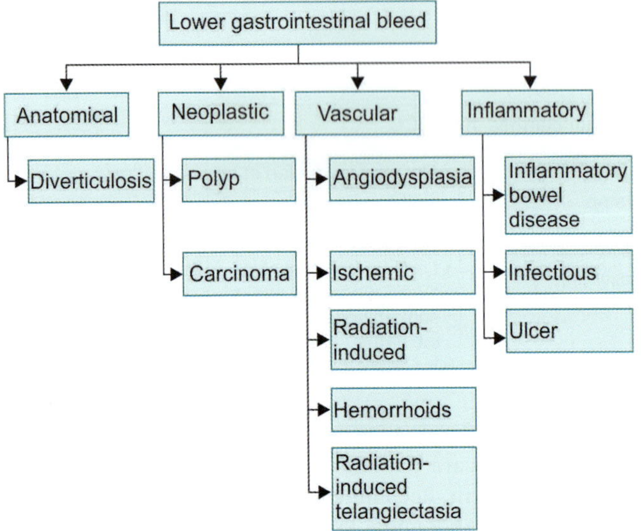


Differential diagnosis and treatment of lower gastrointestinal bleed are given in **Table 1**.

**TABLE 1:** Differential diagnosis and treatment of lower gastrointestinal bleed.

| *Diagnosis* | *Features* | *Treatment* |
|---|---|---|
| Angiodysplasia | Recurrent painless bleeding and age >60 years | Colonoscopy with argon plasma coagulation |
| Colon cancer | Slow chronic blood loss with change in bowel habit | Colonoscopy with endoscopic therapy |
| Diverticular bleeding | Acute, severe, and painless bleeding | Colonoscopy with endoscopic therapy |
| Hemorrhoids | Bleeding with bowel movements | Fiber supplement and banding or photocoagulation |
| Infectious colitis | Bloody diarrhea with fever | Antibiotics according to pathogen |
| Inflammatory bowel disease | Bloody diarrhea with acute lower abdominal pain with weight loss | Colonoscopy with biopsy and fecal calprotectin |
| Ischemic colitis | Bloody diarrhea with acute lower abdominal | Management of underlying vascular disease |

## EVALUATION OF PATIENT WITH HEMATOCHEZIA

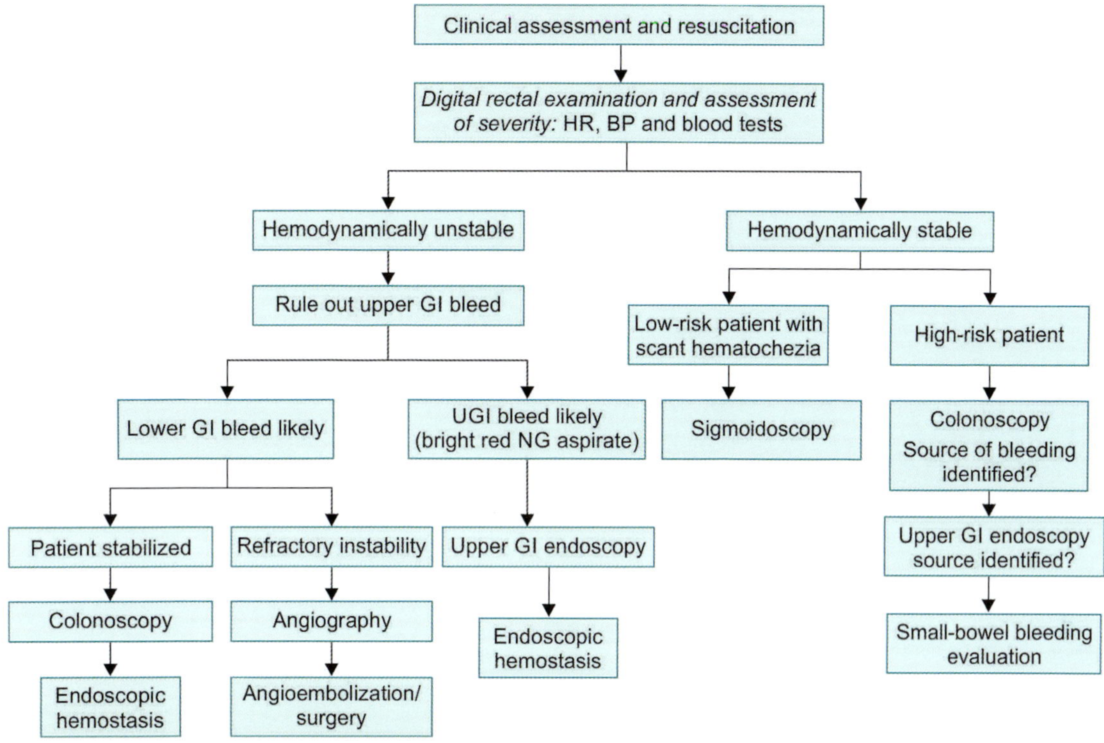


(BP: blood pressure; GI: gastrointestinal; HR: heart rate)

**BOX 1:** Antiplatelet and anticoagulation in lower gastrointestinal bleed.

- Hold aspirin if given for primary prophylaxis
- Continue aspirin, if giving for secondary prophylaxis
- Dual antiplatelet to be held and resumed within 7 days
- Warfarin reversal if life-threatening bleed or supratherapeutic INR with PCC/FFP
- Reversal of dabigatran with idarucizumab in life-threatening bleed or use of dabigatran in last 24 hours
- Reversal of apixaban/rivaroxaban with Adnexa-alfa in life-threatening bleed or use of dabigatran in last 24 hours
- Transfuse to maintain Hb >7 gm/dL in noncardiac patients and >9–10 gm/dL in cardiac patients
- Avoid using antifibrinolytics, e.g., tranexamic acid
- Platelet transfusion to maintain platelet count >30,000 ×109/L in severe lower GI bleed and 50,000, if endoscopic procedure is noted

*Hemodynamically unstable:* HR >100 bpm, SBP <115 mm Hg, pallor, capillary refill >3 seconds, >2 comorbid conditions

In hemodynamically stable patient, colonoscopy is to be done after preparation with PEG solution 4–6 L over 3–4 hours until rectal effluent is clear of blood and stool.

Antiplatelet and anticoagulation process in lower gastrointestinal bleed is detailed in **Box 1**.

## SUGGESTED READING

1. Hawks MK, Svarverud JE. Acute lower gastrointestinal bleeding: Evaluation and management. Am Fam Physician. 2020;101(4):206-12.
2. Sengupta N, Feuerstein JD, Jairath V, Shergill AK, Strate LL, Wong RJ, et al. Management of patients with acute lower gastrointestinal bleeding: An Updated ACG Guideline. Am J Gastroenterol 2023;118(2):208-31.
3. Strate LL, Gralnek IM. ACG Clinical guideline: Management of patients with acute lower gastrointestinal bleeding. Am J Gastroenterol. 2016;111(5):755
4. Zakko L, Rustagi T, Douglas M, Laine L. No benefit from platelet transfusion for gastrointestinal bleeding in patients taking antiplatelet agents. Clin Gastroenterol Hepatol. 2017; 15(1):46-52.

# PART 5

# RENAL

***Editor:*** Kanwalpreet Sodhi
***Associate Editor:*** Neeru Sahni

CHAPTER

# 68 Acute Kidney Injury

## INTRODUCTION

*Patient presenting with acute kidney injury (AKI):*

- Rise in creatinine >0.3 mg/dL over 48 hours, or
- Rise in serum creatinine 1.5 times baseline over 7 days; or
- Reduction in urine output <0.5 mL/kg/h over 6 hours

## HISTORY AND PHYSICAL EXAMINATION

| ***Volume loss*** | | ***Cardiorenal syndrome*** | ***Hepatorenal syndrome*** |
|---|---|---|---|
| *History:*<br>• Vomiting<br>• Diarrhea<br>• Burns<br>• Hemorrhage<br>• Diuretic overdose<br>*Signs:*<br>• Poor skin turgor<br>• Tachycardia<br>• Hypotension | *Causes:*<br>• Sepsis<br>• Hemorrhage<br>• Burns<br>• Acute Gastroenteritis<br>• Heat stroke | *Signs of congestive heart failure:*<br>• Shortness of breath<br>• Dilated neck veins<br>• Presence of S3<br>• Peripheral edema<br>• Pulmonary rales | • Ascites<br>• Caput medusae<br>• Spider angiomas |

## PRERENAL

| ***Acute tubular necrosis*** | ***Glomerular diseases*** | ***Interstitial nephritis*** | ***Vascular causes*** |
|---|---|---|---|
| • H/o drug exposure<br>– Herbal medications<br>– Illicit drugs<br>– Gym diets/supplements<br>– Radio contrast agents<br>– Vancomycin<br>– Aminoglycosides<br>• Rhabdomyolysis<br>– Trauma<br>– Myalgias<br>– Excessive exercise<br>– Heat stroke<br>• Hypotension<br>• Mismatched blood | • Systemic lupus Erythematosus—H/O RASH and arthritis<br>• Infections<br>• Hematuria<br>• Cough/sinusitis<br>• Hemoptysis<br>• Foamy urine with<br>– Pedal edema<br>– Periorbital edema<br>– Rash<br>– Oral ulcers | • H/o medication use<br>– Antibiotics<br>– Proton pump Inhibitors with<br>• H/o fever<br>– Rash<br>– Arthralgia<br>• Infectious diseases | • H/o nephrotic syndrome<br>• Trauma<br>• H/o flank pain<br>• Atheroembolic disease<br>• Vascular surgery<br>• Presence of<br>– Abdominal bruit<br>– Livedo reticularis<br>• Signs of malignant hypertension on fundus examination |

## RENAL

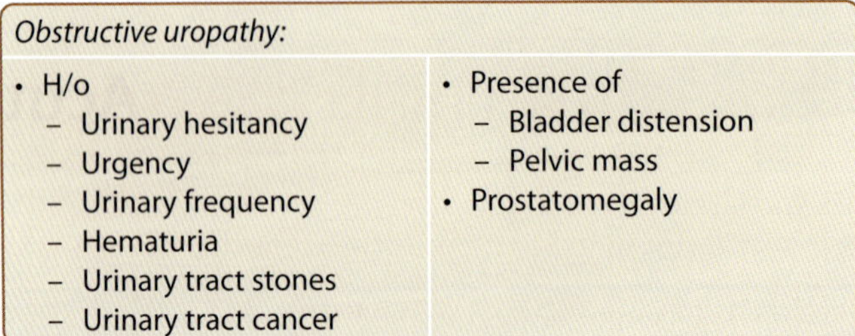


## POSTRENAL

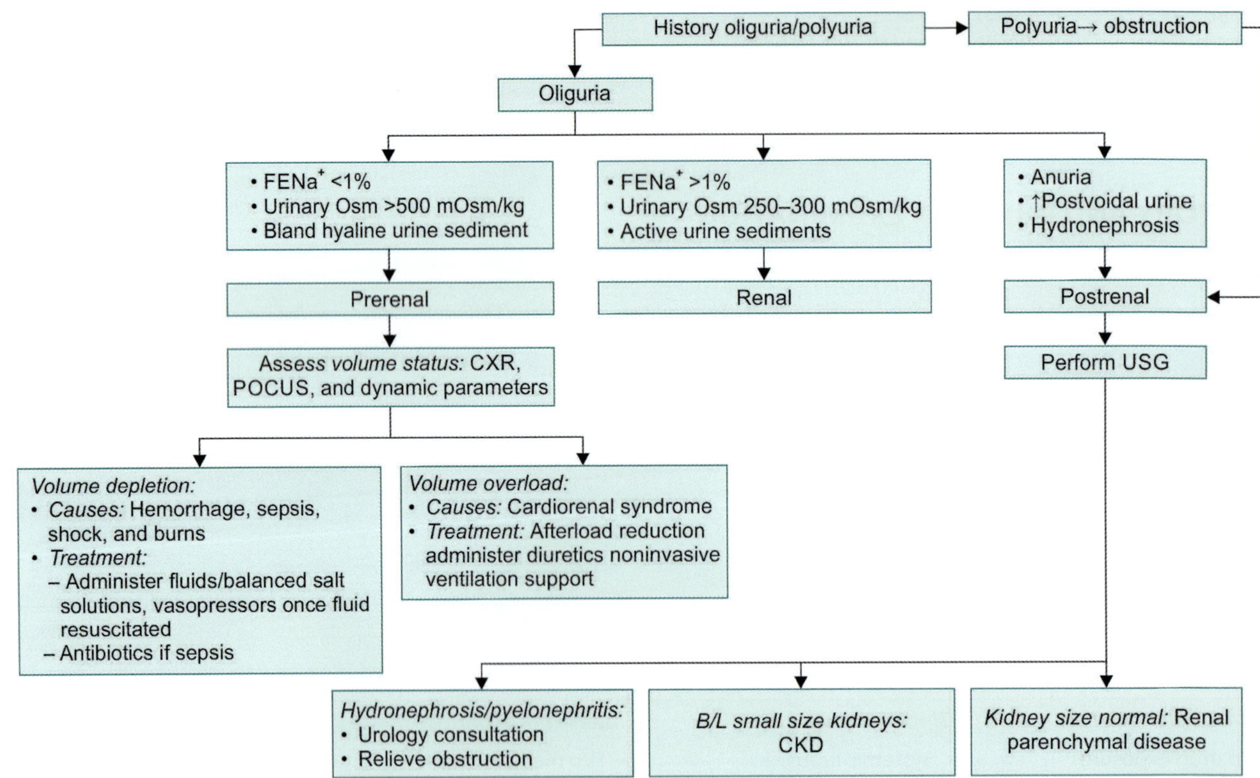


## RENAL: URINE ANALYSIS

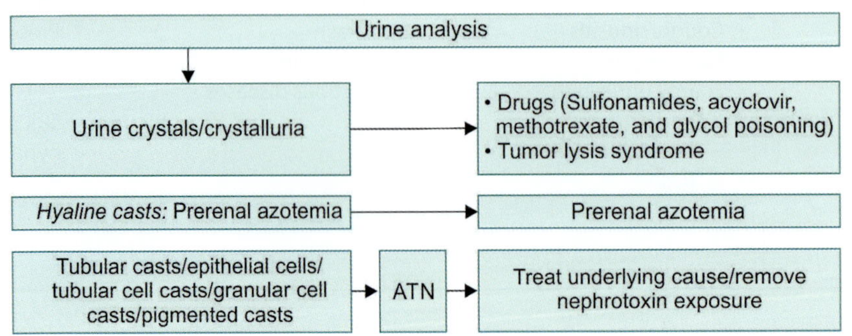


*Contd...*

*Contd...*

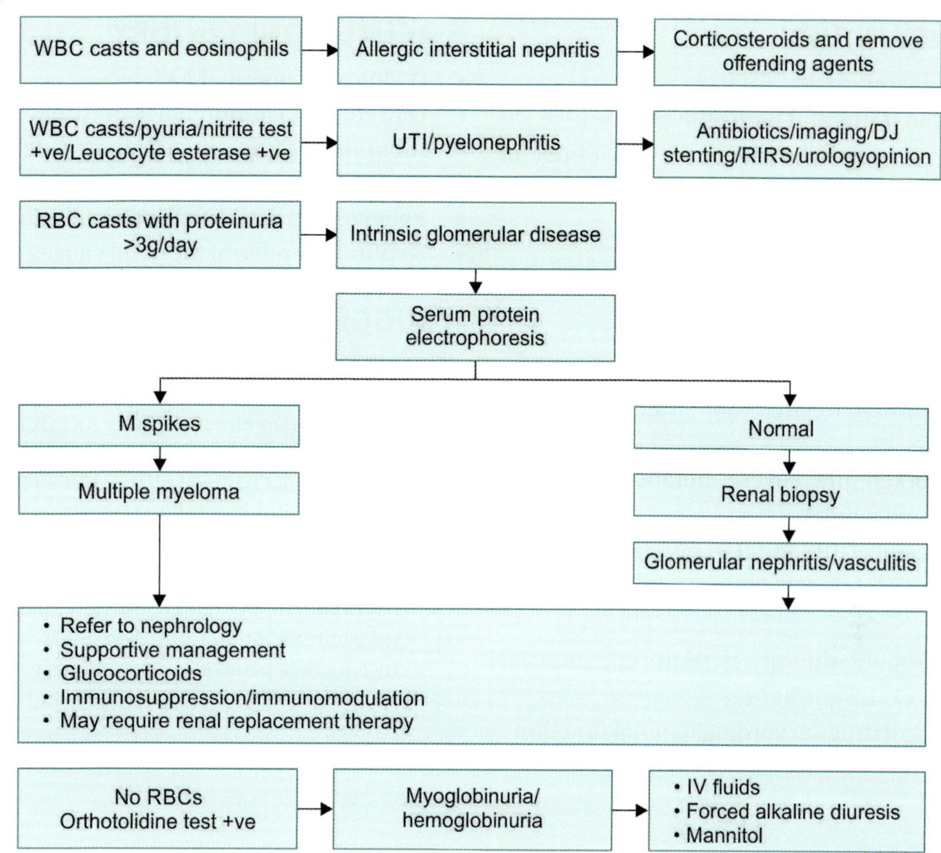
WBC casts and eosinophils
Allergic interstitial nephritis
Corticosteroids and remove offending agents
WBC casts/pyuria/nitrite test +ve/Leucocyte esterase +ve
UTI/pyelonephritis
Antibiotics/imaging/DJ stenting/RIRS/urologyopinion
RBC casts with proteinuria >3g/day
Intrinsic glomerular disease
Serum protein electrophoresis
M spikes
Multiple myeloma
Normal
Renal biopsy
Glomerular nephritis/vasculitis
• Refer to nephrology
• Supportive management
• Glucocorticoids
• Immunosuppression/immunomodulation
• May require renal replacement therapy
No RBCs Orthotolidine test +ve
Myoglobinuria/ hemoglobinuria
• IV fluids
• Forced alkaline diuresis
• Mannitol

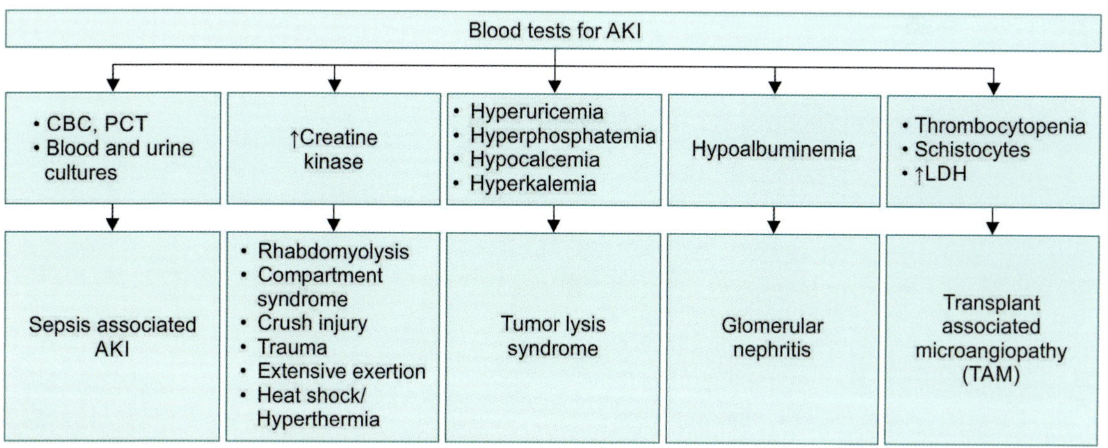
Blood tests for AKI
• CBC, PCT
• Blood and urine cultures
↑Creatine kinase
• Hyperuricemia
• Hyperphosphatemia
• Hypocalcemia
• Hyperkalemia
Hypoalbuminemia
• Thrombocytopenia
• Schistocytes
• ↑LDH
Sepsis associated AKI
• Rhabdomyolysis
• Compartment syndrome
• Crush injury
• Trauma
• Extensive exertion
• Heat shock/ Hyperthermia
Tumor lysis syndrome
Glomerular nephritis
Transplant associated microangiopathy (TAM)

## GENERAL MANAGEMENT OF ACUTE KIDNEY INJURY

- HDU/ICU admission
- Optimize volume status and perfusion pressure
- Avoid diuretics except in patients with evidence of volume overload
- Functional hemodynamic monitoring
- Monitoring urine output and serial serum creatinine
- Cumulative fluid balance recording
- Optimize hemodynamics
- Stop all nephrotoxic drugs
- *Avoid radiocontrast agents:* Consider alternative tests
- Watch for hyperkalemia, severe metabolic acidosis, and uremic complications
- Avoid hyperglycemia (RBS 110–150 mg/dL)
- *Nutrition:* Calorie intake 25–30 kcal/kg/day, protein: 0.8–1gm/kg/day
- If renal replacement therapy is required, increase protein intake to 1–1.5 gm/kg/day.
- Dynamic dosing of drugs according to renal function

## TREATMENT OF CAUSE OF ACUTE KIDNEY INJURY

- IV fluids for prerenal AKI
- Diuretics for cardiorenal syndrome
- Albumin/terlipressin for hepatorenal syndrome
- Antibiotics for sepsis-associated AKI
- Relieve obstruction for postrenal causes
- Nephrology referral for renal causes

## SUGGESTED READING


1. Griffin BR, Liu KD, Teixeira JP. Critical care nephrology: Core curriculum 2020. Am J Kidney Dis. 2020;75(3):435-52.
2. Kellum JA, Lameire N; KDIGO AKI Guideline Work Group. Diagnosis, evaluation, and management of acute kidney injury: a KDIGO summary (Part 1). Crit Care. 2013;17(1):204.
3. Moore PK, Hsu RK, Liu KD. Management of acute kidney injury: Core curriculum 2018. Am J Kidney Dis. 2018;72(1): 136-48.
4. Ostermann M, Bellomo R, Burdmann EA, Doi K, Endre ZH, Goldstein SL, et al. Controversies in acute kidney injury: conclusions from a kidney disease: Improving Global Outcomes (KDIGO) Conference. Kidney Int. 2020;98(2): 294-309.

CHAPTER 69

# Acute-on-Chronic Kidney Disease

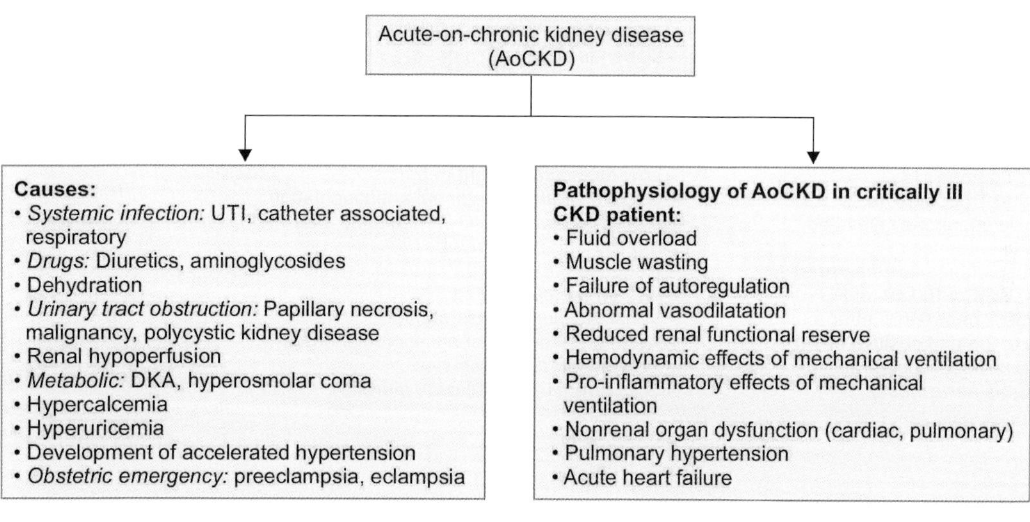

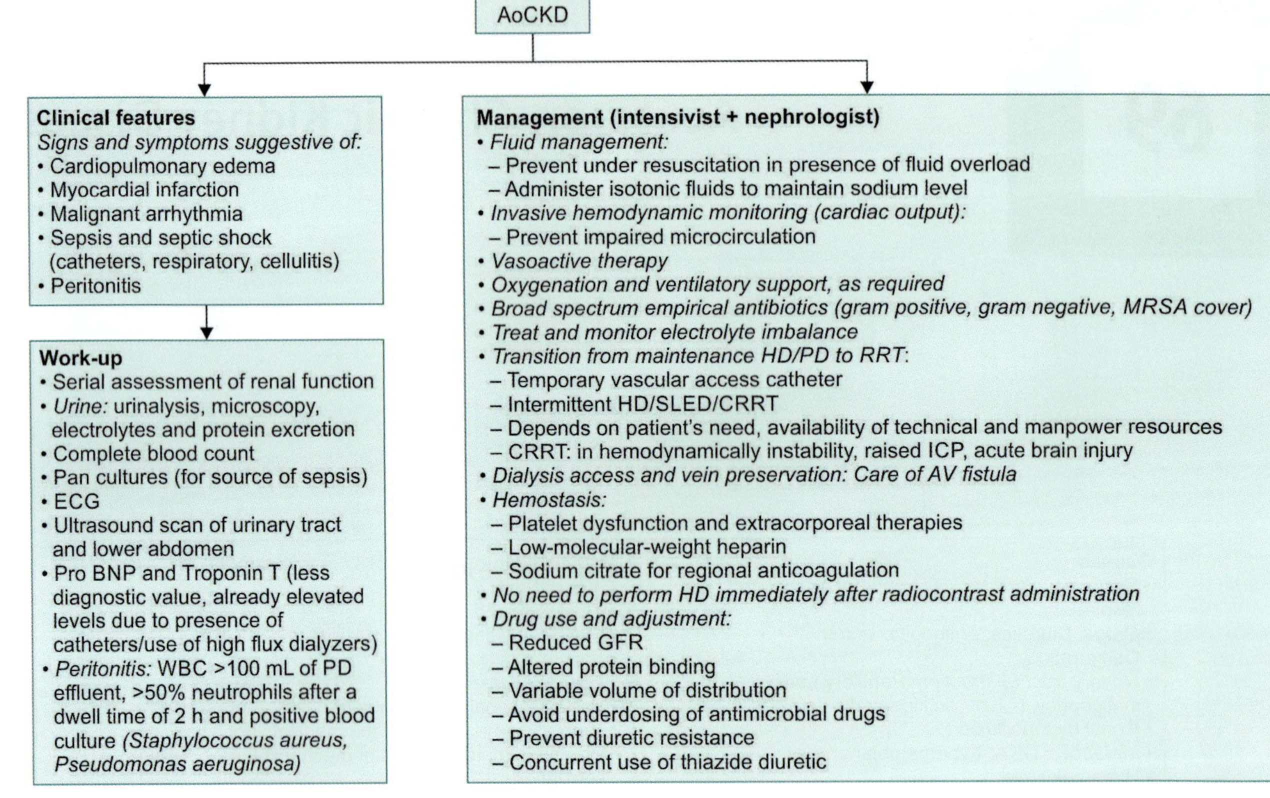


## SUGGESTED READING

1. Abdalrahim MS, Khalil AA, Alramly M, Alshlool KN, Abed MA, Moser DK. Pre-existing chronic kidney disease and acute kidney injury among critically ill patients. Heart Lung. 2020;49(5):626-9.
2. Chawla LS, Eggers PW, Star RA, Kimmel PL. Acute kidney injury and chronic kidney disease as interconnected syndromes. N Engl J Med. 2014;371(1):58-66.
3. De Rosa S, Samoni S, Villa G, Ronco C. Management of chronic kidney disease patients in the intensive care unit: Mixing acute and chronic Illness. Blood Purif. 2017; 43(1-3):151-62.
4. Ferenbach DA, Bonventre JV. Acute kidney injury and chronic kidney disease: From the laboratory to the clinic. Nephrol Ther. 2016;12(Suppl 1):S41-8.
5. Hsu RK, Hsu CY. The role of acute kidney injury in chronic kidney disease. Semin Nephrol. 2016;36(4):283-92.

CHAPTER 70

# Pyelonephritis

## APPROACH TO PATIENTS WITH PYELONEPHRITIS

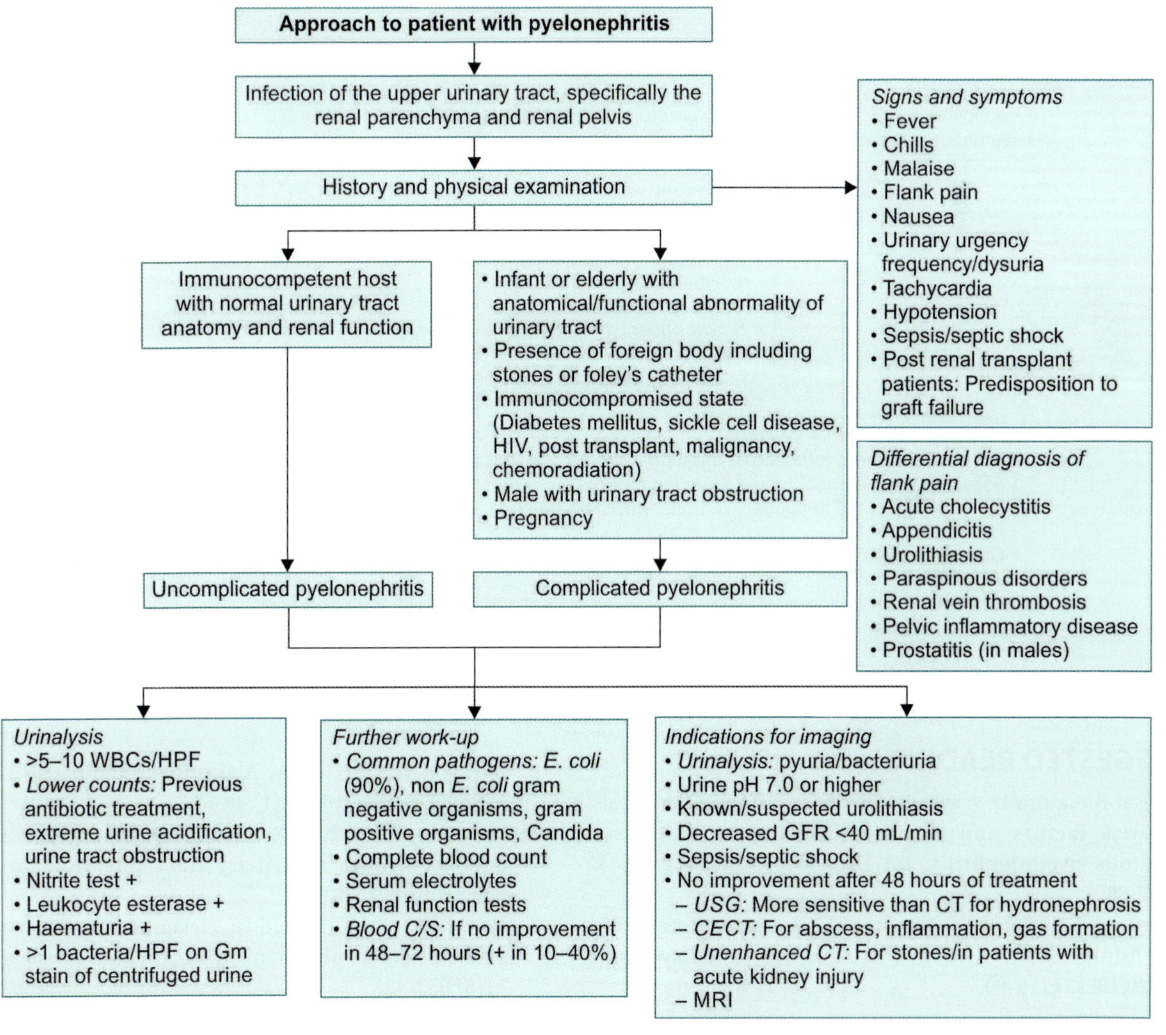

## MANAGEMENT

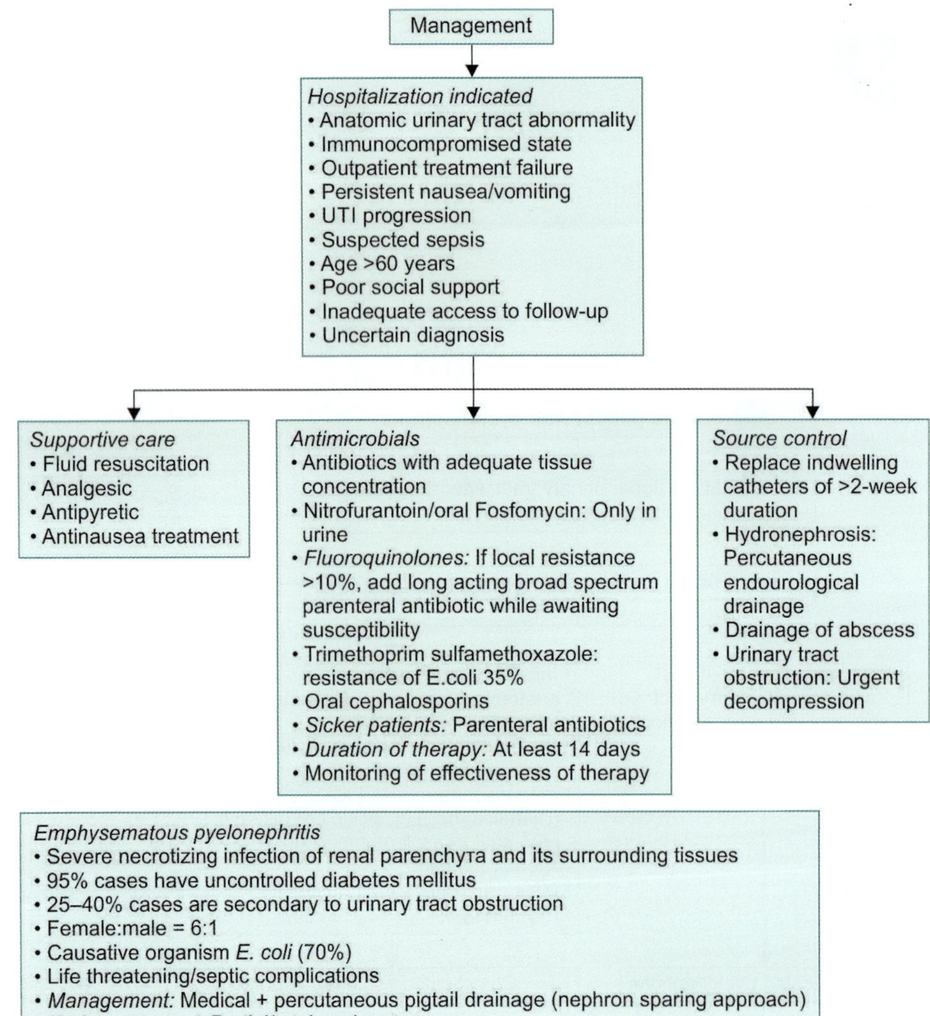


## SUGGESTED READING


1. Desai R, Batura D. A systematic review and meta-analysis of risk factors and treatment choices in emphysematous pyelonephritis. Int Urol Nephrol. 2022;54(4): 717-36.
2. Herness J, Buttolph A, Hammer NC. Acute Pyelonephritis in Adults: Rapid Evidence Review. Am Fam Physician. 2020;102(3):173-80.
3. Johnson JR, Russo TA. Acute Pyelonephritis in Adults. N Engl J Med. 2018;378(1):48-59.
4. Pietrucha-Dilanchian P, Hooton TM. Diagnosis, treatment, and prevention of urinary tract infection. Microbiol Spectrum. 2016;4(6).
5. Ramakrishnan K, Scheid DC. Diagnosis and management of acute pyelonephritis in adults. Am Fam Physician. 2005; 71(5):933-42.

CHAPTER 71

# Urinary Tract Infection

## DEFINITION

American Urological Association Core curriculum defines UTI as single organism in symptomatic patient ≥1,000 CFU/mL.

## SIGNS/SYMPTOMS OF URINARY TRACT INFECTION

*Local signs:*

- Dysuria
- Polyuria
- ↑Frequency
- Hematuria
- Flank pain
- Itching

*Systemic signs:*

- Fever ≥ 38°C (100.8°F) with rigors
- ↑TLC >10,800/mm$^3$
- Malaise/Lethargy
- Confused behavior (especially in elderly)
- Suprapubic tenderness
- Costovertebral angle pain/tenderness

## HISTORY AND PHYSICAL EXAMINATION

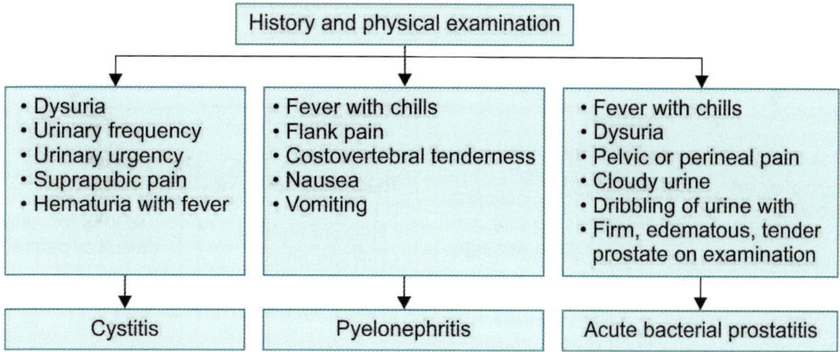

## URINARY TRACT INFECTION WORKUP

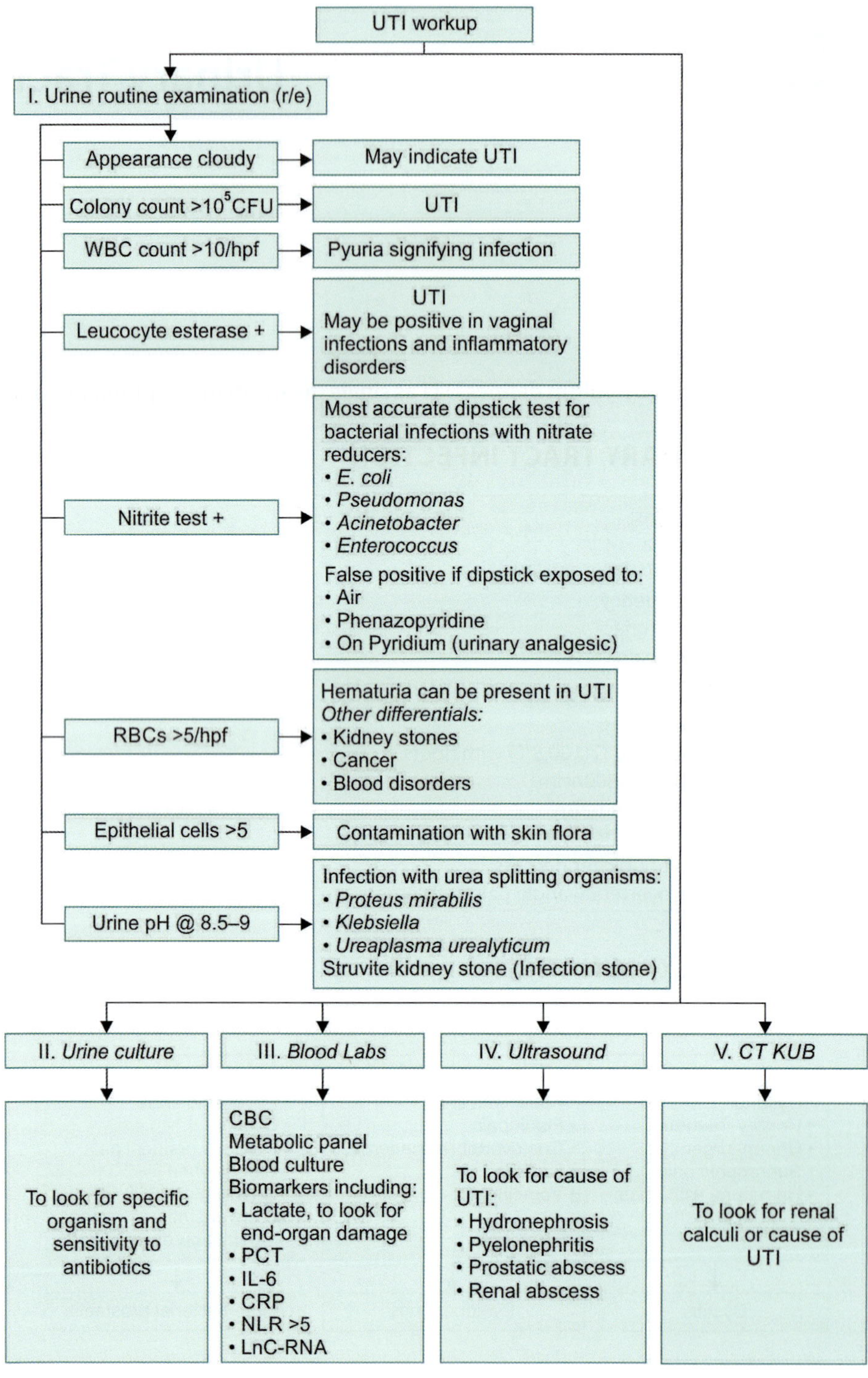

## TREATMENT OF URINARY TRACT INFECTION

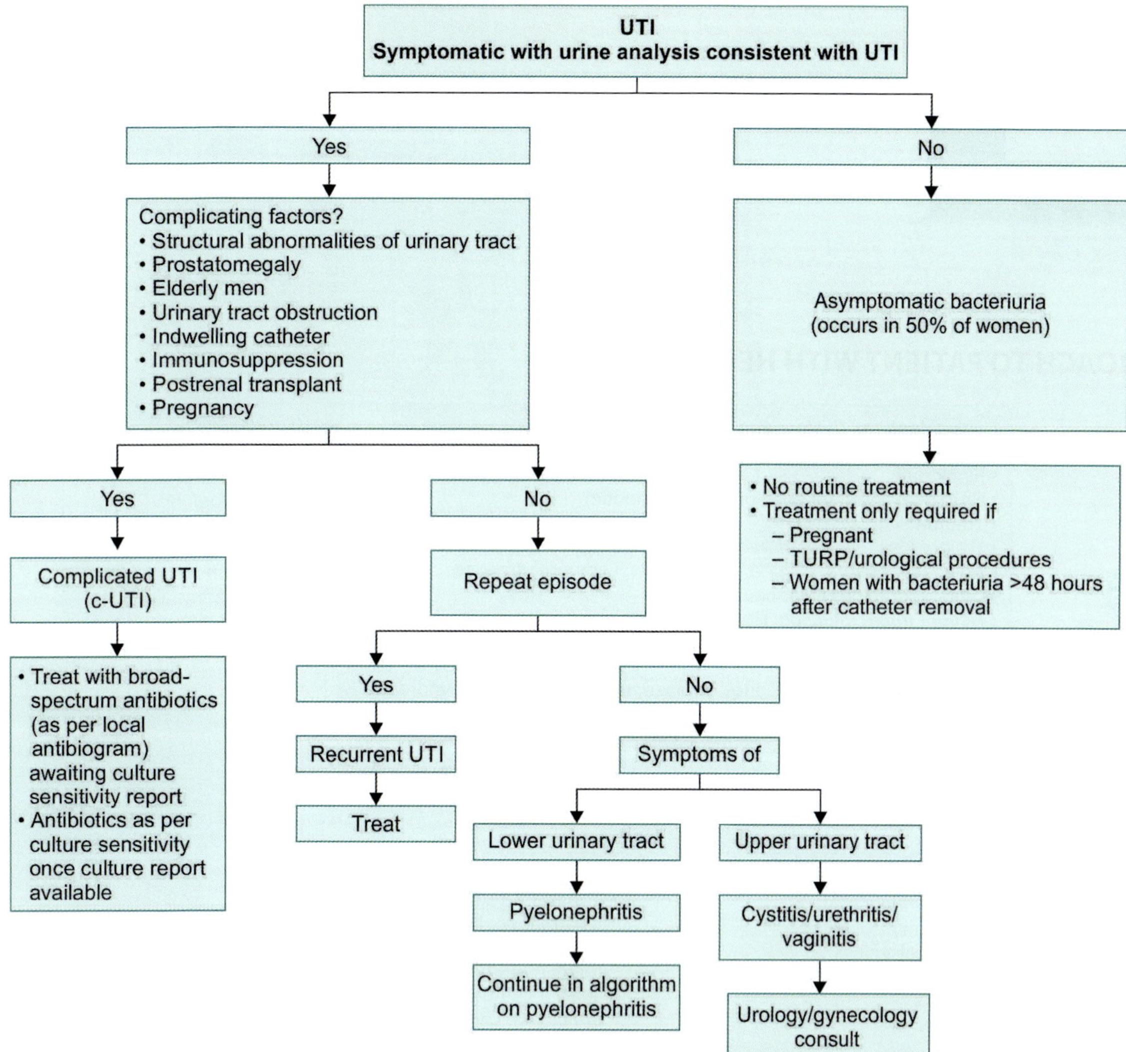


### Types of Treatment

*Cause-directed:*

- Antibiotics
- Elimination of focus of infection

*Supportive treatment:*

Hemodynamic and respiratory stabilization:

- IV fluids
- Vasopressors
- Noninvasive or invasive ventilatory support

*Adjunctive therapy:*

Hemodynamic and respiratory stabilization:

- Corticosteroids in septic shock
- Insulin to maintain euglycemia

## SUGGESTED READING


1. Geerlings SE. Clinical presentations and epidemiology of urinary tract infections. Microbiol Spectr. 2016;4(5).
2. Long B, Koyfman A. The emergency department diagnosis and management of urinary tract infection. Emerg Med Clin North Am. 2018;36(4):685-710.
3. McLellan LK, Hunstad DA. Urinary tract infection: Pathogenesis and outlook. Trends Mol Med. 2016;22(11):946-57.
4. Pietrucha-Dilanchian P, Hooton TM. Diagnosis, treatment, and prevention of urinary tract infection. Microbiol Spectr. 2016;4(6).

CHAPTER

# 72 Hematuria

## APPROACH TO PATIENT WITH HEMATURIA

*Clinical features (history and presentation):*
- *Fever, LUTS, Suprapubic pain:* Urinary tract infection (UTI)
- Flank pain
- Drug intake (anti-platelet or anti-thrombotic)
- Trauma
- *Weight loss, history of (h/o) smoking:* Tumor
- *Puffiness, edema, oliguria, weight gain:* Glomerular cause
- Clots: Extraglomerular cause
- *Recent throat infection:* Postinfectious glomerulonephritis
- *Joint pain, skin rash, fever:* Collagen vascular disease, SLE, Henoch–Schönlein Purpura
- *Family h/o:* Polycystic kidney disease, urolithiasis, alport syndrome

*Urological:*
- Upper tract
- Lower tract

*Nonurological:*
- Medical
- Pseudohematuria (not due to hemoglobin, causes: medication, myoglobimuria, food)

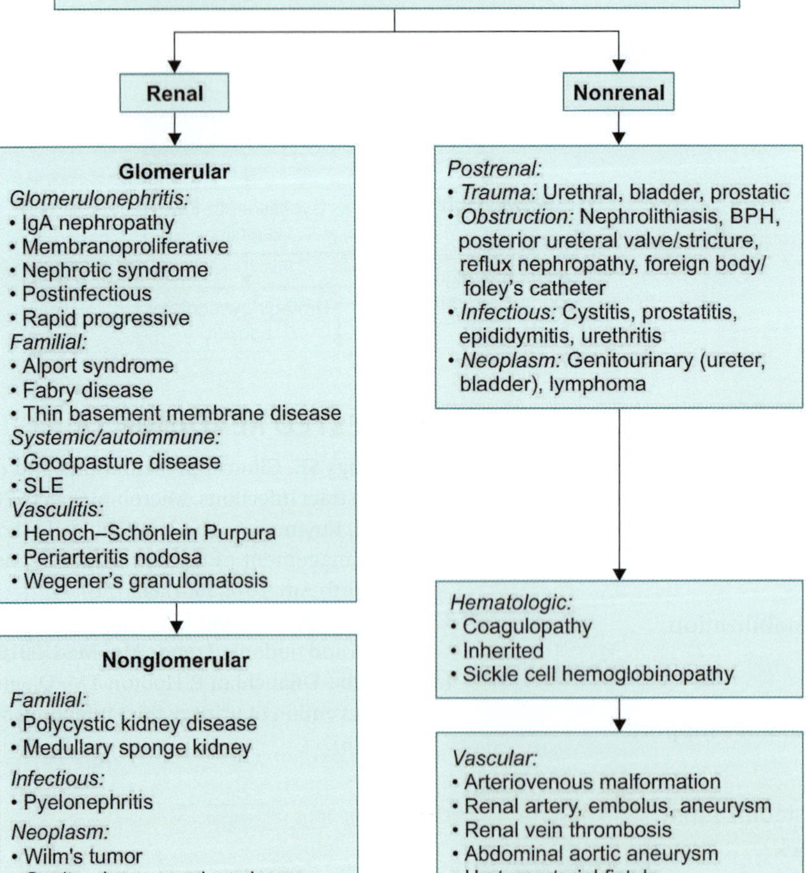

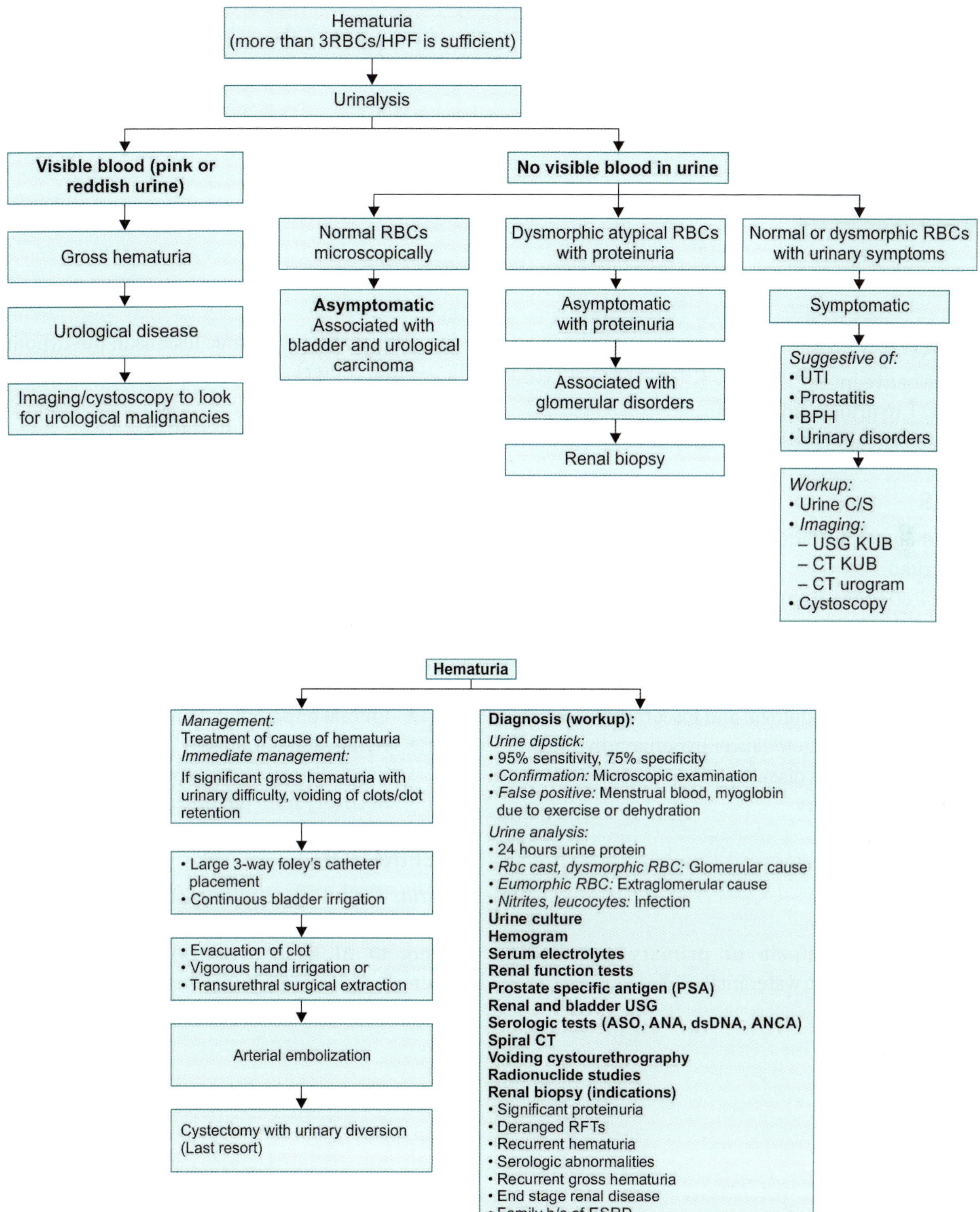


## SUGGESTED READING


1. Barocas D, Boorjian S, Alveraz J. et al. Microhematuria: AUA/SUF Guideline 2020. Diagnosis, evaluation and follow-up of asymptomatic microhematuria (AMH) in Adults: AUA Guideline. American Urological Association (AUA); 2020. [online] Available from: https://www.auanet.org/guidelines/microhematuria. [Last accessed March, 2025]
2. Moloney F, Murphy KP, Twomey M, O'Connor OJ, Maher MM. Haematuria: an imaging guide. Adv Urol. 2014;2014:414125.
3. Willis GC, Tewelde SZ. The approach to the patient with hematuria. Emerg Med Clin North Am. 2019;37(4):755-69.

CHAPTER 73

# Polyuria

## HISTORY

Differentiate between:

- *Polyuria:* ↑ in urine production
- *Frequency:* frequent passage of small amounts of urine

## CAUSES

- Central diabetes insipidus (decreased ADH secretion)
  - Inherited
  - Acquired (due to injury and tumors)
- Nephrogenic diabetes insipidus (decreased peripheral ADH sensitivity)
  - Amyloidosis
  - Drugs (lithium, cidofovir, and foscarnet)
  - Hypercalcemia (due to cancer, hyperparathyroidism, or granulomatous disease)
  - Inherited disorders
  - Hypokalemia
  - Obstructive uropathy
  - Sickle cell disease
  - Sjögren's syndrome
- Psychogenic polydipsia or primary polydipsia (sustained increase in water intake)
  - Primary (hypothalamic lesions in the hypothalamic thirst center)
  - Psychogenic
- Solute or osmotic diuresis due to
  - Hyperglycemia (diabetes mellitus)
  - Electrolyte washout [usually measured by a sodium salt (often chloride)]
    - Excessive administration of saline solution
    - Intravenous sodium bicarbonate administration
    - Excessive salt intake
    - Use of loop diuretics
  - Not mediated by electrolytes in patients who are catabolizing a large quantity of protein due to:
    - Enteral or parenteral nutrition
    - Hypercatabolic states
    - Resolution of obstructive uropathy
    - Recovery from oliguric acute kidney injury

## DEFINITION

*Polyuria:* A clinical condition characterized by a urine output that is inappropriately high (more than 3 L in 24 hours or 40 mL/kg in 24 hours) for the patient's blood pressure and plasma sodium levels.

## ALGORITHMIC APPROACH TO PATIENT WITH POLYURIA

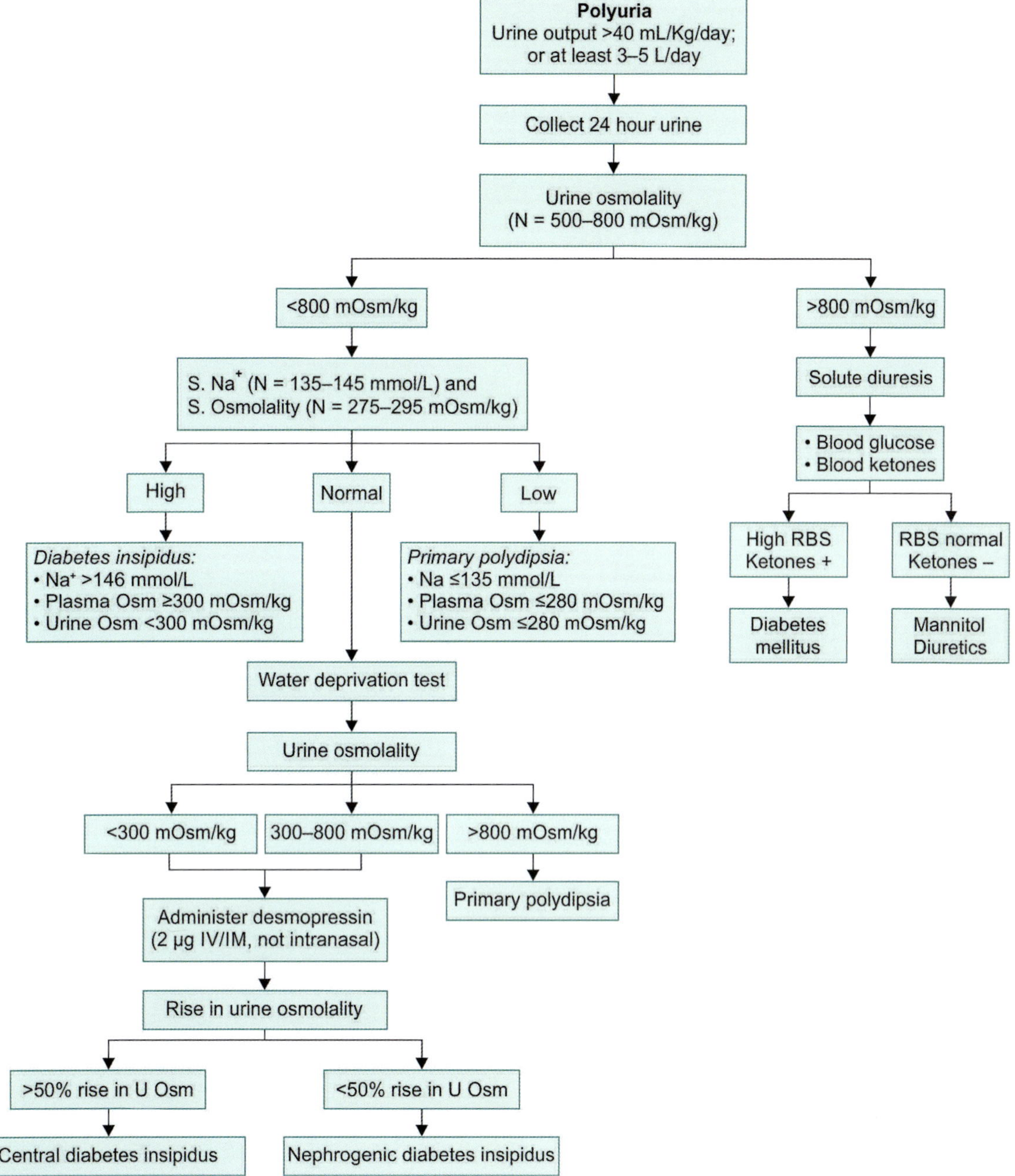


## SUGGESTED READING


1. Nigro N, Grossmann M, Chiang C, Inder WJ. Polyuria-polydipsia syndrome: a diagnostic challenge. Intern Med J. 2018;48(3):244-53.
2. Ramírez-Guerrero G, Müller-Ortiz H, Pedreros-Rosales C. Polyuria in adults. A diagnostic approach based on pathophysiology. Rev Clin Esp (Barc). 2022;222(5):301-8.
3. Rosen CJ, Ingelfinger JR. A reliable diagnostic test for hypotonic polyuria. N Engl J Med. 2018;379(5):483-4.
4. Tomkins M, Lawless S, Martin-Grace J, Sherlock M, Thompson CJ. Diagnosis and Management of central diabetes insipidus in adults. J Clin Endocrinol Metab. 2022;107(10):2701-15.

# PART 6

# TRAUMA

**Editors:** Sunil Karanth, Niraj Tyagi

**Associate Editors:** Vinay K, S Maniraj, Srinivasan Muthusamy, Dileep N

CHAPTER 74

# Polytrauma

## BERLIN CRITERIA FOR DEFINING POLYTRAUMA

| ***Anatomic characteristics (both present)*** | ***Physiological characteristics (one of five present)*** |
|---|---|
| AIS severity ≥3<br>AIS body regions >1<br><br>(Abbreviated Injury Scale score of ≥3 in ≥2 body regions (2AIS ≥3) | *Hypotension:* SBP ≤90 mm Hg<br>*Acidosis:* Base excess < 6 mmol/L<br>*Age:* ≥70 years<br>*Cognitive state:* GCS ≤ 8<br>*Coagulopathy:* INR ≥1.4, or aPTT ≥40 sec |
| (AIS: abbreviated Injury Scale; aPTT: activated partial thromboplastin time; GCS: Glasgow coma scale; INR: international normalized ratio; SBP: systolic blood | |

## MANAGING POLYTRAUMA PATIENTS

The advanced trauma life support (ATLS) (American College of Surgeons) approach focuses on the issues of immediate aid and classifying priorities.

*Initial evaluation:* Take no longer than 2 minutes.

Aim to identify any injuries that endanger the patient's life and/or limbs if they are not treated immediately.

*Resuscitation (ABCDE)*

A. Airway, clear (with the cervical spine under control)
B. Breathing
C. Circulation and control of hemorrhages (identify stage of hemorrhagic shock and response to fluid)
D. Disability, initial neurological assessment
E. Exposure, complete removal of patient's clothing

## TRAUMA SHOCK (HEMORRHAGIC) CLASSIFICATION

| ***Parameter*** | ***Class I*** | ***Class II (mild)*** | ***Class III (moderate)*** | ***Class IV (severe)*** |
|---|---|---|---|---|
| Blood loss (mL) and %<br>Based on 70 kg adult male | < 750<br><15% | 750–1499<br>15–30% | 1,500–2,000<br>30-40% | >2,000<br>> 40% |
| Heart rate (bpm) | <100 | 100–120 | 121-140 | >140 |
| BP | Normal | Decreased | Decreased | Decreased |
| Pulse pressure | Normal or ↑ | ↓ | ↓↓ | ↓↓↓ |
| Respiratory rate | 14–20 | 21–29 | 30–35 | >35 |
| Urine output (mL/hour) | Normal >30 | Oliguric 20–30 | Oliguric 5–19 | Anuric negligible |
| Neurological status GCS | Normal | Agitated | Confused<br>decreased (<15) | Lethargic<br>decreased (<15) |
| Base deficit (mmol/L) | <2.0 | 2–6 | 6–10 | >10 |
| Type of fluid | Crystalloid | Crystalloid | Crystalloid | Crystalloid |
| | | | Blood (crossmatched) | Blood (uncrossmatched) |
| | | | | Massive transfusion protocol |

## HEMODYNAMIC ASSESSMENT INDICES

**Shock index:** HR/SBP Normal <1 and >1.5 predicts massive transfusion need

**Modified shock index:** HR/MAP mSI > 1.3 hypodynamic status

**ROPE Index:** HR/pulse pressure > 2.2, early predictor of volume loss

## RESPONSE TO INITIAL FLUID RESUSCITATION

| | *Rapid response* | *Transient response* | *Minimal or no response* |
|---|---|---|---|
| **Vital signs** | Returns to normal | Transient improvement, recurrence of decreased blood flow and increased heart rate | Low BP and high heart rate |
| **Estimated blood loss** | Minimal (<5%) | Moderate and ongoing (5–40%) | Severe (>40%) |
| Need for blood | Low | Moderate-to-high | Immediate |
| **Blood preparation** | Type and cross-match | Type specific | Emergency blood release |
| **Need for operative/ intervention radiology** | Possibly | Likely | High likely |

## PRIMARY SURVEY

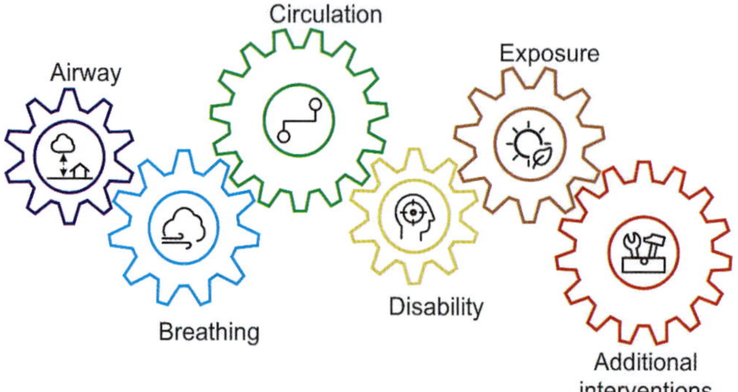


**Adjuncts to primary survey.**

- ECG monitoring
- Urinary catheter
- Gastric catheter
- Lateral cervical X-rays and E-FAST, and diagnostic studies

| **Key components of damage control resuscitation** | *Early hemorrhage control:* Prioritize the identification and control of bleeding sources through direct pressure, tourniquets, or surgical intervention | *Balanced resuscitation:* Administer a balanced ratio of crystalloids and blood products to restore blood volume and improve coagulation. Aim for a 1:1:1 ratio of PRBCs, FFP, and platelets to minimize dilutional coagulopathy | *Minimize crystalloid use:* Limit the use of crystalloids to reduce the risk of dilutional coagulopathy and avoid fluid overload. Use crystalloids judiciously, primarily for initial resuscitation before transitioning to blood products |
|---|---|---|---|
| **Early use of tranexamic acid (TXA):** Administer TXA as soon as possible in cases of significant hemorrhage to reduce mortality associated with trauma-related bleeding | *Monitoring and targets:* Use of a restricted volume replacement strategy with a target systolic blood pressure of 80–90 mm Hg (mean arterial pressure 50–60 mm Hg) until major bleeding has been stopped without clinical evidence of brain injury and/or spinal injury.<br>In patients with severe TBI (GCS £ 8), a mean arterial pressure ≥80 mm Hg to be maintained | *Temperature management:* Prevent hypothermia by using warming blankets, heated IV fluids, and maintaining a warm environment | |

## SECONDARY SURVEY

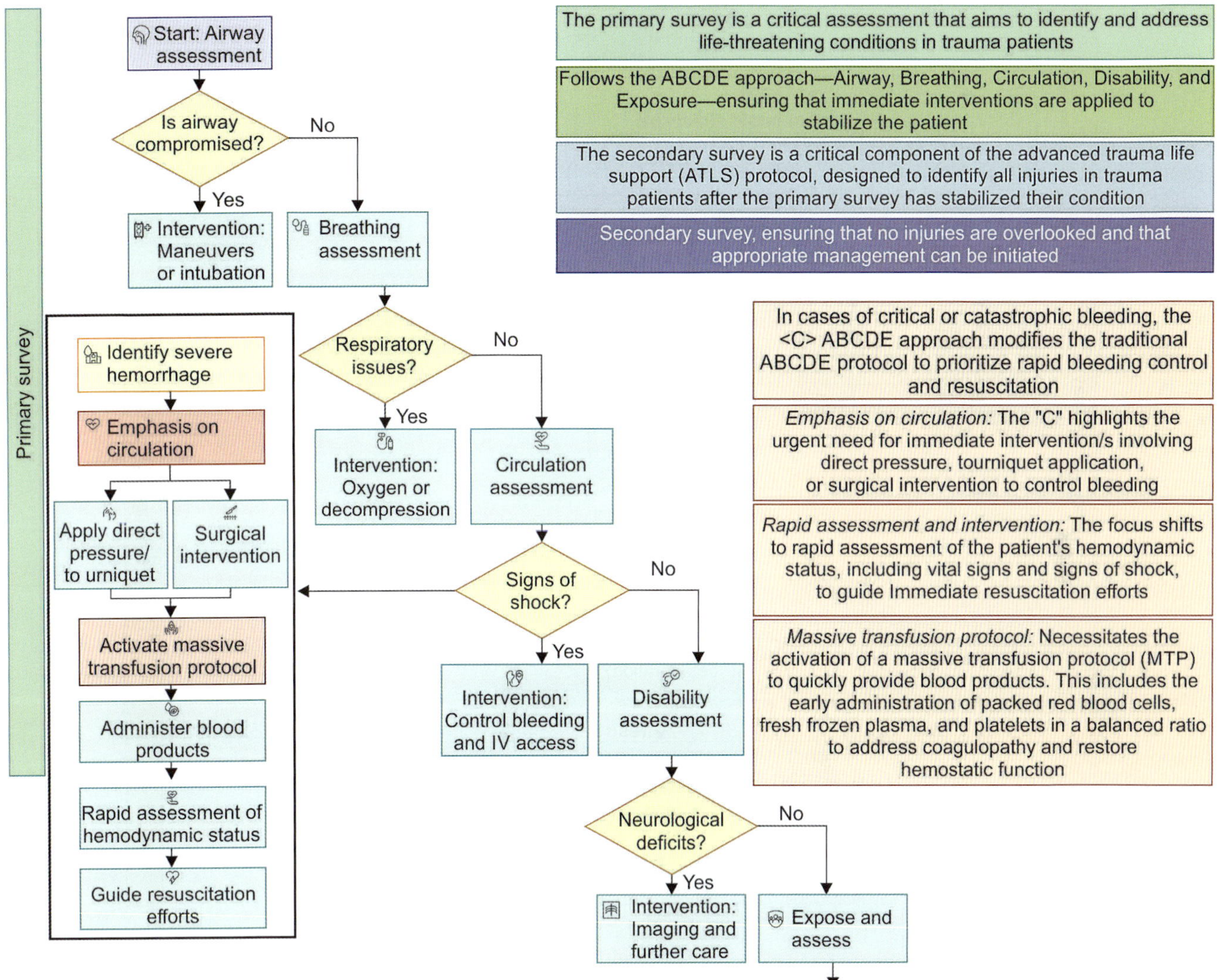


*Contd...*

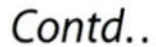

*Contd...*

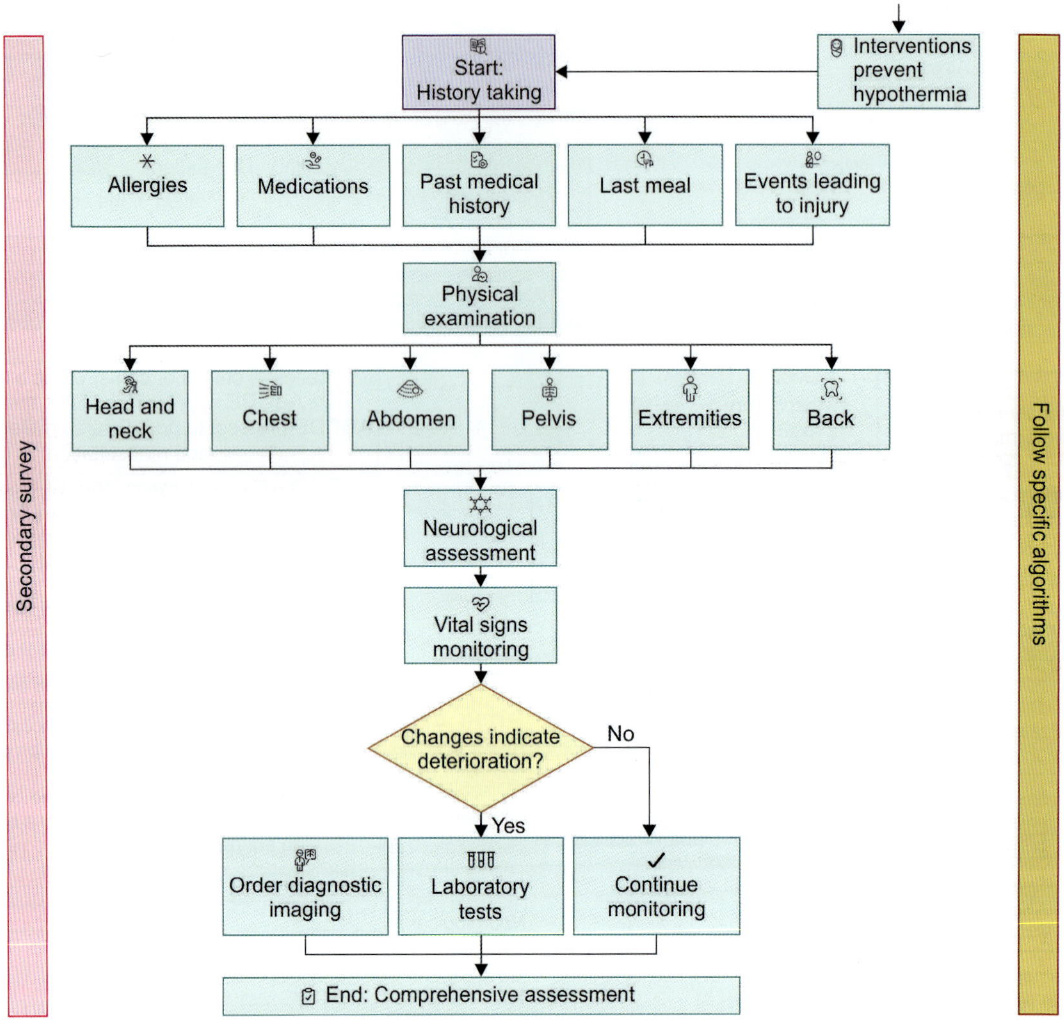

Secondary survey

Interventions prevent hypothermia

Start: History taking

Allergies

Medications

Past medical history

Last meal

Events leading to injury

Physical examination

Head and neck

Chest

Abdomen

Pelvis

Extremities

Back

Neurological assessment

Vital signs monitoring

Changes indicate deterioration?

No

Yes

Order diagnostic imaging

Laboratory tests

Continue monitoring

End: Comprehensive assessment

Follow specific algorithms

CHAPTER

# 75 Chest Trauma

**High-risk mechanisms of injury for blunt thoracic trauma**

- Falls from >6 m
- Motor vehicle collisions with partial or complete ejection, intrusion into the vehicle or death of a passenger in the same compartment of the vehicle
- Collision with a pedestrian or bicyclist
- Motorcycle collisions >32 kph (20 mph)

**What are the potential criteria of gravity for thoracic trauma?**

- Age >65 years old
- Previous cardiopulmonary diseases
- Coagulation diseases or acquired coagulation disorders (anticoagulant or antiplatelet treatments)
- High velocity trauma and penetrating trauma
- More than 2 ribs fracture especially for patients more than 65-year-old
- Respiratory distress with respiratory rate >25/min or hypoxemia (pulse oximetry <90% on air or <95% with oxygen)
- Circulatory failure [systolic arterial pressure (SAP) <110 mm Hg, or more than 30% decrease in SAP]

**Key facts about thoracic trauma**

- Road traffic collisions are the predominant cause of major blunt injury, exceeding contributions from falls, violence, and recreational injuries.
- Thoracic trauma is frequently accompanied by neurological and abdominal trauma.
- A structured 'C-ABCDE' primary survey, emphasizing teamwork and bedside imaging, identifies most life-threatening thoracic injuries.
- The CT trauma survey has added value in identifying life-threatening injuries that are difficult to diagnose clinically or with bedside imaging.
- Potentially life-threatening injuries, such as blunt cardiac injury, might be identified in the secondary survey and require careful assessment, evaluation and multidisciplinary input
- Priorities in cardiac arrest resulting from blunt trauma include recognition and management of reversible causes, including airway control, resuscitation with fluids and bilateral pleural decompression.

## BLUNT THORACIC TRAUMA

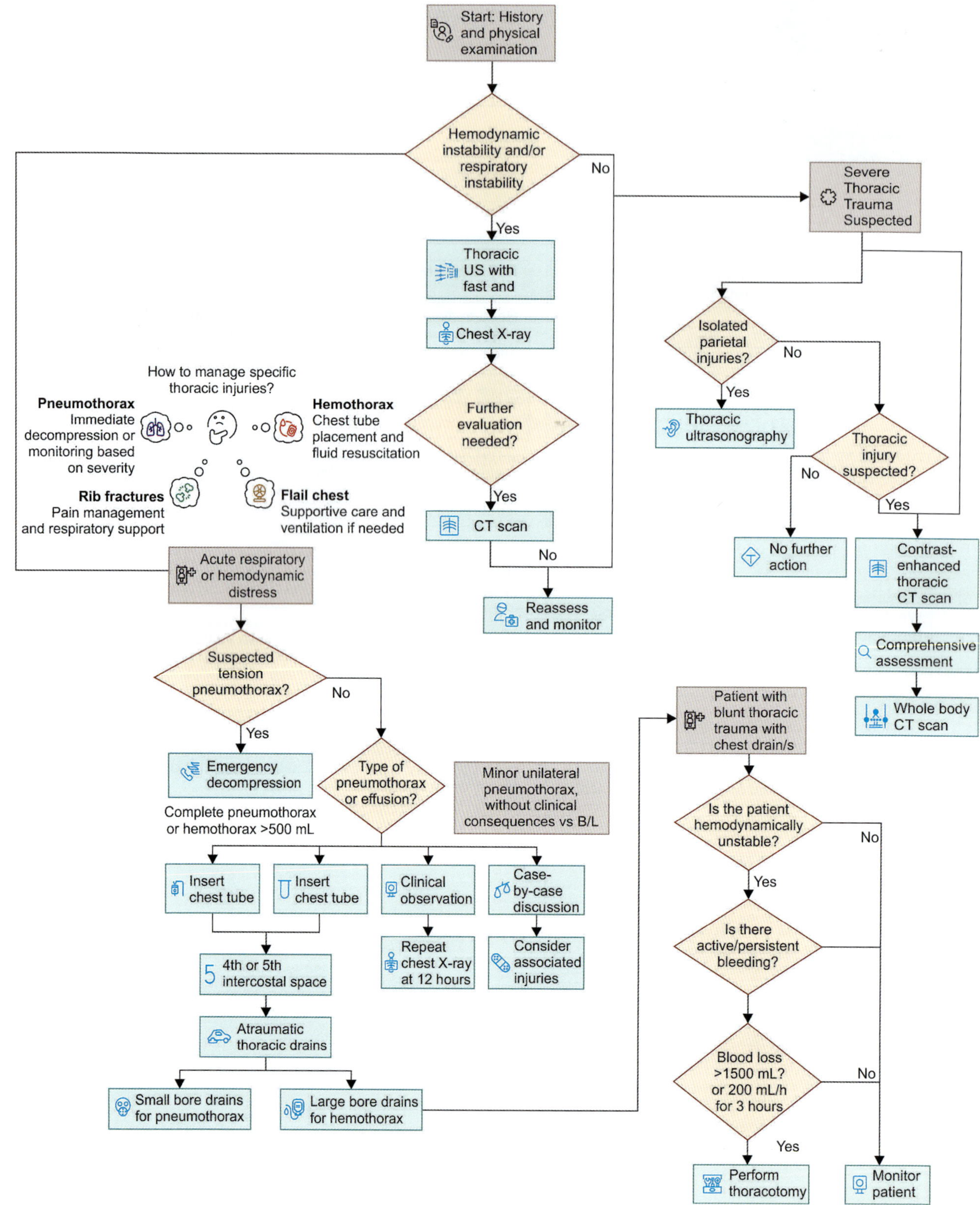

CHAPTER 76

# Penetrating Abdominal Trauma

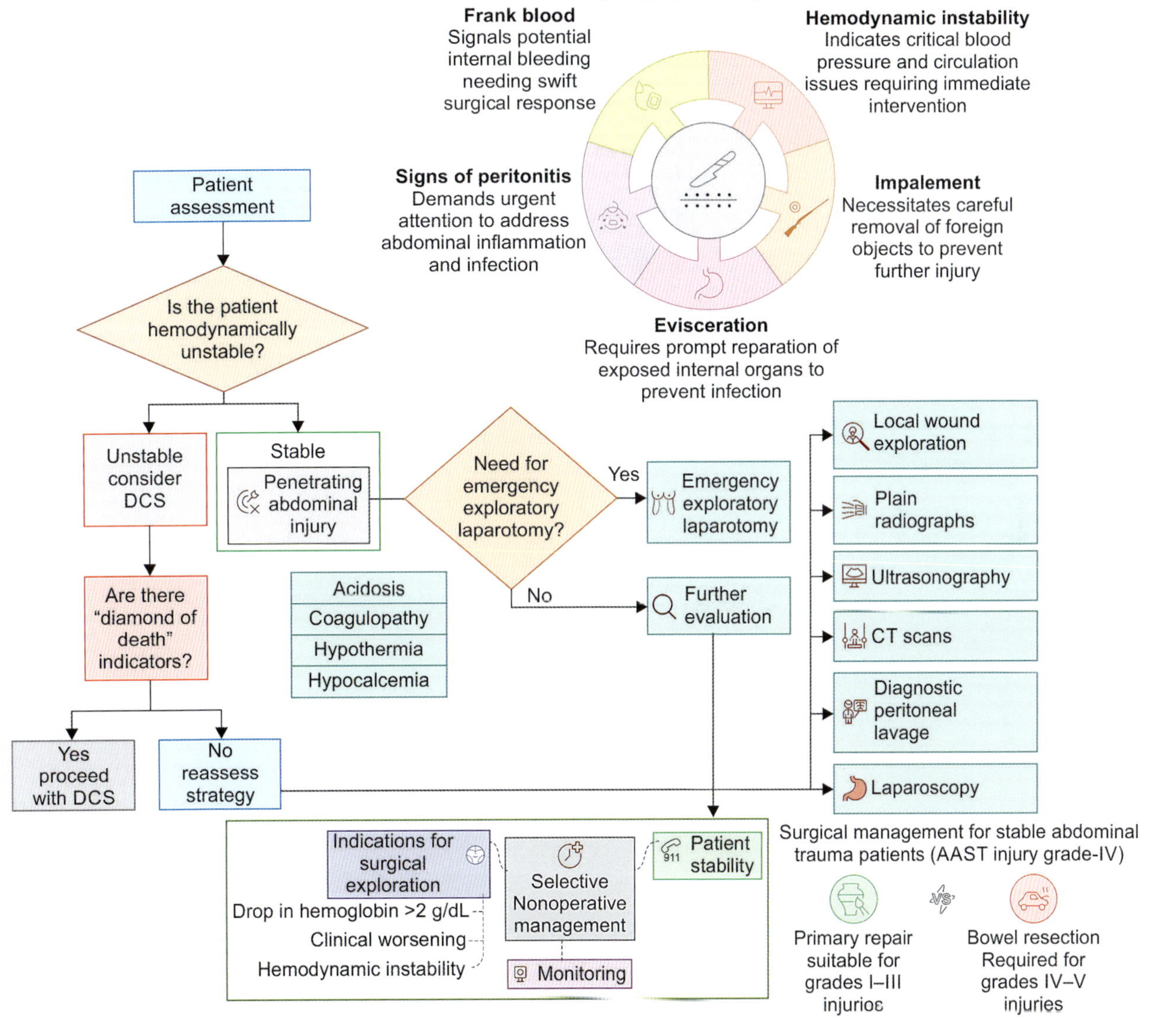

**Managing penetrating abdominal trauma**

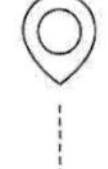

*Selective nonoperative management*
Monitor stable patients to avoid unnecessary surgeries

*Definitive surgical management*
Address anatomical issues in stable patients with structured options

*Damage control surgery*
Prioritize correcting physiology over anatomy in unstable patients

**Key facts about penetrating abdominal trauma:**

***Frequency:*** Penetrating abdominal trauma accounts for less than 15% of all trauma-related admissions

***Common causes:*** Stab injuries are more common than gunshot wounds in the civilian population
Gunshot wounds are less frequent but still important in trauma care

***Commonly affected organs and structures:***
Hollow viscus organs (e.g., intestines) are most commonly injured.
Diaphragm, liver, spleen, mesentery, great vessels (like the aorta and vena cava), and pancreas can also be affected.

***Most common injury locations:*** The left upper quadrant is most frequently injured, followed by the left lower quadrant and then the right side

***Flank wounds:*** These are commonly associated with injuries to retroperitoneal structures, including: kidneys, aorta, inferior vena cava, colon

Approximately 17–34% of cases involve multiple injuries

About 30% of penetrating abdominal trauma cases involve the diaphragm

***Diagnosis:*** A high index of suspicion is crucial in cases of penetrating trauma, especially if there are signs of peritonitis, shock, or massive bleeding

***Management:*** Approach generally involves surgery, and the goal is to control bleeding, repair damaged organs, and prevent further contamination or complications (e.g., sepsis)

CHAPTER 77

# Nonpenetrating Abdominal Trauma

## STABLE NONPENETRATING ABDOMEN TRAUMA ALGORITHM

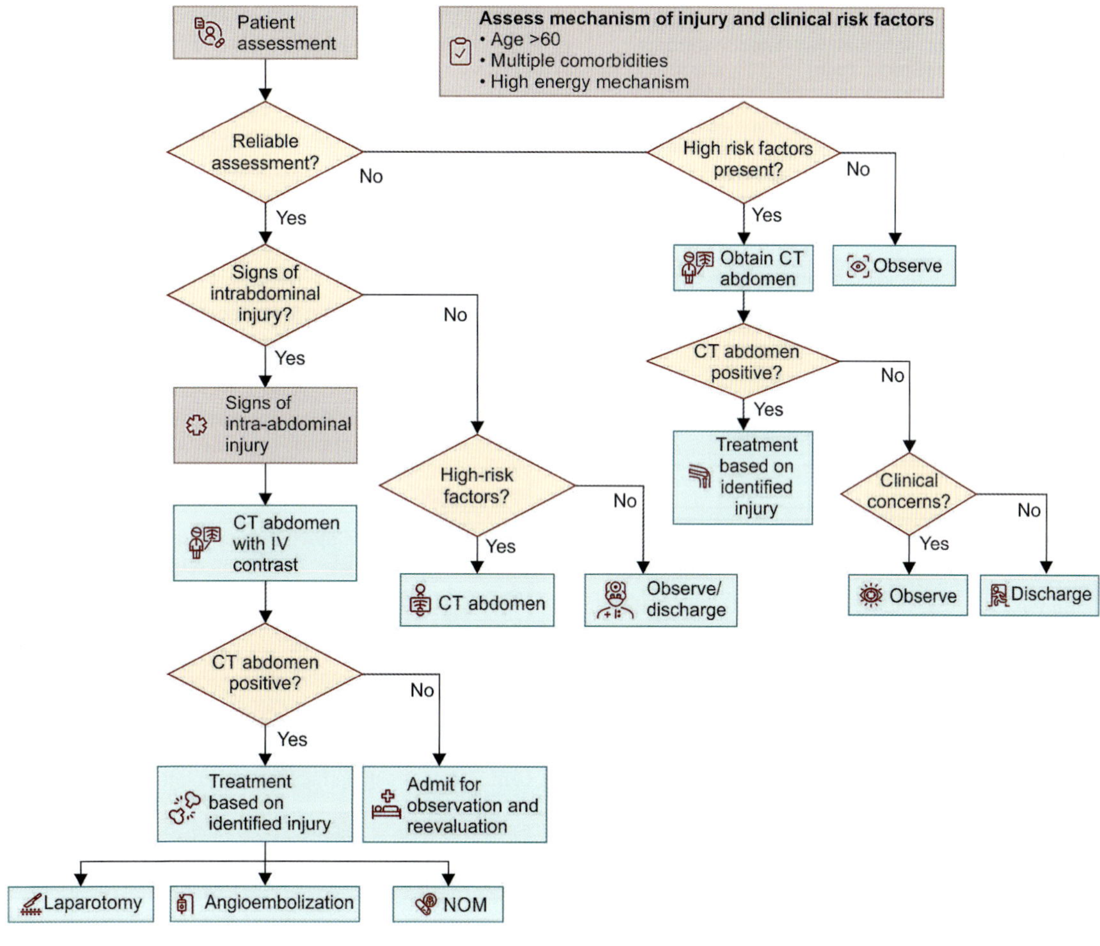

**WSES recommendations (world society of emergency surgery)**

Management of the awake and oriented blunt abdominal trauma patient starts with the primary survey, E-FAST physical examination and the secondary survey, blood chemistry, vital signs followed by contrast-enhanced abdominal CT. (Grade: High)

In patients not clinically evaluable, the diagnosis of hollow viscus injuries relies on injury pattern, vital signs, inflammatory markers trends and follow-up CT. (Grade: Moderate)

The presence of a seatbelt sign should prompt a CT scan and a high index of suspicion for bowel injury. (Grade: High)

Patients with high-risk mechanisms (i.e., handlebar, seatbelt sign) and non-specific CT findings should be admitted for observation including serial clinical examination. (Grade: Moderate)

The presence of highly specific CT findings such as extraluminal air, extraluminal oral contrast, or bowel-wall defects warrants prompt surgical exploration. (Grade: High)

The presence of highly sensitive CT findings such as free fluid in the absence of solid organ injury, abnormal enhancement of bowel wall, and mesenteric stranding can be used as an adjunct to the clinical picture but should not solely determine management. (Grade: Moderate)

Scoring systems that include radiologic, biochemical, and clinical signs can guide management in difficult scenarios. (Grade: Moderate)

**High-risk features according to the ACEP (American College of Emergency Physicians) to get CT Abdomen done**

- Hypotension
- Abdominal or costal margin tenderness
- Altered mental status (GCS <14)
- Abnormal chest radiograph
- Hematocrit <30%
- Hematuria

How to manage blunt abdominal trauma?

**Primary survey and CT**
Initiate with primary survey and E-FAST, followed by CT to assess injuries

**Seatbelt sign**
Perform CT and suspect bowel injury if seatbelt sign is present

**High-Risk mechanisms**
Admit for observation with serial examinations for high-risk patients

**Specific CT findings**
Proceed to surgical exploration if specific CT findings are present

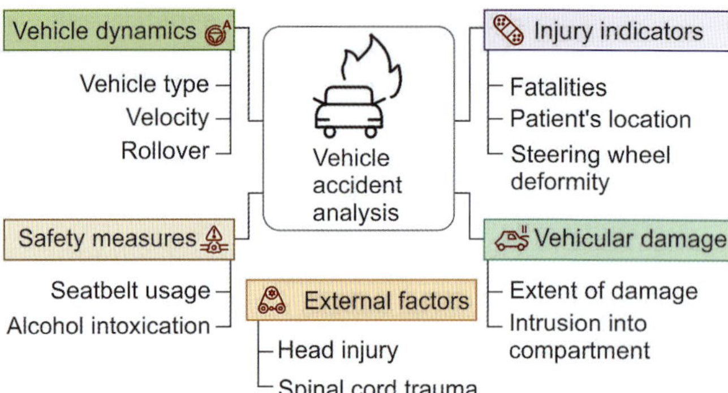


**Laboratory tests:** An adjunct to diagnosis and never a substitute for clinical or radiologic assessment in BAT

Hematocrit, (Hct <30% increases the likelihood of significant intra-abdominal injury in the setting of BAT). Anemia must be interpreted considering the clinical context including the timing and extent of hemorrhage, and the volume of exogenous fluids administered

***Leucocyte count:*** Catecholamine release due to trauma may demarginate the WBCs and cause an elevation with a left shift.

***Pancreatic enzymes:*** Elevated concentrations raise the possibility of pancreatic injury

***Liver function tests:*** Elevations of transaminases may be seen in hepatic injury and there is some evidence to say that higher elevations are associated with severe injuries.

***Urinalysis:*** Gross hematuria may suggest genitourinary trauma.

***Base deficit and Lactates:*** Non-specific. Higher lactates and a larger base deficit may be markers of significant intra-abdominal hemorrhage

## UNSTABLE NONPENETRATING/BLUNT ABDOMINAL TRAUMA

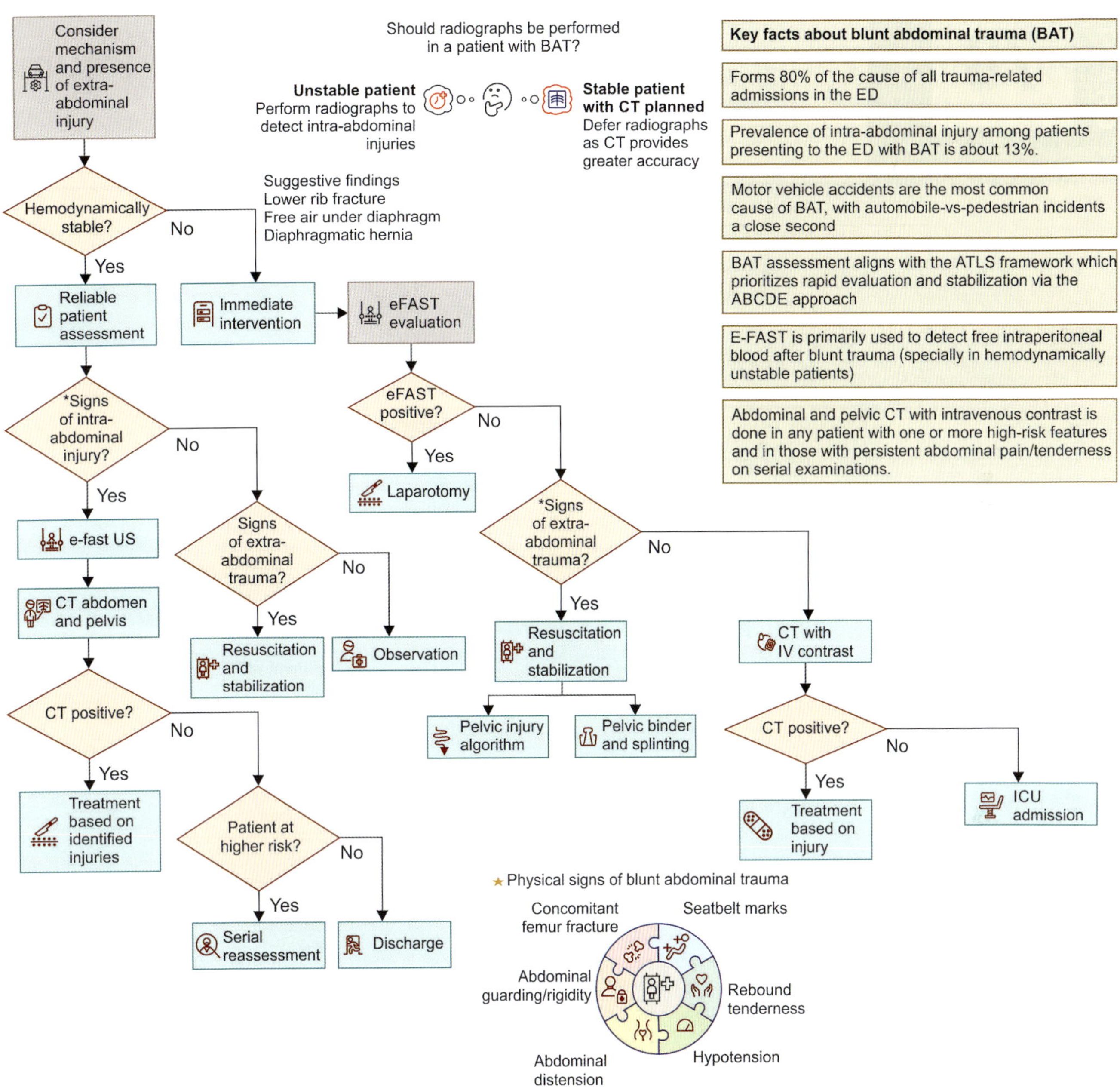


| Key facts about blunt abdominal trauma (BAT) |
|---|
| Forms 80% of the cause of all trauma-related admissions in the ED |
| Prevalence of intra-abdominal injury among patients presenting to the ED with BAT is about 13%. |
| Motor vehicle accidents are the most common cause of BAT, with automobile-vs-pedestrian incidents a close second |
| BAT assessment aligns with the ATLS framework which prioritizes rapid evaluation and stabilization via the ABCDE approach |
| E-FAST is primarily used to detect free intraperitoneal blood after blunt trauma (specially in hemodynamically unstable patients) |
| Abdominal and pelvic CT with intravenous contrast is done in any patient with one or more high-risk features and in those with persistent abdominal pain/tenderness on serial examinations. |

CHAPTER 78

# Cervical Trauma

**Spine stabilization**
- Place semi-rigid C-collar; immobilize entire patient on long spine board
- Maintain C-spine precautions

**Evaluable patient** (must fulfill all criteria)
- Glasgow Coma Scale score = 15
- Not intoxicated
- No distracting injury (preventing patient's full concentration on exam)
- Reliable/cooperative clinical exam

**Non-evaluable patient** (any of the following)
- Glasgow Coma Scale <15
- Intoxicated
- Distracting injury (preventing patient's full concentration on exam)

Determine if patient has neurological deficits and/or C-spine bony tenderness (not soft tissue)

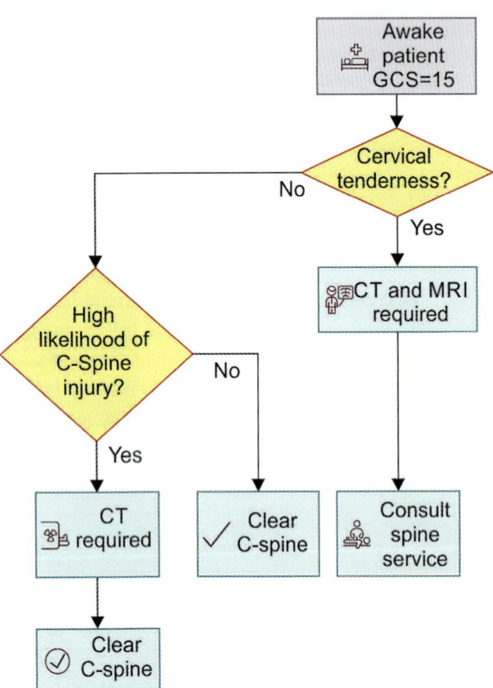


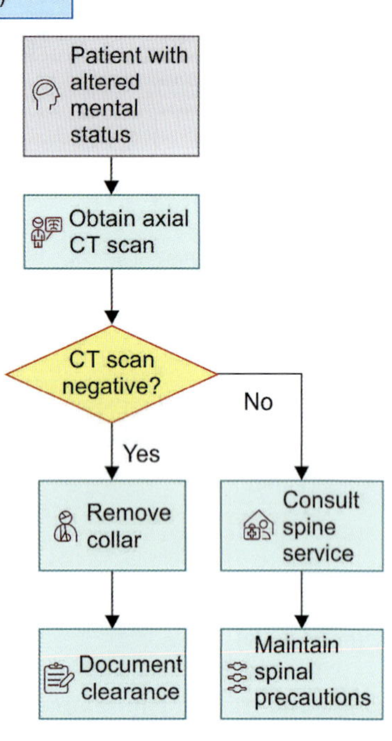

**Evaluating C-Spine injuries using NEXUS criteria**

**No Distracting Injury**
No other injuries that could obscure assessment

**No Tenderness**
Absence of pain along the spine's midline

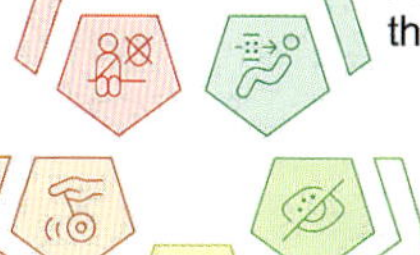

**No Neurologic Deficit**
No signs of nerve function impairment

**No Intoxication**
Clear absence of substance influence

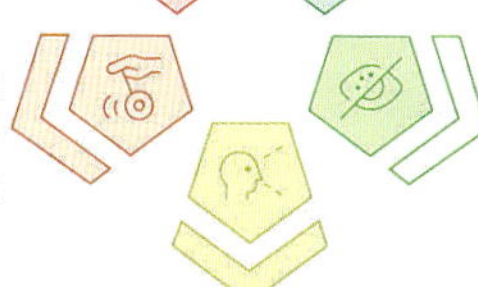

**Alertness**
The patient is fully aware and responsive

Patients should be considered to have a possible cervical spine injury if they present with any of the following conditions:

- A history of blow to the head or neck.
- Traumatic brain injury and/or skull fracture.
- Facial trauma such as fractures, tooth loss, or severe lacerations

- Pain in the cervical spine or paraspinous muscles.
- Pain to palpation of the cervical spine

Neurologic deficits in torso, legs, or arms not explained by peripheral nerve injuries

Age >65

Dangerous mechanism (Fall >3ft/5 stairs; axial load to head; High speed MVC >45mph with roll-over or ejection; bicycle or pedestrian struck)

Previous C-spine surgery

Acute paralysis

CHAPTER 79

# Pelvic Trauma

## YOUNG AND BURGESS CLASSIFICATION OF PELVIC RING FRACTURES

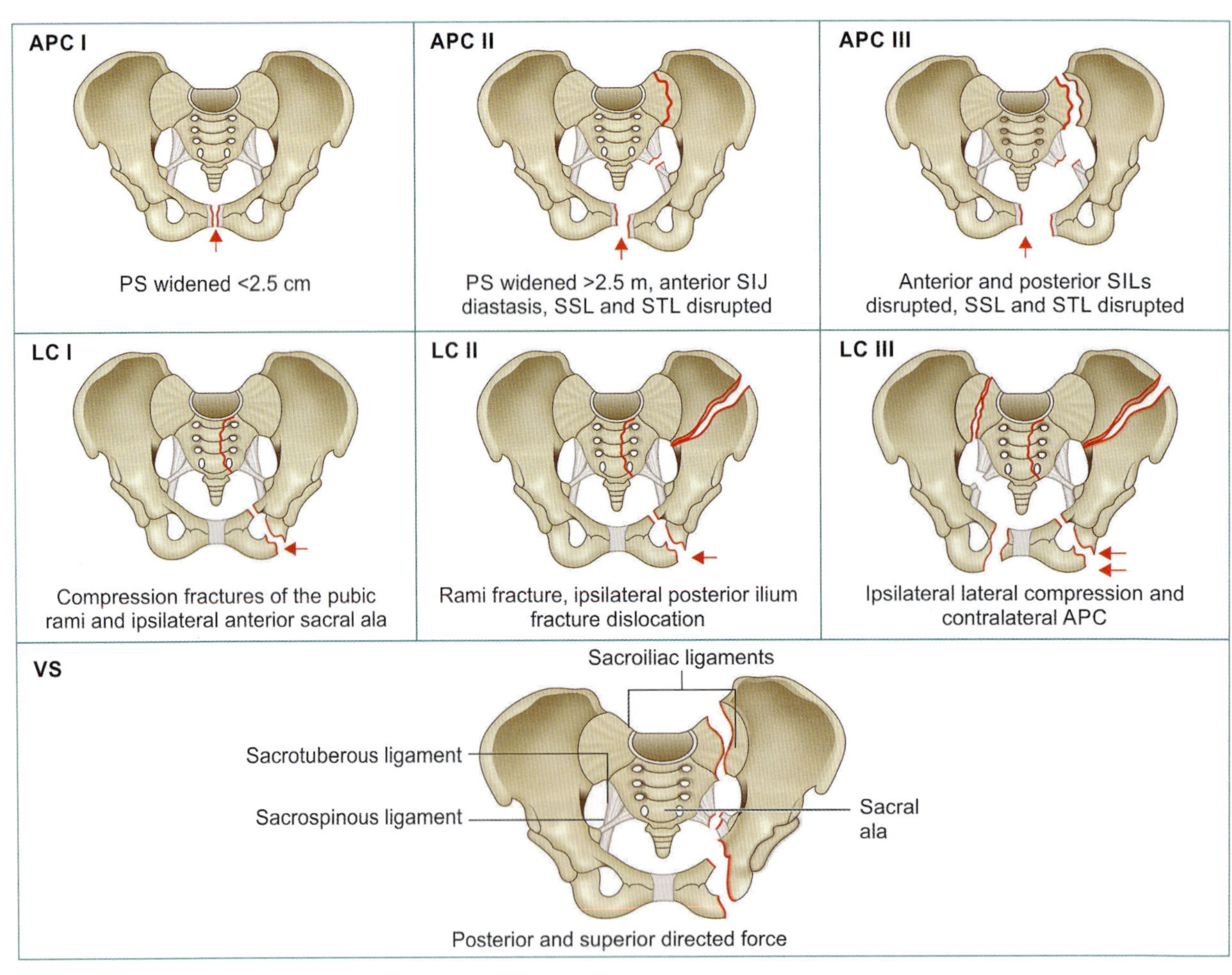

## KEY POINTS REGARDING PELVIC TRAUMA MANAGEMENT

- The management of pelvic trauma has markedly changed throughout the last decades with a significant improvement in outcomes, due to improvements in diagnostic and therapeutic tools.
- In determining the optimal treatment strategy, the hemodynamic status should be supplemented by anatomical lesions classification and associated injuries.
- The anatomical description of pelvic ring lesions is fundamental in the management algorithm but, in clinical practice the first decisions are based mainly on the clinical conditions and the associated injuries, and less on the pelvic ring lesions.
- 10–15% of patients with pelvic fractures arrive to the ED in shock with mortality rate of 32%.
- The causes of dying in the majority is part uncontrolled bleeding and by patients physiologic exhaustion.
- Bleeding from pelvic fractures can occur from veins (80%) and from arteries (20%).
- High-grade injuries often involve thoraco-abdominal trauma (80%) and can also include bladder, urethra (1.6–25%), vaginal, nerve, sphincter, and rectal injuries (18–64%), as well as soft tissue damage (up to 72%). These should be suspected, especially in patients with perineal hematoma or significant soft-tissue disruption.

| **Management Overview** | Initial management involves hemorrhage control and fluid resuscitation | Serum lactates and base deficit are diagnostic markers to estimate the extent of traumatic hemorrhagic shock and to monitor response to resuscitation | TEG or ROTEM if available are recommended to determine the presence of coagulopathy and to provide targeted resuscitation with blood products | *E-FAST and pelvic X-ray:* Recommended in hemodynamic and mechanic unstable patients with pelvic trauma |
|---|---|---|---|---|
| *Hemodynamically stable patients:* Multiphasic CT scan with IV contrast to exclude pelvic hemorrhage | Pelvic hematoma >500 $cm^3$, an arterial injury should be suspected even in the absence of a visible contrast blush | Presence of local perineal hematoma and pelvic disruption at pelvic X-ray: Retrograde urethrogram/ urethrocystogram with contrast CT scan | • *Suspected rectal injuries:* Perineal and digital rectal examination should be done<br>• *Positive rectal examination:* Proctosopy | |

The evaluation of pelvic trauma should be based on the mechanism of injury (particularly in case of high energy impact and blunt trauma), should begin with:

- Physical examination to search a pelvic ring deformity or instability
- A pelvic or perineal hematoma
- A rectal/urethral bleeding

- Role of angioembolization in hemodynamically stable pelvic fractures
- Patients with CT-scan demonstrating arterial contrast extravasation in the pelvis may benefit from pelvic angiography/ angioembolization regardless of hemodynamic status.
- Elderly patients with pelvic fractures should be considered for pelvic angiography/angioembolization regardless of hemodynamic status.

## PELVIC TRAUMA

*Mechanisms of Pelvic injuries*

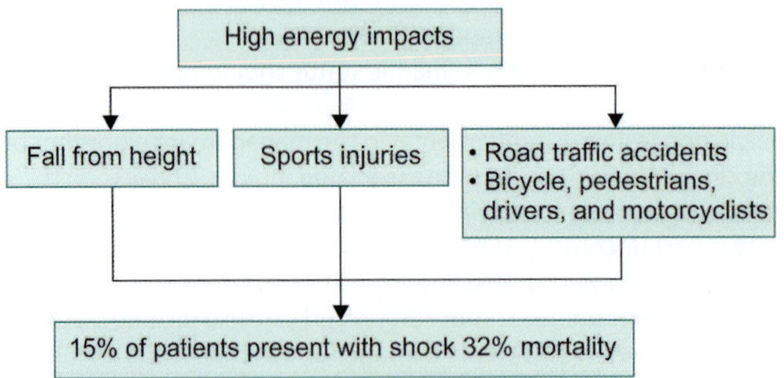


*Injury assessment techniques:*

- Supine pelvic X-ray (adjunct to primary survey)
- Focused assessment with sonography in trauma

Restricted efficacy in isolated pelvic trauma
Risk of false-positive free fluid with a large retroperitoneal hematoma

When to suspect isolated pelvic trauma?

- Mechanism of injury
- Physical examination indicating pelvic injury
- Bleeding from rectum or urethra
- Large hematoma altering the shape of the perineum

Total body spiral computerized tomography offers the most sensitive diagnostic imaging

## MANAGEMENT PRINCIPLES

*Key points:*

- Complex and critical
- Generally caused by high-energy impact
- Index of suspicion is needed to suspect isolated pelvic injury.
- Most often associated with multisystem injury needing a multidisciplinary approach.

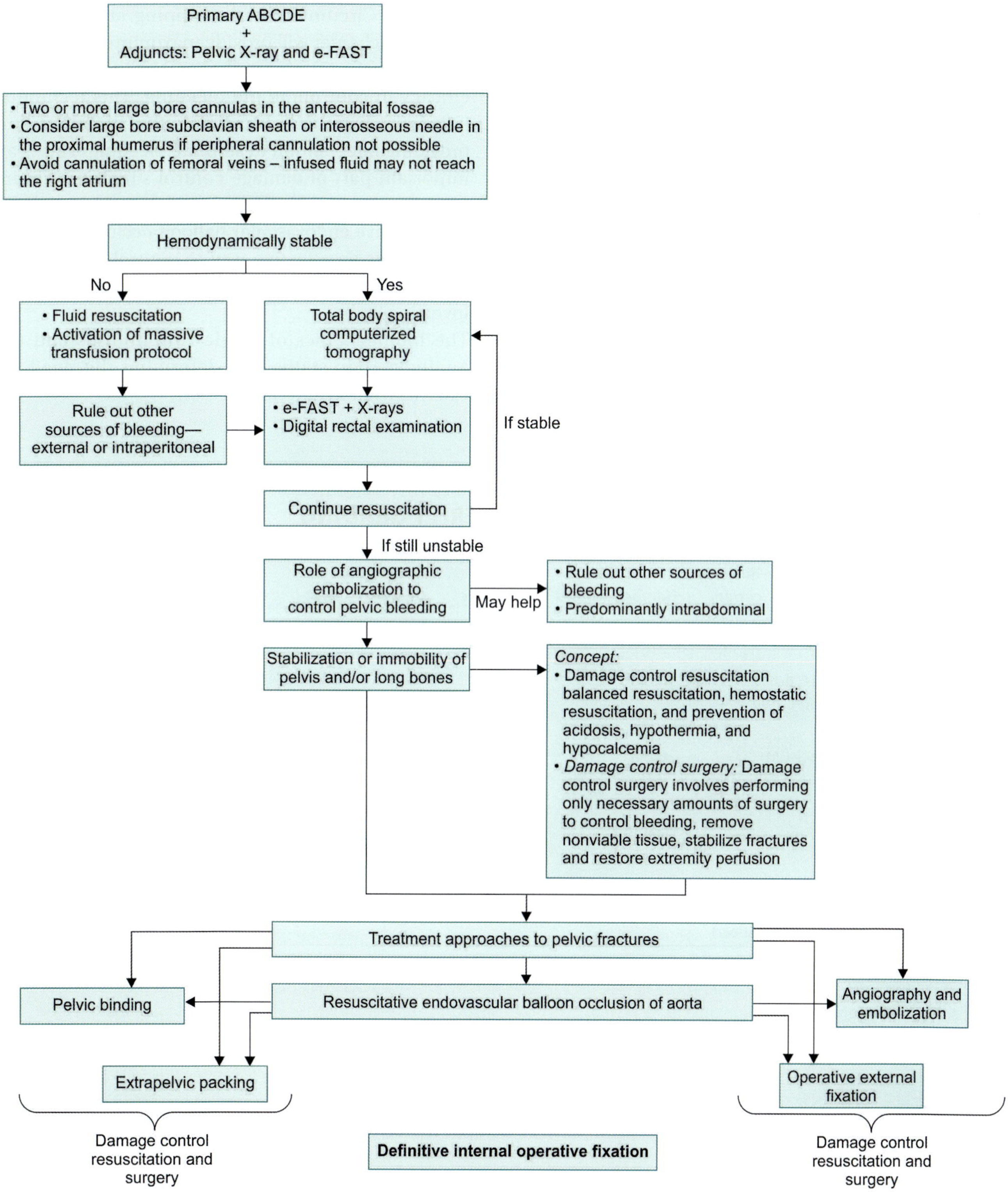

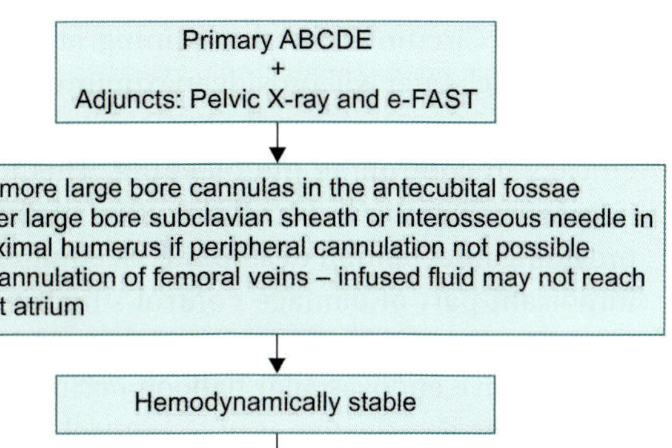

## INJURY ASSESSMENT TECHNIQUE IN PELVIC FRACTURES:

- CT scan most sensitive and relevant imaging modality
- If hemodynamically unstable-practically may not be feasible
  - Use indirect clues to suspect
  - Pelvic fractures on X-ray
  - Negative e-FAST
  - No other injury to explain the hemodynamic instability
  - Perineal hematoma
  - Bleeding per rectum or periurethral

## MANAGEMENT PRINCIPLES OF SEVERE PELVIC FRACTURES

- CT is the most sensitive modality to diagnose and assess pelvic injuries.
- If patient is very unstable, high index of suspicion is needed to suspect pelvic injuries.
- E-FAST and X-rays may only help to rule out non-pelvic abdominal injuries. In fact, a positive E-FAST may mislead and may enhance the risk of missing a pelvic injury.
- Pelvic binder is the simplest and an effective method to provide pelvic stabilization by preventing pelvic movements, reducing volume and decreasing bleeding. Circumferential wrapping at the level of greater trochanter will provide maximum efficacy.
- Transcatheter arterial embolization has a 81–100% efficacy in controlling the bleeding. This technique helps in diagnosis, localizing the bleeding and providing intervention to stop the bleeding. This is an important part of damage control surgery in severe pelvic trauma.
- Resuscitative endovascular balloon occlusion of aorta (REBOA) is an effective way to control hemorrhage in pelvic injuries, despite documented complications involving limbs.
- The biomechanics of pelvic ring injuries and the hemodynamic status will determine the need for external fixation and stabilization.

## MANAGEMENT OF PELVIC TRAUMA AS PER SEVERITY GRADING

| | *WSES grade* | *Young-Burgees classification* | *Hemodynamics* | *Mechanic* | *CT-scan* | *First-line treatment* |
|---|---|---|---|---|---|---|
| Minor | WSES grade I | APC I–LC I | Stable | Stable | Yes | Nonoperative management, |
| Moderate | WSES grade II | LC II/III<br>APC II/III | Stable | Unstable | Yes | Pelvic binder in the field ±<br>Angioembolization (if blush at CT-scan)<br>OM–anterior external fixation |
| | WSES grade III | VS-CM | Stable | Unstable | Yes | Pelvic Binder in the field ±<br>Angioembolization (if blush at CT-scan)<br>OM-C-Clamp |
| | WSES grade IV | Any | Unstable | Any | No | Pelvic Binder in the field Preperitoneal Pelvic Packing ± Mechanical fixation ±<br>REBOA ± Angioembolization |

(APC: anteroposterior compression; CM: combined mechanism; LC: lateral compression; REBOA: resuscitative endo-aortic balloon; OM: operative management; VS: vertical shear)

CHAPTER 80

# Vascular Injuries Management

## ETIOLOGY

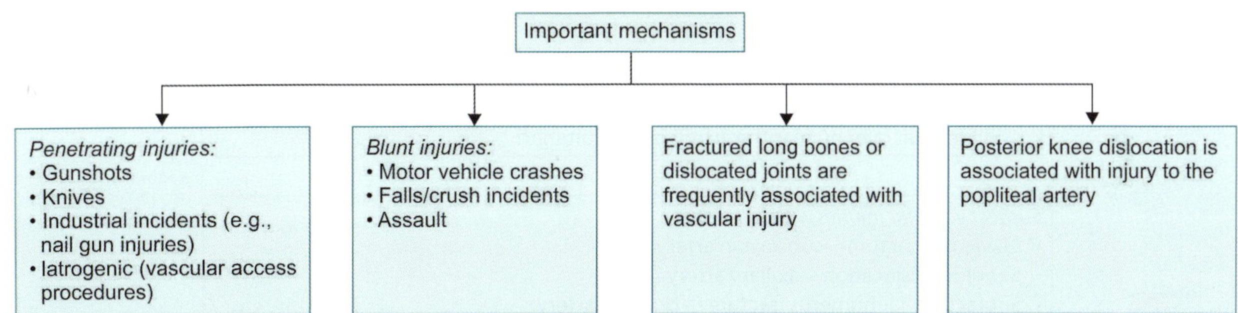


## PATHOPHYSIOLOGY OF VASCULAR INJURIES

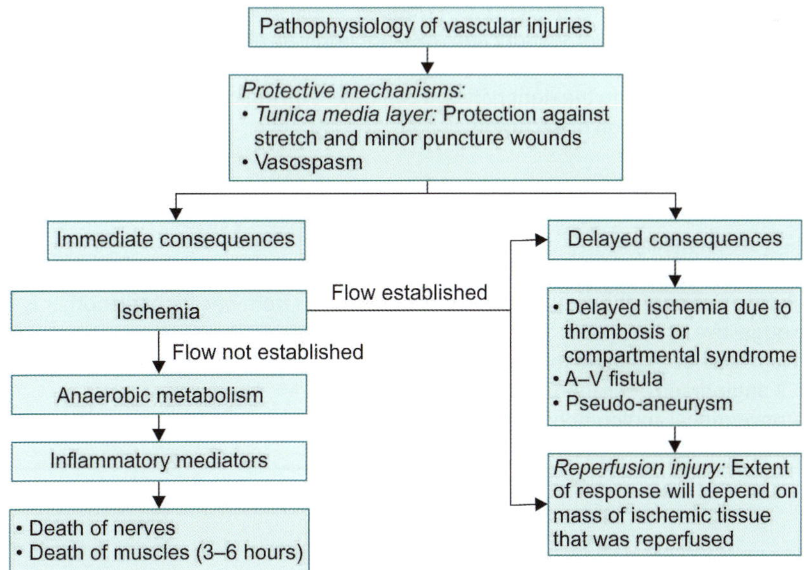

## DIAGNOSIS

*Soft signs:*
- *Which may create suspicion, but need further evaluation:*
- A history of significant hemorrhage at the scene
- Proximity of the penetrating wound, bony injury, or blunt trauma to a major artery
- Decreased pulse compared with the uninjured extremity
- Peripheral nerve deficit
- Small nonpulsatile hematoma
- *Ankle:* Brachial index <0.9
- Abnormal flow-velocity waveform on Doppler ultrasound
- Shock that is not the result of other injuries

*Hard signs:*
- Observed pulsatile bleeding
- Visible expanding hematoma
- Signs of distal ischemia (absent distal pulses; cold and pale limb)
- Palpable thrill (vibration) by manual palpation
- Audible bruit over or near the artery by auscultation

*Suspect vascular injuries with following:*
- Clavicular fracture—subclavian artery
- Shoulder dislocation—axillary artery
- Supracondylar humerus fracture— brachial artery
- Femur fracture—superficial femoral artery
- Posterior knee dislocation—popliteal artery

*Diagnostic adjuncts:*
- *Doppler ultrasound:* The presence of a Doppler signal in a pulseless limb can provide a false sense of security and does not imply an absence of significant vascular injury
- *Duplex ultrasound:* In the right hands, it can detect the following:
  - Arterial disruption or occlusion
  - Intimal flaps
  - Venous occlusion
  - Hematoma
  - Pseudoaneurysm
  - Arteriovenous fistula
- Pulse oximetry—the reduction in oximeter readings from one limb to another is suggestive
- Plain films determining the presence of fractures and foreign bodies
- CT angiography—diagnosis of choice
- Conventional angiography—gold standard, and can be used for therapeutic interventions

## MANAGEMENT

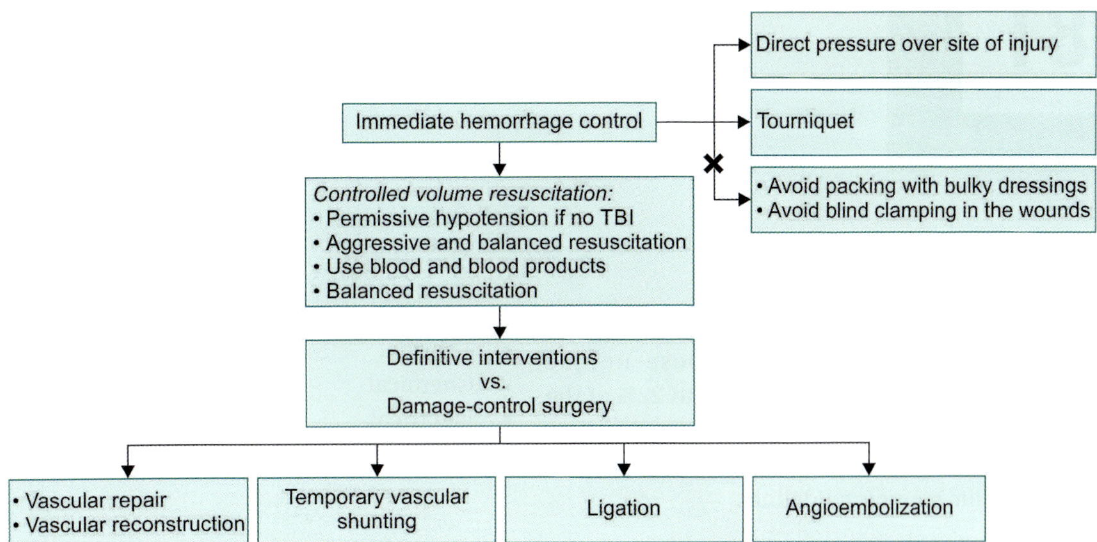


## IMPORTANT CONSIDERATIONS

- Angiography can be considered as gold standard for identification and characterization of vascular injury. Compared to CT Angiographic images are less impacted by the presence of foreign bodies and also provide real-time indication of flow patterns in the imaged arterial segment, while providing access for therapeutic endovascular techniques.
- Hemorrhage controls a very important first step in resuscitation.
- Vascular reconstruction (or restoration of flow with shunting) that occurs within three hours of injury is generally accepted to have the best outcome.
- Control is best achieved by vessel loops passed twice around the vessel or using atraumatic forceps.
- Selected use of balloon tamponade is useful for temporary control of hemorrhage from junctional or deep, difficult-to-access areas.
- Large veins should be repaired (or shunted), and small veins can be ligated.
- Temporary vascular shunting is a damage control technique that should be considered as a temporizing measure.
- Occasionally, it will be impossible or impractical to shunt or repair a vessel, and that vessel may require ligation to control life-threatening hemorrhage.
- Vessels in which ligation may be tolerated include the following:
    - Common and external carotid arteries
    - Subclavian artery (as long as ligated distal to thyro-cervical trunk)
    - Axillary artery
    - Brachial artery (distal to profunda branch)
    - Ulnar or radial artery individually
    - Celiac trunk
    - Internal iliac artery
- Vessels in which ligation may be, poorly tolerated:
    - Internal carotid artery (15–20% incidence of stroke)
    - Superior mesenteric artery
    - External iliac artery
    - Common femoral artery
    - Popliteal artery
- Different options for vascular repair include:
    - Lateral arteriorrhaphy or venorrhaphy
    - Patch angioplasty
    - Resection with end-to-end anastomosis
    - Resection with interposition graft (vein, PTFE/Dacron, CryoVein, Artegraft, etc.)
    - Bypass graft
    - Extra-anatomic bypass
    - Stent-graft repair

CHAPTER 81

# Burns

## INTRODUCTION

Burns as a pathophysiological entity pose unique challenges in critical care management. Up to 22% of the burn's patients attending the emergency-room requires ICU admission. Burns should be evaluated as per the Advanced trauma life support guidelines.

*Modes of burns:*

- Thermal
- Chemical
- Electrical

## INITIAL ASSESSMENT

| Primary survey | Secondary survey |
|---|---|
| • ABCDE assessment including adjuncts to primary survey<br>• *Secure IV access:* Peripheral and/or central access<br>• If obtunded, rule out coexisting carbon monoxide, cyanide toxicity, and CT brain<br>• Temperature control and exposure in the warm environment<br>• If any adherent materials clothes, watches, etc. including the contact lenses should be removed<br>• If any ongoing burns-irrigation with warm water | • History ("AMPLET"—allergies, medications, past medical history, last meal, events leading to presentation, and tetanus immunization history)<br>• Head to toe assessment: Severity and extent of burns<br>• Patients with electrical burns prone to rhabdomyolysis, arrythmias, and compartment syndrome<br>• Closed space burns are prone for inhalational injuries<br>• Circumferential burns are prone for vascular compromise, identify and treat early |

## GRADING OF BURNS

Thickness can be measured by histological staining, thermography, laser Doppler analysis, etc. However, clinical method is most commonly employed.

- Epidermal (superficial, first degree): Involves only the epidermal layer of skin
- Partial-thickness burns (second degree) involve the epidermis and portions of the dermis. They are characterized as either superficial or deep-superficial partial thickness burns.
- Full-thickness burns (Third degree) extend through and destroy all layers of the dermis, often injuring the underlying subcutaneous tissue-Deep partial thickness burns.
- Deep burn injury (fourth degree) extends into underlying soft tissue and can involve muscle and/or bone.

## EXTENT OF BURNS

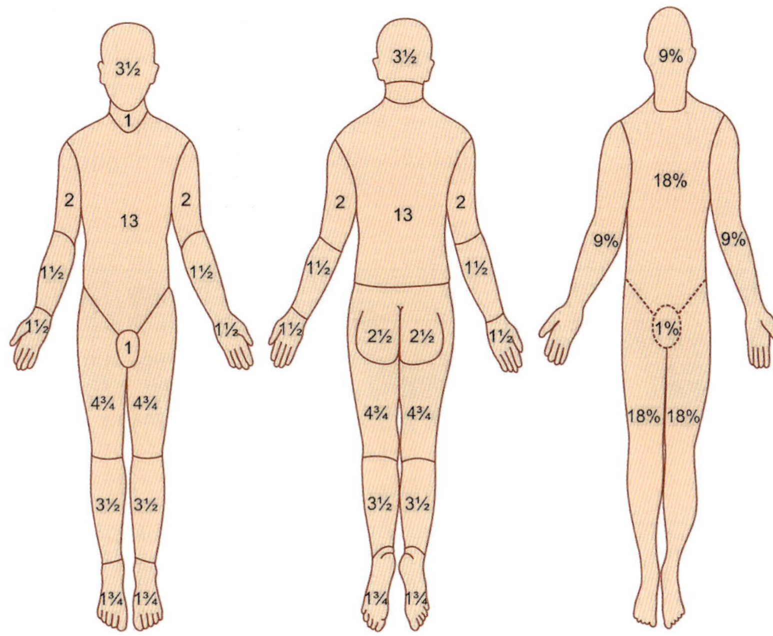


- *Lund and Browder:* Slightly complex but provides more precise information regarding the total body surface area involved
- *Wallace rule of Nine:* Simplified version and easier to recall. Hands 9, front torso-18, back torso-18, legs each-18, head front and back-9, perineum-1
- *Palm method:* Outstretched Patient's palm represents 1 percent of TBSA. Ideal for assessment of scattered burns

## MAJOR BURNS AND REFERRAL CRITERIA

Major burns need to be referred to burns center that comprises of multi-disciplinary team and they are:

- Involving ≥20% of TBSA (excluding 1st degree) in adults or
- ≥10% (<14 years and >60 years).
- Associated with inhalational injury/chemical/electrical injuries or major trauma.
- Circumferential burns with impending neurovascular compromise or
- Burns involving the face, eyes, ears, and perineum.

Patients in the range of 25–70% TBSA should receive the priority of transfer rather than patients with >70% of burns, who have lower overall chances of survival.

## MANAGEMENT

### Airway and Breathing Management

- Upper airway/supraglottic injury easily detected on physical examination and subglottic injury is occult. Any degrees of respiratory distress/stridor are an emergent indication for early intubation.
- Should be considered as difficult airway and should follow AIDAA algorithm and note to avoid succinylcholine as NMB in Rapid sequence intubation.
- If co-existent inhalational injury is suspected Bronchoscopy examination within 24 hours is mandatory and if proven role of nebulized heparin, N-acetyl-cysteine, short acting B2 agonists and corticosteroids to be considered.
- Coexistent CO intoxication may lead to tissue hypoxia. Co-oximetry confirms the diagnosis of Carboxyhemoglobin levels. Severe toxicity -COHb levels >20% in adults and >15% in children. T½ of CO in ambient air is 250 minutes. Reduced to 60 minutes with 100% oxygen and with 2–3 atm hyperbaric oxygen therapy T½ reduced to 30 minutes.
- Cyanide toxicity with industrial, polymer, rubber industry, etc. related fire accidents, clothing must be removed quickly, Use of hydroxocobalamin to reduce the incidence of respiratory infections and mechanical ventilator days. Other options include inducing methemoglobinemia with nitrites and detoxification by converting into non-toxic thiocyanate with sodium thiosulphate.

- Lactates can be an indicator of COHb and cyanide toxicity, also is an independent predictor of mortality in burns.

## Fluids and Hemodynamics

- Optimum fluid management improves mortality and extension of the burn depth. Of the three zones of coagulation, stasis and hyperemia, early adequate perfusion improves zone of stasis and reduces the expansion of coagulation zone in the Jackson's pathophysiological model.
- The goal is to maintain euvolemia and all the patients >20% TBSA burns should undergo protocolized fluid resuscitation. The resuscitation phase lasts for 24–36 hours. Before assessing the extent of burns fluids are started at 10 mL/kg/hr.

<table>
<tr><th>Drug</th><th>Dose and duration</th><th>De-escalation</th></tr>
<tr>
<td>• Crystalloids are preferred.<br>• NS may cause hyperchloremia and AKI<br>• RL: Lower sodium content, may aggravate SIADH and also calcium may be harmful in burns<br>• PlasmaLyte and other balanced solutions are devoid of these issues and are preferred<br>• Colloids are sparingly indicated mainly in subsequent phases.<br>• Dextrose solutions have role in pediatric resuscitation of burns<br>• Hypertonic saline and fresh frozen plasma have been other resuscitative fluids in certain studies</td>
<td>
<table>
<tr><th rowspan="2">Formula</th><th colspan="2">First 24 hours</th><th rowspan="2">Next 24 hours</th></tr>
<tr><th>Choice of fluid</th><th>Volume</th></tr>
<tr><td>Parkland</td><td>Ringer's Lactate</td><td>4 mL/kg/%- first half in 8 h second half in 16 h</td><td>• Colloids only.<br>• No crystalloids</td></tr>
<tr><td>Modified Parkland</td><td>Ringer's Lactate</td><td>4 mL/kg/%- first half in 8 h, second half in 16 h</td><td>5% albumin</td></tr>
<tr><td rowspan="3">Brooke</td><td>Ringer's Lactate</td><td>1.5 mL/kg/%</td><td>Ringer's Lactate</td></tr>
<tr><td>Colloids</td><td>0.5 mL/kg/%</td><td>Colloids</td></tr>
<tr><td>5% D</td><td>2,000 mL</td><td>Dextrose 5%</td></tr>
<tr><td>Modified Brooke</td><td>Ringer's Lactate</td><td>2 mL/kg/%</td><td>Colloids</td></tr>
<tr><td rowspan="3">Evans</td><td>Crystalloid</td><td>1 mL/kg/%</td><td>Crystalloid</td></tr>
<tr><td>Colloid</td><td>1 mL/kg/%</td><td>Colloid</td></tr>
<tr><td>5% D</td><td>2,000 mL</td><td>2,000 mL</td></tr>
</table>
</td>
<td>• Endpoints of Resuscitation<br>• Target urine output (0.3 mL/kg/h)<br>• Use of dynamic indices of fluid resuscitation<br>• POCUS guided assessment<br>• Hypotensive resuscitation and "Permissive hyperlactatemia" (up to 4–5 mmol/L) is accepted in initial phases to avoid fluid creep and multi-organ dysfunction</td>
</tr>
</table>

*De-resuscitation:* Over-resuscitation leads to destruction of glycocalyx and endothelium leading to fluid creep. Resuscitation exceeding 250 mL/Kg increases the risk if Intrabdominal syndrome, organ dysfunction and is termed as Ivy's Index. Use of VExUS, multi-organ POCUS and IAP measurement is of very essential to optimize organ perfusion pressure and improve organ function. WSACS algorithm to be followed to optimize fluid status.

| Nutrition | Sepsis and wound care |
|---|---|
| • Harrison benedict equation or weight-based equations (25 kcal/kg) are used, the final value is multiplied by the stress factor based on TBSA burns assessment. (1.2 for less than 10% TBSA, 1.3 for 10–20% TBSA, 1.5 for 20–40% TBSA, 1.7 for 40–60% TBSA, and 2 for >60% TBSA)<br>• The Curreri formula as follows (40 kcal × TBSA) + (25 kcal × ideal body weight in kilograms)<br>• Indirect calorimetry is used in intubated patients.<br>• 1.5–2 gm/kg of proteins, reduced levels of fat content - no more than 15–30% of total calories due to reduced utilization of lipids and pro-inflammatory mediators<br>• Patients with burns >10% of TBSA should receive standard doses of multivitamins, vitamin C, vitamin E, zinc, and selenium<br>• Evidence suggests early high-dose IV vitamin C (1.5 g every 6 hours) stabilizes the endothelium, reduces capillary leak and resuscitation requirements by 30%. Glutamine supplementation 0.3 g/kg/day for up to two weeks<br>• *Brain induced hypermetabolism* leads to net negative nitrogen balance. Prevent strategies like maintaining ambient temperature, early debridement and grafting if indicated, deep wound coverage, adequate pain control and early ambulation. Pharmacological interventions include propranolol and anabolic steroids (oxandrolone) | • Early infections are by gram-positive skin commensals and beyond 72 hours its by gram negative *Enterobacteriaceae, Pseudomonas, Acinetobacter,* etc.<br>• Higher incidence of MRSA and Candidemia later during the course of illness<br><br>*Wound care:*<br>Goals of care include to keep the wound clean is by debridement, facilitate removal of the slough, prevent secondary infection and facilitate healing. |

| Superficial burns | Partial thickness burns | Full thickness burns |
|---|---|---|
| **Clean + Dress + Debride** | | |
| Topical antimicrobial and non-adherent dressing | Decision at the end of 14 days of dressing and debridement | • Escharotomy<br>• Fasciotomy Skin-grafting (Autograft, Xenograft)<br>• Biological dressing |

Advantages of skin grafting:
- Reduces insensible water loss
- Reduces infection rates
- Maintains temperature
- Reduces the pain
- Prevents hypercatabolic state

Multiorgan compartment syndromes due to resuscitation:
- Thoracic eschar syndrome, affecting lung compliance
- Extremity eschar syndrome, leading to neurovascular compromise needing escharotomy
- Extremity compartment syndromes, addressed by fasciotomy.
- Abdominal compartment syndrome—Ivy index
- Orbital compartment syndrome—lateral canthotomy and cantholysis

- Thromboprophylaxis is mandatory due to higher incidence of VTE at 40% in comparison to general ICU cohort at 2.1%.
- Stress ulcer prophylaxis to prevent Curling's ulcer.
- *Analgesia and sedation in ICU:* Well validated standard ICU scales for pain and sedation can be employed. Multi-modal analgesic approach comprising of paracetamol, NSAIDs, pregabalin or gabapentin, low-dose ketamine, dexmedetomidine or clonidine, and intravenous lignocaine are useful along with opioids. Patient controlled analgesia can be another option for optimization of pain.

## PROGNOSTICATION

- Revised Baux score, which included a separate representation for Inhalational injury and ranges from 0 to 160. rBaux score = Age + Percent Burn + 17 × (inhalation injury, 1 = yes, 0 = no). SMR is calculated based on the rBaux.
- FLAMES (Fatality by Longevity, APACHE II score, Measured Extent of burn, and Sex) is an integrated complex index for prediction of mortality in burns.
- These scores can help on deciding the outcomes and aids in decision for regarding the palliation in severe burns scenarios.

CHAPTER **82**

# Inhalational Injury

## INTRODUCTION

Inhalational injury when associated with the burns adds to the mortality in an already inherently complex clinical entity. Inhalational injury is an independent risk factor and when present with burns adds to the mortality by a factor of 20%, which increase even further when co-existent pneumonia. The injury can be either direct insult or consequent to the damages leading local and systemic complications. Early recognition is essential to prevent catastrophic airway compromise due to airway oedema. Identification needs high index of suspicion:

## SUSPECTING INHALATIONAL INJURY IN BURNS PATIENTS

| *History and symptoms* | *Signs* |
|---|---|
| • Closed spaces fire<br>• Industrial fire accidents<br>• Fires in rubber, tanning, and plastic industries<br>• Loss of consciousness<br>• Combativeness and agitation<br>• Shortness of breath<br>• Voice changes<br>• Facial and neck burns<br>• Requirement if CPR at the scene and bystander causalities | • Wheeze/stridor<br>• Respiratory distress<br>• Hypoxia<br>• Increased secretions<br>• Flu like symptoms (CO toxicity)<br>• Altered mental status<br>• Carbonaceous sputum/ secretions<br>• Soot in nares and pharynx<br>• Singed facial and nasal hairs<br>• Hyperlactatemia<br>• Erythema and blistering of the oral cavity |

## PATHOPHYSIOLOGY OF INHALATIONAL INJURY

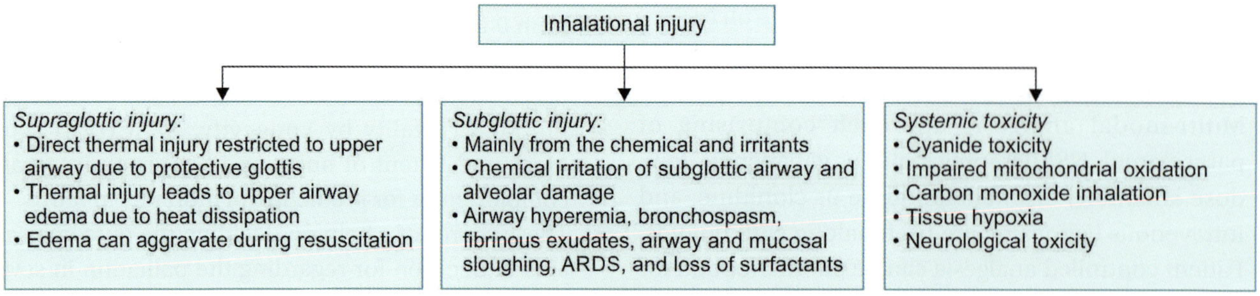

Inhalational injury

*Supraglottic injury:*
- Direct thermal injury restricted to upper airway due to protective glottis
- Thermal injury leads to upper airway edema due to heat dissipation
- Edema can aggravate during resuscitation

*Subglottic injury:*
- Mainly from the chemical and irritants
- Chemical irritation of subglottic airway and alveolar damage
- Airway hyperemia, bronchospasm, fibrinous exudates, airway and mucosal sloughing, ARDS, and loss of surfactants

*Systemic toxicity*
- Cyanide toxicity
- Impaired mitochondrial oxidation
- Carbon monoxide inhalation
- Tissue hypoxia
- Neurololgical toxicity

## DIAGNOSIS AND MANAGEMENT

All the burns patients are evaluated as per the ATLS primary and secondary survey scheme.

*Supraglottic injury:*

- Direct visual and physical examination
- Laryngoscopy and bronchoscopy are used for upper airway injury.
- Visualization of edema—prompt early airway securement before worsening of edema and resuscitation as it can lead to catastrophic airway compromise.
- In case of ingestion of scalding liquids, oropharyngeal scald burns might be seen.

*Subglottic injury and alveolar damage:*

- Physical examination and history have limited role in diagnosing subglottic and lower respiratory injury.
- Fiberoptic bronchoscopy (FOB) is gold standard diagnosis of both supraglottic as well as subglottic injuries.
- FOB is a must and its helpful for grading of inhalational injury and for therapeutic frequent bronchoalveolar lavage.
- FOB is repeated at 48 hours to identify the worsening of existent lesions and/or new onset ARDS, especially in patients with extensive cutaneous burns as part of secondary ARDS due to the inflammatory mediators.
- Chest X-ray and CT scans may also be used for the diagnosis.

## FIBEROPTIC BRONCHOSCOPY GRADING-ABBREVIATED INJURY SCALE

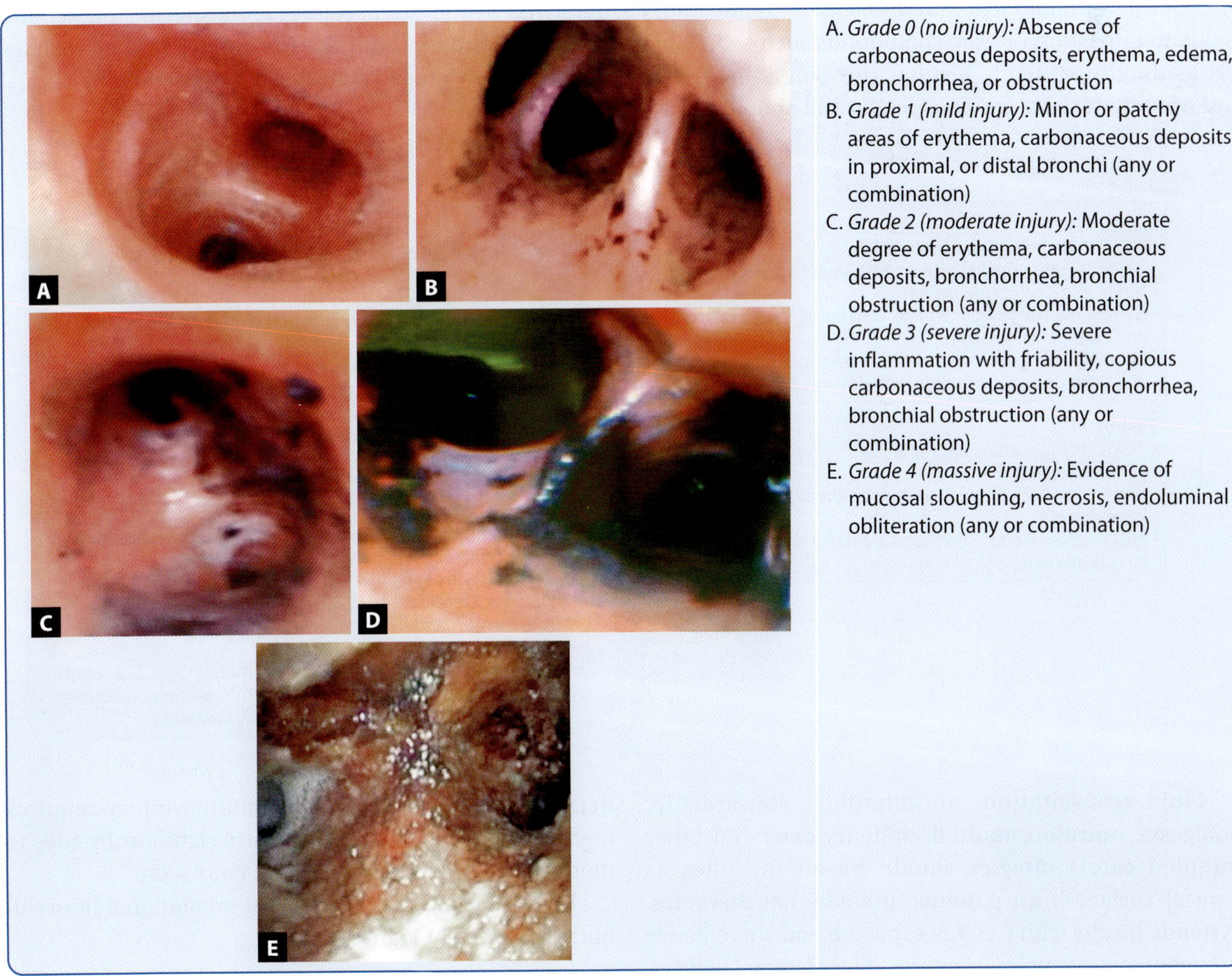


A. *Grade 0 (no injury):* Absence of carbonaceous deposits, erythema, edema, bronchorrhea, or obstruction
B. *Grade 1 (mild injury):* Minor or patchy areas of erythema, carbonaceous deposits in proximal, or distal bronchi (any or combination)
C. *Grade 2 (moderate injury):* Moderate degree of erythema, carbonaceous deposits, bronchorrhea, bronchial obstruction (any or combination)
D. *Grade 3 (severe injury):* Severe inflammation with friability, copious carbonaceous deposits, bronchorrhea, bronchial obstruction (any or combination)
E. *Grade 4 (massive injury):* Evidence of mucosal sloughing, necrosis, endoluminal obliteration (any or combination)

## MANAGEMENT OF SUPRAGLOTTIC AND SUBGLOTTIC INJURY

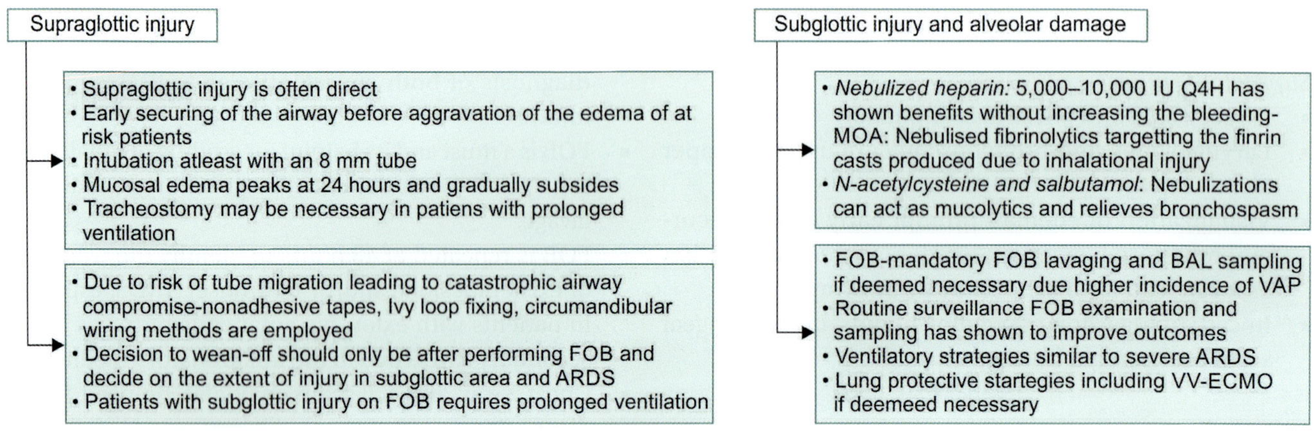


## SYSTEMIC INJURIES DUE TO INHALATION

*Mechanisms of injury and management:* Systemic injury is due to inhalation of toxic compounds such as CO and CN leading to systemic insults. The symptoms COHb and cyanide toxicity are nonspecific and should always be suspected in case of inhalational injuries, until otherwise disproved. Lactate is a nonspecific marker and can be elevated in both the toxicities. Elevated lactates independently predict mortality in burns and Inhalational injury.

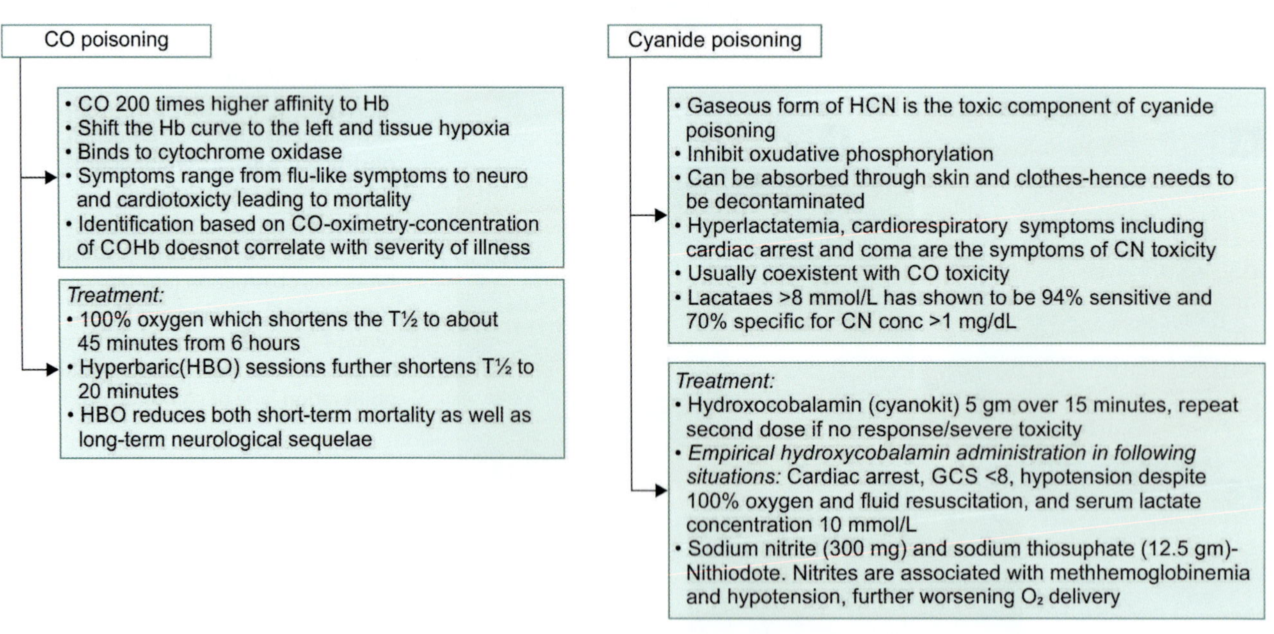


Fluid resuscitation, antimicrobial stewardship, analgesia, nutrition, multidisciplinary care, and other bundled care strategies should be on the lines as care of surface burn patients. Inhalational therapies, systemic insults with CO, CN exposure and surveillance bronchoscopy are unique features of inhalational injuries. Recognition of coexistent inhalational injury requires high index of suspicion and presence significantly adds to mortality as evident on the revised Baux score.

Diagnosis and management of inhalational injury in burns are given in **Figure 1**.

*Patient at risk of BII:*
- Loss of consciousness
- CPR requirement at scene
- Known fatalities in same incident
- Exposure to fire within closed space
- Prolonged duration of exposure

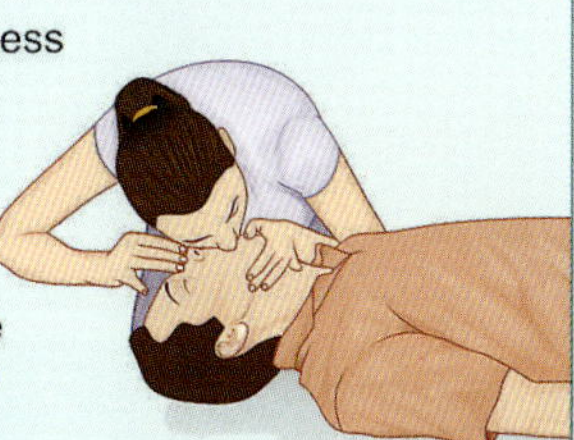

*Physical examination findings suggestive of BII:*
- Facial or neck burns
- Singed facial of nasal hair
- Carbonaceous sputum
- Increased secretions
- Accessory muscle use
- Altered consciousness
- Edema, erythema or blistering of oral cavity
- Stridor, coughing, wheezing, hoarseness or dyspnea

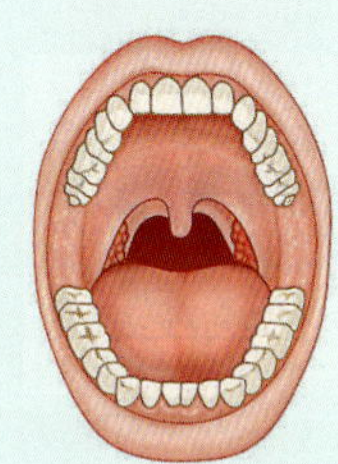

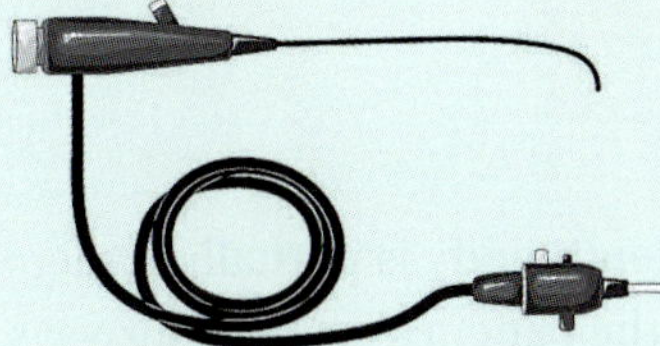

*Fiberoptic bronchoscopy:*
Fiberoptic bronchoscopy may be considered for
- Assessing mortality risk based on bronchoscopy severity grading
- Initial therapeutic lavage for moderate-severe BII
- Serial therapeutic lavage for severe BII
- Serial surveillance of the airways for severe BII

Serial therapeutic tavage should be avoided in nonsevere BII

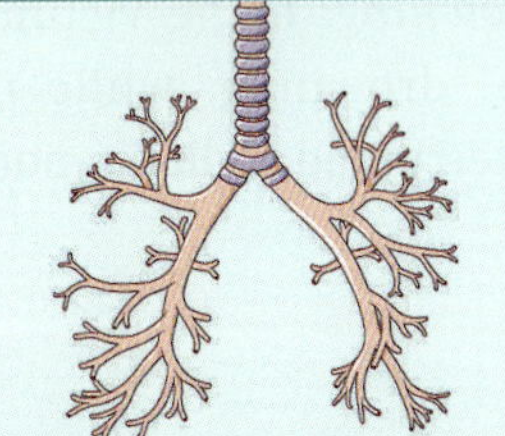

*Airway management strategies:*
- Initial intubation should be with an uncut tracheal tube of internal diameter ≥8.0 mm where possible
- Consider tracheostomy for patients anticipated to require endotracheal intubation exceeding 7 days
- Repeated reintubation should be avoided where possible and tracheostomy performed instead

*Patients at risk of hydrogen cyanide toxicity:*
- Exposure to fire within closed space
- High serum lactate
- Cardiac dysfunction
- Altered consciousness
- Seizures
- Cardiac or respiratory arrest

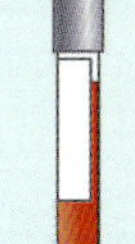

*Treatment of suspected systemic toxicity:*
- High fractional inspired oxygen for suspected CO or HCN toxicity
- Hydroxycobalamin for HCN toxicity
- Hydroxycobalamin administration should not be delayed for laboratory confirmation in the presence of high clinical suspicion of HCN toxicity

*Mechanical ventilatory modes and adjuncts:*
- Lung protective strategies maintaining tidal volumes <6 mL/kg and plateau pressures <30 $cmH_2O$
- Refer for ECMO If clinically indicated, even if requiring patient transfer away from flums center
- Nonprotective strategies, high frequency oscillatory ventilation and high frequency perssussive ventilation should be avoided
- Consider prone positioning, recruitment manoeuvres, inhaled prostacyclin analogues, inhaled nitric oxide and neuromuscular blocking agents for refractory hypoxaemia
- Airway pressure release ventilation may be considered for Bi-ARDS patients if deemed clinically appropriate

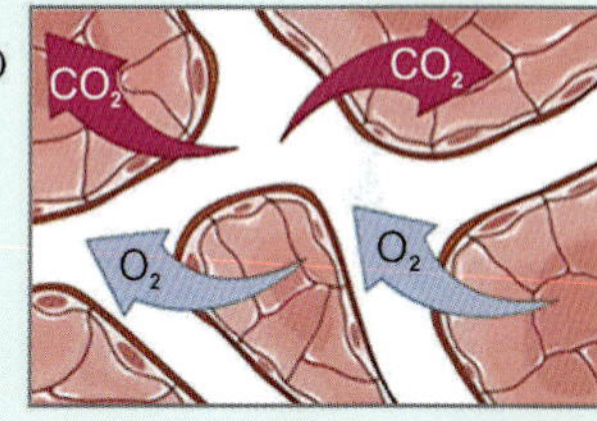


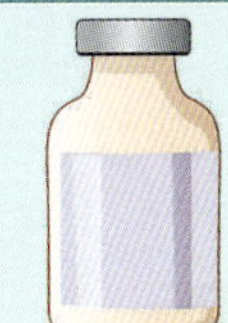

*Pharmacological adjuncts:*
- 5,000 1U nebulized heparin for moderate-severe BII
- Nebulized *N*-acetylcysteine for moderate BII
- Nebulized salbutamol for moderate-severe BII
- Prophylactic antibiotics and corticosteroids should be avoided
- The safety and efficacy of nebulized heparin, *N*-acetylcysteine and salbutamol for mild BII currently uncertain and thus is not recommended

**Fig. 1:** Infographic representing the diagnosis and management of Inhalational injury in burns.
*Source:* Milton-Jones H, Soussi S, Davies R, Charbonney E, Charles WN, Cleland H, et al. An international RAND/UCLA expert panel to determine the optimal diagnosis and management of burn inhalation injury. Crit Care. 2023;27(1):459.

CHAPTER

# 83 Drowning

## IMPORTANT DEFINITIONS

- Drowning is the process of experiencing respiratory impairment from submersion or immersion in liquid.
- *Submersion versus immersion:*
  - *Submersion:* Entire body of the patient is under water including face and airway.
  - *Immersion:* Patient's body is partially under water, which includes the patient's face and airways.
- *Fatal versus nonfatal drowning:* If the victim dies at any time this is fatal drowning, while if the process of drowning is interrupted, called a nonfatal drowning.

## PATHOPHYSIOLOGY

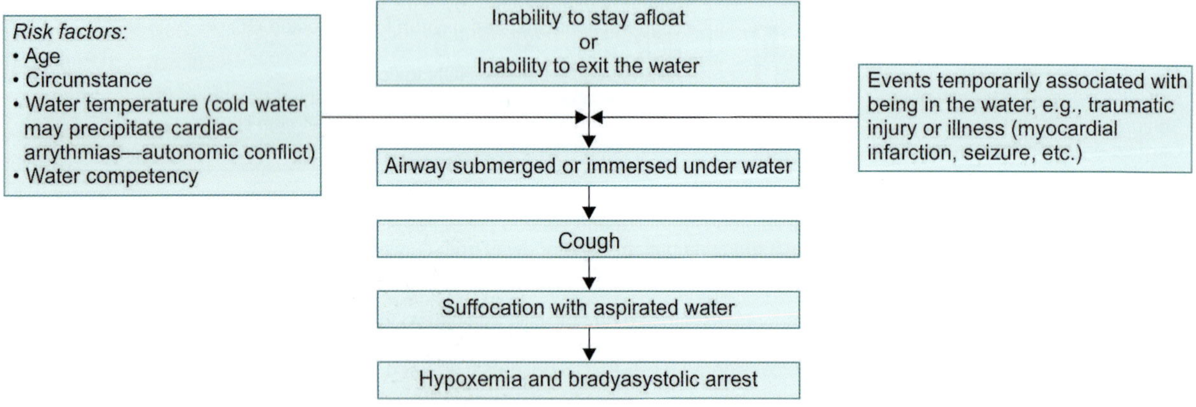


## PREHOSPITAL CARE

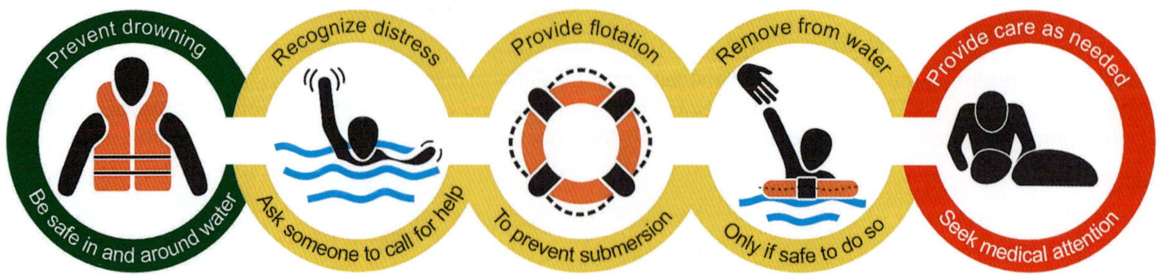


- Safety of caregiver important
- Immediate in-water ventilation *only* if *feasible*
- Basic and advanced life support

## CLASSIFICATION OF DROWNING

| *Grade* | *Symptoms respiratory* | *Symptoms hemodynamic* | *Treatment* | *Destination* | *Mortality (%)* |
|---|---|---|---|---|---|
| 0 | No cough or dyspnea | Palpable radial pulses | Release at scene, education | No transport | 0 |
| 1 | Cough, normal auscultation | Palpable radial pulses | Rest, rewarm, reassure, and release | no transport | 0 |
| 2 | Rales and small amount of foam | Palpable radial pulses | Oxygen via nasal cannula, observe for 6–24 hours | *Transport for observation:* ED or overnight | 0.6 |
| 3 | Acute pulmonary edema | Palpable radial pulses | Oxygen nonrebreathing mask and ACLS | Transport for admission and observation | 5.2 |
| 4 | Acute pulmonary edema | Hypotension | Possible ETT and fluids for blood pressure support, ACLS | Rapid transport ICU stay | 19 |
| 5 | Respiratory arrest | Hypotension | Load and go, ACLS | Rapid transport ICU | 44 |
| 6 | Cardiopulmonary arrest | | ACLS | Rapid transport ICU | 93 |

## INITIAL RESUSCITATION ON LAND

- Call for help and encourage patient to move away from danger.
- Place the patient parallel to the shoreline so that the head and feet are at the same level.
- *CPR:* Airway, breathing, circulation (not CAB due to respiratory impact of drowning)
- If unconscious and not breathing, begin with 5 rescue breaths (ABC rather than CAB), then continue with 30:2 (compressions: rescue breaths). Five breaths are used initially because water in the airways can interfere with effective alveolar expansion initially.
- A drowning patient with only respiratory arrest usually responds after a few rescue breaths
- Cardiac arrest from drowning is due primarily to lack of oxygen. Ventilation support with available tools (oxygen, bag valve mask (BVM), etc.)
- Prepare for vomiting: 65–88% of may develop vomiting

## IN-HOSPITAL MANAGEMENT OF PATIENTS WITH DROWNING

*When to initiate CPR and when to stop:*

| | |
|---|---|
| In whom to begin? | • Give ventilatory support for respiratory distress/arrest to avoid cardiac arrest<br>• Start CPR in all submersions <60 minutes who do not present with obvious physical evidence of death (rigor mortis, body decomposition or dependent lividity) |
| When to discontinue? | • Basic life support should continue unless signs of life re-appear, rescuers exhaustion or advanced life support take over<br>• Advanced life support should be ongoing until patient has been rewarmed (if hypothermic) and asystole persist for more than 20 minutes |

*Who will need evaluation?*

- Anyone who required resuscitation
- Anyone unresponsive in the water
- Anyone exhibiting distress (shortness of breath, persistent cough, anxiety, tachypnea, syncope, foam in the mouth or nose, change in vital signs, abnormal breath sounds, or hypotension)

## INTENSIVE CARE UNIT MANAGEMENT

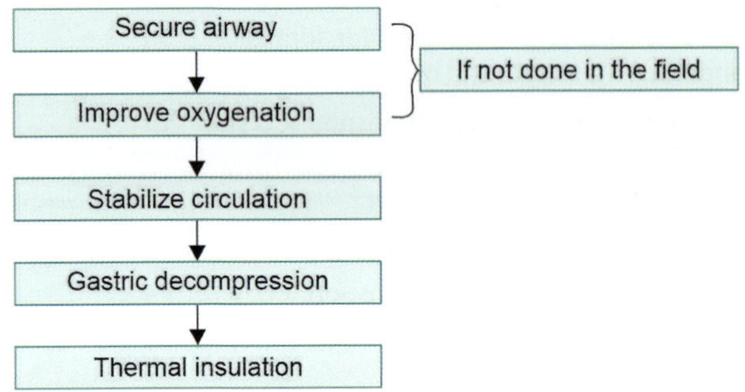


## NEUROLOGIC CARE

- *Assess GCS:* Secure airway if low
- Cervical spine assessment and clearance
- *Post-CPR:* Neuroprotective measures

## RESPIRATORY CARE

- Lung protective ventilation as in ARDS
    - Persist for at least 48 hours prior to weaning (Surfactant waah out will take 2-4 days for replacement)

## CARDIOVASCULAR SYSTEM

- Management of arrhythmias
- Correction of electrolytes
- Correction of hypothermia

## MANAGEMENT OF METABOLIC ABNORMALITIES

### High-quality Intensive Care

*Care for victim who remains comatose or unresponsive after successful CPR or deteriorates neurologically:*

- Raise the head of the bed by 30 degrees (if there is no hypotension)
- Maintain adequate mechanical ventilation by using drugs if necessary to obtain ventilation—patient synchrony
- Ensure appropriate respiratory toilet
- Treatment of seizures
- Avoid sudden metabolic corrections
- Prevent interventions that increase intracranial pressure (ICP), including pain, hypotension, hypercapnia, hypoxemia

*Probability of neurologically intact survival to hospital discharge, based on duration of submersion:*

| ***Duration of submersion*** | ***Death or severe neurological impairment*** |
|---|---|
| 0–<5 minutes | 10% |
| 5–<10 minutes | 56% |
| 10–<25 minutes | 88% |
| >25 minutes | 100% |

Note in these data how 5 more minutes of submersion in the 5–<10 minutes group which increases mortality by over 6 times as compared to less than 5 minutes group

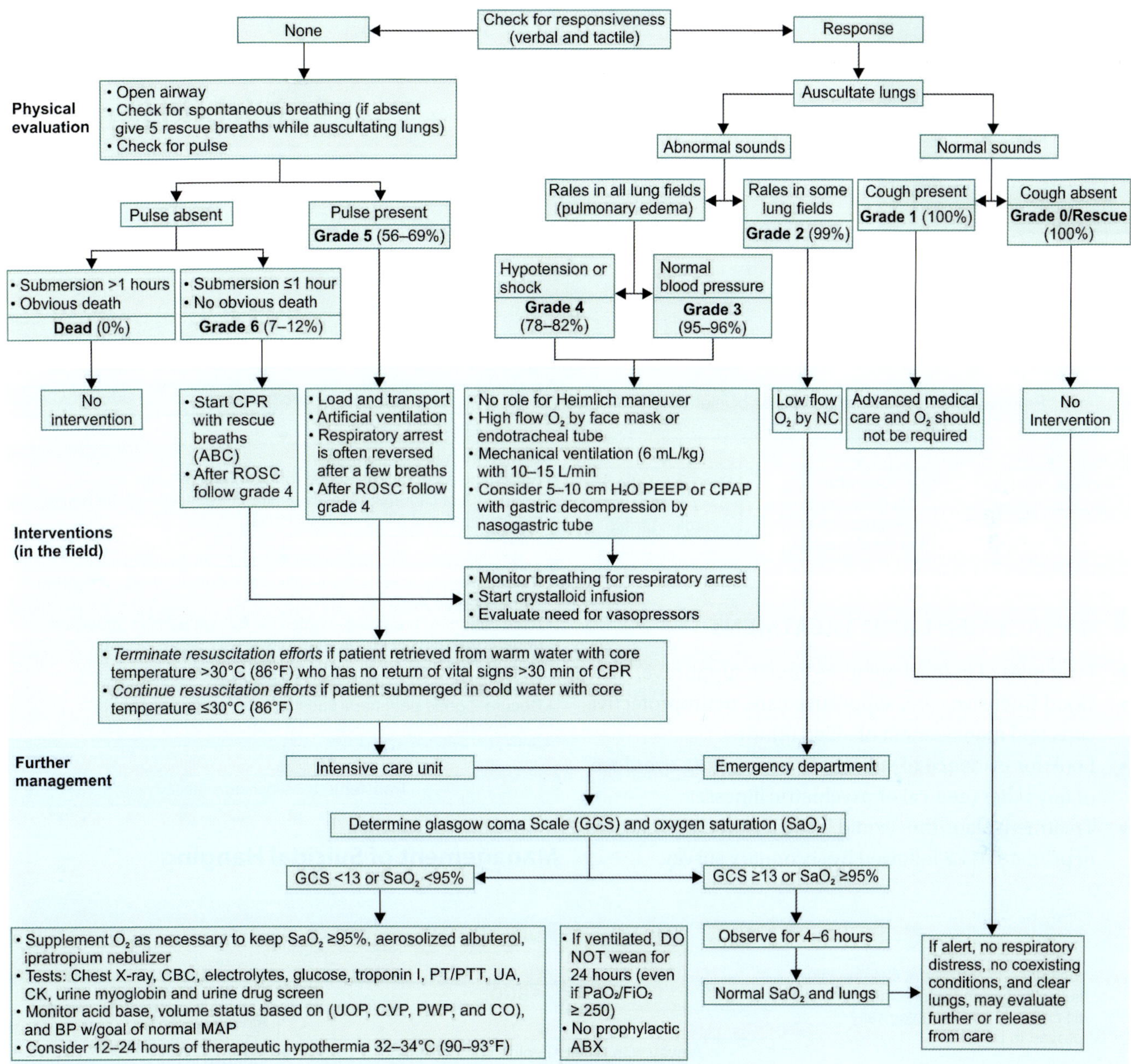


*Source:* LT Parenteau, integrating figure New England Journal of Medicine. 366(22):2102-10 with Tintinalli's Emergency Medicine Manual, 7th Edition and Auerbach's Wildemess Medicine.

CHAPTER 84

# Suicidal Hanging

## PATHOPHYSIOLOGY

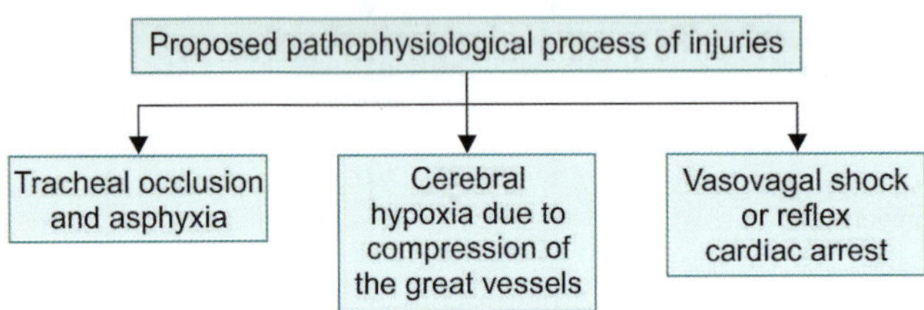


## MANAGEMENT AND TREATMENT

- Principles of management are largely supportive.
- Good Intensive care, supportive care, neuroprotective care, and management of allied injuries
- Look for evidence of substance abuse, drug overdose, or any other medical or psychiatric illnesses.
- Treatment algorithm would be based on the principles of primary ATLS followed by secondary survey.

## Prehospital Care

Prehospital care

↓

Release from the ligature after:
- Assessing safety at the scene for the medical team
- Collection of circumstantial evidence at the scene of the act for medicolegal and allied clinical issues

↓

- Primary Airway assessment—secure definitive airway if needed and expertise available
- Assessment of breathing—watch for foreign body in airway or upper/lower airway injuries
- Immobilization of cervical spine with hard collar and manual in-line stabilization for any necessary procedure
- Secure 2 good peripheral lines
- Cardiopulmonary resuscitation if complicated by cardiac arrest

↓

Transfer to a critical care facility

## Management of Suicidal Hanging

Incidence of significant C-spine injury is low, but keep the precautions on till clinically and radiologically proven to be safe

Hemorrhage control may not be relevant if there are no other injuries

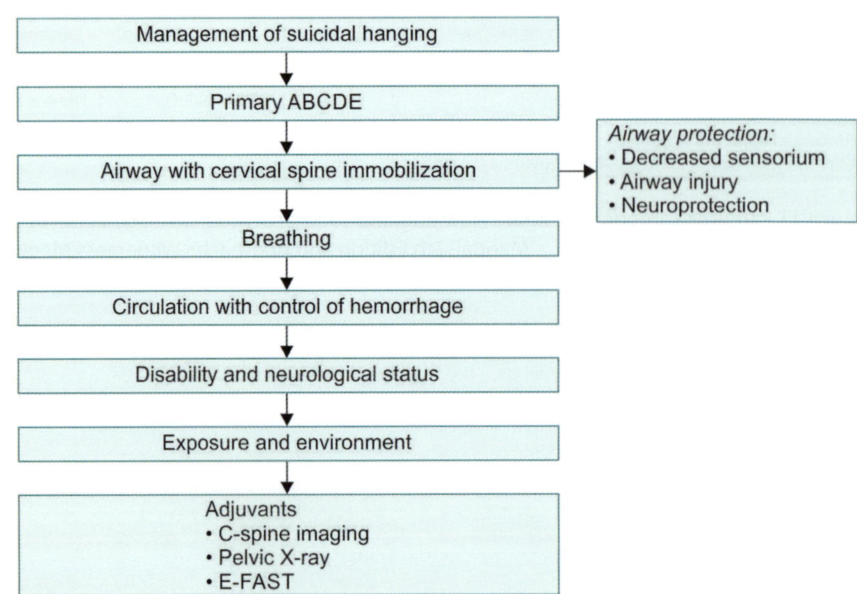

## Intensive Care Unit Management

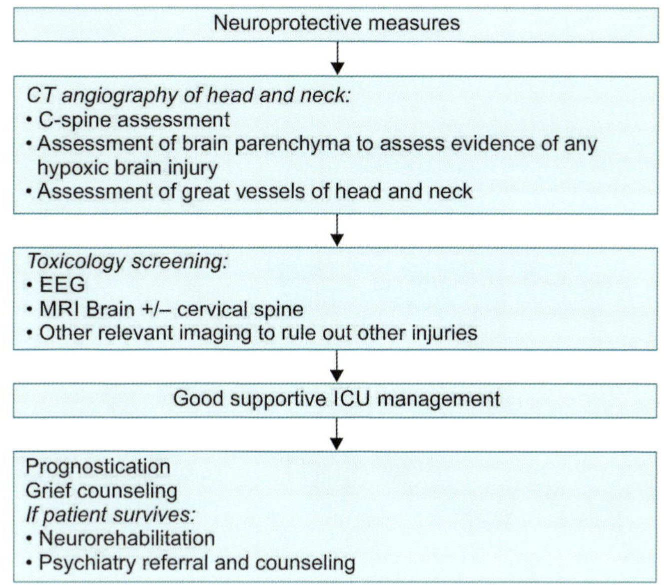

# PART 7

# METABOLIC ISSUES

***Editors:*** Aklesh Tandekar, Ravindra Ghawat

***Associate Editors:*** Suvadeep Sen, Rajan Bhupesh Pandya, Ashwini Ajay Yadav, Divya Rajasekaran, Jasmine Nathani, Shailesh Hiraman Chouksey, Subhra Sen

CHAPTER 85

# Hyponatremia

## INTRODUCTION

Hyponatremia is a condition characterized by an abnormally low concentration of sodium in the blood, typically defined as a serum sodium level of less than 135 mEq/L. Sodium is a crucial electrolyte that helps regulate water balance, nerve function, and muscle activity.

**TABLE 1:** Signs and symptoms.

| ***Severity*** | ***Serum sodium level*** | ***Signs and symptoms*** | ***Adverse effects*** | ***Diagnosis*** |
|---|---|---|---|---|
| Mild hyponatremia | 130–135 mEq/L | • Nausea<br>• Headache<br>• Fatigue<br>• Dizziness<br>• Mild confusion | • Subtle cognitive impairment<br>• Increased fall risk in the elderly | • *Serum sodium:* 130–135 mEq/L<br>• Evaluate volume status (e.g., hypovolemic, euvolemic, hypervolemic) |
| Moderate hyponatremia | 120–129 mEq/L | • More pronounced confusion<br>• Muscle cramps<br>• Lethargy<br>• Disorientation | • Increased risk of falls<br>• Risk of seizures with rapid progression | • *Serum sodium:* 120–129 mEq/L<br>• Check for medications (e.g., diuretics, SSRIs, antipsychotics) |
| Severe hyponatremia | <120 mEq/L | • Severe lethargy<br>• Seizures<br>• Coma<br>• Vomiting<br>• Profound confusion | • Cerebral edema<br>• Brain herniation<br>• Seizures<br>• Death | • *Serum sodium:* <120 mEq/L<br>• Urine osmolality, urine sodium, and serum osmolality for further classification |
| Acute hyponatremia | Any level with rapid onset | • Sudden severe symptoms like seizures<br>• Nausea and vomiting<br>• Respiratory distress | • Brain swelling<br>• Risk of brain herniation and death | • Sudden drop in serum sodium<br>• Typically seen in post-operative patients or those with rapid fluid shifts |
| Chronic hyponatremia | Slow onset at any level | • Milder symptoms<br>• Cognitive changes<br>• Impaired concentration<br>• Gait disturbances | • Increased risk of fractures in elderly<br>• Cognitive decline | • Chronic low serum sodium<br>• Typically associated with heart failure, liver disease, or SIADH |

**BOX 1:** Clinical approach to hyponatremia.

- Confirm the patient truly has a hypo-osmolar state by checking serum osmolality
- Assess for serious signs or symptoms suggesting cerebral edema
- Determine the duration of development of hyponatremia (less or more than 48 hours)
- Assess the patient's extracellular fluid volume status using clinical examination and laboratory testing (spot urine sodium, serum uric acid)
- Check the urine osmolality to see if the urine is appropriately dilute (<100 mOsm/kg) or inappropriately concentrated (≥100 mOsm/kg)
- Assess for underlying causes of hyponatremia that may correct rapidly with treatment (e.g., hyponatremia induced by thiazide diuretics)
- Assess the patient's medications (intravenous antibiotics, infusions) and nutritional intake (total parenteral nutrition, tube-feeding) for sources of water
- Look for drugs the patient is taking that potentiate antidiuretic hormone action

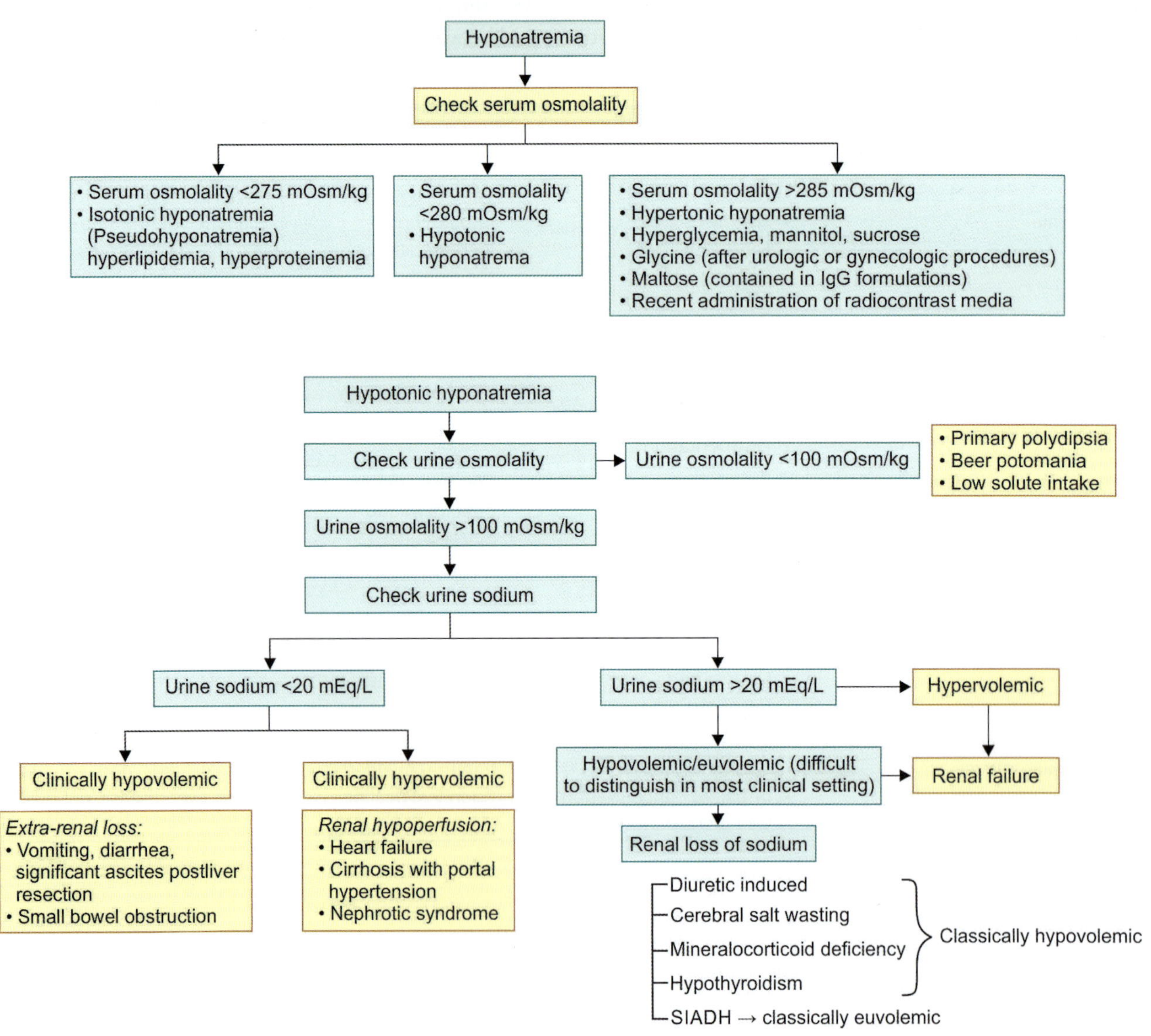

**BOX 2:** Diagnostic Criteria for SIADH.

*Essential criteria:*
- Effective serum osmolality <275 mOsm/kg (true hyponatremia)
- Urine osmolality >100 mOsm/kg at some level of decreased effective osmolality
- Clinical euvolemia
- Urine sodium concentration >30 mmol/l with normal dietary salt and water intake
- Absence of adrenal, thyroid, pituitary, or renal insufficiency
- No recent use of diuretic agents

*Supplemental criteria:*
- Serum uric acid <0.24 mmol/l (<4 mg/dL)
- Serum urea <3.6 mmol/l (<21.6 mg/dL)
- Failure to correct hyponatremia after 0.9% saline infusion
- Fractional sodium excretion >0.5%
- Fractional urea excretion >55%
- Fractional uric acid excretion >12%
- Correction of hyponatremia through fluid restriction

| *Category* | *SIADH* | *CSW* |
|---|---|---|
| Mechanism | Water retention due to elevated vasopressin (ADH) | Excess excretion of sodium and water |
| Volume status | Clinically euvolemic/ hypervolemic | Volume-depleted state and sodium-wasting state |
| Clinical signs | No sign of dehydration | Appears dehydrated |
| Plasma BUN/ creatinine<br>Hematocrit | ↓<br>Unchanged | ↑ or normal<br>↑ or normal |
| Urine sodium<br>Urine osmolality<br>Serum uric acid<br>Urine specific gravity | >20 meq/L<br>>100 mEq/L<br>Low<br>>1.010 (concentrated) | >20 mEq/L<br>>100 mEq/L<br>Low<br>>1.010 (concentrated) |
| Urine output | Normal | Increased |
| Fractional excretion of PO4 | Low | Elevated |
| Fractional excretion of urate (after correction of sodium) | Normal | High |
| Treatment of choice | Free water restriction, Hypertonic saline | Fluid replacement with isotonic solutions, Fludrocortisone |

*Contd...*

*Contd...*

## SUGGESTED READING


1. Adrogué HJ, Madias NE. Hyponatremia. N Engl J Med. 2000;342(21):1581-9.
2. Ellison DH, Berl T. The syndrome of inappropriate antidiuresis. N Engl J Med. 2007;356(20):2064-72.
3. Hoorn EJ, Zietse R. Diagnosis and Treatment of Hyponatremia: Compilation of the Guidelines. J Am Soc Nephrol. 2017;28(5):1340-9.
4. Sterns RH, Nigwekar SU, Hix JK. The treatment of hyponatremia. Semin Nephrol. 2009;29(3):282-99.
5. Verbalis JG, Goldsmith SR, Greenberg A, Korzelius C, Schrier RW, Sterns RH, et al. Diagnosis, Evaluation, and Treatment of Hyponatremia: Expert Panel Recommendations. Am J Med. 2013;126(10 Suppl 1):S1-42.

CHAPTER 86

# Hypernatremia

## INTRODUCTION

Hypernatremia is a condition characterized by an abnormally high concentration of sodium in the blood, typically defined as a serum sodium level of greater than 145 mEq/L. Sodium is a key electrolyte that helps regulate fluid balance, nerve function, and muscle contraction.

**TABLE 1:** Signs and symptoms.

| ***Severity*** | ***Serum sodium level*** | ***Signs and symptoms*** | ***Adverse effects*** | ***Diagnosis*** |
|---|---|---|---|---|
| Mild hypernatremia | 146–150 mEq/L | • Thirst<br>• Dry mouth<br>• Restlessness<br>• Fatigue | • Dehydration<br>• Mild neurological symptoms | • *Serum sodium:* 146–150 mEq/L<br>• *Physical exam:* Dry mucous membranes, orthostatic hypotension<br>• Urine osmolality and electrolytes to assess dehydration |
| Moderate hypernatremia | 151–160 mEq/L | • Lethargy<br>• Irritability<br>• Muscle weakness<br>• Nausea and vomiting | • Neurological symptoms due to brain cell shrinkage (confusion, agitation) | • *Serum sodium:* 151–160 mEq/L<br>• Assess volume status (hypovolemic, euvolemic, hypervolemic)<br>• Rule out causes such as diabetes insipidus, diuretics |
| Severe hypernatremia | >160 mEq/L | • Severe confusion<br>• Seizures<br>• Coma<br>• Twitching<br>• Hyperreflexia | • Cerebral edema (if corrected too rapidly)<br>• Brain hemorrhage<br>• Seizures<br>• Coma | • *Serum sodium:* >160 mEq/L<br>• Immediate brain imaging if seizures or neurological symptoms<br>• Rapid electrolyte testing to guide correction |
| Critical hypernatremia | >170 mEq/L | • Profound weakness<br>• Respiratory arrest<br>• Severe muscle twitching<br>• Unresponsiveness (coma) | • Death from severe dehydration or brain injury<br>• Cardiac arrest | • *Serum sodium:* >170 mEq/L<br>• Emergency neurological and cardiac evaluation<br>• Requires immediate correction of sodium levels |

## CLINICAL APPROACH TO HYPERNATREMIA

*Step 1:* Consider history. Most patients presenting with hypernatremia are at their extremes of age
- Clinical assessment of volume status
- Hematocrit level depends on volume status

**Take history**

- Try to assess volume status: Following patients are at risk of either euvolemic or hypovolemic
- History of GI loss (diarrhea, vomiting, NG loss, loss from enteric fistula)
- Persistent fever, burn, excessive sweating
- Elderly patients, with dementia or prolonged bedridden state, incapable of taking care of themselves self-low water intake
- Patient on ventilator or NIV without humidifier
- Excessive and prolonged administration of normal saline in the ICU or in the ward
- History of polyuria, polydipsia favors diabetes insipidus
- Drug history like Lithium, amphotericin B, aminoglycosides, and colchicine favors nephrogenic diabetes insipidus
- History of brain trauma, pituitary surgery, and tumor indicates
- Administration of mannitol, excess diuretics

**Clinical examination**

- Try to assess volume status: dry skin, dry tongue,
- Most patients with hypernatremia are either dehydrated or in euvolemic state
- Some patients may be clinically hypervolemic
- Features of cushing syndrome

*Step 2:* Check urine osmolality and urine sodium. Urine osmolality and urine sodium concentration help differentiate renal causes from extrarenal causes

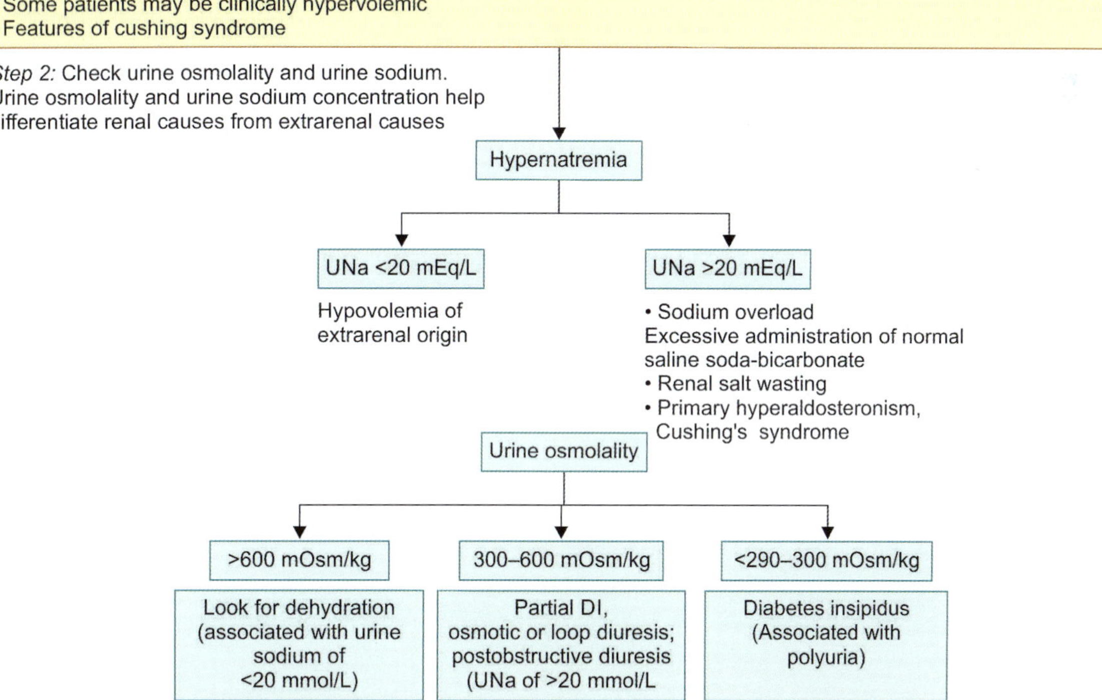


*Step 3:* If the patient has DI, determine the type using the initial Uosm and its response to the administration of desmopressin. Once DI is diagnosed, the ddAVP test (response to desmopressin) differentiates central from nephrogenic DI

**Signs and symptoms of hyponatremia according to severity:**

| *Severity* | *Neurological* | *Physical examination* | *Muscular* | *Other symptoms* |
|---|---|---|---|---|
| Mild | Thirst, irritability, restlessness | Dry skin, dry mucous membranes | – | Polydipsia |
| Moderate | Confusion, fatigue, headache | Decreased skin turgor, orthostatic hypotension | – | – |
| Severe | Seizures, stupor, coma | Edema, hypertension, jugular venous distention | Weakness, hyperreflexia | Polyuria |

## MANAGEMENT OF HYPERNATREMIA

| *Condition* | *Initial treatment* | *Ongoing management* | *Special considerations* |
|---|---|---|---|
| Hypovolemic hypernatremia | Isotonic fluids (e.g., normal saline) | Follow with hypotonic fluids | Monitor for signs of fluid overload |
| Euvolemic hypernatremia | Increase water intake or hypotonic fluids<br>Plain water or 5% dextrose | Treat underlying cause (DI) | Monitor for response to treatment |
| Hypervolemic hypernatremia | Fluid restriction, diuretics | Treat underlying cause (e.g., hyperaldosteronism) | Monitor sodium and fluid balance |

Treatment of diabetes insipidus:

| *Type of Diabetes Insipidus* | *Primary Treatment* | *Adjunctive/Alternative Treatments* | *Monitoring and Support* |
|---|---|---|---|
| Central DI | Desmopressin (DDAVP) | Vasopressin, Chlorpropamide (less common) | Monitor serum sodium, osmolality, and hydration status |
| Nephrogenic DI | Thiazide diuretics | Low-salt diet, Indomethacin, Amiloride (specific cases) | Ensure adequate fluid intake, monitor renal function |

## SUGGESTED READING


1. Adrogué HJ, Madias NE. Hypernatremia. N Engl J Med. 2000;342(20):1493-99.
2. Ayus JC, Arieff AI. Hypernatremia Induced Neurological Damage in Humans. J Am Coll Nutrition. 1995;14(4):337-46.
3. Bennani SL, Abouqal R, Zeggwagh AA, Madani N, Abidi K. Incidence, Causes, and Prognosis of Hypernatremia in Critically Ill Patients. Am J Kidney Diseas. 2003;41(2):429-32.
4. Hoorn EJ, Zietse R. Diagnosis and treatment of hypernatremia. Kidney Internat. 2017;92(1):103-8.
5. Verbalis JG, Goldsmith SR, Greenberg A, Schrier RW, Sterns RH. Diagnosis, Evaluation, and Treatment of Hypernatremia: Expert Panel Recommendations. Am J Med. 2013;126(10 Suppl 1):S24-7.

CHAPTER 87

# Hypokalemia

## INTRODUCTION

Hypokalemia is characterized by an abnormally low concentration of potassium in the blood, typically defined as a serum potassium level of less than 3.5 mEq/L. Potassium is an essential electrolyte that is critical in maintaining normal cell function, nerve transmission, muscle contraction, and heart function.

| ***Severity*** | ***Serum potassium level*** | ***Signs and symptoms*** | ***Adverse effects*** | ***Diagnosis*** |
|---|---|---|---|---|
| Mild hypokalemia | 3.0–3.5 mEq/L | • Fatigue<br>• Muscle weakness<br>• Cramps<br>• Constipation | • Minimal symptoms<br>• Slight muscle weakness or fatigue | • *Serum potassium:* 3.0–3.5 mEq/L<br>• Assess for diuretic use, vomiting, or diarrhea<br>• ECG may be normal or show slight changes |
| Moderate hypokalemia | 2.5–3.0 mEq/L | • Muscle cramps<br>• Muscle weakness<br>• Palpitations<br>• Polyuria<br>• Nausea | • Increased risk of arrhythmias<br>• ECG changes: Flattened T waves, U waves | • *Serum potassium:* 2.5–3.0 mEq/L<br>• *ECG:* Flattened T waves, ST depression<br>• Evaluate for metabolic alkalosis or renal potassium losses |
| Severe hypokalemia | <2.5 mEq/L | • Severe muscle weakness<br>• Paralysis<br>• Hyporeflexia<br>• Respiratory depression<br>• Confusion | • Life-threatening arrhythmias (ventricular tachycardia, ventricular fibrillation)<br>• Rhabdomyolysis | • *Serum potassium:* <2.5 mEq/L<br>• ECG: U waves, ST-segment depression, T wave inversion<br>• Evaluate for gastrointestinal, renal, or medication-related potassium loss |
| Critical hypokalemia | <2.0 mEq/L | • Respiratory failure<br>• Paralysis<br>• Severe arrhythmias (ventricular fibrillation, asystole) | • Cardiac arrest<br>• Death due to refractory arrhythmias or respiratory muscle paralysis | • *Serum potassium:* <2.0 mEq/L<br>• Immediate clinical and cardiac evaluation<br>• Emergency treatment required |

## CLINICAL APPROACH TO HYPOKALEMIA

*Step 1:* Take history providing clues to diagnosis and etiology of hypokalemia

1. Weakness, palpitation
2. Previous episodes of a typical history of sporadic sudden paralysis after strenuous exercise in young adolescents suggest familial hypokalemic periodic paralysis
3. *Detection of hypertension at a young age:* Raises suspicion of hyperaldosteronism or renal artery stenosis
4. History of vomiting, NG aspirates, diarrhea
5. *Drug history:* Loop or thiazide diuretics, osmotic diuretics, aminoglycosides, steroids, theophylline, insulin use, amphotericin B

*Step 2:* Biochemical parameters

- Exclude pseudohypokalemia in patients with acute leukemia when blood is stored at room temperature for a long before evaluation.
- *Serum magnesium:* Uncorrected serum magnesium leads to refractory hypokalemia.
- *Check spot urine potassium:* Provides information about whether potassium loss is renal origin or extra-renal. Urine spot potassium <20 mEq/L is associated with extrarenal loss of potassium. While high urinary potassium means renal potassium loss.
- Arterial blood gas to detect alkalosis or acidosis: provides a differential diagnosis
- Calculate TTKG: to determine whether the renal response to or hypokalemia is appropriate. Estimates the degree of renal potassium excretion in the distal nephron. During hypokalemia, the TTKG should be less than 4; greater values suggest renal potassium wasting.

TTKG < 2 usually means increased tubular flow due to any reason.

$$\text{TTKG} = \frac{\text{Urine potassium}}{\text{Serum potassium}} \div \frac{\text{Urine osmolality}}{\text{Plasma osmolality}}$$

- Check spot urine chloride when hypokalemia is associated with alkalosis and high TTKG

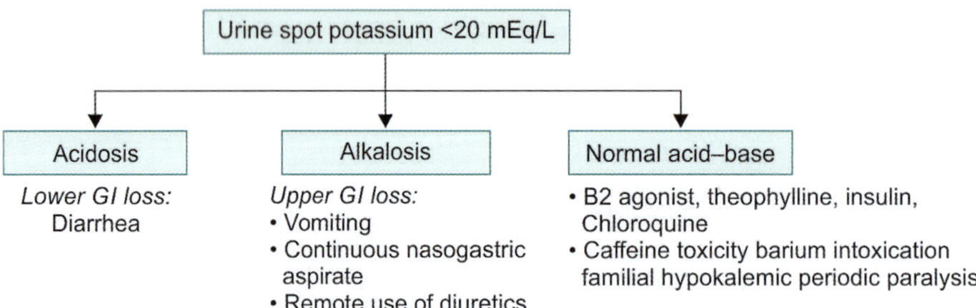

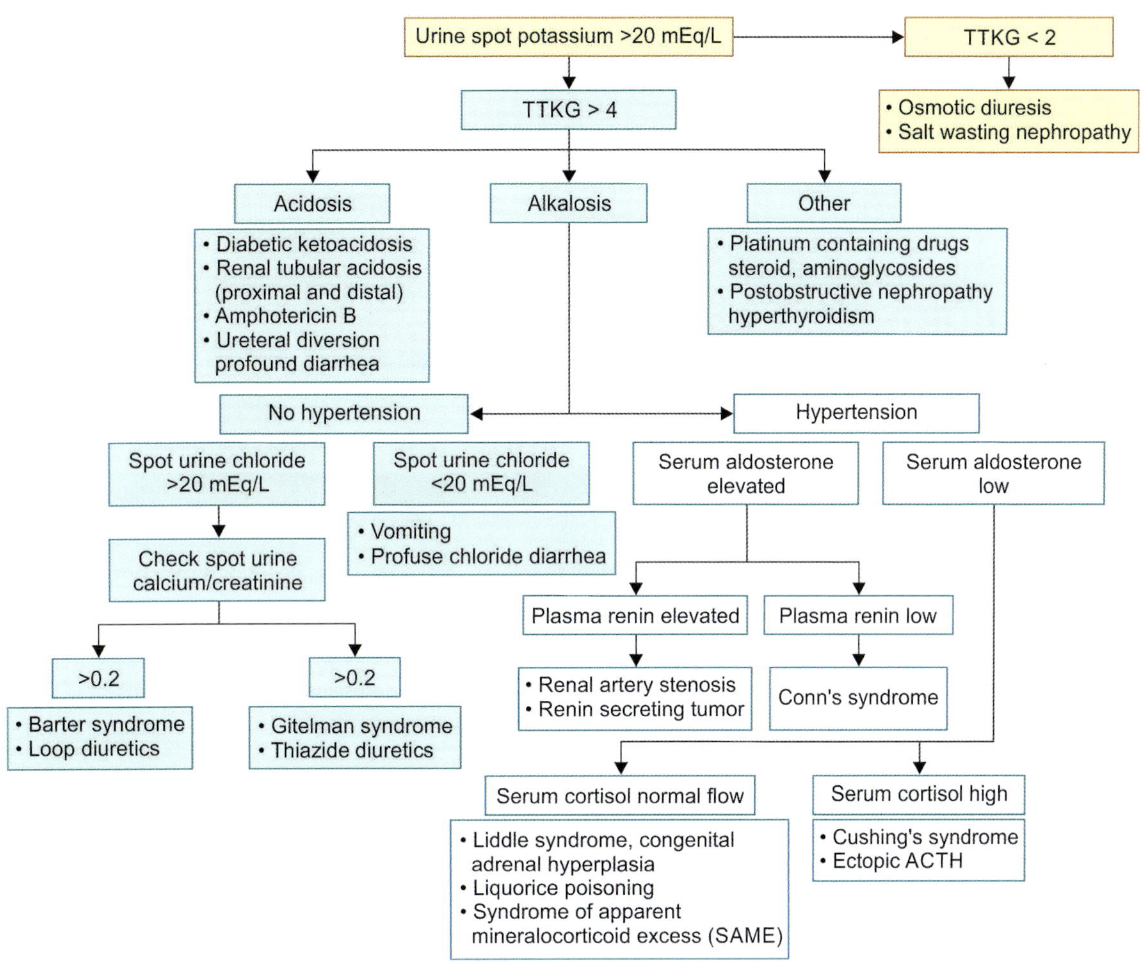


## MANAGEMENT OF HYPOKALEMIA

| *Severity* | *Treatment* | *Monitoring* | *Prevention and management* |
|---|---|---|---|
| Mild hypokalemia | Oral potassium supplements | Check serum potassium levels | Dietary potassium, medication review |
| Moderate hypokalemia | Oral potassium supplements | Regular serum potassium monitoring | Address underlying causes |
| Severe hypokalemia | Intravenous potassium replacement | Continuous monitoring, ECG | Prevent recurrence with dietary and medication management |

Different formulations of potassium salts:

| *Formulation* | *Forms* | *Uses* | *Dosage/Administration* | *Special considerations* |
|---|---|---|---|---|
| Oral potassium chloride (KCl) | Tablets, extended-release, oral solutions, powders | Mild to moderate hypokalemia | 20-40 mEq/day, with food | Monitor for gastrointestinal irritation |
| Potassium bicarbonate | Tablets, oral solutions | Hypokalemia with metabolic acidosis | Varies with needs | Used also for acidosis correction |
| Potassium citrate | Tablets, oral solutions | Hypokalemia, kidney stones prevention | Adjust based on needs | Also used for metabolic acidosis |

*Contd...*

*Contd...*

| Different formulations of potassium salts: | | | | |
|---|---|---|---|---|
| ***Formulation*** | ***Forms*** | ***Uses*** | ***Dosage/Administration*** | ***Special considerations*** |
| Potassium gluconate | Tablets, oral solutions | Hypokalemia, less GI irritation | Typically, lower doses | May be preferred in sensitive patients |
| Intravenous KCl | Concentrated solutions | Severe hypokalemia | 10-20 mEq in 100–500 mL fluid; up to 20 mEq/h in critical care | Monitor closely for ECG changes |
| Potassium phosphate | IV solutions | Hypokalemia with hypophosphatemia | Based on patient needs | Monitor phosphate levels closely |
| Potassium acetate | IV solutions | Alternative to KCl, less acidic form | Adjust based on needs | Consider for specific patient needs |

| IV potassium supplementations: | |
|---|---|
| ***Step*** | ***Details*** |
| Indications | Severe or symptomatic hypokalemia, inability to tolerate oral potassium, need for rapid correction |
| Preparation | Dilute potassium chloride in 100–500 mL of IV fluid (normal saline or dextrose) |
| Dosage & Rate | Initial dose: 10–20 mEq; Infusion rate: max 10–20 mEq/h; up to 20 mEq/h in ICU setting |
| Monitoring | Continuous ECG monitoring in critical settings, frequent serum potassium checks, vital signs |
| Safety Measures | Avoid rapid infusion, use proper dilution, and monitor for complications |

## SUGGESTED READING


1. Einhorn LM, Zhan M, Hsu VD, Walker LD, Moen MF, Seliger SL, et al. The frequency of hyperkalemia and its significance in chronic kidney disease. Arch Intern Med. 2009;169(12):1156-62.
2. Gennari FJ. Hypokalemia. N Engl J Med. 1998;339(7): 451-8.
3. Knochel JP. Hypokalemia and Skeletal Muscle. Kidney International. 1982;22(5):513-20.
4. Terlizzi V, Pitinca T, Lamberti A, Ferraguti G, Bertelli M. Pathophysiology of hypokalemia and hyperkalemia. J Clin Med. 2020;9(9):2953.
5. Weiner ID, Wingo CS. Hypokalemia--consequences, causes, and correction. J Am Soc Nephrol. 1997;8(7):1179-88.

CHAPTER

# 88 Hyperkalemia

## INTRODUCTION

Hyperkalemia is a condition characterized by an abnormally high concentration of potassium in the blood, typically defined as a serum potassium level greater than 5.0 mEq/L. Potassium is a critical electrolyte that plays a key role in maintaining normal muscle function, nerve transmission, and heart rhythm.

If there are any warning signs or ECG changes, start treatment before any evaluation for the cause.

## SIGNS AND SYMPTOMS

| *Severity* | *Serum potassium level* | *Signs and symptoms* | *Adverse effects* | *Diagnosis* |
|---|---|---|---|---|
| Mild hyperkalemia | 5.1–5.5 mEq/L | • Often asymptomatic<br>• Fatigue<br>• Muscle weakness<br>• Paresthesia (tingling) | • Mild ECG changes (peaked T waves) | • Serum potassium: 5.1–5.5 mEq/L<br>• ECG may show early changes: Peaked T waves<br>• Review medications (e.g., ACE inhibitors, potassium-sparing diuretics) |
| Moderate hyperkalemia | 5.6–6.5 mEq/L | • Muscle weakness<br>• Paresthesia<br>• Nausea<br>• Palpitations<br>• Decreased deep tendon reflexes | • ECG changes: Peaked T waves, prolonged PR interval, wide QRS complexes | • Serum potassium: 5.6–6.5 mEq/L<br>• ECG: Peaked T waves, widened QRS, prolonged PR<br>• Check renal function and metabolic acidosis |
| Severe hyperkalemia | >6.5 mEq/L | • Severe muscle weakness<br>• Paralysis<br>• Hyporeflexia<br>• Shortness of breath<br>• Chest pain | • Life-threatening arrhythmias: Ventricular fibrillation, asystole<br>• Cardiac arrest | • Serum potassium: >6.5 mEq/L<br>• ECG: Absent P waves, sine wave pattern, ventricular tachycardia/fibrillation<br>• Immediate evaluation of renal function, potassium intake |
| Critical hyperkalemia | >7.0 mEq/L | • Profound muscle paralysis<br>• Respiratory failure<br>• Cardiac arrest<br>• Coma | • Death from refractory arrhythmias or cardiac arrest | • Serum potassium: >7.0 mEq/L<br>• ECG: Sine wave pattern leading to ventricular fibrillation or asystole<br>• Requires immediate emergency treatment |

## CLINICAL APPROACH FOR EVALUATION OF HYPERKALEMIA

### Initial Assessment

- History:
  - *Review medications:* Potassium supplements, ACE inhibitors, ARBs, potassium-sparing diuretics, NSAIDs, etc.
  - *Assess for conditions causing potassium retention:* Chronic kidney disease (CKD), heart failure, adrenal insufficiency.
  - Check for recent trauma, burns, or rhabdomyolysis (tissue breakdown).
  - Ask about dietary potassium intake and use of salt substitutes.
- Physical Examination:
  - Look for signs of muscle weakness, flaccid paralysis, or cardiac abnormalities like irregular pulse.
  - Assess volume status: dehydration (hypovolemia) or fluid overload (hypervolemia) can indicate underlying conditions like kidney dysfunction or heart failure.

### Diagnostic Evaluation

- Serum potassium level:
  - Confirm hyperkalemia with a serum potassium level >5.0 mEq/L.
- ECG (electrocardiogram):
  - Check for ECG changes such as:
    - Peaked T waves (early sign),
    - Prolonged PR interval,
    - Flattened or absent P waves,
    - Widened QRS complex,
    - Sine wave pattern (pre-terminal sign).
  - These changes are critical to determine the urgency of treatment, even if the serum potassium is only moderately elevated.
- Serum electrolytes and renal functions:
  - Creatinine and BUN to assess renal function and GFR for kidney disease.
  - Serum bicarbonate to check for metabolic acidosis (often seen in renal failure).
  - Serum sodium, calcium, and chloride to identify associated electrolyte imbalances.
- Blood Gas (ABG or VBG):
  - Check for acidosis, as it can exacerbate hyperkalemia by shifting potassium from cells into the bloodstream.
- Urine Potassium and Electrolytes:
  - Measure urine potassium to differentiate between renal and non-renal causes.
  - Low urine potassium suggests impaired renal excretion.

**BOX 1:** Diagnostic algorithm of hyperkalemia.

If there is no life-threatening clinical or ECG sign, proceed for evaluation.

*Step 1:* Exclude pseudohyperkalemia:
- Hemolysis
- Collection error: tourniquet use, fist clenching, difficult venepuncture
- Taking sample from same line administering potassium

↓

*Step 2:* Identify medications or conditions that can cause hyperkalemia from increased potassium load or transcellular shift (redistribution hyperkalemia) or reduced excretion
- Potassium containing medications (penicillin G potassium)
- Oral potassium supplementation (medication or food)
- Heparin and low molecular weight heparin
- Cotrimoxazole, succinylcholine, beta blocker, somatostatin
- NSAIDs
- ACE-Inhibitors, ARBs, potassium-sparing diuretics, lithium and calcineurin inhibitors
- Digoxin toxicity
- Uncontrolled diabetes mellitus, insulin resistance, severe acidosis
- Red blood transfusion, tumor lysis syndrome, rhabdomyolysis

*Contd...*

*Contd...*

↓

*Step 3:* Assess renal function and urine output: Estimate GFR:
- Acute kidney injury and chronic kidney disease Hyperkalemia is uncommon unless GFR ≤ 15 mL/min.
- If GFR > 15 mL/min:

*Hyporeninemic hypoaldosteronism:* (characterized by hyperkalemic, hyperchloremic metabolic acidosis) is usually associated with mild or moderately advanced renal insufficiency.
- Type 4 renal tubular acidosis
- Diabetic nephropathy, Interstitial nephritis, obstructive nephropathy, systemic lupus erythematosus [SLE] nephropathy, sickle cell nephropathy

*Hyperreninemic hypo-aldosteronism:*
Sometimes, in critically ill patients, post adrenalectomy, when there is delayed recovery of the contralateral gland, sudden discontinuation of drugs having mineralocorticoid activity.

↓

*Step 4:* further evaluation of hyperkalemia in the presence of normal renal function
*Condition with low serum aldosterone:*
- *Addison's disease:* Check random cortisol level and do a cosyntropin stimulation test
- Congenital adrenal hyperplasia
- Primary hypoaldosteronism
- Drugs causing adrenal suppression

*Condition with aldosterone resistance:*
- Autosomal dominant or recessive pseudo-hypoaldosteronism (PHA AD)
- Urinary tract infection (UTI) and obstructive uropathy (resistance to aldosterone synthase)
- Assessment of urinary electrolytes is sometimes helpful. In a healthy patient, high potassium intake is associated with a high urinary potassium excretion rate; in the presence of hyperkalemia, low urinary potassium is prima facie evidence of inadequate renal potassium excretion.

## *Management Based on Severity*

Management of hyperkalemia depends on the severity and presence of ECG changes.

*Mild Hyperkalemia (5.1–5.5 mEq/L, no ECG changes)*
- *Dietary modification:* Restrict dietary potassium and avoid high-potassium foods (e.g., bananas, oranges, potatoes).
- *Medication review:* Discontinue or reduce medications that contribute to hyperkalemia (e.g., potassium-sparing diuretics, ACE inhibitors).
- *Potassium-binding resins:* Oral agents like patiromer or sodium polystyrene sulfonate (Kayexalate) to reduce potassium levels over time.

*Moderate Hyperkalemia (5.6–6.0 mEq/L, mild ECG changes)*
- *IV Calcium:* If ECG changes are present, give IV calcium gluconate (1 g IV over 5–10 minutes) to stabilize the cardiac membrane. This does not lower potassium but protects the heart.
- *Shift Potassium into Cells:*
  - *Insulin and glucose:* Administer 10 units of regular insulin IV with 25–50 g of glucose to shift potassium into cells.
  - *Beta-agonists:* Nebulized albuterol (10–20 mg) can also drive potassium into cells.
  - *Sodium bicarbonate (if metabolic acidosis is present):* 50–100 mEq of sodium bicarbonate IV may help shift potassium into cells in cases of acidosis.
- *Loop diuretics* (e.g., furosemide) may promote urinary potassium excretion if renal function allows.

*Severe Hyperkalemia (>6.0 mEq/L or significant ECG changes)*
- *Immediate ECG monitoring:* Continuous cardiac monitoring is required due to the high risk of arrhythmias.
- *IV Calcium Gluconate:* Administer immediately if there are significant ECG changes.
- *Insulin and Glucose:* Continue to shift potassium into cells.

- *Dialysis:* Emergency hemodialysis may be necessary in patients with severe renal failure or life-threatening hyperkalemia that is not responsive to medical therapy.
- Loop diuretics (if kidney function allows) to promote potassium excretion.
- Potassium-binding resins to help eliminate excess potassium via the GI tract.

*Identify and treat the underlying cause*

- *Renal failure:* In cases of acute or chronic kidney disease, adjust medications, manage fluid balance, and consider long-term potassium-lowering strategies.
- *Medications:* Stop or adjust medications that impair potassium excretion (e.g., ACE inhibitors, ARBs, NSAIDs, potassium-sparing diuretics).
- *Adrenal insufficiency:* In cases of Addison's disease or hypoaldosteronism, replacement therapy with mineralocorticoids (e.g., fludrocortisone) may be necessary.
- *Tissue damage:* In patients with rhabdomyolysis, burns, or crush injuries, manage the underlying condition and monitor potassium closely.

*Monitoring and follow-up*

- *Serial potassium measurements:* Regular monitoring of serum potassium levels to ensure response to treatment and avoid recurrence.
- *ECG monitoring:* Continue ECG monitoring until potassium levels normalize and the patient is stable.
- *Renal function and electrolytes:* Follow-up to assess renal function and ensure electrolyte balance.

Here are key references regarding hyperkalemia, including its causes, clinical implications, and management strategies:

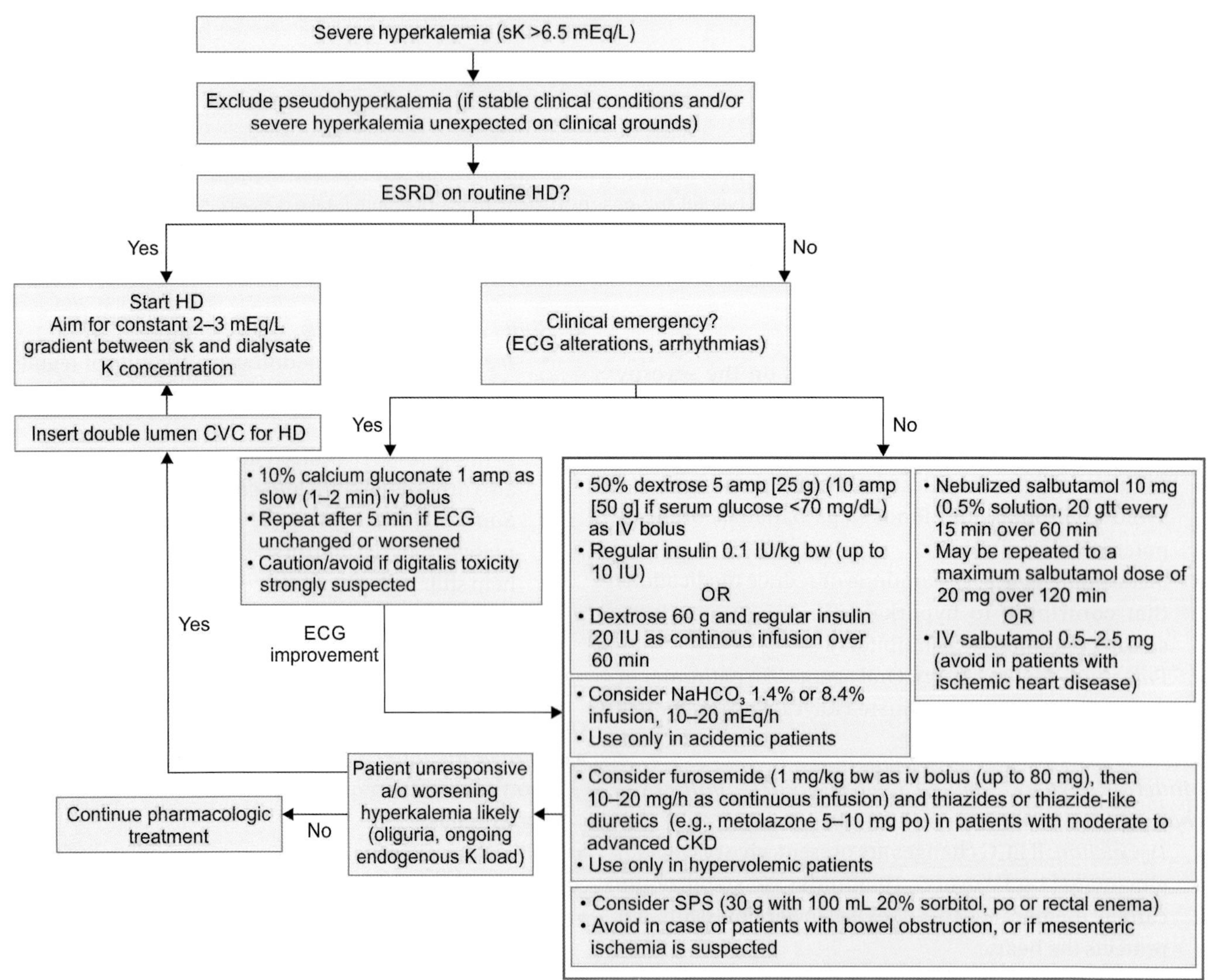

## SUGGESTED READING

1. Einhorn LM, Zhan M, Hsu VD, Walker LD, Moen MF, Seliger SL, et al. The Frequency of Hyperkalemia and Its Significance in Chronic Kidney Disease. Arch Intern Med. 2009;169(12):1156-62.
2. Kovesdy CP, Appel LJ. Management of Hyperkalemia: An Update for the practicing clinician. J Am Med Assoc. 2017;318(8):804-14.
3. Sica DA. Clinical Pharmacology of Potassium and the Management of Hypokalemia and Hyperkalemia in Hypertension. J Clin Hypertension. 2005;7(9):464-8.
4. Sterns RH, Perazella MA. Hyperkalemia: An Updated Review of Clinical Manifestations, Diagnosis, and Treatment. J Am Soc Nephrol. 2021;32(1):158-68.
5. Weiner ID, Wingo CS. Hyperkalemia: A Critical Review. Journal of the American Society of Nephrology. 1997;8(5): 1140-48

CHAPTER 89

# Hypocalcemia

## CALCIUM METABOLISM

- Normal serum calcium: 8–10 mg/dL
- 40% of this is bound to albumin
- 50–55% ionized form, which is physiologically active and lies within a narrow range of 4.6 to 5.1 mg/dL
- Remaining calcium is attached with other anions like phosphates, lactate, bicarbonate, sulfate, and citrate.
- Corrected total serum calcium in hypoalbuminemia: Add 1 mg/dL to serum calcium for each 1 gm/dL reduction in serum albumin below 4 gm/dL

## REGULATION

| Thyroid gland | | Calcitonin |
|---|---|---|
| HIGH | | Decrease Calcium |
| Blood calcium level | | |
| Increase calcium | | LOW |
| PTH | | Parathyroid gland |
| Stimulates bone resorption | Activates Vit D to active form 1,25 $(OH)_2D_3$ | Increase renal Ca reabsorption |
| • Increase intestinal Ca absorption<br>• Bone reabsorption | | |

## DEFINITION

- Hypocalcemia is a condition that happens when the level of calcium in serum is less than 8.5 mg/dl or ionized calcium is less than 1.05 mmol/L.
- It is often caused by abnormal levels of parathyroid hormone (PTH) or vitamin D in the body.

## ETIOLOGY

| *Low parathyroid hormone levels (Hypoparathyroidism)* | *High parathyroid hormone levels (Secondary Hyperparathyroidism)* |
|---|---|
| • *Parathyroid agenesis:*<br>– Isolated<br>– DiGeorge's syndrome<br>• *Parathyroid destruction:* Surgical, Radiation, metastases or systemic diseases, Autoimmune<br>• *Reduced parathyroid function:*<br>– Hypomagnesemia<br>– Autosomal dominant hypocalcemia | • *Vitamin D deficiency or impaired 1,25(OH)2D production/action:*<br>– Nutritional vitamin D deficiency (poor intake or absorption)<br>– Renal insufficiency with impaired 1,25(OH)2D production<br>– Vitamin D resistance, including receptor defects<br>• *Parathyroid hormone resistance syndromes:*<br>– PTH receptor mutations<br>– Pseudohypoparathyroidism (G protein mutations) |
| *Drugs:*<br>• Calcium chelators<br>• Inhibitors of bone resorption (bisphosphonates, plicamycin)<br>• Altered vitamin D metabolism (phenytoin, ketoconazole) | *Miscellaneous causes:*<br>• Acute pancreatitis<br>• Acute rhabdomyolysis<br>• Hungry bone syndrome after parathyroidectomy<br>• Osteoblastic metastases with marked stimulation of bone formation (prostate cancer) |

## CLINICAL MANIFESTATIONS

| ***Symptoms*** | ***Signs*** |
|---|---|
| • Muscle cramps<br>• Carpopedal spasms<br>• Seizures<br>• Paresthesia tingling sensation around mouth and toes<br>• Tetany<br>• Laryngospasm, stridor | • Prolong QT interval<br>• Chvostek's sign<br>• Trousseau's sign |

## PATHOPHYSIOLOGY

Decrease extracellular calcium

↓

Membrane potential outside the cell wall becomes less negative

Amount of depolarization required to initiate action potential is less

Increased excitability of muscle and nerve tissue

### Approach to Hypocalcemia

| Hypocalcemia (adjusted for albumin) | | | |
|---|---|---|---|
| ***Serum PTH*** | | | |
| ***Low*** | | ***Normal*** | ***High*** |
| • Creatinine normal<br>• $PO_4$ normal or high | | • Creatinine normal<br>• $PO_4$ normal or high<br>• Mg normal | |
| *Magnesium (Mg)* | | Low albumin | |
| *Low* | *Normal* | *Hypoalbuminemia* | |
| *Mg deficiency* | *Hypoparathyroidism* | | |
| | | • Creatinine normal<br>• $PO_4$ normal or low<br>• Mg normal | • Creatinine high<br>• $PO_4$ normal or high<br>• Mg normal |
| | | 25-hydroxyvitamin D | Pseudohypoparathyroidism (rare) |
| | | Vitamin D deficiency | Renal disease |

### Treatment of Hypocalcemia

| Symptomatic hypocalcemia or calcium <1.9 mmol/l | | |
|---|---|---|
| To correct rapidly | | To correct slowly |
| Intravenous calcium gluconate 10 mL of 10% solution over 10 min | | Vitamin D treatment |
| If persistent, infusion of 10 ampuls of calcium gluconate or 900 mg of calcium in 1 L of 5% dextrose or 0.9% sodium chloride administered over 24 h | Parathyroid hormone deficient | Parathyroid hormone intact |
| | • Vitamin D analog<br>• Calcitriol start dose of 0.5–1 mg/day can increase every 4–7 days | Cholecalciferol typical dose of 50,000 IU each weekly orally for 8 weeks |

## SUGGESTED READING


1. Cooper MS, Benson K. Management of Acute Hypocalcemia. In: Brandi M, Brown E (Eds). Hypoparathyroidism. Milano: Springer.
2. Cooper MS, Gittoes NJ. Diagnosis and management of hypocalcaemia. BMJ (Clinical Research ed.). 2008; 336(7656):1298-302.
3. In: Jameson JL (Ed). Harrison's Principles of internal medicine, 21st edition. New York: McGraw-Hill Education; 2022.

CHAPTER 90

# Hypercalcemia

## CALCIUM METABOLISM

- Normal serum calcium: 8–10 mg/dL
- 40–45% of this is bound to albumin
- 45–50% ionized form, which is physiologically active and lies within a narrow range of 4.6–5.2 mg/dl (1.16–1.31 mmol/lit)
- Remaining (approximately 10–15%) calcium is attached with other anions like phosphates, lactate, bicarbonate, sulfate, and citrate.
- Corrected total serum calcium in hypoalbuminemia: add 0.8–1 mg/dl to serum calcium for each 1 gm/dl reduction in serum albumin below 4 g/dL.
- *Pseudohypocalcemia*: Serum calcium low, ionized calcium normal (e.g., volume overload, chronic illness, malnutrition, nephrotic syndrome)
- Acidosis reduces while alkalosis enhances the binding of the albumin calcium complex

## REGULATION

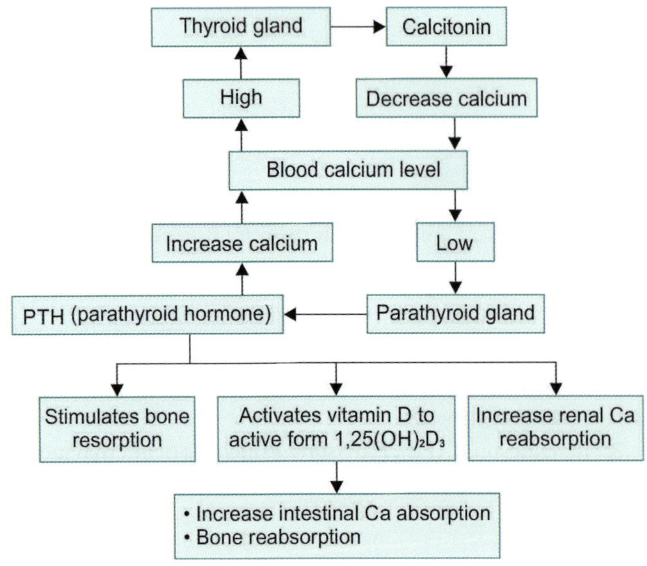


Hypercalcemia

| | ***Total Ca (mg/dL)*** | ***Ionized Ca (mg/dL)*** |
|---|---|---|
| Mild | 10.5–11.9 | 5.6–8 |
| Moderate | 12–13.9 | 8–10 |
| Hypercalcemic crisis | 14–16 | 10–12 |

## ETIOLOGY

*Excessive PTH production*
- Primary hyperparathyroidism (adenoma, hyperplasia, rarely carcinoma)
- Tertiary hyperparathyroidism (long-term stimulation of PTH secretion in renal insufficiency)
- FHH –Familial Hypocalciuric Hypercalcemia
- Ectopic PTH secretion

*Hypercalcemia of malignancy*
- Overproduction of PTHrP (parathyroid hormone-related protein)
- Lytic skeletal metastases (breast and myeloma)

*Excessive calcium intake:*
- Total parenteral nutrition
- Milk-alkali syndrome

*Primary increase in bone resorption:*
- Hyperthyroidism
- Immobilization

*Excessive 1,25(OH)$_2$D production*
- Granulomatous diseases (sarcoidosis, tuberculosis, silicosis)
- Lymphomas
- Vitamin D intoxication

*Endocrine disorders*
- Adrenal insufficiency
- Pheochromocytoma

*Medications:*
- Thiazides
- Vitamin A
- Antiestrogens

## CLINICAL FEATURES

| *System* | *Symptoms* | *Signs* |
|---|---|---|
| CNS | • Weakness<br>• Confusion<br>• Altered mentation | • Stupor<br>• Coma |
| GIT | • Nausea<br>• Vomiting<br>• Anorexia<br>• Constipation<br>• Abdominal pain | • Peptic ulcer disease<br>• Pancreatitis |
| Renal | • Polyuria<br>• Nocturia | • Nephrolithiasis<br>• Nephrogenic Diabetes insipidus<br>• Renal tubular acidosis<br>• Acute kidney injury<br>• Chronic kidney disease |
| Skeletal | Bone pain | Fractures |
| CVS | | • Shortened QT interval<br>• Ventricular arrhythmias |

## DIAGNOSIS

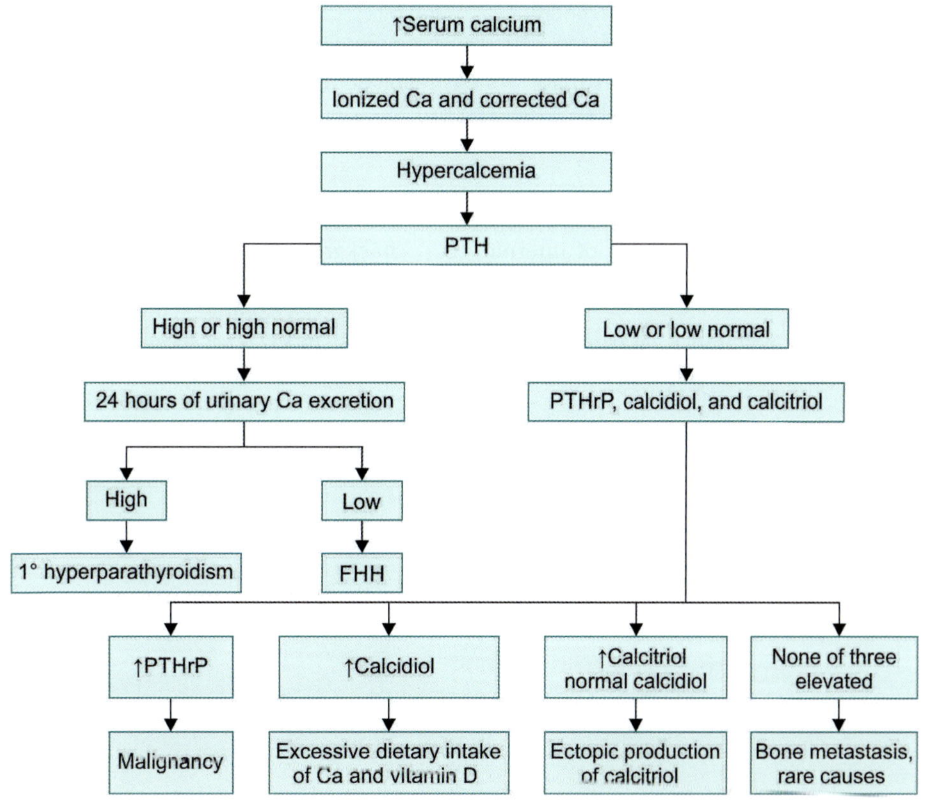

## TREATMENT

| *Drug* | *Dose* | *Onset of action* | *Mode of action* | *Comments* |
|---|---|---|---|---|
| Isotonic saline | 4–6 L/day | Hours | Restores intravascular volume<br>Increase urine Ca excretion | Caution in elderly and heart failure patients |
| Frusemide | 20–160 mg IV 8 hrly after volume expansion | Hours | Inhibit Ca reabsorption in the loop of Henle and Increase urine Ca excretion | Avoid dehydration, hypokalemia and hypomagnesemia |
| Hemodialysis | | Hours | Removes Ca | Severe hypercalcemia |
| Bisphosphonate<br>Pamidronate<br>Zoledronate | 60–90 mg IV over 2–4 hours<br><br>4 mg IV over 15 mins | 24–72 hours | Inhibit bone resorption | Caution in renal insufficiency |
| Calcitonin | 4–8 IU/kg IM/SC 6–12 hourly | 4–6 hours | Inhibit bone resorption<br>Increase urine Ca excretion | Useful for urgent therapy |
| Gallium nitrate | 100–200 mg/m$^2$/day continuous infusion × 5 days | 2–6 days | Inhibits ostoclastic activity | Risk of nephrotoxicity |
| Glucocorticoids<br>Hydrocortisone<br>Oral<br>Prednisolone | <br>100–300 mg IV daily<br>40–60 mg daily | 2–5 days | Decrease intestinal Ca absorption<br>In granulomas and lymphomas, decrease vit D3 production | Effective in vit D intoxication, malignancies, sarcoidosis |
| Oral phosphate | 67 mg PO 6 hourly | 4–6 hours | Inhibits Ca absorption and promotes Ca deposition | Serum $pO_4 < 3$ mg/dL and normal renal function |
| Denosumab | 60–120 mg SC | 4–10 days | Inhibit bone resorption | Risk of hypocalcemia and infection |

## SUGGESTED READING

1. In: Jameson JL (Ed). Harrison's principles of internal medicine. 21st edition. New York: McGraw-Hill Education; 2022.
2. In: Vincent JL, Moore FA, Bellomo R, Marini JJ (Eds). Textbook of Critical Care. Amsterdam: Elsevier Health Sciences; 2022.
3. Lederer E. Hypophosphatemia: Practice essentials, background, pathophysiology and etiology. [Online] Available from https://emedicine.medscape.com/article/242280overview?&icd=login_success_email_match_fpf#a2 [Last accessed February, 2025].
4. Sharma S, Hashmi MF, Castro D. Hypophosphatemia. In: Treasure Island (FL): StatPearls Publishing; 2020.

CHAPTER 91

# Hypophosphatemia

## INTRODUCTION

- Phosphate is an essential electrolyte in the human body as it constitutes about 1% of the TBW
- Most phosphorus in the human body is complexed with oxygen as $PO_4$, which is a major intracellular anion
- The phosphate anion ($PO_4^-$) is basically phosphoric acid ($H_3PO_4$)
- It has three pKas (2.2, 7.2, and 12.4) and can exist as ($PO_4^-$), ($PO_4^{2-}$), and ($PO_4^{3-}$), though at body fluid pH, it is usually a mixture of ($PO_4^-$) and ($PO_4^{2-}$).
- Main regulators of phosphate homeostasis

> - Parathyroid hormone
> - Calcitriol
> - Number of peptides collectively known as the "phosphatonins," of which fibroblast growth factor-23 (FGF-23)

## ABSORPTION OF $PO_4$

- 40 mmol/day is normal oral intake; plus another 5 mmol/day is generated in the metabolism of phospholipids and proteins
- The transient pool of extracellular inorganic phosphate originates from multiple sources. Much of it is a byproduct of the metabolism of bone hydroxyapatite, and some is being absorbed from the gut and recirculated from the kidneys. The size of this pool is therefore regulated by:
    - Regulation of bone metabolism
    - Regulation of gut absorption
    - Regulation of renal reabsorption

> *Bone phosphate metabolism*
> - *Calcitriol* increases the absorption of phosphate from bone
> - *PTH* increases the absorption of phosphate from bone and stimulates the production of calcitriol

> *Intestinal phosphate absorption:*
> - Dietary sodium: It is a co-factor necessary for active phosphate transport in the gut
> - Phosphate concentration in the gut (a high concentration is necessary for passive transport)
> - *Calcitriol* increases the absorption of phosphate (and conversely, a low phosphate stimulates the synthesis of calcitriol).
> - *PTH* does not seem to have direct control over phosphate reabsorption in the gut, but it increases the synthesis of calcitriol, which in turn increases phosphate reabsorption. So, indirectly, PTH increases gut absorption of phosphate.

> *Renal phosphate reabsorption:*
> - *PTH*, which decreases the proximal tubular reabsorption. In the absence of PTH, reabsorption is greater. When PTH release is stimulated by hypocalcemia, renal expression of apical sodium-potassium cotransporters decreases.
> - *Calcitriol* increases the reabsorption of phosphate in the proximal tubule
> - *PTH* does not seem to have direct control over phosphate reabsorption in the gut, but it increases the synthesis of calcitriol, which in turn increases phosphate reabsorption. So, indirectly, PTH increases gut absorption of phosphate.

## DISTRIBUTION OF $PO_4$

| | |
|---|---|
| (600 g = 20 mol) bone as crystalline hydroxyapatite | 85% |
| Soft tissues, mostly intracellularly as a component of organic compounds, such as nucleic acids, cell membrane phospholipids, ATP, red blood cell, 2,3-DPG, and phosphoproteins | 14% |
| Extracellular fluid | 15% |

## ECF $PO_4$ DISTRIBUTION

| | |
|---|---|
| Free serum $PO_4$ ionized | 45% |
| Complexed with Na, Ca, Mg | 40% |
| Bound with albumin | 15% |

- Serum laboratory analyses measure the free inorganic phosphate ions $H_2PO_4^-$ and $HPO_4^{2-}$ their ratio is pH dependent; at 7.4, the ratio is 1:4.

## ELIMINATION OF $PO_4$

- 30 mmol is excreted renally
- 15 mmol is lost via stool

## ROLE OF $PO_4$

| | |
|---|---|
| Structural role | • Bone mineral<br>• Phospholipid of cell membrane<br>• Incorporated into DNA and RNA molecules |
| Regulatory role | • Secondary messenger (IP3)<br>• Protein activity is turned on and off by phosphorylation and dephosphorylation |
| Metabolic role | • Co-factor in oxygen transport (as 2,3-DPG)<br>• Trapping glucose in cells (as glucose-6-phosphate)<br>• Synthesis of ATP (it's the P in ATP)<br>• Acid-base regulation (urinary and intracellular buffering) |

## HYPOPHOSPHATEMIA

Serum phosphate level of less than 2.5 mg/dL (0.8 mmol/L)

| | |
|---|---|
| Mild | 2–2.5 mg/dL |
| Moderate | 1–2 mg/dL |
| Severe | < 1 mg/dL |

Abnormalities in serum magnesium, calcium, and potassium levels may also seen.

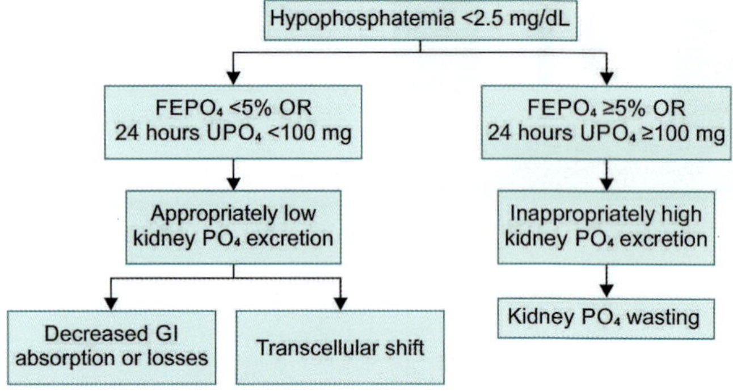


$$FEPO_4 = (UPO4 \times PCr \times 100)/(PPO_4 \times UCr)$$

| ***Decreased GI absorption or losses*** | ***Transcellular shift*** |
|---|---|
| Aluminum and magnesium-containing antacids | Recovery from starvation and acidosis |
| Malnutrition | Refeeding syndrome |
| Nasogastric suctioning | Acute respiratory alkalosis |
| Diarrhea | IV Glucose |
| Vomiting | Prolong insulin therapy |
| Vitamin D deficiency | Catecholamines |
| Irritable bowel syndrome | Rapid cellular proliferation, e.g., GF therapy, intensive erythropoietin therapy, leukemic blast crisis |
| Chronic alcoholism | Hypo Mg/ hypo K |
| | Burns |

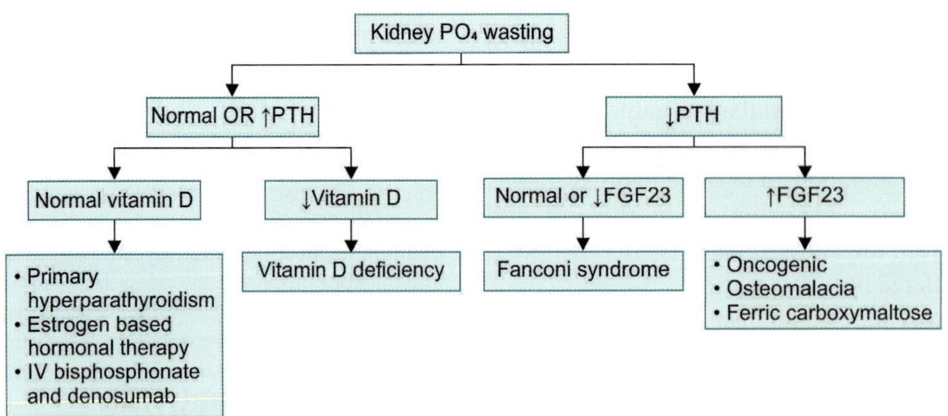

| | |
|---|---|
| *Respiratory*<br>• Worsened respiratory failure<br>• Dependence on ventilator | *Cardiovascular*<br>• Impaired myocardial contractility<br>• Cardiac rhythm disturbance (supraventricular and ventricular tachycardia).<br>• Heart failure. |
| *Hematologic*<br>• Hemolysis<br>• Thrombocytopenia<br>• Affected phagocytosis and chemotaxis | *Neurologic*<br>• Irritability<br>• Confusion<br>• Dysarthria<br>• Altered mental status<br>• Seizures<br>• Coma<br>• Ataxia<br>• Paresthesia<br>• May promote the development of central pontine myelinolysis. |
| *Muscular*<br>• Muscular weakness<br>• Rhabdomyolysis | *Other*<br>• Insulin resistance |

## TREATMENT

Possible losses should be identified and stopped.

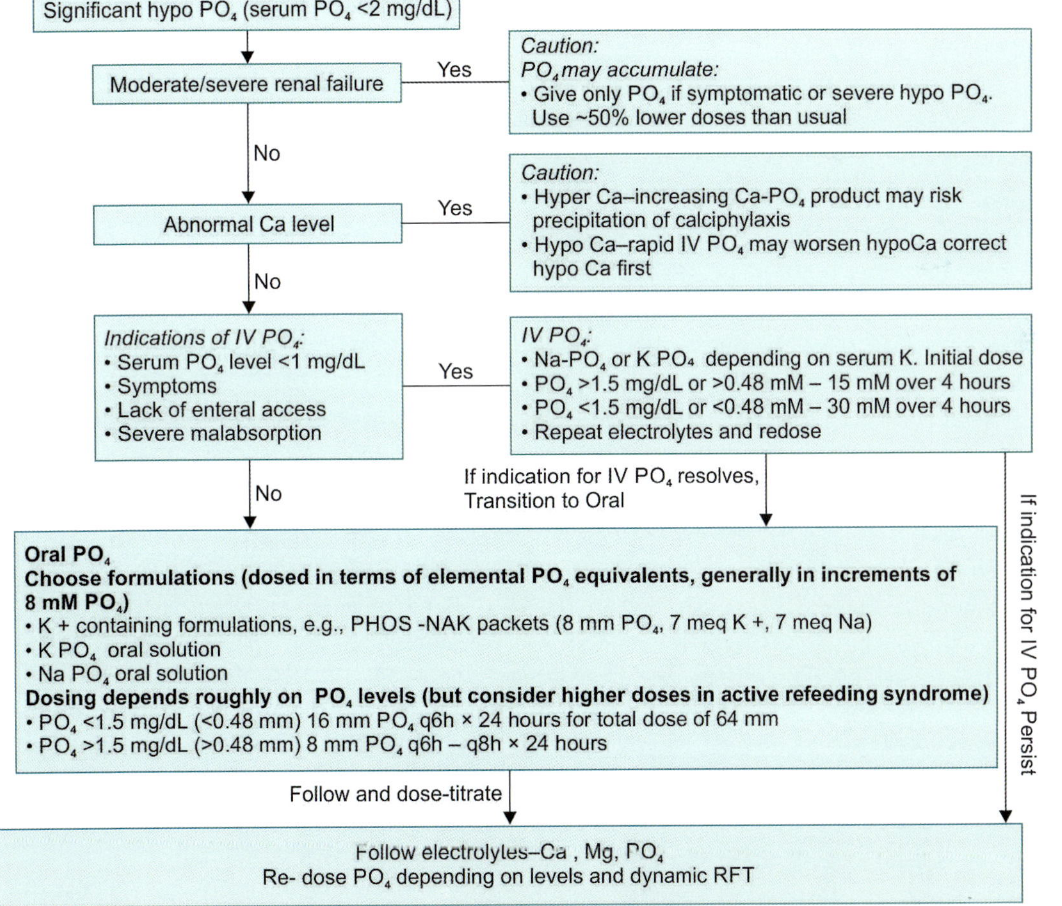


In patients greater than 130% of their ideal body weight, adjusted body weight should be used to calculate the doses.

## ADVERSE EFFECTS

Adverse effects of intravenous phosphate repletion

- Metastatic calcification
- Hypocalcemia
- Hyperkalemia associated with potassium-containing supplements
- Volume excess
- Hypernatremia associated with sodium-containing supplements
- Metabolic acidosis
- Hyperphosphatemia

## SUGGESTED READING


1. In: Jameson JL (Ed). Harrison's principles of internal medicine. 21st edition. New York: McGraw-Hill Education; 2022.
2. In: Vincent JL, Moore FA, Bellomo R, Marini JJ (Eds). Textbook of Critical Care. Amsterdam: Elsevier Health Sciences; 2022.
3. Lederer E. Hypophosphatemia: Practice essentials, background, pathophysiology and etiology. [Online] Available from https://emedicine.medscape.com/article/242280overview?&icd=login_success_email_match_fpf#a2 [Last accessed February, 2025].
4. Sharma S, Hashmi MF, Castro D. Hypophosphatemia. In: Treasure Island (FL): StatPearls Publishing; 2020.

CHAPTER 92

# Hypomagnesemia

## INTRODUCTION

*Hypomagnesemia* is a condition characterized by low levels of magnesium in the blood, typically defined as a serum magnesium concentration less than 1.7 mg/dL (0.7 mmol/L). Magnesium is an essential mineral involved in various physiological processes, including nerve function, muscle contraction, and maintaining normal heart rhythm.

**TABLE 1:** Signs and symptoms.

| *Severity* | *Serum magnesium level* | *Signs and symptoms* | *Adverse effects* | *Diagnosis* |
|---|---|---|---|---|
| Mild hypomagnesemia | 1.2–1.7 mg/dL | • Fatigue<br>• Nausea<br>• Muscle cramps<br>• Weakness | • Subtle neuromuscular irritability | • Serum magnesium: 1.2–1.7 mg/dL<br>• Check for associated hypokalemia or hypocalcemia |
| Moderate hypomagnesemia | 0.9–1.1 mg/dL | • Muscle twitching<br>• Tremors<br>• Hyperreflexia<br>• Confusion | • ECG changes: Prolonged QT interval<br>• Increased risk of arrhythmias | • Serum magnesium: 0.9–1.1 mg/dL<br>• Assess kidney function<br>• Evaluate for malabsorption or alcohol use |
| Severe hypomagnesemia | <0.9 mg/dL | • Seizures<br>• Tetany<br>• Carpopedal spasm<br>• Confusion<br>• Cardiac arrhythmias (torsades de pointes) | • Life-threatening arrhythmias<br>• Respiratory muscle paralysis<br>• Refractory hypokalemia and hypocalcemia | • Serum magnesium: <0.9 mg/dL<br>• ECG: Prolonged QT, PR, and QRS intervals<br>• Assess gastrointestinal losses (e.g., diarrhea, vomiting) |
| Critical hypomagnesemia | <0.5 mg/dL | • Severe muscle weakness<br>• Respiratory depression<br>• Coma<br>• Cardiac arrest | • Cardiac arrest<br>• Death due to refractory arrhythmias | • Serum magnesium: <0.5 mg/dL<br>• Immediate neurological and cardiac evaluation<br>• Emergency treatment required |

## CLINICAL APPROACH TO HYPOMAGNESEMIA

### Initial Assessment

*History and Risk Factors*

Assess for conditions that may lead to magnesium loss or inadequate intake, such as:

- Chronic alcoholism
- Malnutrition or poor dietary intake
- Malabsorption syndromes (e.g., Crohn's disease, celiac disease)
- Prolonged diarrhea or vomiting
- Renal loss (e.g., use of diuretics, uncontrolled diabetes)
- Medications (e.g., diuretics, proton pump inhibitors, aminoglycosides)

### Diagnostic Evaluation

*Serum Magnesium Levels*

Confirm hypomagnesemia with serum magnesium levels typically <1.7 mg/dL (0.7 mmol/L).

*Electrolyte Panel*

Check for hypokalemia (low potassium) and hypocalcemia (low calcium), as they frequently coexist with hypomagnesemia.

*Renal Function Tests*

Assess serum creatinine and BUN to evaluate kidney function, especially if renal losses are suspected.

*ECG (Electrocardiogram)*

Look for ECG changes such as prolonged QT interval, ST-segment depression, or ventricular arrhythmias in more severe cases.

Most of the causes of hypomagnesemia do not require detailed biochemical evaluation.

History itself provides clues to diagnosis.

*For biochemical evaluation:*

*Step 1:* Check fractional excretion of magnesium (FEMg):

$$100 \times \frac{\text{UrineMg} \times \text{PlasmaCr}}{0.7 \times \text{PlasmaMg} \times \text{UrineCr}}$$

*Step 2:* If FEMg is < 2-2.5% (or 24-hour urine magnesium < 10 gm/day). → suggests nonrenal magnesium wasting

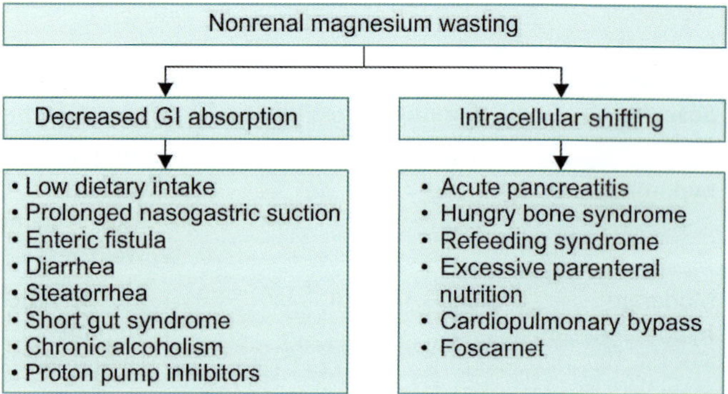


*Step 3:* If FEMg is > 2-2.5% or 24-hour urinary magnesium is > 10 gm/day

It suggests renal magnesium wasting.

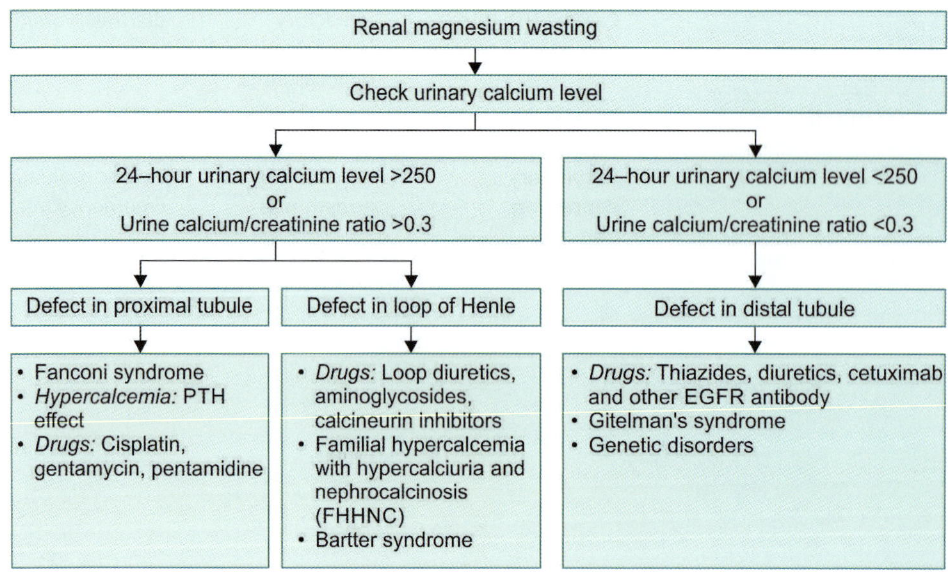

## MANAGEMENT OF HYPOMAGNESEMIA

Management of hypomagnesemia depends on its etiology. Magnesium is usually supplemented parenterally. IV magnesium sulfate should be administered slowly, as rapid administration may lead to vasodilatation.

Oral magnesium is less commonly available and is reserved only in selected cases.

Hypomagnesemia is commonly associated with other electrolyte abnormalities. As for example:

1. Hypercalcemia and hyperphosphatemia act as a potential cause of hypomagnesemia.
2. Hypokalemia and hypocalcemia occur as a result of hypomagnesemia, and correction of serum magnesium is required for correction of serum potassium and calcium levels.

## SUGGESTED READING


1. Alfrey AC. Dialysis and magnesium. Kidney Intern. 1987;32(6):912-9.
2. Cundy T, Dissanayake A. Severe hypermagnesemia due to laxative use. Lancet. 2008;371(9627):1596-7.
3. Kopple JD. Magnesium Homeostasis and Hypermagnesemia. Clin J Am Soc Nephrol. 2017;12(6):1015-20.
4. Perazella MA, Moe SM. Hypermagnesemia: A Clinical Perspective. Am J Kidney Dis. 2013;62(3):622-30.
5. Rasmussen HS, McNair P. Magnesium metabolism in chronic renal failure. Magnesium. 1986;5(3-4):216-27.
6. Whang R, Ryder KW, Dyckner T. Magnesium and Potassium Interactions in Cardiac Arrhythmias. Magnesium Res. 1990;7(4):373-81.

CHAPTER 93

# Hypermagnesemia

## INTRODUCTION

*Hypermagnesemia* is a condition characterized by elevated levels of magnesium in the blood, typically greater than 2.5 mEq/L (1.25 mmol/L). It is relatively rare and often associated with conditions that impair renal function or with excessive intake of magnesium-containing medications.

The symptoms of hypermagnesemia can vary depending on the severity of the condition **(Table 1)**.

**TABLE 1:** Signs and symptoms of hypermagnesemia.

| ***Severity*** | ***Serum magnesium level*** | ***Signs and symptoms*** | ***Adverse effects*** | ***Diagnosis*** |
|---|---|---|---|---|
| Mild hypermagnesemia | 2.5–4 mEq/L | • Nausea and vomiting<br>• Flushing (skin warmth)<br>• Lethargy<br>• Muscle weakness | • Hypotension<br>• Decreased reflexes | • *Serum magnesium:* 2.5–4 mEq/L<br>• Routine blood test showing elevated magnesium |
| Moderate hypermagnesemia | 5–12 mEq/L | • Decreased deep tendon reflexes<br>• Muscle weakness<br>• Bradycardia<br>• Drowsiness<br>• ECG changes (prolonged PR interval) | • Risk of worsening hypotension<br>• Cardiac arrhythmias | • *Serum magnesium:* 5–12 mEq/L<br>• ECG showing prolonged PR interval or bradycardia |
| Severe hypermagnesemia | >12 mEq/L | • Complete loss of deep tendon reflexes<br>• Paralysis (including respiratory)<br>• Coma<br>• Hypotension | • Cardiac arrest<br>• Respiratory failure<br>• Asystole or complete heart block | • *Serum magnesium:* >12 mEq/L<br>• Immediate ECG showing severe arrhythmias or asystole |
| Critical hypermagnesemia | >15 mEq/L | • Respiratory failure<br>• Cardiac arrest<br>• Unresponsiveness<br>• Severe bradycardia or asystole | Death from cardiac or respiratory arrest | • *Serum magnesium:* >15 mEq/L<br>• Immediate clinical evaluation for emergency resuscitation |

## CLINICAL APPROACH TO HYPERMAGNESEMIA

- Evaluate for *renal impairment* (acute or chronic kidney disease), as it is the most common cause.
- Assess for excessive use of *magnesium-containing medications* (antacids, laxatives, supplements) or iatrogenic causes (intravenous magnesium sulfate, especially in obstetric patients).
- Look for associated conditions like *hypothyroidism, Addison's disease, or adrenal insufficiency*
- Check *calcium, potassium,* and *phosphate* levels, as magnesium imbalances can affect these.
- Serum *creatinine* and *blood urea nitrogen (BUN)* levels to assess renal function.
- Continuous ECG monitoring if there are significant arrhythmias or conduction abnormalities.

## DIAGNOSIS OF HYPERMAGNESEMIA

1. *History and physical examination:*
    - Evaluate for underlying renal disease, medications (e.g., antacids or laxatives containing magnesium), or iatrogenic causes (such as intravenous magnesium sulfate administration).
    - Assess for signs and symptoms of hypermagnesemia.
2. *Laboratory tests:*
    - *Serum magnesium levels:* Elevated magnesium levels (>2.5 mEq/L) confirm hypermagnesemia.
    - *Renal function tests:* Evaluate serum creatinine blood urea nitrogen (BUN) to assess kidney function.
    - *Electrolytes:* Check calcium, potassium, and phosphate levels, as hypermagnesemia can be associated with other electrolyte abnormalities.
    - *Electrocardiogram (ECG):* Look for ECG changes like prolonged PR interval, QRS widening, or heart block.
3. *Identify the underlying cause:*
    - Renal failure (acute or chronic)
    - Excessive intake of magnesium (e.g., overuse of supplements, laxatives, or antacids)
    - Addison's disease
    - Hypothyroidism

## MANAGEMENT ALGORITHM FOR HYPERMAGNESEMIA

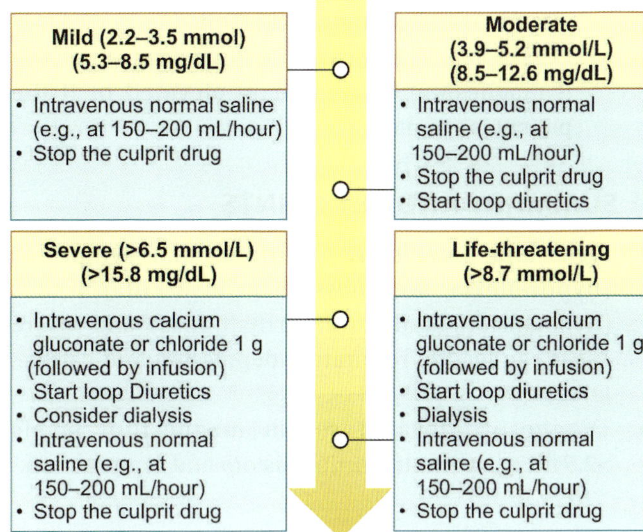


1. *Mild-to-Moderate Hypermagnesemia (asymptomatic or mild symptoms, 2.5–4 mEq/L):*
    - *Discontinue magnesium-containing medications:* Stop any exogenous magnesium intake, such as supplements, antacids, or laxatives.
    - *Hydration:* Administer intravenous fluids (e.g., normal saline) to enhance renal excretion of magnesium.
    - *Loop diuretics:* If the patient has normal or near-normal kidney function, furosemide (Lasix) can promote renal excretion of magnesium.
2. *Moderate to Severe Hypermagnesemia (symptomatic, >4 mEq/L):*
    - *Calcium gluconate:* Administer 1–2 g of calcium gluconate intravenously to counteract the neuromuscular and cardiovascular effects of hypermagnesemia (especially if there are ECG changes or muscle weakness).
    - *Dialysis:* For patients with renal failure or life-threatening hypermagnesemia (magnesium >6 mEq/L), hemodialysis is the most effective method to remove magnesium.
    - *Mechanical ventilation:* If there is respiratory muscle paralysis, mechanical ventilation may be required.

3. *Ongoing monitoring:*
   - *Serum magnesium* levels should be monitored closely, especially if the patient is receiving treatment with dialysis or calcium.
   - *ECG monitoring* for cardiac arrhythmias, especially if magnesium levels remain elevated or if the patient is symptomatic.

## SUMMARY AND KEY POINTS

- *Signs and Symptoms:* Neuromuscular symptoms (hyporeflexia, weakness), cardiovascular issues (hypotension, bradycardia, arrhythmias), and severe cases can lead to respiratory depression and cardiac arrest.
- *Diagnosis:* Elevated serum magnesium levels >2.5 mEq/L with supporting history and examination.
- *Management:* Discontinuation of magnesium intake, hydration, diuretics, calcium gluconate for symptomatic relief, and dialysis for severe cases.

## SUGGESTED READING


1. Alfrey AC. Dialysis and magnesium. Kidney Intern. 1987;32(6):912-9.
2. Cundy T, Dissanayake A. Severe hypermagnesemia due to laxative use. Lancet. 2008;371(9627):1596-7.
3. Kopple JD. Magnesium Homeostasis and Hypermagnesemia. Clin J Am Soc Nephrol. 2017;12(6):1015-20.
4. Perazella MA, Moe SM. Hypermagnesemia: a clinical perspective. Am J Kidney Dis. 2013;62(3):622-30.
5. Rasmussen HS, McNair P. Magnesium metabolism in chronic renal failure. Magnesium. 1986;5(3-4):216-27.
6. Whang R, Ryder KW, Dyckner T. Magnesium and potassium interactions in cardiac arrhythmias. Magnesium Res. 1990; 7(4):373-81.

CHAPTER

# 94 Hyperammonemia

## DEFINITION

A condition characterized by elevated levels of ammonia in the blood, often leading to neurological impairment such as encephalopathy.

## METABOLISM

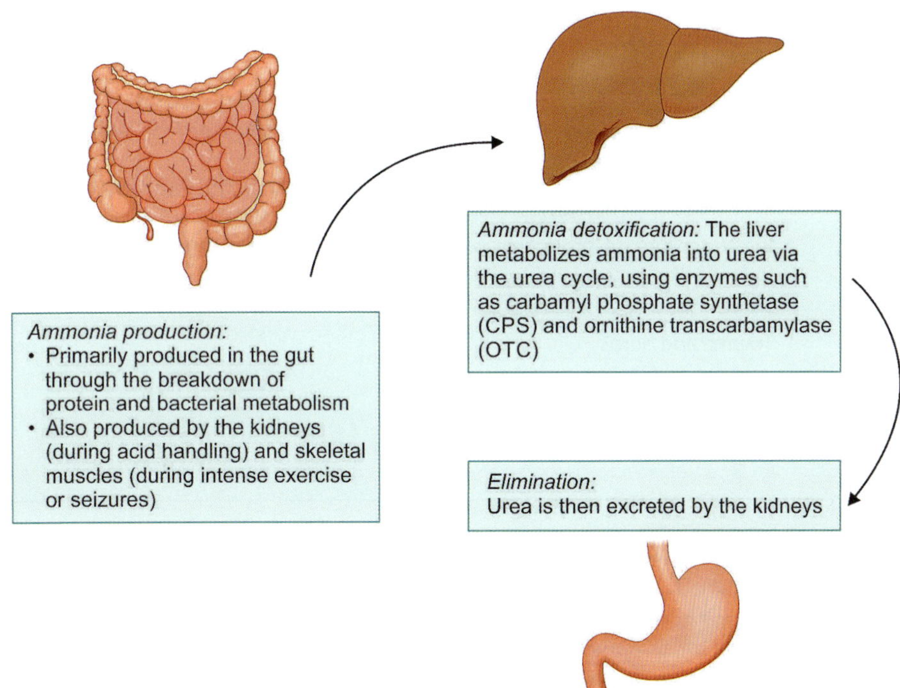

## PATHOPHYSIOLOGY OF HYPERAMMONEMIA

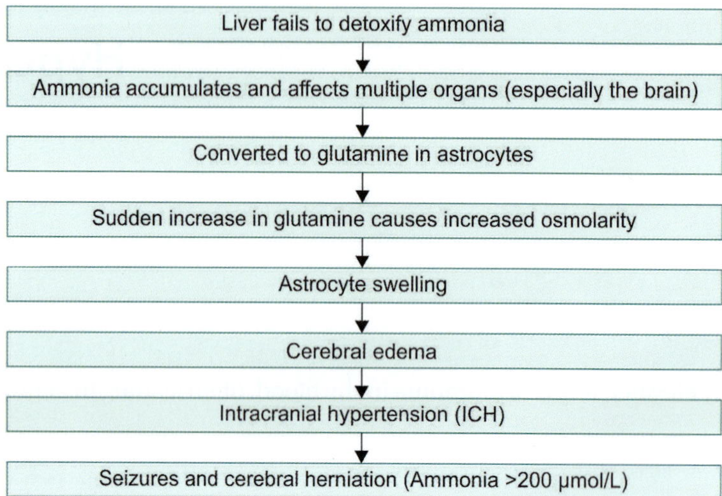


## CAUSES OF HYPERAMMONEMIA

| ***Liver failure*** | ***Increased ammonia production*** | ***Inborn errors of metabolism (IEMs)/Urea cycle disorders (UCDs)*** | ***Drugs*** |
|---|---|---|---|
| Acetaminophen overdose | Gastrointestinal (GI) bleeding | OTC deficiency | Valproate |
| Hepatitis A, E and other viruses | Total parenteral nutrition (TPN) | Citrullinemia | Glycine |
| Toxins- Amanita phalloides, Alcohol | Infections (urease-producing bacteria like Proteus and Klebsiella | Carbamyl phosphate synthetase deficiency | Salicylates |
| Autoimmune disease | Trauma and burns | | Chemotherapy agents |
| Vascular diseases, e.g., Budd–Chiari syndrome | | | |
| Metabolic disease—Wilson's disease, NASH | | | |

## DIAGNOSIS

| ***Laboratory tests*** | ***Imaging*** |
|---|---|
| *Ammonia levels:* Direct measurement is the key diagnostic tool | *Ultrasound or CT:* To assess liver damage or portal vein thrombosis |
| *Liver function tests:* To rule out or confirm hepatic causes | |
| *Serum amino acids, urine orotic acid:* Used to diagnose UCDs or other IEMs | |
| *Acetaminophen levels, viral serology:* To investigate drug-induced or viral hepatic failure | |

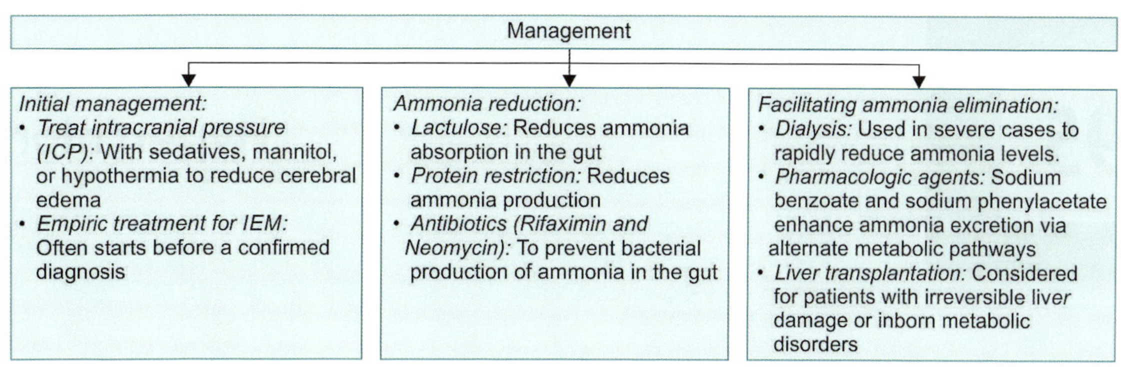


## SUGGESTED READING


1. Clay AS, Hainline BE. Hyperammonemia in the ICU. Chest. 2007;132:1368-78.
2. Machado, MC, Pinheiro da Silva, F. Hyperammonemia due to urea cycle disorders: a potentially fatal condition in the intensive care setting. J Intensive Care. 2014;2(22).
3. Shah NJ, Royer A, John S. Acute Liver Failure. In: StatPearls [Internet]. Treasure Island (FL): StatPearls Publishing; 2024.

CHAPTER

# 95

# Hyperchloremia

## PHYSIOLOGY OF CHLORIDE

- Chloride is the second most abundant electrolyte in the extracellular fluid.[1]
- Molecular weight of 35.5 and contributes to 70 percent of the total extracellular anion content
- Distribution—predominant extracellular base[1]
- The chloride distribution in the three major body fluid compartments—plasma, interstitial fluid (ISF), and intracellular fluid
- Plasma, the chloride concentration is 104 mmol/L, and in the interstitial fluid, it is 117 mmol/L.[2]
- Normal serum chloride concentration is 97–107 mEQ/L, which may vary from lab to lab
- The chloride concentration of cerebrospinal fluid is higher than that of plasma because of the absence of organic anions.[2]

## CONDITIONS ASSOCIATED WITH HYPERCHLOREMIA[3]

| *Cause* | *Examples* | *Mechanism* |
|---|---|---|
| Chloride infusion and administration of chloride-rich fluids | Sodium 0.9% (normal saline), albumin, $NH_4Cl$ (ammonium chloride), arginine HCl, lysine HCl, total parenteral nutrition (TPN) | Direct increase in serum chloride due to chloride-rich infusions |
| Water loss (Excessive water loss or chloride retention) | Skin loss (sweating due to exercise, dehydration, fever), gastrointestinal loss (diarrhea), burns | Relative increase in chloride concentration due to water depletion |
| Renal conditions and increased tubular chloride reabsorption | Central diabetes insipidus, nephrogenic diabetes insipidus, osmotic diuresis, post-obstructive diuresis, intrinsic renal disease, diuretics | Enhanced chloride reabsorption or loss of water relative to chloride |

*Contd...*

*Contd...*

## REGULATION OF CHLORIDE

Chloride is mainly regulated by the kidneys, which filter large amounts daily, reabsorbing over 99%. In the *proximal convoluted tubule (PCT)*, more than 60% of chloride is reabsorbed, mostly passively, due to a rising concentration gradient. The *loop of Henle* reabsorbs chloride via the NKCC2 co-transporter, with chloride exiting through basolateral channels. In the *distal convoluted tubule (DCT)*, chloride reabsorption is influenced by sodium movement through ENaC channels.[4]

Chloride plays a role in *acid-base balance,* influencing the anion gap. *Hyperchloremic metabolic acidosis* occurs when bicarbonate is replaced by chloride, maintaining a normal anion gap. Chloride depletion can also lead to *metabolic alkalosis.*

In the *gastrointestinal tract*, chloride secretion creates an osmotic gradient that drives water movement into the intestines, regulated by CFTR, CaCC.

| Aspect | Details |
|---|---|
| Kidney regulation of chloride | The kidneys filter large amounts of chloride daily, reabsorbing over 99%. |
| Proximal convoluted tubule (PCT) | Over 60% of chloride is reabsorbed, mostly passively, due to a rising concentration gradient |
| Loop of henle | Chloride is reabsorbed via the NKCC2 co-transporter and exits through basolateral channels |
| Distal convoluted tubule (DCT) | Chloride reabsorption is influenced by sodium movement through ENaC channels |
| Role in Acid-base balance | Chloride affects the anion gap and acid-base balance. Hyperchloremic metabolic acidosis occurs when bicarbonate is replaced by chloride, maintaining a normal anion gap. Chloride depletion can lead to metabolic alkalosis |
| Gastrointestinal tract function | Chloride secretion in the GI tract creates an osmotic gradient for water movement, regulated by CFTR, CaCC, and ClC-2 channels |

## APPROACH TO PATIENTS WITH HYPERCHLOREMIA

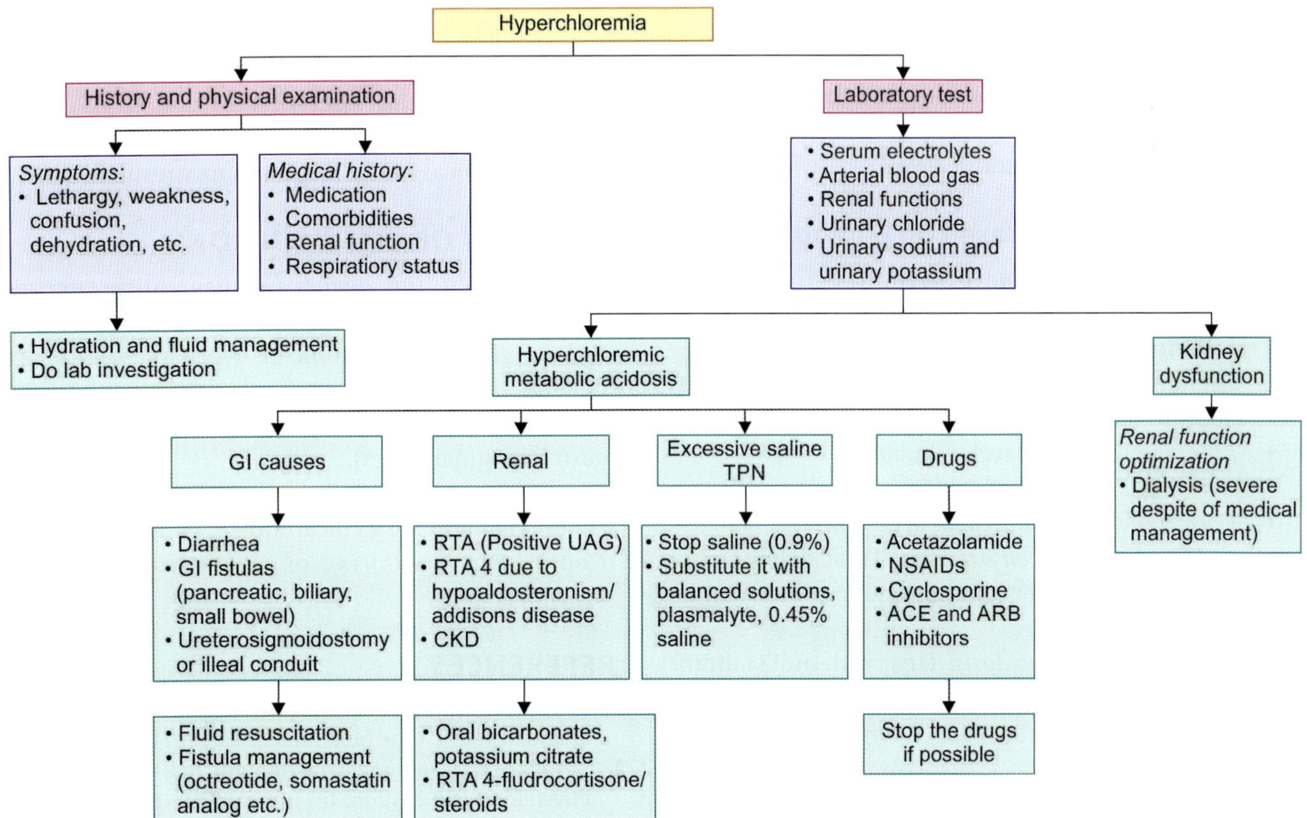


### Initial Assessment

- *History and physical examination*
  - Assess for symptoms (e.g., lethargy, weakness, confusion, hyperventilation, dehydration).
  - Review medical history (medications, comorbidities, renal function, and respiratory status).
- *Laboratory tests*
  - Serum chloride levels.
  - Serum sodium levels (to assess hypernatremia or hyponatremia).
  - Arterial blood gas (ABG) to check for metabolic acidosis or alkalosis.
  - Serum bicarbonate ($HCO_3^-$) levels.

- Renal function tests (BUN, creatinine).
- Urinary sodium potassium and chloride concentration.
- Urinary anion gap (UAG) = (Urine $Na^+$ + Urine $K^+$) – Urine $Cl^-$
- Positive UAG >0 suggest RTA while negative UAG suggest GI cause

## Identify the Underlying Cause

- *Hyperchloremic metabolic acidosis*
  - *Common causes:* Diarrhea, renal tubular acidosis (RTA), overuse of saline fluids (0.9% NaCl), acetazolamide, or gastrointestinal fistulas.
- *Kidney dysfunction*
  - Check for renal insufficiency or failure, acute kidney injury, or chronic kidney disease.
- *Medications*
  - Review the use of saline infusions, corticosteroids, carbonic anhydrase inhibitors, or other medications that may increase chloride levels.

## Treatment Approach Based on Etiology

- *If due to excessive IV saline (0.9% NaCl)*
  - *Action:* Stop or reduce saline administration.
  - *Substitute fluids* with a balanced solution (e.g., Lactated Ringer's, Plasmalyte) or 0.45% NaCl if appropriate.
  - *Monitor* electrolyte levels regularly.
- *If associated with metabolic acidosis*
  - *Correct the underlying cause of acidosis:*
    - *Diarrhea-induced acidosis:* Treat diarrhea by providing oral rehydration solutions or IV fluids with bicarbonate.
    - *Renal tubular acidosis:* Treat with oral sodium bicarbonate or potassium citrate.
    - *RTA 4:* Fludrocortisone (steroids—minerelo-corticoids)
    - *High output fistula:* Treat underlying cause (octreotide, somatostatin analog)
  - *Monitor and adjust* bicarbonate levels as needed.
- *If associated with kidney dysfunction*
  - *Acute or chronic renal failure:*
    - Optimize renal function and treat underlying renal disease.
    - *Consider dialysis* if severe hyperchloremia or acidosis persists despite other treatments.
  - *Monitor* renal function and manage fluid and electrolyte balance carefully.

## Symptomatic Treatment

- *Hydration and fluid management*
  - Ensure adequate hydration to support renal clearance of chloride.
- *Monitor ABG and electrolytes*
  - Check for improvements in chloride, sodium, bicarbonate, and pH levels.
  - Adjust fluid or bicarbonate therapy based on lab values.

## Monitor and Follow-up

- Regularly check serum electrolytes, ABG, renal function, and clinical symptoms.
- Adjust treatment based on ongoing evaluation of the patient's clinical status and laboratory results.

# SUMMARY OF INTERVENTIONS

- *Stop contributing agents* (excess saline, certain medications).
- *Balance fluids:* Use isotonic or hypotonic solutions if needed.
- *Treat underlying conditions* (e.g., acidosis, renal issues, gastrointestinal losses).
- *Correct electrolyte imbalances* with appropriate supplementation (e.g., bicarbonate, potassium).
- *Continuous monitoring* of electrolytes and renal function.

# REFERENCES


1. Koch SM, Taylor RW. "Chloride ion in intensive care medicine.," Crit. Care Med., 1992;20(2):227-40.
2. Schultz SG. The internal environment. In Essential Medical Physiology, 3rd edition. In: Johnson LR, Byrne JH (Eds). San Diego: Academic Press; 2003. pp. 4-6.
3. Berend K, Van Hulsteijn LH, Gans ROB. Chloride: The queen of electrolytes? Eur J Intern Med. 2012;23(3): 203-11.
4. Yunos NM, Bellomo R, Story D, Kellum J. Bench-to-bedside review: Chloride in critical illness. Crit Care. 2010;14(4):1-10.

CHAPTER

# 96 Hypothermia

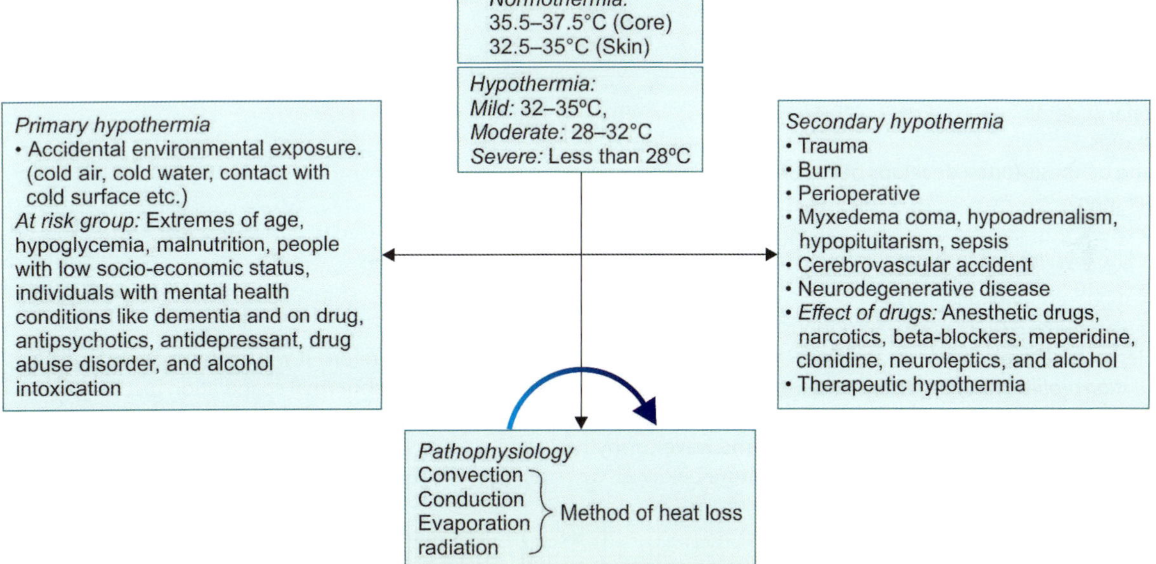


- Method of heat preservation by vasoconstriction and shivering is overwhelmed by cold
- Decreased depolarization of cardiac pacemaker cells, causing bradycardia. It is resistant to atropine as it is not vagal-mediated
- Mean arterial pressure and cardiac output decrease
- Atrial and ventricular arrhythmias. Below 28ºC, the chance of ventricular fibrillation increases
- Progressive decrease in CNS function linearly with hypothermia. At 19ºC-20ºC, EEG mimics brain death
- Decrease in metabolic rate at lower temperatures, a greater hemoglobin affinity for oxygen coupled with impaired oxygen extraction of hypothermic tissues
- Decrease in ADH secretion as a result of renal cell dysfunction can lead to diuresis and loss of fluid to interstitium leading to hypovolemia, masked by vasoconstriction, will lead to circulatory collapse, and shock during rewarming phase due to vasodilatation

**Diagnose and assess for signs, symptoms, and complications.**

*Diagnose hypothermia:* Measure core temperatures using a low-reading esophageal (unconscious with protected airway) in lower third of esophagus, rectal, or bladder thermometer.

Look for signs and symptoms of hypothermia
- Intense shivering occurs → ceases below about 30°C → body temperature drops more precipitously.
- *CNS:* Assess with GCS scoring. Lethargy and clumsiness followed by confusion, irritability, sometimes hallucinations → coma
- *Pupils:* Unreactive
- *Reflexes:* Hyporeflexia
- *Chest:* Pulmonary congestion, later bradypnea
- *Renal:* diuresis → oliguria
- *Cardiac:* Hypotension, bradycardia resistant to atropine or cardiac pacing, slow atrial fibrillation, the terminal rhythm is ventricular fibrillation or asystole

*Watch for complications:*
- Cardiac arrhythmias at temperatures below 30–32°C
- Infection
- Aspiration pneumonia
- Pulmonary edema
- Pancreatitis
- Bleeding diathesis (often develops below 34°C)
- Bladder atony
- Frostbite
- Electrolyte (hyperkalemia, hypoglycemia), hematocrit, coagulation study abnormalities

*Send investigations simultaneously:*
- *ABG:* If warmed to 37°C may reveal spuriously high $O_2$ and $CO_2$ and a lower pH
- *CBC:* Hematocrit levels may increase by 2% for each 1°C drop in core temperature therefore, it will be deceptively high
- *Coagulation profile:* This may not be evident on a kinetic test as it is done at 37°C. An abnormal coagulation test may reveal DIC hypofibrinogenemia
- *ECG:* Prolongation of PR, QRS, QT, J wave (Osborne wave), arrhythmia: more common with core temperature below 30°C, ventricular arrhythmia more with core temperature below 22°C

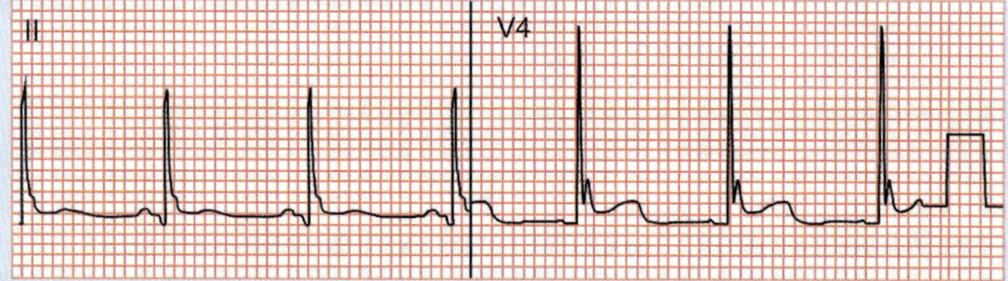


- *Serum electrolyte:* Hypokalemia (chronic hypothermia), hypomagnesemia. Or hyperkalemia due to cell lysis. Classic ECG changes of hyperkalemia may be absent or diminished. A value of more than 10 mmol/L is an indicator of poor prognosis.
- *Chest X-ray:* Pulmonary edema
- *Fingerstick glucose:* Acute hypothermia: hyperglycemia; chronic: hypoglycemia
- *BUN, creatinine:* Renal failure ensues with moderate to severe hypothermia
- *Diagnosis of the underlying cause:* Thyroid function test, serum cortisol, other injuries in case of trauma, serum lactate, creatinine kinase, troponin, toxicology screen

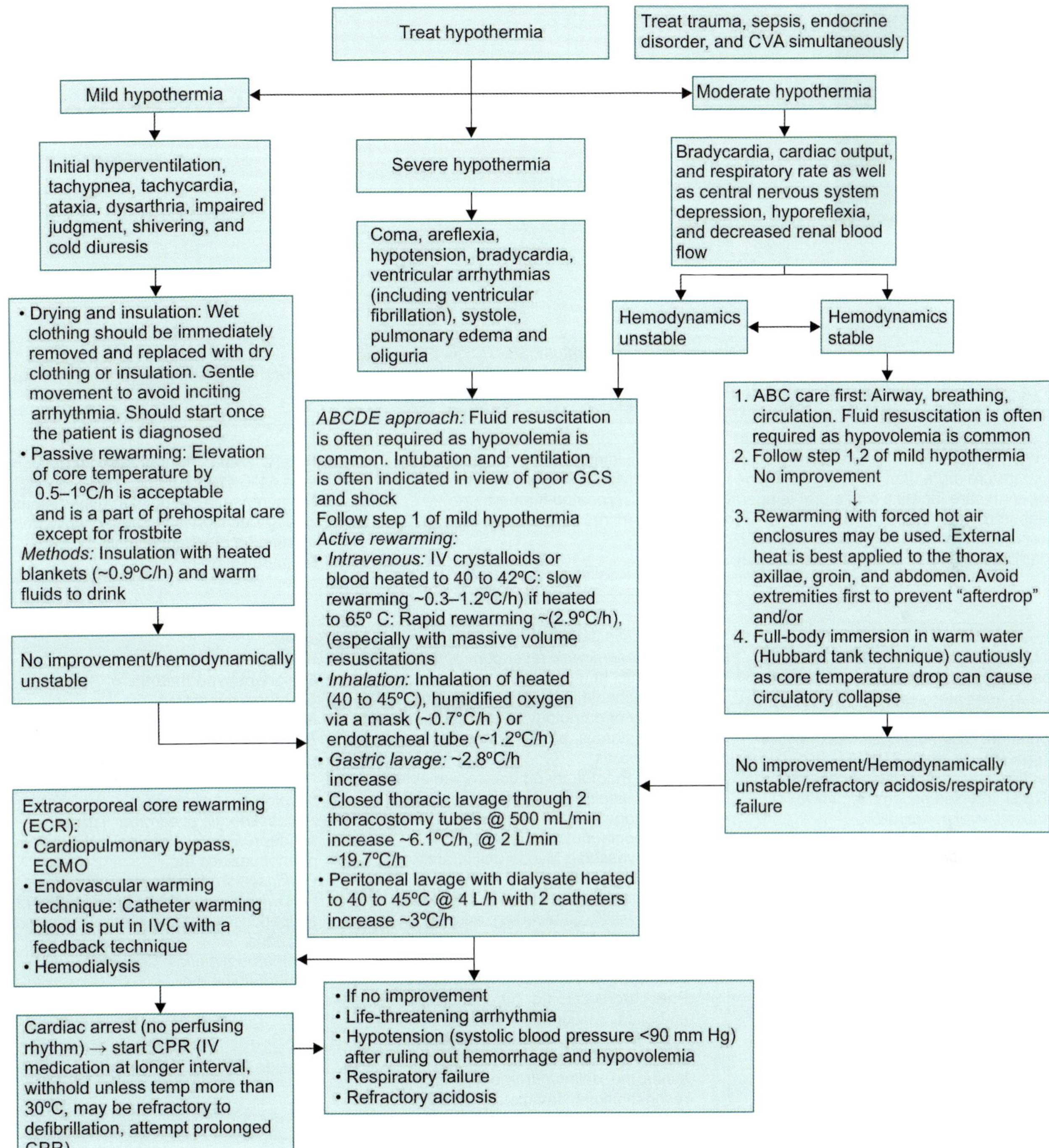


## SUGGESTED READING

1. Crit Care. Pharmacodynamics in hypothermia. 2012 Jun 7;16(Suppl 2):A6. doi: 10.1186/cc11264.
2. Internet Book Of Critical Care. Hypothermia.October 1, 2021 by Josh Farkas.
3. Temperature management in critically ill patients. Matthew Faulds, BMedSci (Hons) MBChB FRCA, Tim Meekings, BMedSci (Hons) MBChB MRCP FRCA DICM FFICM; Continuing Education in Anaesthesia Critical Care & Pain, Volume 13, Issue 3, June 2013, Pages 75–9, https://doi.org/10.1093/bjaceaccp/mks063.Published:18 January 2013.

CHAPTER 97

# Hyperthermia

*Normal body temperature:* 36–37.5°C (96.8–99.5°F)
*Diurnal variation:* (0.5°C –1°C (0.9–1.8°F) (body temperature typically decreases in early morning and increases in afternoon/evening and also during menstrual period)

- *Fever:* Temperature increase more than 38.3°C (101°F), immunocompromized patient temperature more than 38°C (100.4°F) for 1 hour. In individuals >65 years old residing in long-term care facilities single oral temperature >37.8°C, repeated temperature measurements >37.2°C (oral) or >37.5°C (rectal), or an increase from baseline >1.1°C
- Increase in thermoregulatory set point of hypothalamus
- Adaptive response remains intact. Antipyretics work

*Infective causes:*
- *CNS:* Meningitis, encephalitis, cerebral abscess, neurosurgical shunt infection
- *Chest:* Ventilator-associated pneumonia, lung abscess, other causes of pneumonia
- *Abdomen: Clostridium difficile,* infective diarrhea
- *Cardiovascular:* Infective endocarditis, CRBSI, infected pacemaker, valve abscess, viral pericarditis
- *Renal:* Pyelonephritis
- *Bone and joint infection:* Septic arthritis, osteomyelitis, abscess etc.

Common drugs causing fever carbamazepine, phenytoin, phenobarbitone; Minocycline, beta lactams, sulfonamides, nitrofurantoin; Allopurinol; Heparin; Amphotericin B; Bleomycin; Paraldehyde; Pentazocine; Routine vaccinations etc.

*Noninfective causes:*
- *CNS (neurogenic fever/central fever):* Ischemic, hemorrhagic stroke, subarachnoid hemorrhage, seizure, surgery or pathology involving the hypothalamus, anti-NMDA receptor encephalitis
- *Chest:* Pulmonary embolism, atelectasis, ARDS, aspiration pneumonitis, BOOP, bronchogenic carcinoma without pneumonia, pulmonary infarction
- *Cardiovascular:* Myocardial infarction, Dressler syndrome
- *Abdomen:* Ischemic bowel, acalculous cholecystitis, GI bleeding, acute pancreatitis
- *Miscellaneous, drugs:* Decubitus ulcer, gout, drug fever, SLE, Thyroid storm, Pheochromocytoma, Adrenal crisis, Fat embolism, Malignancy, Stevens-Johnson syndrome, HLH, transfusion reaction, alcohol, BZD, opiate withdrawal syndrome, delirium tremens, immune reconstitution inflammatory syndrome, transplant rejection, tumor lysis etc.

- *Hyperthermia:* Temperature increase more than 41°C (105.8°F)
- No increase in set point in hypothalamus. Heat production is increased while heat dissipation mechanism fails
- Antipyretics do not work

*Causes:*
- Heat stroke
- Malignant hyperthermia
- Serotonin syndrome
- Neuroleptic malignant syndrome
- *Endocrine:* Thyrotoxicosis (most common) pheochromocytoma, and adrenal crisis
- *Propofol infusion syndrome:* 30% can develop hyperthermia
- *Anticholinergic syndrome:* Tricyclic antidepressants, atropine, antihistamines, phenothiazines etc.
- *Parkinsonism hyperpyrexia syndrome:* Following the reduction or cessation of antiparkinsonian drug therapy, especially levodopa
- *Sympathomimetics:* Cocaine, amphetamine etc.

## PATHOPHYSIOLOGY OF HYPERTHERMIA/FEVER

*Exogenous stimuli* → production of IL1,IL6,TNF Alpha → acts on Organum vasculosum of Lamina Terminalis → production of PGE2 → increase in cAMP → reset of hypothalamus thermoregulatory set point → fever → dehydration, nausea, vomiting, hypotension,tachycardia,acidosis

*Heat stroke* → rhabdomyolysis → disseminated intravascular coagulation, renal and liver failure, hypoglycemia, lactic acidosis, and hyperkalemia (common feature of hyperthermia)

*Malignant hyperthermia* → inherited mutations in the ryanodine receptor → inhalational anesthetics or depolarizing paralytic medications → large influx of calcium → depletion of ATP → myocyte injury → muscle rigidity, hyperthermia, and acidosis → acute kidney injury, DIC

*Neuroleptic malignant syndrome* → centrally-acting dopamine antagonists (typical antipsychotics such as haloperidol and fluphenazine, antinauseant medications such as metoclopramide → blockade of heat loss pathways in the hypothalamus and the heat production from the muscle rigidity (*insidious onset*) (intracellular calcium influx similar to MH) → hyperthermia, and mental status changes

*Serotonin syndrome* → supra-therapeutic serotonin levels in the synapses of the brain (SSRIs, monoamine oxidase inhibitors (MAOIs), TCAs, venlafaxine, trazodone, tramadol, linezolid, MDMA, etc. common culprits) → rapid onset of hyperthermia, autonomic instability (tachycardia, mydriasis, and diaphoresis), cognitive (agitation, confusion, hallucinations, coma), and neuromuscular changes (tremor, hyperreflexia, and clonus)

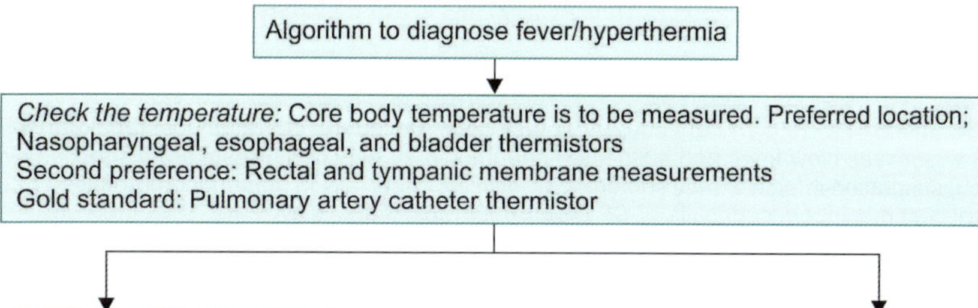


*History :*

*Typical history of hyperthermia syndrome:*
- Exposure of older, chronically ill and debilitated individuals to heat waves
- Exposure to inhalational, depolarizing agents with often positive family history of hyperthermia
- Exposure to offending drugs that increases Serotonin, Catecholamines, Acetyl-choline etc.

*Presence of factors for nosocomial infection:*
- Invasive lines
- Broad spectrum antibiotic use with diarrhea
- Presence of ET, TT with risk of VAP, nasopharyngeal tube with risk of sinusitis
- Presence of implants, implantable devices like AICD, PPI, EVD, shunt, prosthetic valves etc.
- Prolonged urinary catheterization with no other source of infection
- Prolonged bedridden state, decubitus ulcer
- Extracorporeal organ support system

Positive history of noninfective diseases that cause inflammation, drugs

History suggestive of systemic infection, chills and rigors strongly suggestive of bacteremia

*Clinical examination:* Watch for....
- *CNS:* Neck rigidity, kernig, brudzinski sign (meningism), pupillary signs, GCS, mini mental status examination score, motor, sensory, cranial nerve examination
- *Chest and ENT:* S/o sinusitis, ear discharge, added sounds in chest auscultation, increased vocal fremitus, resonance, reduced breath sound, pleural rub
- *Cardiac:* New onset murmurs, arrhythmia, pericardial rub Abdomen: S/o peritonitis, renal angle tenderness, right hypochondrial tenderness, tenderness at Mc Burney point, suprapubic tenderness
- *Skin:* The presence of rashes, thrombophlebitis, cellulitis, vasculitis, necrotizing fasciitis, skin mottling, meningococcal purpura, variation in acral skin temperature, the typical skin manifestation of infective endocarditis, erythema nodosum, ecthyma gangrenosum, erythema multiforme, purpura fulminans, etc.
- *Joints and muscles:* Gas gangrene, warm, swollen, and painful joint, s/o rheumatoid arthritis, gout.
- *Eye:* Endophthalmitis common in fungal, gram-positive bacterial sepsis, CMV retinitis. Choroid tubercle in tuberculosis, retinal hemorrhage in hypertensive urgency with CVA, s/o hypertensive, diabetic retinal disease

Simultaneously do investigations as relevant and interpret with history and symptoms/signs

↓

**Routine investigations**

- *CBC:* Polymorphonuclear leukocytosis, thrombocytopenia, neutropenia s/o infection
- *Coagulation profile:* Deranged INR, hypofibrinogenemia may suggest DIC, Gi hemorrhage in chronic liver disease
- *Renal function test:* Uremia, AKI, serum electrolyte abnormality (hyperkalemia in hyperthermia syndrome)
- *Liver function test:* Cholestasis, increased liver enzymes may suggest drug induced liver injury, hyperbilirubinemia may suggest hemolysis besides indicative of acute/chronic liver failure
- *Arterial blood gas:* Hypoxemia, hypercarbia may point towards acute/chronic respiratory failure in the patient's history s/o respiratory, cardiac etiology. Metabolic acidosis is common in hyperthermia as well as s/o renal failure, metabolic causes like Diabetic keto acidosis, drug abuse. A lactate level of >2 mmol/liter is indicative of septic shock.
- X-ray: CXR in patients with suspected respiratory cause of fever, to differentiate tracheobronchitis from fever, abdominal X-ray for suspected intestinal perforation, obstruction

**Specific investigations**

*Blood culture:*

- Patent with central line catheter in situ and with no other obvious source simultaneous culture from blood and at least 2 lumens of CVC (Avoid drawing blood from needleless connector to avid contamination) is to be sent and ask for differential time to positivity
- Patient clinically unstable with new onset sepsis and septic shock
- In patients with high risk of bacteremia including infective endocarditis/endovascular infection, catheter-associated bloodstream infection, vertebral discitis/osteomyelitis, epidural abscess, meningitis, native joint septic arthritis and intermediate risk including acute pyelonephritis severe CAP, VAP, cholangitis, severe cellulitis or cellulitis in patients with comorbidities, rigor
- Blood culture is to be collected preferably by peripheral venipuncture at the same time from 2 anatomical sites.
  - *Rapid molecular testing of blood including NAAT:* For new fever of unknown origin concomitantly with blood culture
  - *Urine culture:*
    - Febrile ICU patients with pyuria (defined as 5–10 WBC/hpf) and in whom urinary tract infection (UTI) from newly placed catheter
    - Patient lacks a Foley catheter and has symptoms of urinary tract infection
    - Neutropenic fever
    - Structural urologic abnormality (e.g., recent surgery or urological procedure, or status post renal transplant)
  - *BioFire (bacterial, viral)/Naat:* New fever and suspected pneumonia, or new upper respiratory infection symptoms (Respiratory panel), suspected infective gastroenteritis, *C. difficile,* especially in immunocompromised patients *(Stool panel),* suspected meningoencephalitis *(CSF BioFire)* for rapid diagnosis
  - *PCT, CRP:* Fever and no clear focus of infection with low to intermediate clinical probability of bacterial infection to stop antibiotics, for discontinuation of antibiotics by serial measurement along with clinical judgement
  - *CPK total:* For hyperthermia syndrome.
  - *Thyroid function test, cortisol:* To diagnose endocrine causes
  - *USG scan:* Patients with abdominal, chest symptoms, signs with abnormal liver function test
  - *CT scan:* Post abdominal, thoracic, pelvic surgery patients with fever, immunocompromised patient with abnormal radiograph, sonography findings. To diagnose noninfective etiologies. To diagnose retroperitoneal pathology, abscess, ischemic bowel (with help of contrast study), source of GI bleeding, hemoptysis with help of angiography
  - *Endoscopic study:* To diagnose certain infectious and non-infectious pulmonary, GI etiologies. Important for immunocompromised patient to diagnose uncommon infection
  - *PET-CT:* Fever in ICU patient where cause is not established after all other diagnostic test

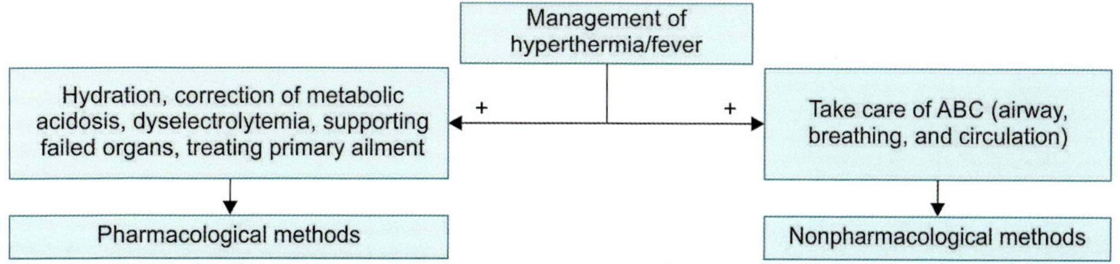


- *Antipyretics:* For neurologic injury (e.g., stroke, anoxic brain injury, TBI), severe fever (e.g., >40°C/104°F), altered mental status (delirium in some at-risk patients), hemodynamic instability or acute myocardial ischemia. Acetaminophen is preferred over NSAIDs
- *Medication for non-infective neurogenic fever:* Bromocriptine, baclofen, chlorpromazine, propranolol, morphine, NSAIDS, e.g.: Indomethacin, ibuprofen, diclofenac in patients with low risk of kidney injury.
- *Drugs for controlling shivering:* IV magnesium repletion, dexmedetomidine, propofol, pain dose ketamine, ondansetron, opiates, e.g., fentanyl is preferred
- *Empirical antibiotics:* After sending appropriate cultures depending on the suspected source of infection. The choice of antibiotic should be individualized according to source, local antibiogram, community/hospital-acquired, patient's immunity status, and previous history of antibiotic use Antibiotics should be deescalated according to culture/sensitivity record or stopped if fever is diagnosed as noninfective. Biomarkers help to discontinue antibiotics
- *Drugs for hyperthermia syndrome:* Withdrawal of offending agent first line of treatment
  For alleviating symptoms, reverse pathophysiology....
- *Heat stroke:* Dantrolene, corticosteroids;
  - *NMS:* dopamine agonists such as bromocriptine and amantadine, in severe cases, dantrolene, refractory cases ECT;
  - *MH:* IV Dantrolene;
  - *Serotonin syndrome:* Diazepam for mild hypertension, tachycardia, cyproheptadine, a 5HT-2A receptor antagonist might help

*External cooling:* Reduce body temperature by enhancing core body heat loss by evaporation and convection

*Methods:* Specialized cooling blankets, sponging and ice packs (application to groin, axillae, neck, and torso), spraying of cold water with use of fans to increase evaporation, wrapping in damp sheets or a combination of these therapies

*Internal cooling:*
- An intravenous infusion of 20 $cm^3$/kg of normal saline at a temperature of 4°C is typically infused over approximately 15 minutes, and leads to a drop in core temperature by approximately 1°C
- Bladder irrigation/gastric lavage with 40°C saline

*Complications:*
- Shivering-to be treated
- Overcorrection to hypothermia–increase chance of coagulopathy, arrythmia
- Skin damage from continuous application of cold ice pack, water-to be monitored and prevented
- Fluid overload with internal cooling method in patients with heart failure, CKD, poor cardiac reserve

## SUGGESTED READING


1. Central fever: a challenging clinical entity in neurocritical care. Keshav Goyal, MD, DM; Neha Garg, MD; Parmod Bithal, MD. J Neurocrit Care. 2020;13(1):19-31.
2. Drug-induced hyperthermia in critical care Edward Walter and Mike Carraretto. Journal of the Intensive Care Society 2015;16(4):306-11.
3. Pyrexia: aetiology in the ICU. Daniel J. Niven and Kevin B. Laupland. Niven and Laupland Critical Care. 2016;20:247.

# PART 8

# ENDOCRINE

***Editor:*** Jaicob Varghese

***Associate Editors:*** Biji Thomas Philip, Melwin George, Nilanjan Umesh, Meenakshy Vijayakumar

CHAPTER 98

# Diabetic Ketoacidosis Management Protocol

## INTRODUCTION

Diabetic ketoacidosis (DKA) is a serious complication of diabetes characterized by a triad of hyperglycemia, ketosis, and acidosis.

## DIAGNOSIS

- All of these three must be present
  1. **D:** Blood glucose >200 mg/dL
  2. **K:** Ketones > 3mmol/L or s ketonuria > 2+ or more
  3. **A:** Bicarbonate concentration <15 mmol/L or pH <7.3
- Anion gap is not included and is used to determine the severity of the disease
- Euglycemic ketoacidosis is a condition where sugar is normal and the treatment is same as hyperglycemic ketoacidosis

## GRADING/SEVERITY

| | *Mild DKA* | *Moderate DKA* | *Severe DKA* |
|---|---|---|---|
| Arterial pH | 7.25–7.3 | 7.0 to <7.24 | <7.0 |
| Serum bicarbonate (mmol/L) | 15–18 | 10 to <15 | <10 |
| Anion gap | >10 | >12 | >10 |
| Mental status | Alert | Alert/drowsy | Stupor/ coma |

## MANAGEMENT

### Immediate Management: 0–60 Minutes

- Obtain large bore intravenous access
- Start on 0.9% sodium chloride solution:
  - *Systolic BP (SBP) below 90 mm Hg:*
    - Most Likely to be due to low circulating volume due to osmotic diuresis, but need to rule out other causes such as heart failure, sepsis, cardiogenic shock, bleeding
    - Give 500 mL of 0.9% sodium chloride solution over 10–15 minutes up to 500–1,000 mL
    - Once SBP is >90 mm Hg, give 1 L 0.9% sodium chloride over the next 60 minutes.
  - *Systolic BP on admission 90 mm Hg and over:*
    - Give 1 L 0.9% sodium chloride over the first 60 minutes
    - Potassium correction is not given if K >5.5 and if K <5.5 need to start on IV correction of potassium
- Start IV insulin infusion at 0.1 units/kg/h (no bolus), 50 units of insulin made up to 50 mL with 0.9% NaCl (if patient normally takes long-acting insulin analog continue at usual dose and time)
- Assess the patient
- *Investigations to be send:* CBC, blood glucose, CXR, ECG, blood cultures, urine routine, S. electrolytes, VBG
- *Monitoring:*
  - Hourly blood glucose
  - Ketones daily
  - VBG/ABG q8h
  - S. electrolytes q8h (if not available in ABG)
  - Continuous cardiac, respiratory, and neurological monitoring in the ICU
- Identify and manage the precipitating cause as early as possible

### 60 Minutes–6 Hours

- *Aim of treatment:*
  - Bicarbonate rise of 3 mmol/L/h or glucose decrease of 3 mmol/L/h
  - Maintain serum K in normal range
  - Avoid hypoglycemia
- Reassess patient and monitor vital signs

- Investigations as described above
- Continue fluid replacement according to urine output, IVC assessment and tissue perfusion
- Add dextrose containing fluid if BG falls to <250 mg/dL, and reduce insulin infusion to 0.05 U/kg/h
- If target not achieved, increase insulin infusion by 1 U/h till target is achieved
- Start DVT prophylaxis

### 6–12 Hours

- Aim of treatment
  - Continue IV fluid replacement
  - Assess for biochemical and clinical improvement
  - Avoid hypoglycemia
  - Assess for complication like fluid overload and cerebral edema
  - Continue treatment of precipitating events
- Reassess and monitor vital signs
- Continue fluid replacement according to urine output, IVC assessment and tissue perfusion
- Add dextrose containing fluid if BG falls to <250 mg/dL, and reduce insulin infusion to 0.05 U/kg/h
- Resolution of DKA is defined as ketone < 0.3 mmol/L or pH >7.3 ( bicarbonate is not used)
- DKA not resolved review insulin infusion dose and look for treating precipitating event.

### 12–24 Hours

- By 24 hours the ketonemia and acidosis should have resolved.
- *Aim of treatment:*
  - Ensure that clinical and biochemical parameters are improved or are normal
  - Continue IV fluid replacement if not eating and drinking
  - Reassess for complications of treatment, e.g., fluid overload, cerebral edema
  - Continue to treat precipitating factors
  - Transfer to subcutaneous insulin if the person is eating and drinking normally and biochemistry is normal
  - Do not discontinue intravenous insulin infusion until 30 minutes after subcutaneous short acting insulin has been given

## BRIDGING TO S/C INSULIN

- Therapeutic daily dose of insulin is calculated by multiplying the individual's weight (in kg) by 0.5–0.75 U.
- 50% of the amount is given as long-acting insulin (glargine), and other 50% is divided into 3 and given before each meal as rapidly acting insulin.

## ALGORITHM

- Blood sugar >200 mg/day
- Ketones >3 mmol/L or significant ketonuria
- Bicarbonate concentration <15 mmol/L or pH < 7.3

↓

- IV access
- Fluid resuscitation with 0.9% saline
- CBC, blood glucose, CXR, ECG, blood cultures, urine routine, *S. electrolytes,* VBG
- Potassium <5.5, start potassium correction 40 mEq and adjust according to repeat K values
- Insulin infusion at 0.1 U/kg/h
- Look for precipitating cause

↓

- Reassess
- Fluid resuscitation according to fluid status
- If sugars <250 mg/dL, add dextrose containing fluid, and decrease insulin to 0.05 U/kg/h
- Maintain normal potassium level
- If sugar level decrease <50 mg/dL/h increase dose of by 1 U/h

↓

- Reassess
- If ketone <0.3 mmol/L or pH >7.3, resolution of DKA
- Maintain normoglycemia
- Change to S/C insulin
- Do not stop insulin infusion until 30 minutes after S/C insulin

## SUGGESTED READING


1. Dhatariya KK; Joint British Diabetes Society for inpatient care. The Management of Diabetic Ketoacidosis in Adults-An updated guideline from the Joint British Diabetes Society for Inpatient Care. Diabet Med. 2022;39(6): e14788.
2. Kitabchi AE, Umpierrez GE, Miles JM, Fisher JN. Hyperglycemic crises in adult patients with diabetes. Diabetes Care. 2009;32:1335-43.
3. Sampson M, Jones C. Joint British Diabetes Societies for Inpatient Care: clinical guidelines and improving inpatient diabetes care. Diabetic Med. 2018;35:988-91.

CHAPTER 99

# Hyperglycemic Hyperosmolar Nonketotic Syndrome

**BOX 1:** Characteristic features.

- Severe hyperglycemia (600–1,200 mg/dL)
- Absence of significant metabolic acidosis or ketones
- Commonly observed in elderly noninsulin-dependent diabetes mellitus
- Severe dehydration (usually 6–9 L)
- Confusion and lethargy
- Cerebral edema is a rare but fatal complication

**Flowchart 1:** Management of HONK.

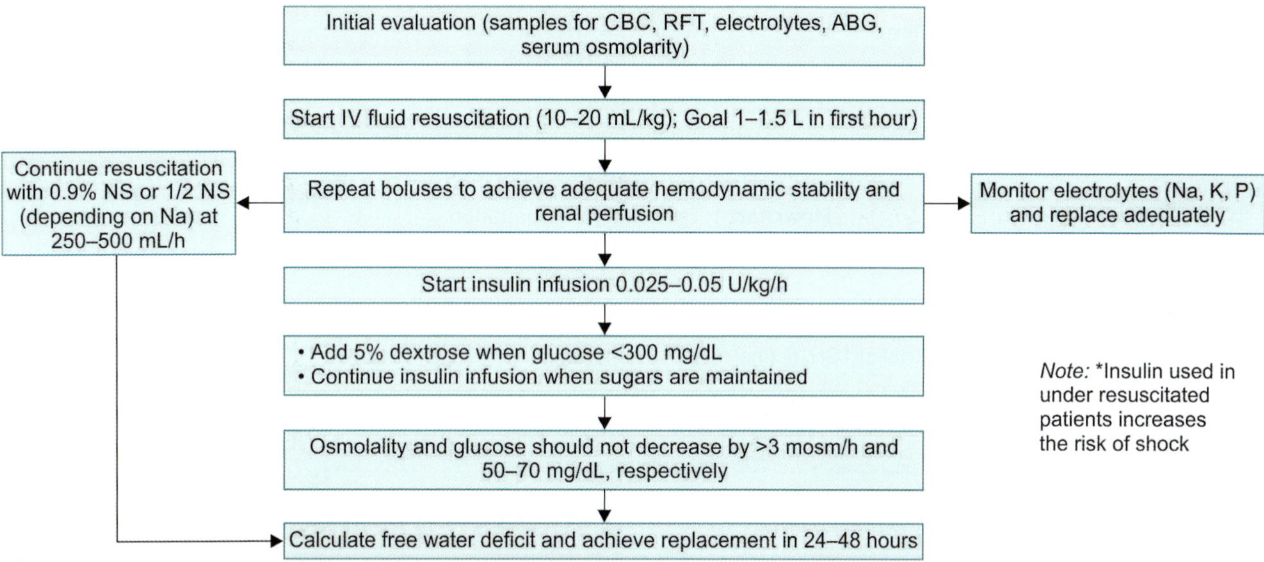


**BOX 2:** Management of cerebral edema in hyperosmolar hyperglycemic state.

- Initiate treatment as soon as cerebral edema is suspected
- Intubate for airway protection and impending respiratory failure
- Avoid hyperventilation, $pCO_2$ <22 mm Hg
- Give mannitol 0.6–1 g/kg IV over 20 minutes and repeat after 1/2 h if necessary
- Reduce the rate of fluid administration by one-third
- Hypertonic saline 5–10 mL/kg over 30 minutes, as an alternative or if no response to mannitol
- Head end elevation
- Imaging after initiation of measures to control cerebral edema

## SUGGESTED READING

1. Kitabchi AE, Guillermo EU, Miles JM, Fisher JN. Hyperglycemic crises in adult patients with diabetes. Diabetes Care. 2009;32:1335-43.
2. Kitabchi AE, Umpierrez GE, Fisher JN, Murphy MB, Stentz FB. Thirty years of personal experience in hyperglycemic crises: diabetic ketoacidosis and hyperglycemic hyperosmolar state. J Clin Endocrinol Metab. 2008;93(5):1541-52.
3. Nyenwe EA, Kitabchi AE. Evidence-based management of hyperglycemic emergencies in diabetes mellitus. Diabetes Res Clin Pract. 2011;94(3):340-51.

CHAPTER 100

# Myxedema Coma

## INTRODUCTION

Myxedema coma is an extreme form of hypothyroidism, which is rare and occurs typically in patients who develop a systemic illness superimposed on a previously undiagnosed or untreated hypothyroidism **(Boxes 1 and 2; Flowcharts 1 and 2)**.

**BOX 1:** Signs and symptoms.

- Comatose
- Hypothermia
- Bradycardia
- Hypoventilation
- Absent or sluggish deep tendon reflexes
- Non pitting pedal edema
- Hypotension
- Hyponatremia
- Pleural or pericardial effusion

**BOX 2:** Predisposing factors.

- Sepsis/infection
- Cerebrovascular disease
- Congestive cardiac failure
- Trauma
- Burns
- Medications (anesthetics, amiodarone, and narcotics)
- Metabolic disturbances (hypoglycemia, hyponatremia, hypercapnia, etc.)

**Flowchart 1:** Laboratory interpretation.

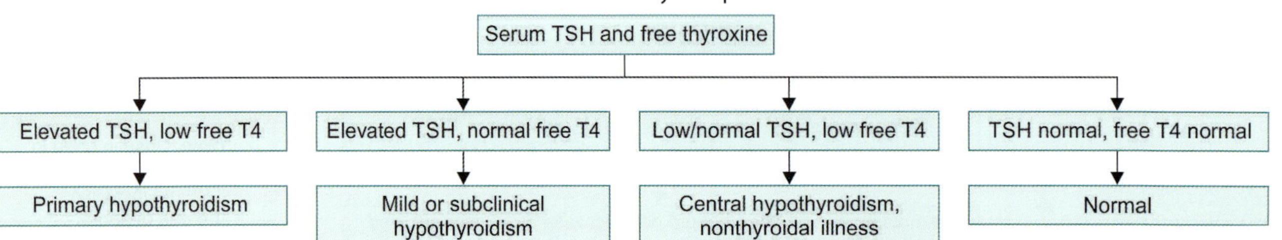


**Flowchart 2:** Treatment of myxedema coma.

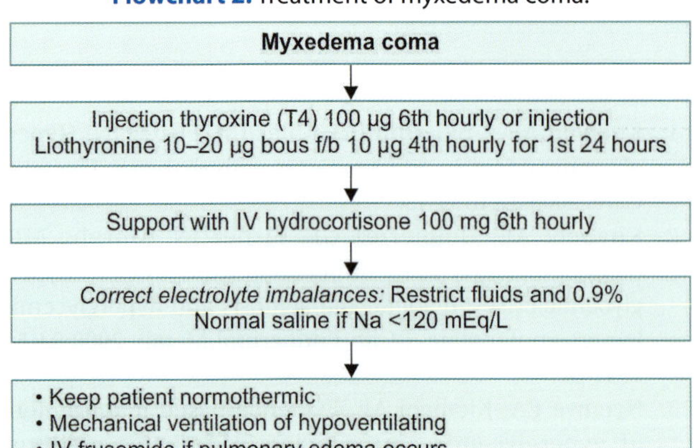


*Note:* Look for hypoadrenalism and panhypopituitarism

## SUGGESTED READING


1. De Sanctis V, Soliman A, Daar S, Di Maio S, Alhumaidi N, Alali M, et al. The Myxedema coma in children and adolescents: A rare endocrine emergency—Personal experience and review of literature. Acta Biomed. 2021;92(5):e2021481.
2. Eipe N, Murto K. Adrenal insufficiency and thyroid replacement therapy. Paediatr Anaesth. 2009;19:422-3.
3. Holvey DN, Goodner CJ, Nikoloff JT, Dowling JT. Treatment of myxedema coma with intravenous thyroxine. Arch Intern Med. 1964;113:139-46.
4. Klubo-Gwiezdzinska J, Wartofsky L. Thyroid emergencies. Med Clin North Am. 2012;96:385-403.

CHAPTER

# 101 Thyrotoxicosis

## INTRODUCTION

Thyrotoxicosis describes disorders of excess thyroid hormone with or without the increased synthesis of thyroid hormone (hyperthyroidism). It can result in a variety of symptoms, including tachycardia, unexplained weight loss, nervousness or anxiety, increased sweating, tremors, heat intolerance, and irregular menstrual cycles in women. The most common cause of thyrotoxicosis is hyperthyroidism, where the thyroid gland produces too much hormone. Other causes can include thyroiditis (inflammation of the thyroid), excessive intake of thyroid hormone supplements, and certain types of thyroid tumors

## CAUSES OF THYROTOXICOSIS

*Thyrotoxicosis associated with hyperthyroidism:*

- Graves' disease
- Toxic multinodular goiter
- Solitary toxic adenoma
- TSH secreting pituitary adenoma
- Neonatal Graves' disease
- Choriocarcinoma
- Hyperemesis gravidarum
- Struma ovarii
- Metastatic follicular thyroid carcinoma
- Iodine or iodine containing drugs

*Thyrotoxicosis is not associated with hyperthyroidism:*

- Painless thyroiditis
- Acute/subacute thyroiditis
- Exogenous thyroid hormone
- Drug induced thyroiditis
- Acute infectious thyroiditis
- Radiation-induced thyroiditis

## SYMPTOMS AND SIGNS OF THYROTOXICOSIS

| | ***Symptoms*** | ***Signs*** |
|---|---|---|
| Cardiovascular | Palpitations, shortness of breath | Tachycardia, hypertension, atrial arrythmia, high output cardiac failure |
| Gastrointestinal | Increased appetite | Weight loss |
| Central nervous system | Emotional lability, poor concentration, agitation | Hyperactivity, agitation |
| Eyes (Graves' disease) | Soreness, grittiness | Periorbital edema, lid retraction and lid lag, conjunctival injection, ophthalmoplegia |
| Thyroid | Neck swelling | Goiter |
| Muscles | Weakness | Tremor, muscle wasting |
| Skin | Sweating, heat intolerance | |
| Hair | Hair thinning, hair loss | |
| Peripheral nervous system | | Hyperreflexia |
| Reproductive system | | Oligomenorrhea. Reduced fertility (women) |

Evaluation of thyrotoxicosis: (1) Thyroid function test, (2) thyroid autoantibodies, and (3) imaging.

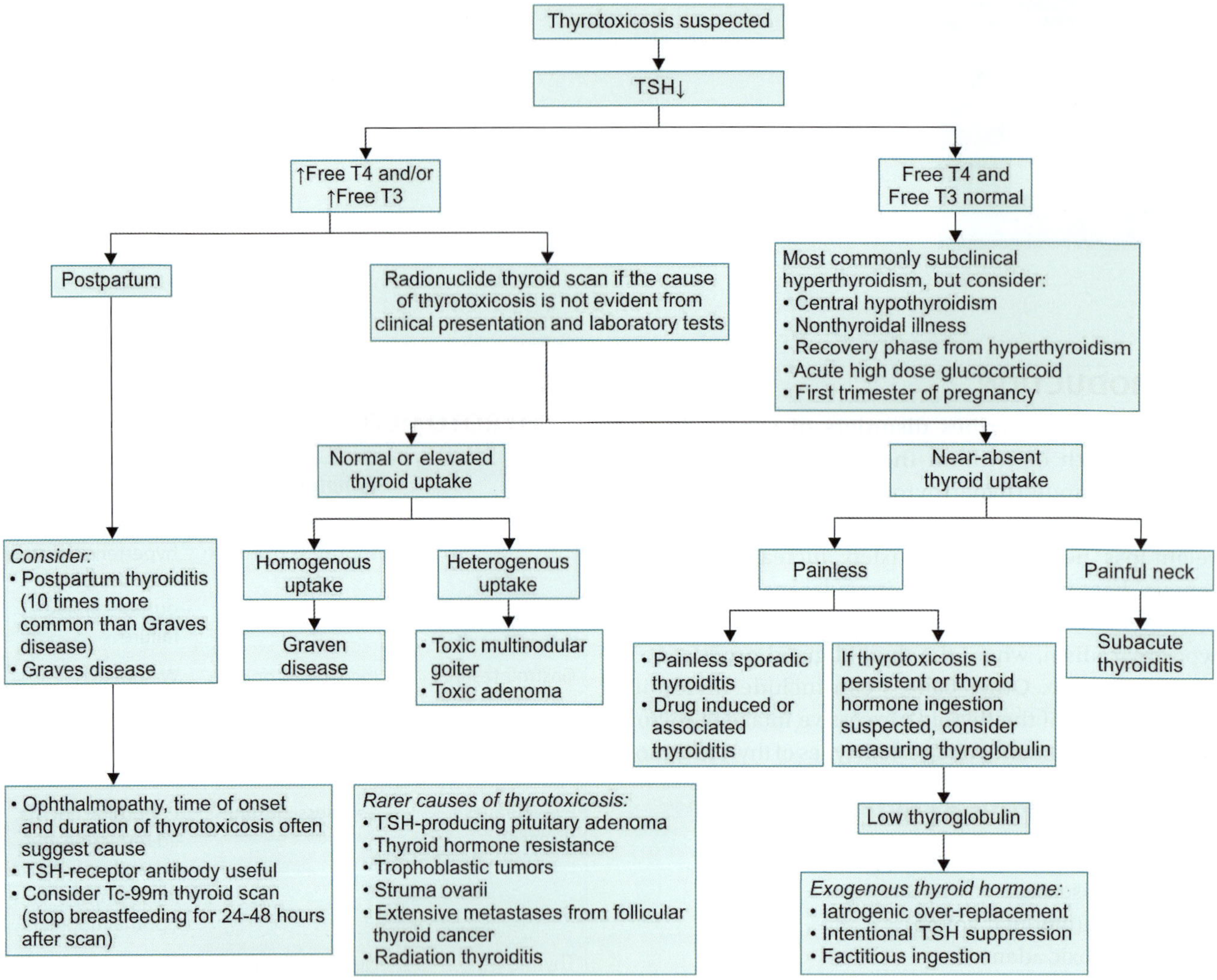

Thyrotoxicosis suspected
→ TSH↓

- ↑Free T4 and/or ↑Free T3
  - Postpartum
    - *Consider:*
      - Postpartum thyroiditis (10 times more common than Graves disease)
      - Graves disease
    - • Ophthalmopathy, time of onset and duration of thyrotoxicosis often suggest cause
      • TSH-receptor antibody useful
      • Consider Tc-99m thyroid scan (stop breastfeeding for 24-48 hours after scan)
  - Radionuclide thyroid scan if the cause of thyrotoxicosis is not evident from clinical presentation and laboratory tests
    - Normal or elevated thyroid uptake
      - Homogenous uptake → Graven disease
      - Heterogenous uptake → • Toxic multinodular goiter • Toxic adenoma
    - Near-absent thyroid uptake
      - Painless
        - • Painless sporadic thyroiditis • Drug induced or associated thyroiditis
        - If thyrotoxicosis is persistent or thyroid hormone ingestion suspected, consider measuring thyroglobulin → Low thyroglobulin → *Exogenous thyroid hormone:* • Iatrogenic over-replacement • Intentional TSH suppression • Factitious ingestion
      - Painful neck → Subacute thyroiditis
- Free T4 and Free T3 normal
  - Most commonly subclinical hyperthyroidism, but consider:
    - Central hypothyroidism
    - Nonthyroidal illness
    - Recovery phase from hyperthyroidism
    - Acute high dose glucocorticoid
    - First trimester of pregnancy

*Rarer causes of thyrotoxicosis:*
- TSH-producing pituitary adenoma
- Thyroid hormone resistance
- Trophoblastic tumors
- Struma ovarii
- Extensive metastases from follicular thyroid cancer
- Radiation thyroiditis

## MANAGEMENT OF THYROTOXICOSIS

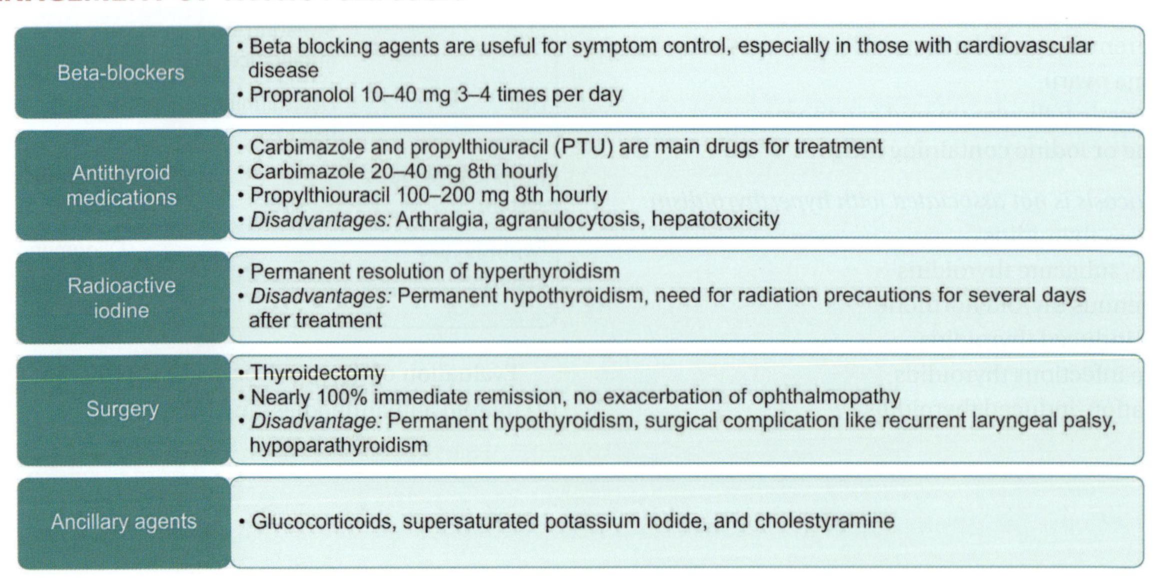

| | |
|---|---|
| Beta-blockers | • Beta blocking agents are useful for symptom control, especially in those with cardiovascular disease<br>• Propranolol 10–40 mg 3–4 times per day |
| Antithyroid medications | • Carbimazole and propylthiouracil (PTU) are main drugs for treatment<br>• Carbimazole 20–40 mg 8th hourly<br>• Propylthiouracil 100–200 mg 8th hourly<br>• *Disadvantages:* Arthralgia, agranulocytosis, hepatotoxicity |
| Radioactive iodine | • Permanent resolution of hyperthyroidism<br>• *Disadvantages:* Permanent hypothyroidism, need for radiation precautions for several days after treatment |
| Surgery | • Thyroidectomy<br>• Nearly 100% immediate remission, no exacerbation of ophthalmopathy<br>• *Disadvantage:* Permanent hypothyroidism, surgical complication like recurrent laryngeal palsy, hypoparathyroidism |
| Ancillary agents | • Glucocorticoids, supersaturated potassium iodide, and cholestyramine |

## BURCH-WARTOFSKY SCORE: DIAGNOSTIC CRITERIA FOR THYROID STORM

| ***Thermoregulatory dysfunction*** | | ***Cardiovascular dysfunction*** | |
|---|---|---|---|
| *Temperature (°F \| °C)* | | *Tachycardia* | |
| 99–99.9 \| 37.2–37.7 | 5 | 99–109 | 5 |
| 100–100.9 \| 37.8–38.2 | 10 | 110–119 | 10 |
| 101–101.9 \| 38.3–38.8 | 15 | 120–129 | 15 |
| 102–102.9 \| 38.9–39.4 | 20 | 130–139 | 20 |
| 103–103.9 \| 39.4–39.9 | 25 | ≥140 | 25 |
| ≥104.0 \| >40.0 | 30 | *Atrial fibrillation* | 10 |
| *Central nervous system effects* | | *Heart failure* | |
| *Mild*<br>• Agitation | 10 | *Mild*<br>• Pedal edema | 5 |
| *Moderate*<br>• Delirium<br>• Psychosis<br>• Extreme lethargy | 20 | *Moderate*<br>• Bibasilar rales | 10 |
| | | *Severe*<br>• Pulmonary edema | 15 |
| *Severe*<br>• Seizure<br>• Coma | 30 | *Precipitant history* | |
| | | • Negative | 0 |
| | | • Positive | 10 |
| *Gastrointestinal-hepatic dysfunction* | | | |
| *Moderate*<br>• Diarrhea<br>• Nausea/vomiting<br>• Abdominal pain | 10 | | |
| *Severe*<br>• Unexplained jaundice | 20 | | |

*Note:* A score of 45 or more is highly suggestive of thyroid storm, a score of 25–44 supports the diagnosis, and a score below 25 makes thyroid storm unlikely.

## MANAGEMENT OF THYROID STORM

| | |
|---|---|
| Reduction of thyroid hormone production and secretion | • *Inhibition of T4 and T3 synthesis:* Propylthiouracil, carbimazole<br>• *Inhibition of T4 and T3 secretion:*<br>– Inorganic iodide (potassium iodide, Lugol's solution)<br>– Radiographic contrast agents (sodium ipodate, iopanoic acid)<br>– Lithium carbonate<br>– Thyroidectomy |
| Therapy directed against systemic disturbances | • *Treatment of fever:* Acetaminophen external cooling<br>• *Correction of volume depletion and poor nutrition:* Intravenous fluid and electrolytes, glucose (calories), vitamins<br>• *Supportive therapy:* Oxygen, vasopressor drugs<br>• Treatment for congestive heart failure (diuretics, digoxin) |
| Amelioration of the peripheral actions of thyroid hormone | • Inhibition of extrathyroidal conversion of T4 to T3<br>– Propylthiouracil<br>– Radiographic contrast agents (sodium ipodate, iopanoic acid)<br>– Glucocorticoids<br>– Propranolol or other β-adrenergic antagonist drugs<br>• *Removal of T4 and T3 from serum:* Cholestyramine, plasmapheresis, hemodialysis, hemoperfusion |
| Treatment of any precipitating or underlying illness | • Trauma, infection, stress, stop acute iodine load, avoid vigorous palpation of the thyroid gland |
| Supportive treatment | • Airway maintenance<br>• Oxygen<br>• IV fluids<br>• Cooling blanket (do not use salicylate to treat fever because salicylates increase free T4 and free T3 levels) |

## SUGGESTED READING


1. Campbell K, Doogue M. (2012). Evaluating and managing patients with thyrotoxicosis. [online] Available from https://www.racgp.org.au/afp/2012/august/evaluating-and-managing-patients-with-thyrotoxicos [Last accessed February, 2025].
2. Gilbert J. Thyrotoxicosis - investigation and management. Clin Med. 2017;17(3):274-7.
3. Kahaly GJ, Bartalena L, Hegedüs L, Leenhardt L, Poppe K, Pearce SH. 2018 European Thyroid Association Guideline for the Management of Graves' Hyperthyroidism. Eur Thyroid J. 2018;7(4):167-86.
4. Kravets I. Hyperthyroidism: Diagnosis and Treatment. Am Fam Physician. 2016;93(5):363-70.
5. Ross DS, Burch HB, Cooper DS, Greenlee MC, Laurberg P, Maia AL, et al. 2016 American Thyroid Association Guidelines for Diagnosis and Management of Hyperthyroidism and Other Causes of Thyrotoxicosis. Thyroid. 2016;26(10):1343-421.
6. Ross DS, Cooper DS, Mulder JE. (2024). Thyroid storm. [online] Available from: https://www.uptodate.com/contents/thyroid-storm?search=thyrotoxicosis%20treatment&source=search_result&selectedTitle=4%7E150&usage_type=default&display_rank=4 [Last accessed February, 2025].

CHAPTER 102

# Adrenal Insufficiency

## INTRODUCTION

The onset of adrenal insufficiency (AI) is often very gradual, and may go undetected until an illness or other stress precipitates adrenal crisis.

Adrenal insufficiency may occur secondary to pathology of- the adrenal gland-primary adrenal insufficiency, PAI),

Hypothalamic or pituitary pathology—secondary AI, SAI),

Suppression of the hypothalamic-pituitary-adrenal (HPA) axis by exogenous glucocorticoid therapy—tertiary AI, TAI

*Symptoms and signs of AI depend on:*

- Rate and extent of loss of adrenal function
- Whether mineralocorticoid production is preserved
- Degree of physical stress

| *Severity* | *Symptoms* |
|---|---|
| Mild | Fatigue, myalgia, loss of appetite, weight loss, skin hyperpigmentation |
| Severe | • Shock out of proportion to severity of current illness<br>• Nausea, vomiting, salt craving<br>• Unexplained hypoglycemia, fever<br>• Dehydration, hypotension,<br>• Abdominal pain -"acute abdomen" |
| Electrolyte abnormalities due to Glucocorticoid deficiency | Hyponatremia, hypoglycemia, hypocalcemia (rare) |
| Findings due to mineralocorticoid deficiency—seen in PAI only | Hyperkalemia , nonanion gap acidosis, Postural hypotension, skin hyperpigmentation |

Diagnostic evaluation in Adrenal failure—Whom to test

- Peripheral vascular collapse—vasodilatory shock
- Unexplained severe hypoglycemia or hyponatremia
- Preoperative—patients on intermediate doses of steroids or who have stopped steroids within 1 year
- Patients on chronic glucocorticoids with symptoms of AI
- Patients with symptoms of AI—fatigue, myalgias, arthralgias, anorexia, weight loss, hyponatremia, salt craving, and skin pigmentation

The diagnosis of AI depends on the demonstration of inappropriately low cortisol production.

- *Basal Serum Cortisol*—within three hours after wakening (e.g., 6–9 AM)
    - *Suspected adrenal crisis*—In *hypotensive patients* considered to be in adrenal crisis a basal *serum cortisol level <18 µg/dL* suggests the *diagnosis of* AI
    - The cortisol does not need to be measured in the early morning in the setting of suspected adrenal crisis.
- *ACTH stimulation test*—Done in patients with equivocal serum cortisol values (3–18 µg/dL)
    - Obtain baseline serum cortisol.
    - Administer cosyntropin (synthetic ACTH) 250 µg IM or IV,
    - Obtain *serum cortisol at 30 and 60 minutes post-injection*

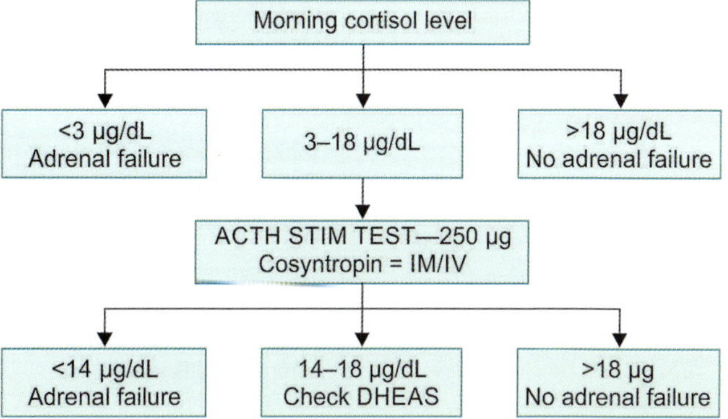

*Stimulated Cortisol level 14 to <18 μg/dL*—varied interpretation according to clinical likelihood of adrenal failure, sent *DHEAS level* for further clarity, normal DHEAS means AI is *unlikely*, low DHEAS means likely adrenal failure (DHEAS—dehydroepiandrosterone sulfate)

- *Plasma ACTH level* can help *distinguish between primary and, secondary* or tertiary AI.

It should be measured along with morning cortisol sample.

*Utility of aldosterone and renin levels:* In early primary AI due to autoimmune adrenalitis, mineralocorticoid deficiency may be more pronounced than cortisol deficiency

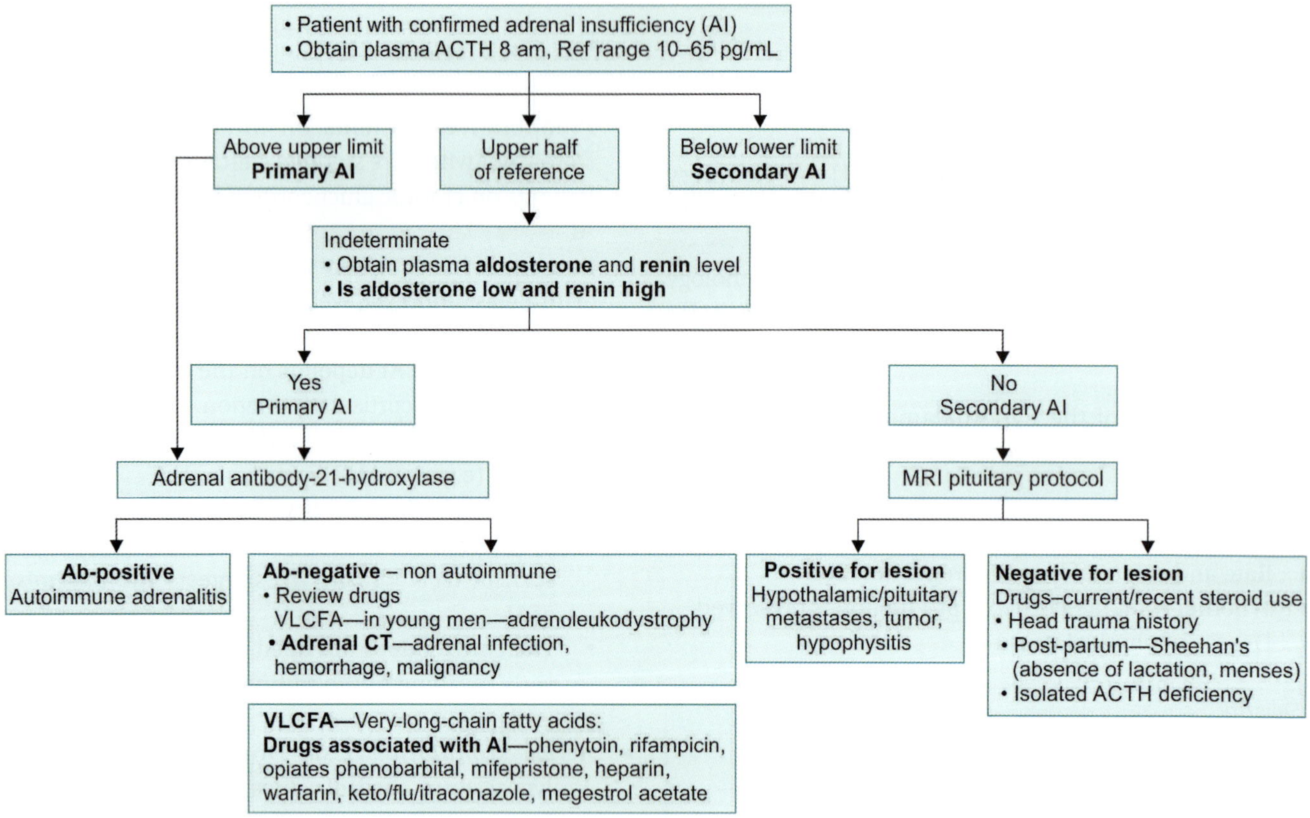

• Patient with confirmed adrenal insufficiency (AI)
• Obtain plasma ACTH 8 am, Ref range 10–65 pg/mL
Above upper limit
Primary AI
Upper half
of reference
Below lower limit
Secondary AI
Indeterminate
• Obtain plasma aldosterone and renin level
• Is aldosterone low and renin high
Yes
Primary AI
No
Secondary AI
Adrenal antibody-21-hydroxylase
MRI pituitary protocol
Ab-positive
Autoimmune adrenalitis
Ab-negative – non autoimmune
• Review drugs
VLCFA—in young men—adrenoleukodystrophy
• Adrenal CT—adrenal infection, hemorrhage, malignancy
Positive for lesion
Hypothalamic/pituitary metastases, tumor, hypophysitis
Negative for lesion
Drugs–current/recent steroid use
• Head trauma history
• Post-partum—Sheehan's (absence of lactation, menses)
• Isolated ACTH deficiency
VLCFA—Very-long-chain fatty acids:
Drugs associated with AI—phenytoin, rifampicin, opiates phenobarbital, mifepristone, heparin, warfarin, keto/flu/itraconazole, megestrol acetate

## TREATMENT OF ACUTE ADRENAL INSUFFICIENCY

Establish IV, draw bloods—Na, K, cortisol, ACTH, RFT, RBS
fluid resuscitation—1 L of DNS, repeat as needed
• Hydrocortisone—100 mg bolus, 50 mg—6th hourly
• Maintenance IV fluids for 24–48 hours
• Search for precipitating causes—infections
• Taper hydrocort to 50 mg 12 hourly after 24–48 hours
• In moderate to severe infections/postoperative continue oral stress dose steroids—3 times the usual daily dose for 3 days
• Taper to maintenance dose 15–25 mg/d, 15 mg morning dose and 10 mg afternoon
• Fludrocortisone 50–100 μg/day is added for patients with primary adrenal insufficiency

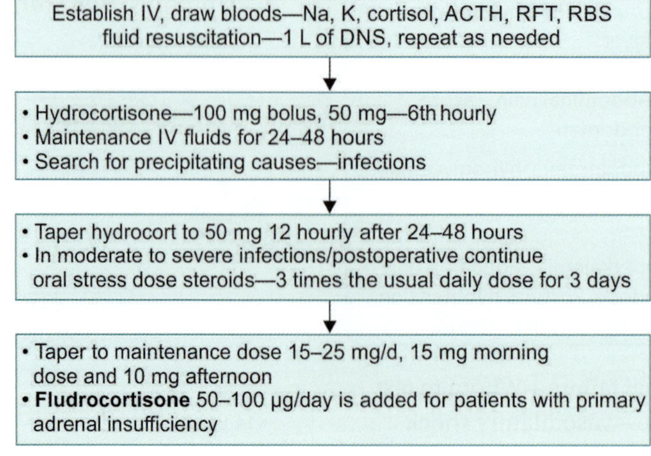

# PART 9

# BLOOD GAS ANALYSIS

***Editors:*** Pragyan Kumar Routray, Dharmajivan Samantaray

CHAPTER

# 103 Arterial Blood Gas

## STEP 1—CHECK THE VALIDITY OF THE ABG

Using the Henderson-Hasselbalch equation:

$$[H^+] = 24(PaCO_2)/[HCO_3^-]$$

If the pH and the $[H^+]$ are inconsistent, the ABG is probably not valid.

| *pH* | *Approximate $[H^+]$ (mmol/L)* |
|---|---|
| 7.00 | 100 |
| 7.05 | 89 |
| 7.10 | 79 |
| 7.15 | 71 |
| 7.20 | 63 |
| 7.25 | 56 |
| 7.30 | 50 |
| 7.35 | 45 |
| 7.40 | 40 |
| 7.45 | 35 |
| 7.50 | 32 |
| 7.55 | 28 |
| 7.60 | 25 |
| 7.65 | 22 |

### Illustration

65 years M with CKD presenting with nausea, diarrhea and acute respiratory distress

*ABG:* 7.22/17/235 on 50% VM

*Na – 123/Cl – 97/$HCO_3$ – 7/BUN – 119/Cr – 5.1/ALB – 4*

*Step 1:* $[H^+]$ = 24[17/7]= 58, 80–58 = 22, last two digits of pH, i.e., =7.22 → Validated

*Step 2:* pH 7.22 → Acidemic

*Step 3:* Metabolic or Respiratory $HCO_3$ = 7, <20 → Metabolic

### Alternate Formula

$H^+$ = 80 – (Last two digits after the decimal point)

## STEP 2

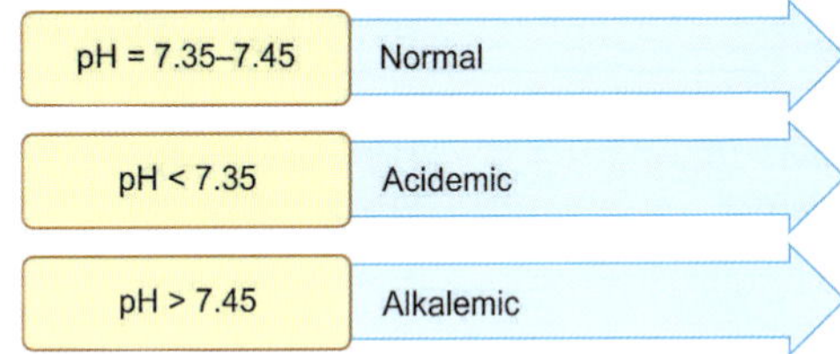


## STEP 3

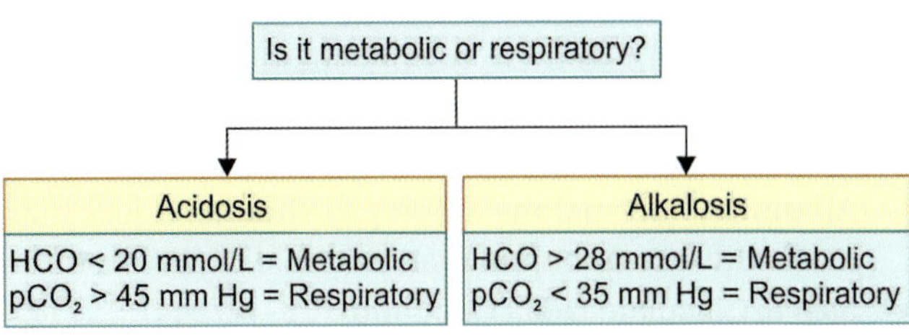

## STEP 4

Algorithm for metabolic acidosis

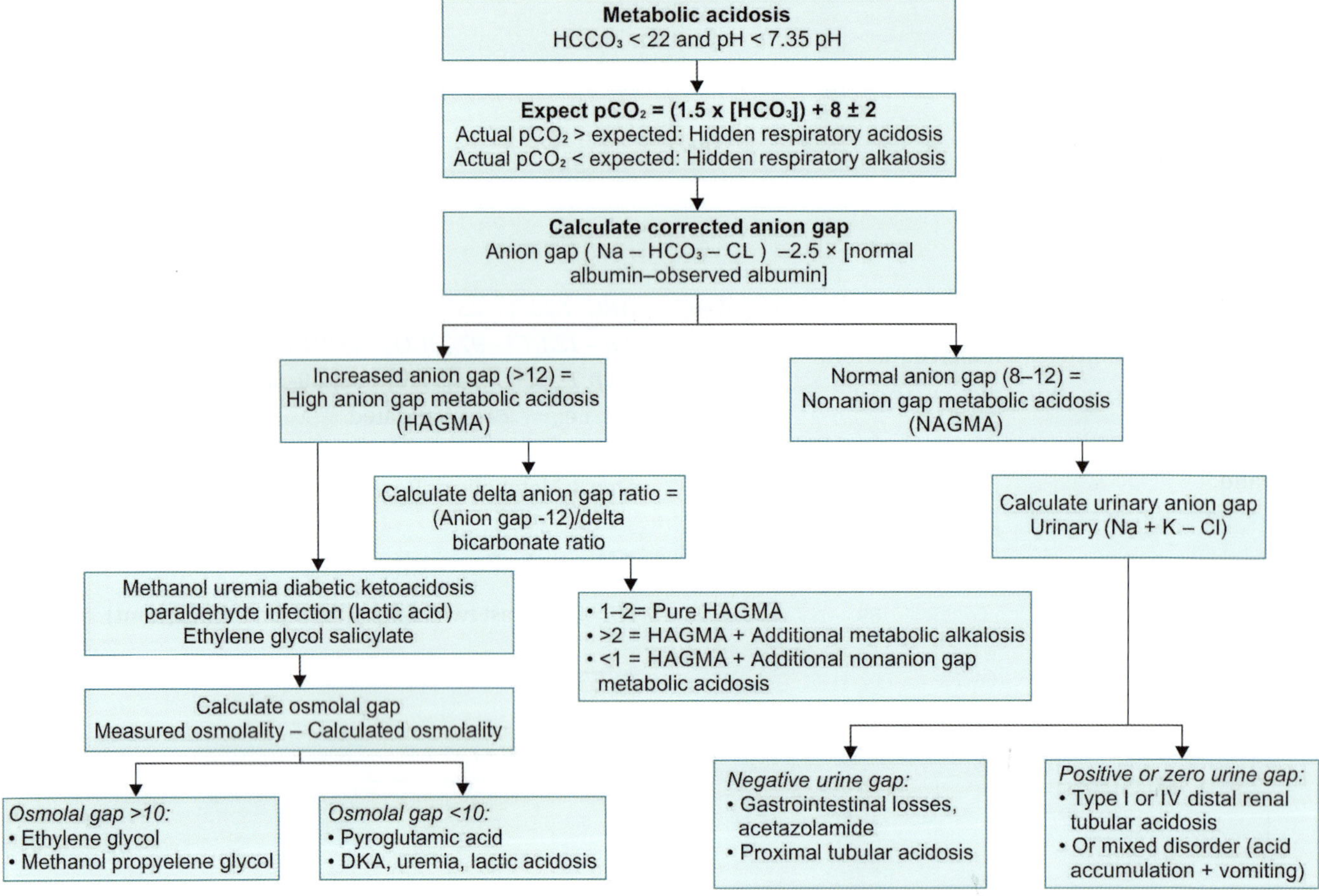


## Illustration

- *Step 4:* Expected $pCO_2$ = (1.5 × 7) + 8 ± 2 = 18.5 (16.5-20.5), Here $pCO_2$ = 17, so there is appropriate compensation so there is only one disorder *Primary metabolic*
- *Step 5:* Calculate Corrected AG = 123–7–97 = 19, As Albumin is normal the anion gap should be less than 12. So this case scenario is an example of *HAGMA*.
- *Step 6:* Calculate Delta Gap ratio = 19–12/24–7 = 7/17 = 0.411, which is <1, so additional *NAGMA* present.
- *Step 7:* What is the differential for the clinical processes? Final Diagnosis is *HAGMA+NAGMA*
- Why HAGMA? Our patient for anion gap portions it is due to BUN of 119 UREMIA, but would still check lactic acid.
- Why NAGMA? Most likely due to diarrhea.
    - While Calculating AG take the value of Corrected $[Na^+] = Na^+$ (RBS mg%–100/100) × 1.4

CHAPTER 104

# Metabolic Alkalosis

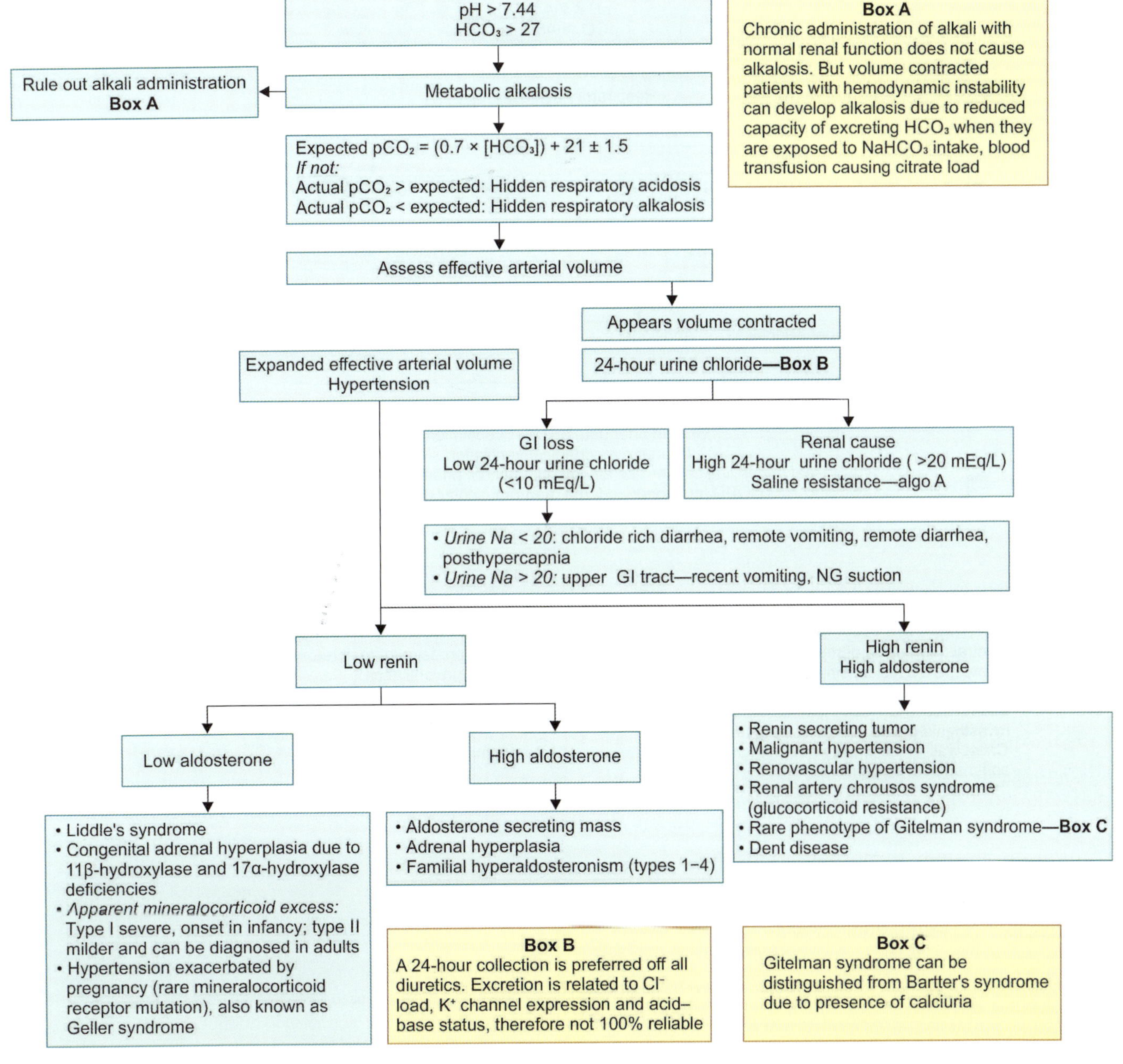

CHAPTER 105

# Respiratory Acidosis

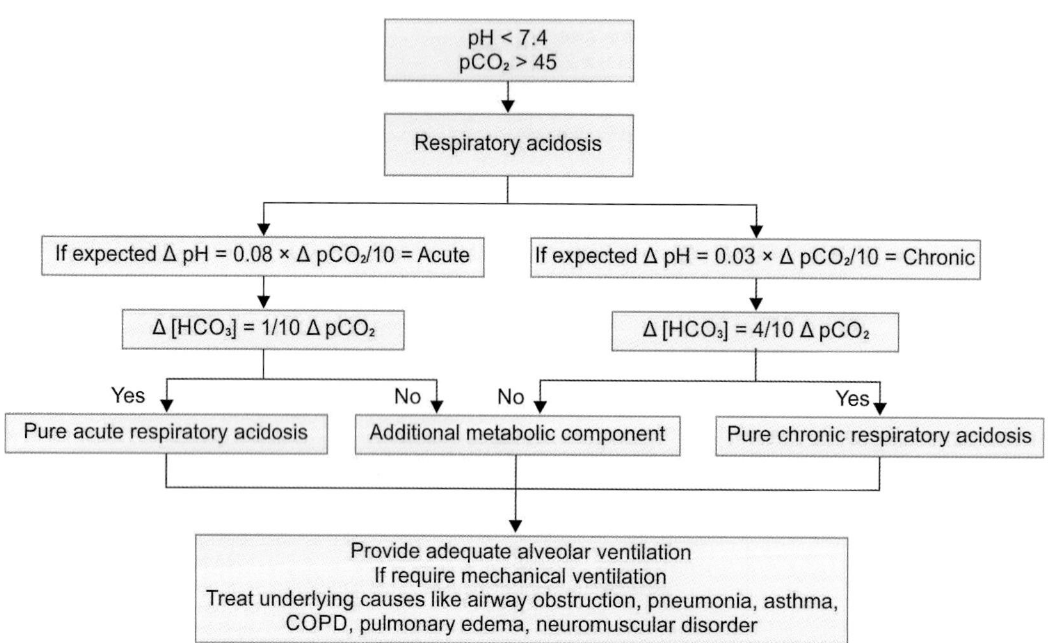


**Causes of acute respiratory acidosis**

- Central depression of respiratory drive—drugs, opiates, CNS lesion, stroke, encephalities
- Neuromuscular—spinal cord lesion, trauma above C4 level, tetanus, ALS, myasthenia gravis, OP poisoning, botulism
- Chest wall—Flail chest, pneumothorax, ARDS, asthma, COPD, sepsis

**Causes of chronic respiratory acidosis**

- Central depression of respiratory drive—primary alveolar hypoventilation
- Neuromuscular—poliomyelitis, malnutrition, electrolyte imbalance
- Chest wall—kyphoscoliosis, obesity
- Parenchyma—ILD, COPD

CHAPTER 106

# Respiratory Alkalosis

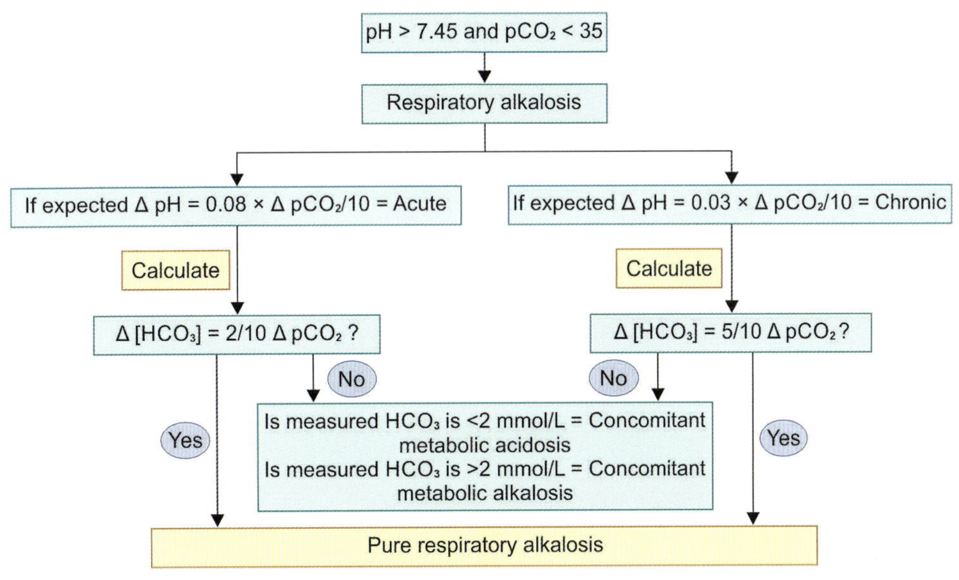


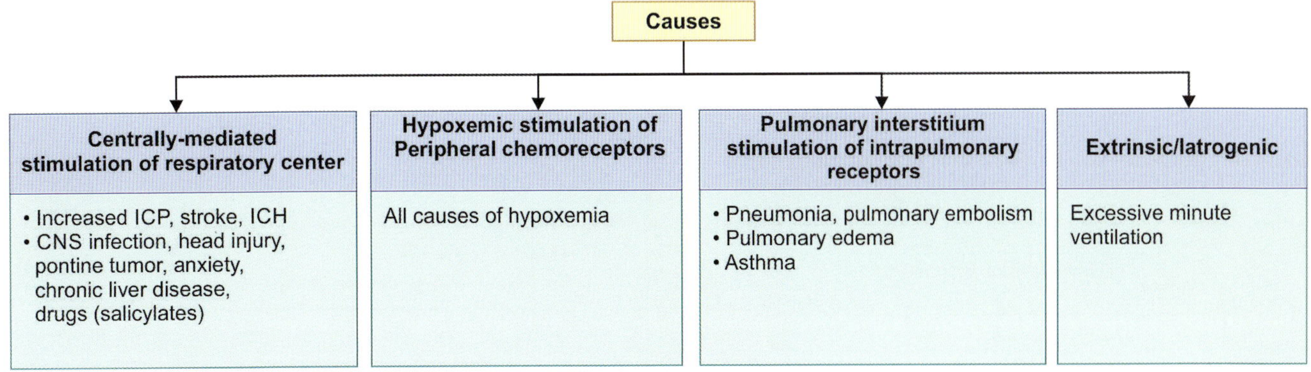

# PART 10

# TOXICOLOGY

***Editor:*** Binila Chacko

***Associate Editors:*** Lovely Thomas, Manoj Job

CHAPTER 107

# Approach to Unknown Poisoning

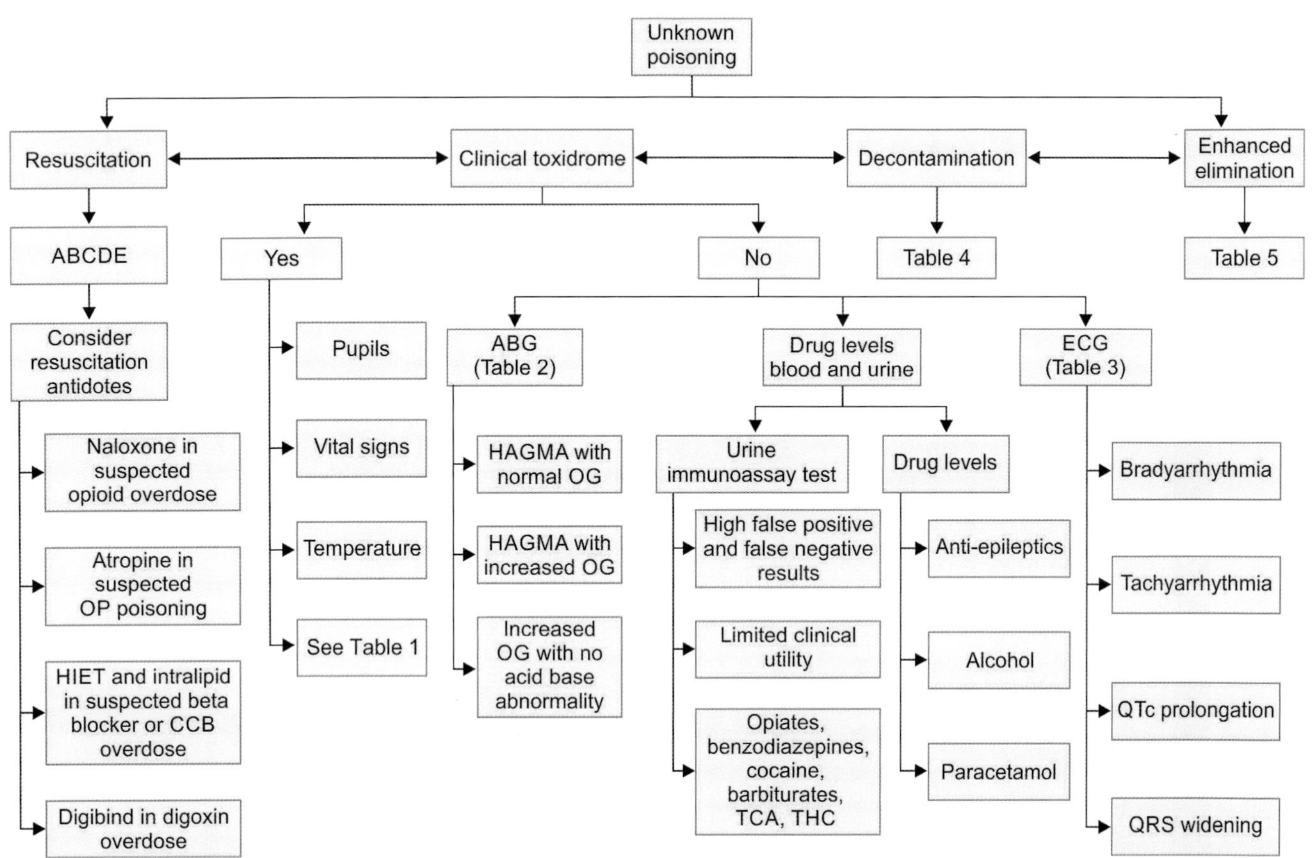


(ABCDE: airway, breathing, circulation, disability and seizure control, exposure and temperature control; HIET: hyperinsulinemic euglycemic therapy; ABG: arterial blood gas; CCB: calcium channel blocker; ECG: electrocardiogram; HAGMA: high anion gap metabolic acidosis; TCA: tricyclic antidepressants; THC: tetrahydrocannabinol; OG: osmolal gap; OP: organophosphorus poison)

**TABLE 1:** Classic toxidromes.

| *Toxidrome* | *Time to clinical presentation* | *Temperature* | *Pupils* | *Vital signs* | *Skin* | *Bowel sounds* | *Other specific points* |
|---|---|---|---|---|---|---|---|
| Cholinergic | <12 hours | Normal | Miosis | • HR and BP low but may be increased in early poisoning<br>• RR decreased or increased | Diaphoresis | Increased | Seizures+/–, SLUDGE symptoms, muscle fasciculations +/– |
| Opioid syndrome | <12 hours | Normal or decreased | Miosis | • Decreased or normal HR and BP<br>• RR bradypnea or apneic | Normal | Decreased | • *Board like rigidity:* Fentanyl<br>• *Seizures:* Meperidine and tramadol<br>• *No miosis:* Meperidine<br>• Reports of non-cardiogenic pulmonary edema |
| Sympatholytics | <12 hours | Normal or decreased | Miosis | • Decreased HR, BP, RR<br>• Hypertension also reported | Normal or dry | Decreased | |
| Sedative hypnotic | <12 hours | Normal or decreased | Normal | • Decreased or normal HR and BP<br>• RR bradypnea or apneic | Normal | Normal | Normal reflexes |
| Anticholinergic | <12 hours | Hyperthermia | Mydriasis | Increased HR, BP, RR | Dry | Decreased | • Lilliputian hallucinations<br>• Reflexes normal |
| Sympathomimetic | <12 hours | Hyperthermia | Mydriasis | Increased HR, BP, RR | Diaphoresis | Increased | • Muscle tone and reflexes normal<br>• Agitation and hyperactive delirium<br>• Seizures +/-<br>• Widened pulse pressure |
| Serotonin syndrome | <12 hours | Hyperthermia | Mydriasis | Autonomic dysfunction | Diaphoresis or normal | Increased | • Agitated, hyperactive delirium, confusion<br>• Tremor, hyperreflexia and clonus predominantly in the lower limbs<br>• Ocular clonus may be present |
| Neuroleptic malignant syndrome | 1 to 3 days after new drug or dose increase | Hyperthermia | Normal | Increased HR, BP, RR | Diaphoresis | Normal | Rigidity and bradyreflexia |

**TABLE 2:** ABG and osmolar gap abnormalities.

| *HAGMA with normal osmolal gap <10 mOsm/kg* | *HAGMA with increased osmolal gap >10 mOsm/kg* | *Increased osmolar gap with normal acid base status* | *Oxygen saturation gap (>5% difference between measured and calculated value on the arterial blood gas)* |
|---|---|---|---|
| • Salicylate overdose (associated respiratory alkalosis)<br>• Alcohol overdose over time<br>• Iron overdose<br>• Metformin overdose<br>• Isoniazid overdose<br>• NSAID overdose<br>• Cellular asphyxiants, e.g., methemoglobinemia or cyanide toxicity | Ethanol, methyl alcohol and ethylene glycol overdose | Isopropyl alcohol overdose | • Carbon monoxide (dichloromethane-paint remover overdose; hookah abuse)<br>• Cyanide (potassium cyanide overdose; illicit phencyclidine overdose, acetonitrile from nail polish removers)<br>• Methemoglobinemia (e.g., nitrate or nitrite overdose, aniline dye overdose)<br>• Sulfhemoglobinemia |

[NSAID: nonsteroidal anti-inflammatory drugs; Osmolal gap: measured serum osmolality – calculated serum osmolality; $Osm_C$ = (2 Na + Urea/6 + Glucose/18) or (2 Na + Urea/6 + Glucose/18 + Ethanol/4.6 + Methanol/3.2 + Ethylene glycol/6.2 + Isopropanol/6)]

**TABLE 3:** ECG clues to the poison.

| *Bradyarrhythmia* | *Tachyarrhythmia* | *Prolonged QT interval* | *QRS widening* |
|---|---|---|---|
| • Beta blocker overdose<br>• Calcium channel blocker overdose<br>• Digoxin overdose<br>• Alpha 2 agonist overdose<br>• Cholinergic overdose<br>• Opioid overdose<br>• Sedative hypnotic overdose | • Sympathomimetic overdose<br>• Anticholinergic overdose<br>• Thyroid hormone overdose<br>• Drug withdrawal states | • Antihistamines<br>• Loratadine<br>• Terfenadine<br>• Anti-psychotics, e.g., Haloperidol, Quetiapine, Risperidone, Chlorpromazine<br>• Chloroquine, Quinine<br>• Antiarrhythmics<br>• Antidepressants<br>• Fluoroquinolones<br>• Tacrolimus | • Antihistamines<br>• Cocaine<br>• Propoxyphene<br>• Sodium channel blockers, e.g., tricyclic antidepressants<br>• β-Adrenergic blocking agents<br>• Calcium channel antagonists |

**TABLE 4:** Role of decontamination.

| *Skin decontamination* | *Gastric lavage* | *Activated charcoal single dose* | *Whole bowel irrigation* |
|---|---|---|---|
| • Remove contaminated clothing<br>• Wash with soap and water (soaps containing 30% ethanol advocated)<br>• No evidence of benefit of cholinesterase sponges | Gastric lavage limited absorption even if used within an hour | Decreases toxin levels by its high adsorption capacity and by interrupting enterohepatic recirculation | • Cleanse the entire bowel of toxin with large volumes of polyethylene glycol electrolyte solution<br>• Caution in patients with ileus and uncontrolled vomiting |
| Important aspect in OP | Not routinely recommended | • Single-dose activated charcoal SHOULD NOT be administered routinely in poisoned patients<br>• Do NOT use in suspected overdose with corrosive acids, alkali, iron, lithium, lead and arsenic | • Sustained release toxins (CCB's, Potassium overdose)<br>• Fe overdose<br>• Pb ingestion<br>• Arsenic<br>• Body packers |

**TABLE 5:** Role of enhanced elimination.

| ***Multiple dose activated charcoal 50 g q4h*** | ***Urinary alkalization >7.5 with isotonic bicarbonate therapy*** | ***Hemodialysis*** | ***Charcoal or resin-based hemoperfusion*** |
|---|---|---|---|
| Charcoal adsorbs toxins that are secreted into the intestine before being reabsorbed | Increases ionization of the toxin and limits tubular re-absorption of the toxin | Small Molecular weight substances (<10000 Da) with a small Volume of Distribution | Toxins which are protein bound and high lipid solubility with a small Volume of Distribution |
| • Toxins that undergo entero-enteric or enterohepatic circulation<br>• Carbamazepine, phenytoin, phenobarbital, dapsone, quinine, salicylate or theophylline | • Acidic toxins<br>• Salicylates, phenobarbital and tricyclic antidepressant overdose | • Li (neurotoxicity + level >2.5 mmol/L)<br>• Metformin lactic acidemia<br>• $K^+$<br>• Salicylates<br>• Theophylline<br>• Toxic alcohols<br>• Valproic acid<br>• Dabigatran | • Antiepileptic overdose-Phenobarbitone, phenytoin and carbamazepine overdose<br>• Aluminum overdose<br>• Paraquat overdose |

CHAPTER 108

# Organophosphorus (OP) Poisoning

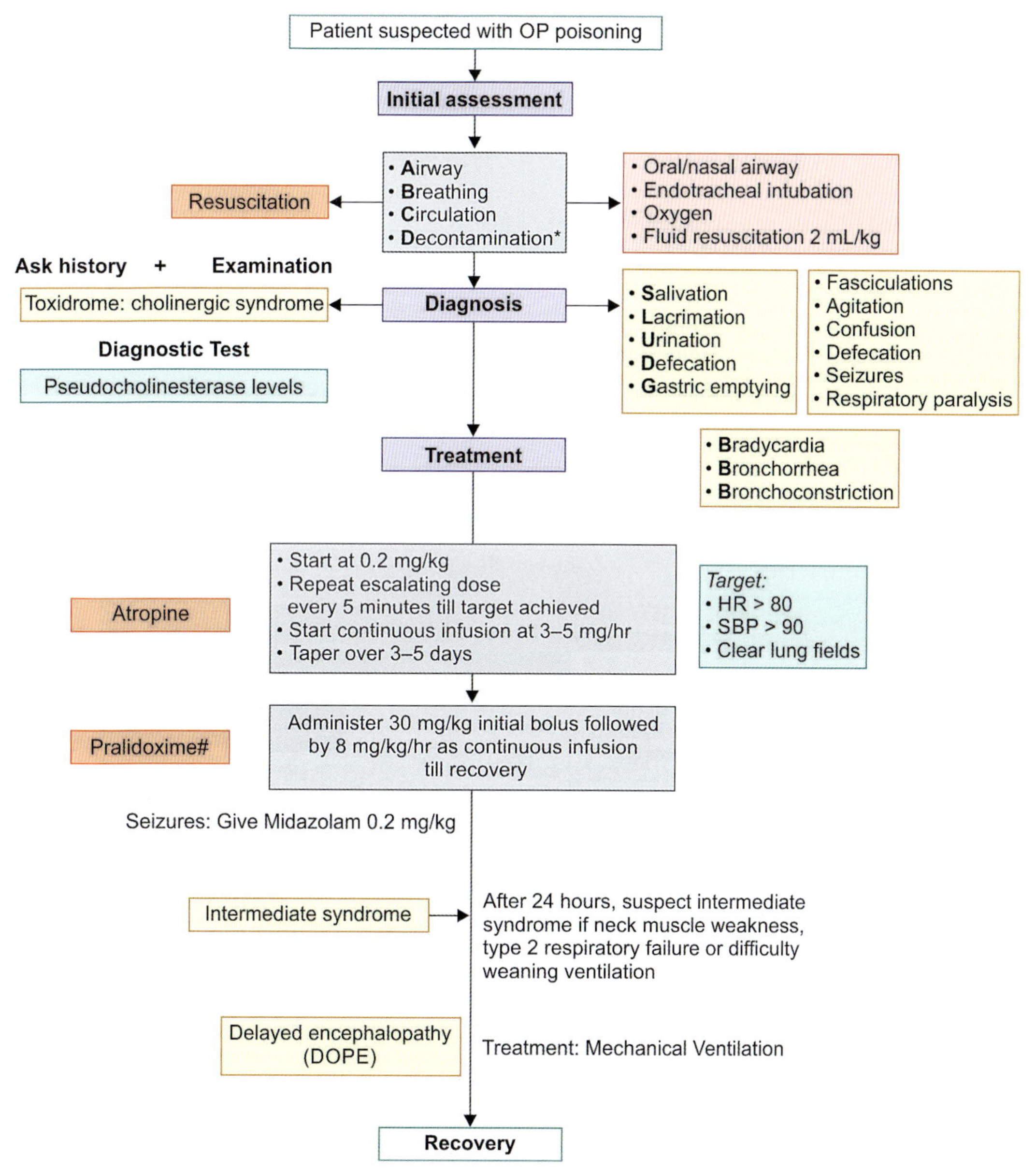


(DOPE: Delayed organophosphorus poisoning: between 4 and 7 days after poisoning, reduced conscious state, pinpoint pupils, may mimic brain death)

CHAPTER 109

# Hair Dye Poisoning: Super Vasmol Overdose

| *Telltale signs* | *Toxic compounds* |
|---|---|
| • Early angio-neurotic edema of face and neck<br>• Hoarseness of voice<br>• Stridor<br>• Dark brown colored urine<br>• Acute kidney injury | • Paraphenylene diamine (PPD) – aromatic amine used for color enhancement<br>• Resorcinol – phenol derivative – has corrosive properties<br>• Propylene glycol – solvent |
| *Note:* A 100-mL Super Vasmol contains 12 g of PPD, minimal dose required to produce systemic features of poisoning is Approximately 3 g. The fatal dose after oral ingestion is 7 g or more. | |
| *Decontamination:*<br>• NO antidote<br>• NO induced emesis/gastric lavage *(PPD with contact with mucosa will worsen edema/resorcinol is a corrosive)*<br>• Doubtful benefit of activated charcoal | |

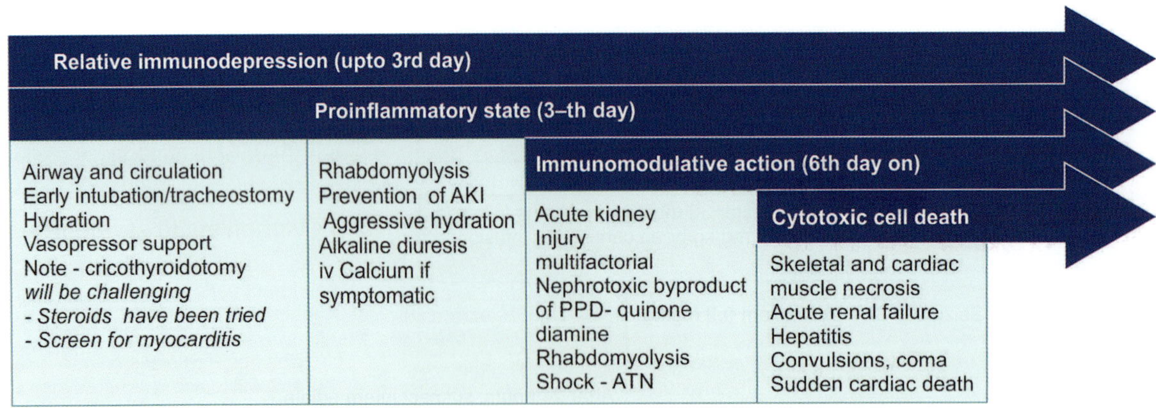


**Fig. 1:** Progressive stages seen in lethal dose of Hair Dye ingestion.

**TABLE 1:** Management of rhabdomyolysis—a cornerstone treatment in hair dye poisoning.

| | | |
|---|---|---|
| • Corrects volume depletion<br>• prevents pre-renal AKI by maintaining renal perfusion<br>• Limits precipitation and formation of intratubular cast<br>• Flushes out myoglobin pigment | • Monitoring of CPK, monitor ELECTROLYTES—Sodium, potassium and calcium<br>• Monitor intake output hourly and for features of fluid overload, monitor arterial pH<br>• Early Nephrology input | AGGRESSIVE HYDRATION<br>Crystalloids, isotonic fluids (NS, Ringer lactate, Plasmalyte) @ 200–1000 mL/h targeting a urine output of 300 mL/h.<br>*Continuous titration of fluid rate based on patient's volume status and urine output* |
| Volume replete with good urine output and no volume overload | | FORCED DIURESIS<br>CONTINUE hydration<br>• To achieve urine output of 200–300 mL/h<br>• Till consistent declining trend of CPK <5,000 U/L |
| Volume replete with oligo-anuria | | DECREASE the hydration<br>• CAUTION - Mannitol* - produces free water loss - can worsen volume status if not adequately hydrated and can worsen hypernatremia<br>• AVOID- Loop Diuretics*<br>• CONSIDER - Dialysis |
| Volume overload | | STOP fluid resuscitation- Dialysis |
| • Prevents intratubular cast formation by decreasing precipitation of heme-protein with Tamm-Horsfall<br>• Decrease the release of free iron from myoglobin responsible for vasoconstriction of renal arterioles<br>• Decrease the risk for tubular precipitation of uric acid | | **ROLE OF SODABICARBONATE:** Urine alkalinization**<br>150 meq $NaHCO_3$ in 1 liter of Dextrose @ 200 mL/h i.e., 30 meq/h of $NaHCO_3$ (titrate the isotonic saline fluids accordingly)<br>Monitor urine pH - target >6.5<br>*Contraindication:*<br>• If arterial ph >7.5<br>• Hypocalcemia<br>• Serum bicarbonate is <30 mEq/L<br>*Discontinue:*<br>• If the urine pH <6.5 after 3-4 hrs, symptomatic hypocalcemia, Or any contraindication mentioned |

*No robust scientific evidence to support their effectiveness over saline diuresis
**No clear evidence to support urinary alkalinization in preventing AKI

CHAPTER 110

# Zinc or Aluminum Phosphide Poisoning

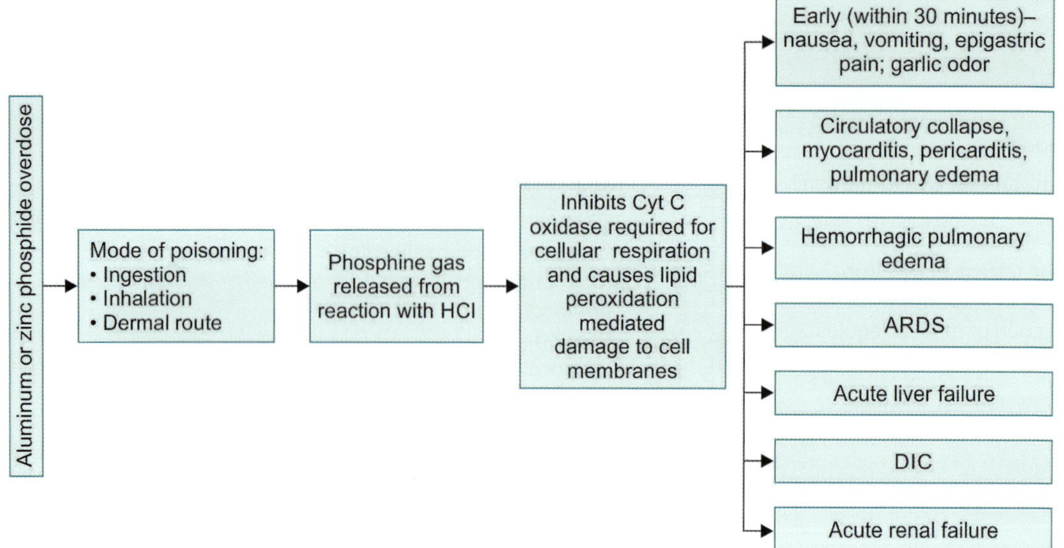


(ARDS: acute respiratory distress syndrome; DIC: disseminated intravascular coagulation; HCl: hydrochloric acid)

## TREATMENT OF ZINC OR ALUMINUM PHOSPHIDE POISONING

### Decontamination

No role-may increase disintegration of poison and increase toxicity

### Supportive Treatment

- Mechanical ventilation
- Organ supportive therapy
- N-acetyl cysteine in patients with acute liver failure (as in paracetamol overdose)
- Possible role of trimetazidine and magnesium sulfate
- Research on role of pralidoxime
- No antidote available

CHAPTER 111

# Corrosive Poisoning

## CORROSIVE POISONING

*Corrosive:* A chemical substance that causes visible destruction or irreversible alterations in living tissue by chemical action at the site of contact.

**TABLE 1:** Common corrosives.

| | *Mechanism of Injury* | *Chemicals agents* | *Common uses* | *Brands* |
|---|---|---|---|---|
| Alkali | Liquefactive necrosis easier to swallow esophageal injury > stomach [stomach acid neutralizes] | • Sodium hydroxide<br>• Potassium hydroxide<br>• Sodium hypochlorite | • Stain removers<br>• Drain cleaner<br>• Soap<br>• Cleaning agents | • Chlorox<br>• Lysol<br>• Drano<br>• Lye Soap |
| Acid | Coagulative necrosis forms eschar stomach > esophagus | • Sulfuric acid<br>• Hydrochloric acid<br>• Nitric acid<br>• Carbolic acid | • Drain cleaner<br>• Car battery<br>• Button battery | Phenol |
| Others | | • Hydrogen peroxide<br>• Potassium permanganate<br>• Mercuric chloride | • Disinfectant<br>• Water softener | |

**TABLE 2:** Endoscopic findings in corrosive poisoning.

| *Grade* | *Endoscopic finding* | *Prognosis* |
|---|---|---|
| 0 | Normal | Complete recovery |
| 1 | Oedema and erythema | Complete recovery |
| 2A | Friability, hemorrhage and superficial ulcerations | Stricture unlikely |
| 2B | Deep ulcerations (discrete or circumferential) | High risk of stricture, low risk of perforation |
| 3A | Small, scattered areas of necrosis | High risk of stricture and perforation |
| 3B | Extensive necrosis | High risk of stricture and perforation |
| 4 | Perforation | Often fatal |

**Flowchart 1:** Corrosive poisoning—an approach.

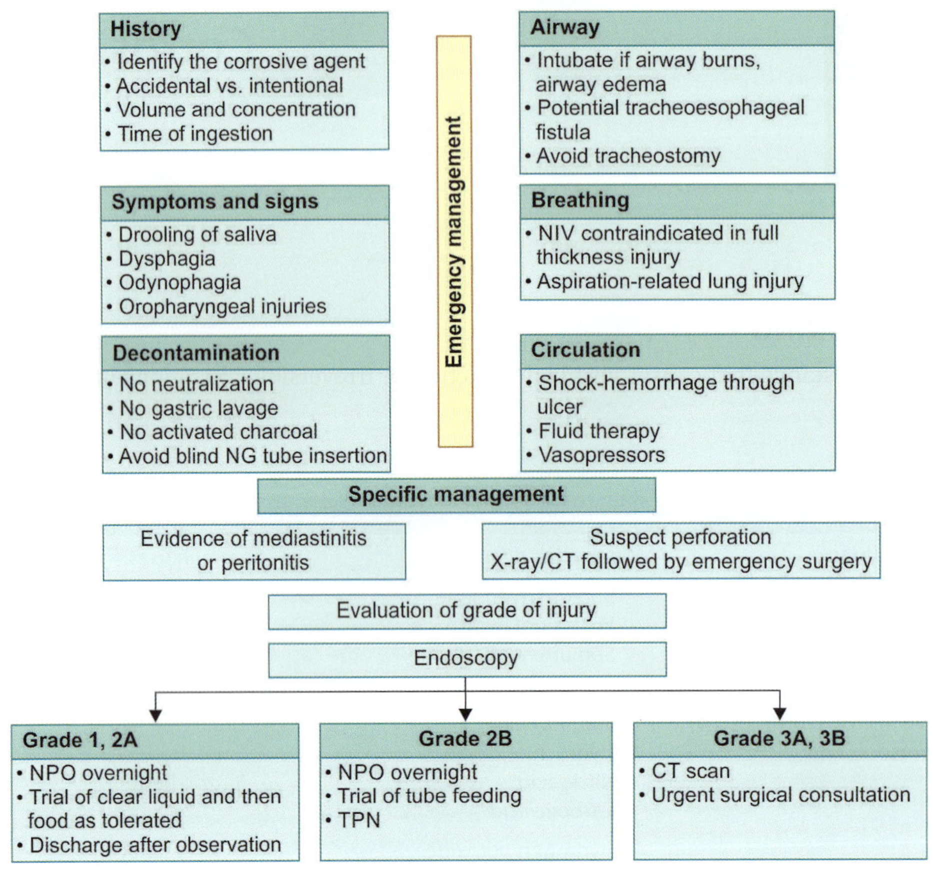


*Presentation within 24 hours of consumption

CHAPTER 112

# Calcium Channel Blocker/ Beta-blocker Toxicity

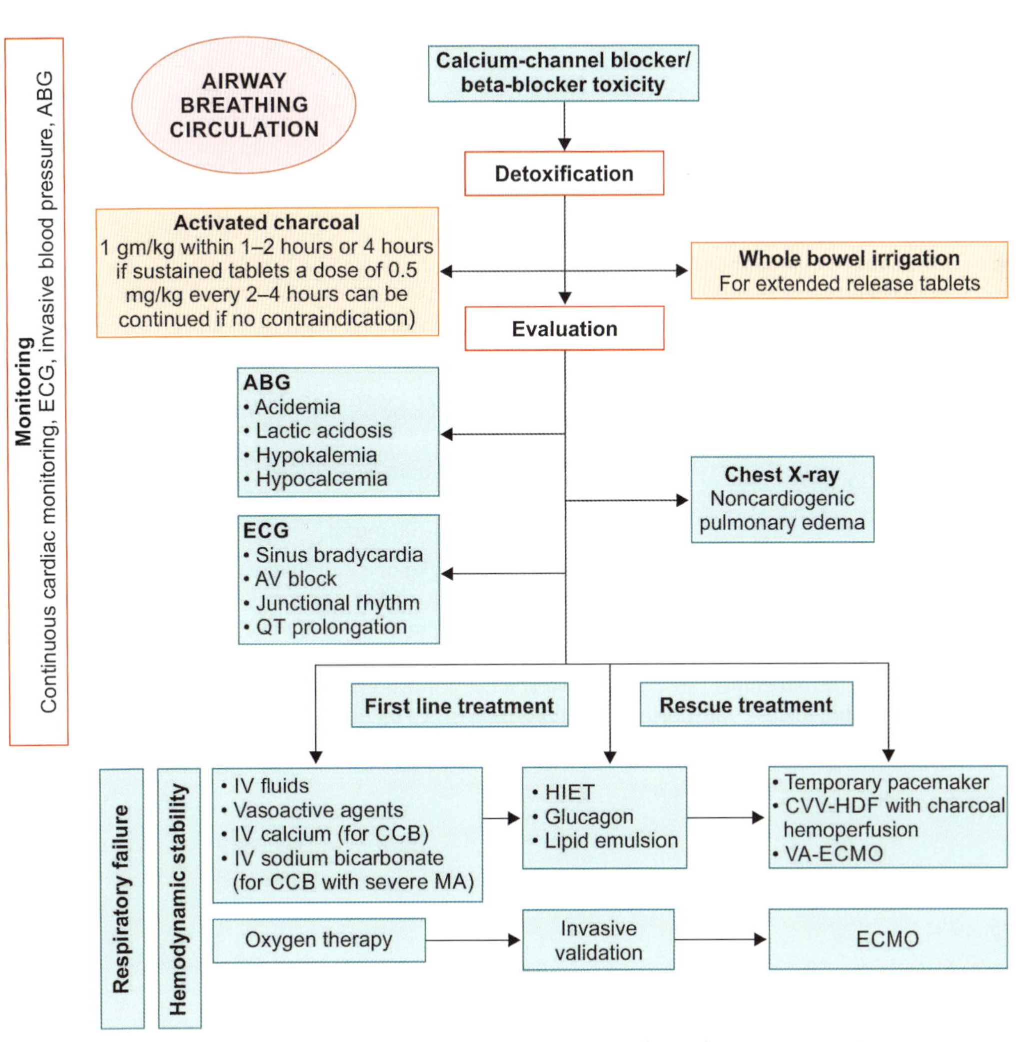


(CCB: calcium channel blocker; ECMO: extra corporeal membrane oxygenation; HIET: hyperinsulinemic euglycemic therapy; MA: metabolic acidosis)

**TABLE 1:** Classification of calcium channel blockers.

| | ***Verapamil (Phenylalkylamines)*** | ***Diltiazem (Benzothiazepines)*** | ***Amlodipine (Dihydropyridines)*** |
|---|---|---|---|
| Macro-circulatory level | | | |
| Negative INOTROPY | +++ | +++ | – |
| Negative CHRONOTROPY | +++ | ++++ | – |
| VASCULAR SMOOTH MUSCLE | Vasodilation +++ | Vasodilation + | Vasodilation +++ |
| Micro-circulatory level – Hyperglycemia, insulin resistance<br>– Interfere with mitochondrial function – increased lactate production and acidosis | | | |

*Note:* With high doses—verapamil and diltiazem cause hypotension with bradycardia, Nifedipine triggers hypotension and reflex sinus tachycardia.

| | ***Mechanism of action*** | ***Dose*** | ***Adverse effects*** |
|---|---|---|---|
| Glucagon* | Increases cAMP increase heart rate<br>*Minimal effects on the mean arterial pressure | 1–5 mg IV push<br>May repeated dose, max dose is 15 mg | Nausea and vomiting |
| Hyper-insulinemic euglycemic therapy **(HIET) | Meets the "metabolic hunger" of the heart by increasing the uptake of glucose and lactate into myocardial cells → improving myocardial function<br>** Treatment effect pronounced in patients with myocardial dysfunction | Insulin bolus @ 1 unit/kg IV +25% dextrose 100 mL (If glucose <200 mg/dL)<br>• Continuous infusion @ 0.5–1 units/kg/h<br>• If no hemodynamic stabilization after 20 mins<br>• Increase insulin by 0.5 units/kg/h q 15 mins<br>• Max dose – 4 units/kg/h<br>• Give dextrose to maintain glucose in the range of 100–200 mg/dL | Electrolyte disturbances (hypoglycemia hypokalemia, hypomagnesemia, hypophosphatemia) |
| Lipid emulsion therapy | "Lipid sink," surrounds a lipophilic drug and renders it ineffective.<br>Fatty acids are a ready "energy source" for heart<br>"Lipid shuttle" effect the encapsulated toxin is transported to target organs for metabolism | Bolus of 1.5 mL/kg of a 20% lipid emulsion sol over 1 mins → If NO response → repeat dose every 3–5 mins (total of *three bolus* doses)<br>Follow it by → infusion of 0.025 mL/kg /min *(max dosing is 12.5 mL/kg in a 24 hrs )* | Hypersensitivity reactions<br>Hyper triglyceridemia<br>Fat embolism<br>Infections |

CHAPTER 113

# Snake Envenomation

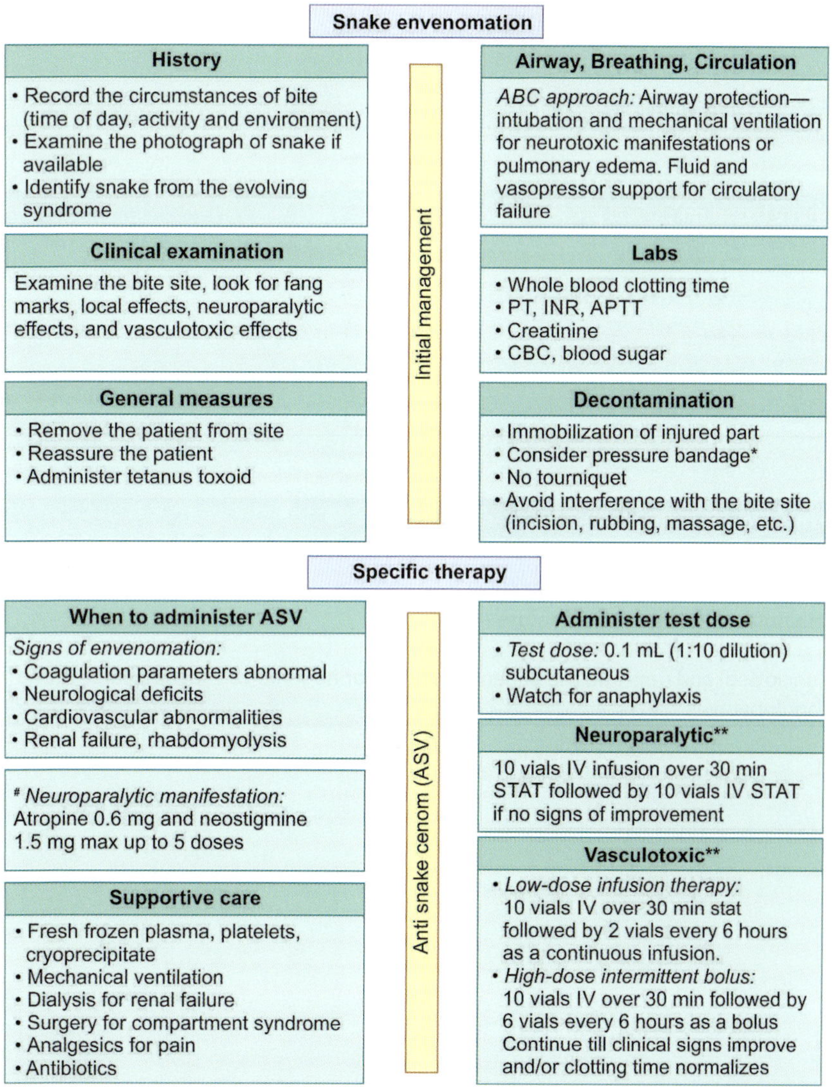

**Snake envenomation**

**History**
- Record the circumstances of bite (time of day, activity and environment)
- Examine the photograph of snake if available
- Identify snake from the evolving syndrome

**Clinical examination**

Examine the bite site, look for fang marks, local effects, neuroparalytic effects, and vasculotoxic effects

**General measures**
- Remove the patient from site
- Reassure the patient
- Administer tetanus toxoid

Initial management

**Airway, Breathing, Circulation**

*ABC approach:* Airway protection—intubation and mechanical ventilation for neurotoxic manifestations or pulmonary edema. Fluid and vasopressor support for circulatory failure

**Labs**
- Whole blood clotting time
- PT, INR, APTT
- Creatinine
- CBC, blood sugar

**Decontamination**
- Immobilization of injured part
- Consider pressure bandage*
- No tourniquet
- Avoid interference with the bite site (incision, rubbing, massage, etc.)

**Specific therapy**

**When to administer ASV**

*Signs of envenomation:*
- Coagulation parameters abnormal
- Neurological deficits
- Cardiovascular abnormalities
- Renal failure, rhabdomyolysis

*# Neuroparalytic manifestation:* Atropine 0.6 mg and neostigmine 1.5 mg max up to 5 doses

**Supportive care**
- Fresh frozen plasma, platelets, cryoprecipitate
- Mechanical ventilation
- Dialysis for renal failure
- Surgery for compartment syndrome
- Analgesics for pain
- Antibiotics

Anti snake cenom (ASV)

**Administer test dose**
- *Test dose:* 0.1 mL (1:10 dilution) subcutaneous
- Watch for anaphylaxis

**Neuroparalytic****

10 vials IV infusion over 30 min STAT followed by 10 vials IV STAT if no signs of improvement

**Vasculotoxic****
- *Low-dose infusion therapy:* 10 vials IV over 30 min stat followed by 2 vials every 6 hours as a continuous infusion.
- *High-dose intermittent bolus:* 10 vials IV over 30 min followed by 6 vials every 6 hours as a bolus Continue till clinical signs improve and/or clotting time normalizes

**Fig. 1:** Snake bite—an approach.

*Pressure bandage retard systemic absorption of venom, but can cause gangrene if applied too tight

#Role in non-intubated respiratory failure patients due to neurotoxic snake bit

**ASV does is the same for children and adults, the total required dose will be 10–25 as each vial neutralizes 6 mg of Russel viper venon. There is no sufficient evidence for low does infusion vs high dose intermittent therapy. There may be no potential benefit in continuing ASV more than 30 vials.

**TABLE 1:** Common snakes.

| *Family* | *Snakes* |
|---|---|
| Elapidae | Cobra, Krait |
| Viperidae | Russell's viper, saw scaled viper, Pit viper |
| Hydrophidae | Sea snake |

**TABLE 2:** Clinical presentation.

| *Syndromes* | *Symptoms* | *Snakes* |
|---|---|---|
| Progressive painful swelling | Local Necrosis, Ecchymosis, Blistering, Painful swelling, Compartment syndrome | Russell's viper |
| Neuroparalytic | Ptosis, Diplopia, Dysarthria, Dysphagia, Dyspnea, Dysphonia, Drooling | Cobra, Krait |
| Vasculotoxic/hematotoxic | Bleeding, DIC | Viper |

**TABLE 3:** Identification of snake based on clinical presentation.

| *Type of snake* | *Local effects* | *Neurotoxic* | *Hemotoxic* | *Cardiac* | *Renal* |
|---|---|---|---|---|---|
| Cobra | ++ | +++ | – | +/– | – |
| Russel vi per | +++ | ++ | +++ | – | ++ |
| Saw-scaled viper | ++ | – | +++ | – | + |
| Krait | – | +++ | +/– | – | – |

**TABLE 4:** How to do whole blood clotting time.

*Whole blood clotting time:*

- Place 2 mL of freshly sampled venous blood in a small, new or heat cleaned, dry, glass vessel
- Leave undisturbed for 20 minutes at ambient temperature
- Tip the vessel once
- If the blood is still liquid (unclotted) and runs out, the patient has hypofibrinogenemia ("incoagulable blood") as a result of venom-induced consumption coagulopathy

CHAPTER 114

# Paracetamol Poisoning

**TABLE 1:** Common brand names of paracetamol.

| *Preparation* | *Common brand names* |
|---|---|
| Immediate release | Paracetamol, Crocin, Dolo, Metacin, Pyrigesic |
| Modified release | Paracetamol SR, Dolowin, Suminat |

**TABLE 2:** Clinical features of paracetamol poisoning based on timing of ingestion.

| | *Timing* | *Clinical features* |
|---|---|---|
| Stage 1 | <24 hours | Asymptomatic or mild nausea, vomiting, lethargy<br>LFT normal |
| Stage 2 | 24–72 hours | Tender hepatomegaly<br>AST/ALT elevated |
| Stage 3 | 72–96 hours | Elevated AST/ALT, Hyperammonemia Hepatic encephalopathy, Coagulopathy, Lactic acidosis, Hyperbilirubinemia, Renal failure |
| Stage 4 | 4 days to 2 weeks | Recovery phase |

**TABLE 3:** N acetyl cysteine (NAC) dosing.

| *NAC regimen* | *Intravenous dosing* | *Oral dosing* |
|---|---|---|
| Loading dose | 150 mg/kg IV over 60 minutes | 140 mg/kg per oral |
| Maintenance dose | 50 mg/kg IV over 4 hours | 70 mg/kg per oral every 4 hours |
| | 100 mg/Kg IV over 16 hours | |

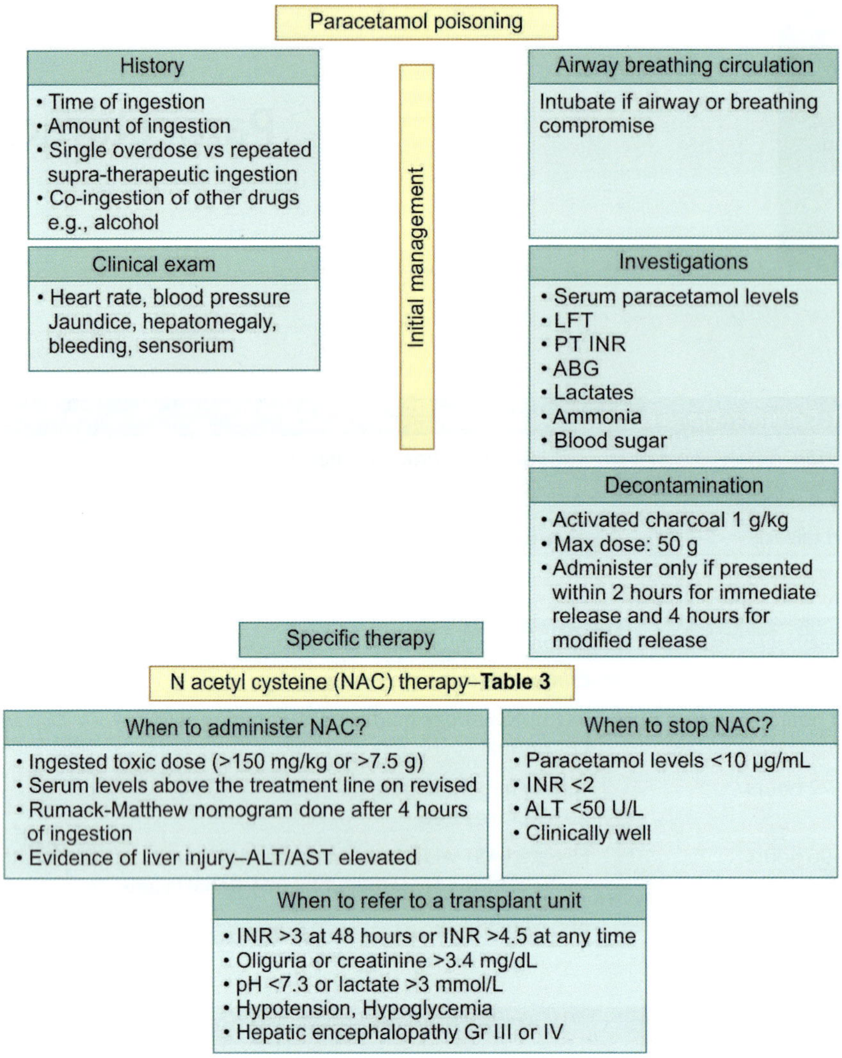

Paracetamol poisoning

Initial management

**History**
- Time of ingestion
- Amount of ingestion
- Single overdose vs repeated supra-therapeutic ingestion
- Co-ingestion of other drugs e.g., alcohol

**Clinical exam**
- Heart rate, blood pressure Jaundice, hepatomegaly, bleeding, sensorium

**Airway breathing circulation**

Intubate if airway or breathing compromise

**Investigations**
- Serum paracetamol levels
- LFT
- PT INR
- ABG
- Lactates
- Ammonia
- Blood sugar

**Decontamination**
- Activated charcoal 1 g/kg
- Max dose: 50 g
- Administer only if presented within 2 hours for immediate release and 4 hours for modified release

Specific therapy

N acetyl cysteine (NAC) therapy–**Table 3**

**When to administer NAC?**
- Ingested toxic dose (>150 mg/kg or >7.5 g)
- Serum levels above the treatment line on revised
- Rumack-Matthew nomogram done after 4 hours of ingestion
- Evidence of liver injury–ALT/AST elevated

**When to stop NAC?**
- Paracetamol levels <10 μg/mL
- INR <2
- ALT <50 U/L
- Clinically well

**When to refer to a transplant unit**
- INR >3 at 48 hours or INR >4.5 at any time
- Oliguria or creatinine >3.4 mg/dL
- pH <7.3 or lactate >3 mmol/L
- Hypotension, Hypoglycemia
- Hepatic encephalopathy Gr III or IV

**Fig. 1:** Acute paracetamol poisoning—approach.

*Note:* Revised Rumack Matthew nomogram is not reliable in repeated supratherapeutic ingestion

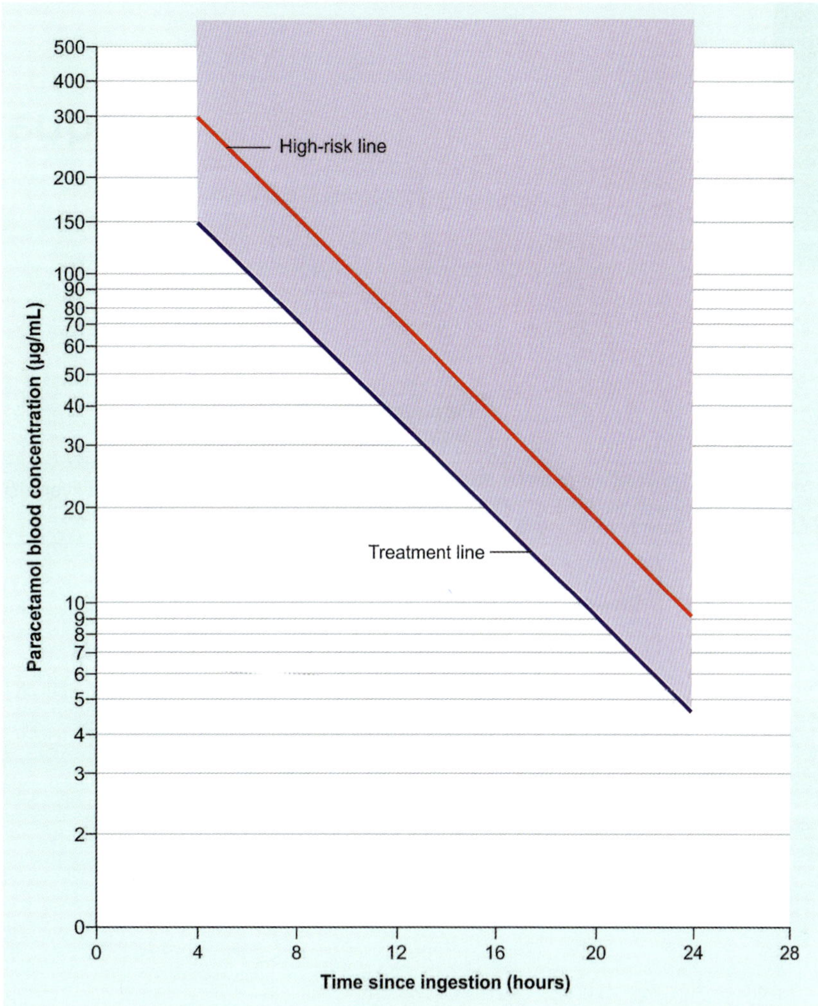


**Fig. 2:** Revised Rumack-Matthew nomogram for the acute ingestion of paracetamol.

CHAPTER 115

# Paraquat Poisoning

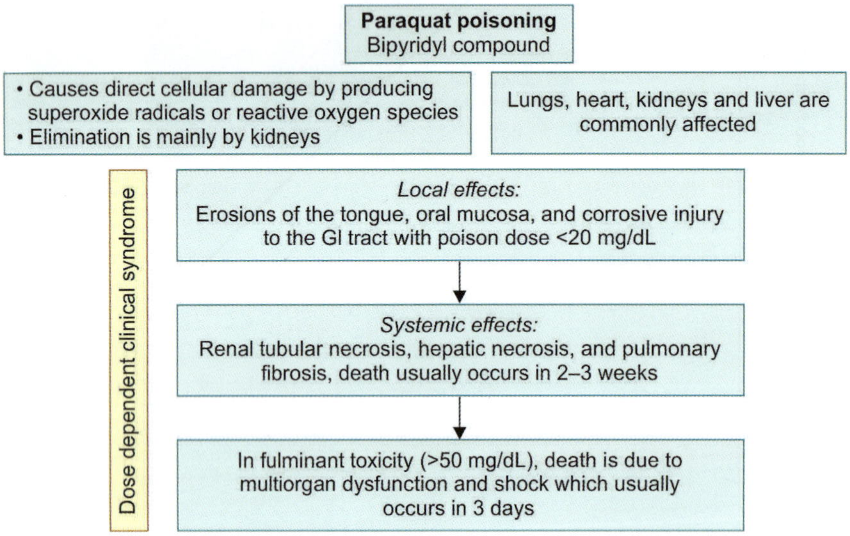

**Paraquat poisoning**
Bipyridyl compound

- Causes direct cellular damage by producing superoxide radicals or reactive oxygen species
- Elimination is mainly by kidneys

Lungs, heart, kidneys and liver are commonly affected

Dose dependent clinical syndrome

*Local effects:*
Erosions of the tongue, oral mucosa, and corrosive injury to the GI tract with poison dose <20 mg/dL

↓

*Systemic effects:*
Renal tubular necrosis, hepatic necrosis, and pulmonary fibrosis, death usually occurs in 2–3 weeks

↓

In fulminant toxicity (>50 mg/dL), death is due to multiorgan dysfunction and shock which usually occurs in 3 days

## MANAGEMENT IN PARAQUAT POISONING

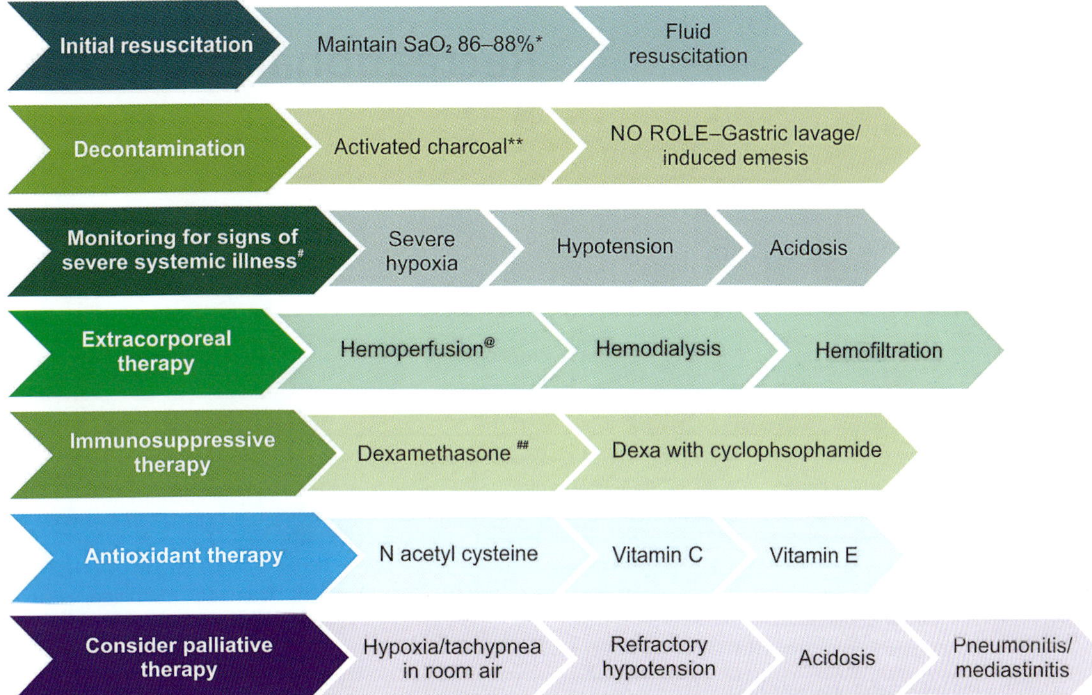


*Note:* There is no definitive antidote or beneficial cocktail of therapy established in Paraquat poisoning.

*OXYGEN supplementation can exacerbate the cellular damage

**Activated charcoal (1 g/kg in water; maximum dose 50 g) - beneficial when given within 2 hours of consumption

#Indicates poor prognosis

@For 4 hours, within 4 hours of consumption and no evidence of systemic effects of poisoning

##Inj Dexamethasone 8 mg IV q8 hours for the first 72 hours

CHAPTER 116

# Recreational Drug Overdose

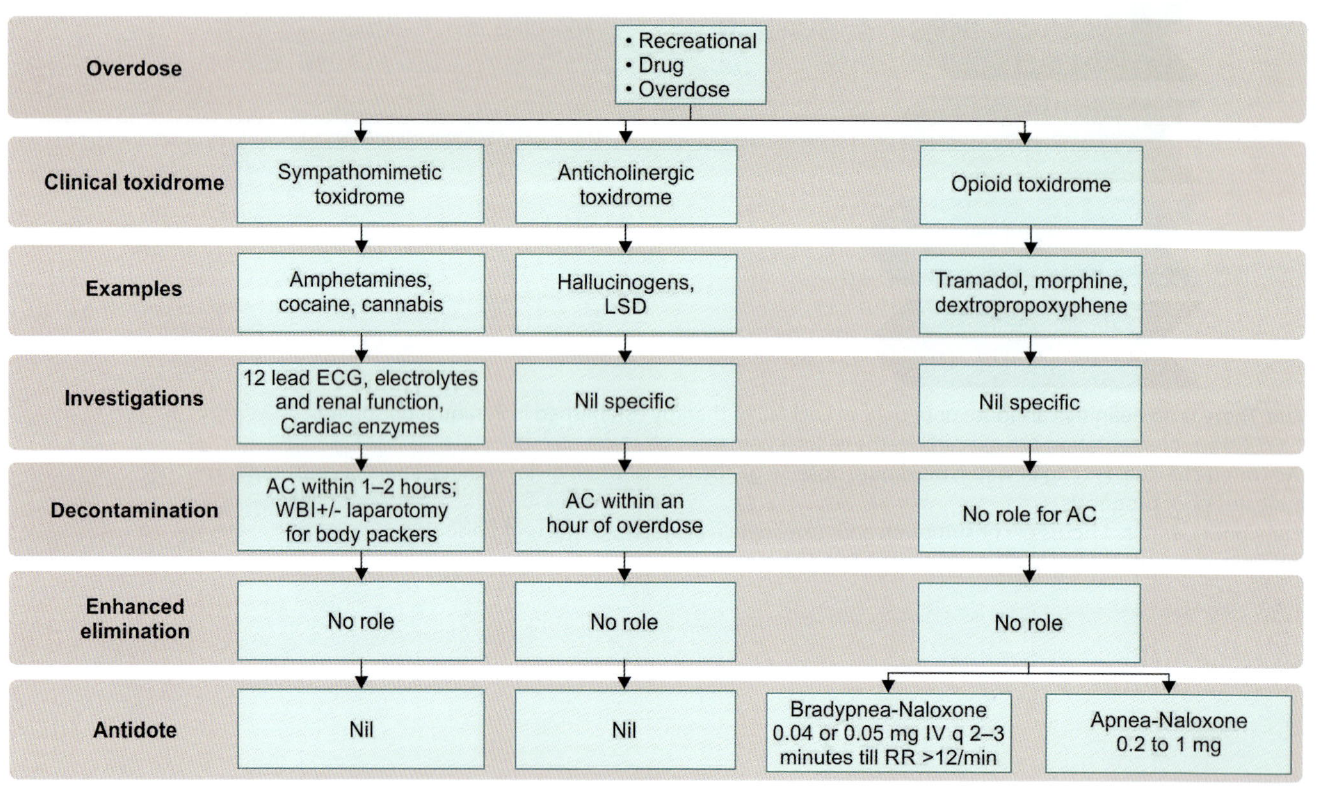


***Important points to consider:***

| *Sympathomimetic overdose* | *Anticholinergic toxidrome* | *Opioid overdose* |
|---|---|---|
| • Agitation control with Benzodiazepines, dexmedetomidine; AVOID haloperidol<br>• Hypertension control with nitrates and phentolamine; AVOID beta blockers as there can be uninhibited alpha agonist action<br>• Seizure control with Benzodiazepines; AVOID phenytoin<br>• Temperature management with active cooling measures | • Benzodiazepines for severe agitation or anxiety<br>• Haloperidol for hallucinations | • Naloxone infusion every hour at 2/3rd the dose required to re-instate breathing may be needed in apneic patients<br>• In the setting of bradypnea<br>• Consider alternate diagnosis if no improvement with 5 mg<br>• Acute respiratory distress syndrome secondary to opiates<br>• Use small doses of naloxone as rapid precipitation of withdrawal in the setting of elevated $PCO_2$ is associated with a surge in catecholamine concentrations, thereby increasing afterload, which causes interstitial edema followed by alveolar filling |

# PART 11

# SKIN AND SOFT TISSUE

***Editor:*** V Dedeepiya Devaprasad

***Associate Editors:*** Sandeep Shyamsundar, A Karthick Ramalingam

CHAPTER 117

# Lupus Flare

## INTRODUCTION

Systemic lupus erythematosus (SLE) is a chronic autoimmune disorder characterized by a broad spectrum of symptoms and manifestations, encompassing almost all organs and tissues. Its clinical course has remissions and exacerbations.

In 2011, a working party organized by the Lupus Foundation of America defined a flare in a lupus patient as: "a measurable increase in disease activity in one or more organ systems involving new or worse clinical signs and symptoms and/or laboratory measurements. It must be considered clinically significant by the assessor and usually there would be at least consideration of a change or an increase in treatment".

Validated instruments to assess clinical disease activity in SLE are enlisted in **Table 1**.

**TABLE 1:** Validated instruments to assess clinical disease activity in SLE.

| *SLEDAI* | *BILAG* | *PGA* |
|---|---|---|
| Global index of 24 weighted variables* | • Global index of 97 variables across 8 organ domains<br>• Each domain scored in an ordinal scale (A to E)<br>• Anchored to intention to treat—nonbinding recommendation for each domain letter grade | • Visual analog scale (VAS) of global disease activity scored by the clinician<br>• 3-inch VAS with anchors at mild, moderate and severe disease |
| Modifications include SELENA-SLEDAI, SLEDAI-2K | BILAG 2004 modifications (9 domains**, glossary modifications) | Normalized to 100 mm VAS in clinical trials |
| Summed to total score 0–105 | Modifications allow summation of domain scores | |
| Activity in preceding 30 days | Activity in the preceding 4 weeks | Activity in the preceding month |
| Each 30-day period scored independently of previous disease activity | *Transitional index:* Each manifestation must be compared to previous 4 weeks—absent, same, improving, worse or new | Each monthly period scored independently of previous disease activity |
| Extensively used and validated | Most comprehensive SLE disease activity instrument to date | Simple and intuitive |

*Contd...*

*Contd...*

| ***SLEDAI*** | ***BILAG*** | ***PGA*** |
|---|---|---|
| *Limitations:* | | |
| • Cannot capture partial worsening or improvement of existing manifestations—poorly sensitive to change<br>• Heavily influenced by renal disease<br>• Some SLE features not scored, others have too low weights<br>• Broad range of disease activity within certain parameters (e.g., rash, vasculitis, arthritis) | • Extensive glossary and scoring rules for each manifestation and organ domain<br>• Scoring time consuming and effort intense, may limit applicability and compromise accuracy<br>• Broad range of disease activity within certain manifestations (e.g., moderate arthritis) | • Increased inter and intra-rater variability<br>• Compression of broad spectrum of disease in small region of the scale problematic, especially when multiple organs involved |

*Seizures, psychosis, organic brain syndrome, visual disturbance, cranial nerve disorder, lupus headache, CVA, vasculitis, arthritis, myositis, urinary casts, hematuria, proteinuria, pyuria, rash, alopecia, mucosal ulcers, pleurisy, pericarditis, low complement, increased DNA binding, fever, thrombocytopenia, leukopenia

**Constitutional, mucocutaneous, neuropsychiatric, musculoskeletal, cardiopulmonary, gastrointestinal, ophthalmic, renal, hematologic

Definitions of SLE flares according to existing validated indices are given in **Table 2**.

**TABLE 2:** Definitions of SLE flares according to existing validated indices.

| | |
|---|---|
| PGA | *Mild/moderate:* Increase by ≥1.0 compared with the previous visit<br>*Severe:* Increase by ≥1.0 to ≥2.5 |
| SLEDAI | *Mild/moderate:* Increase by >3<br>*Severe:* Increase by >10 |
| SFI | *Mild/moderate:* (1) Increase of SLEDAI by ≥3 points; and/or (2) new/worse skin, stomatitis, serositis, arthritis, fever; and/or (3) increase in PGA by ≥1.0; and/or (4) treatment intensification: increase in prednisone <0.5 mg/kg or added NSAIDs or hydroxychloroquine. Sever: (1) Increase of SLEDAI by >12; and/or (2) new/worse CNS involvement, vasculitis, glomerulonephritis, myositis, platelet counts 0.5 mg/kg; and/or (3) need for hospitalization due to SLE; and/or (4) any manifestation requiring prednisone >0.5 mg/kg or new immunosuppressive therapy; and/or (4) increase in PGA to >2.5 |
| BILAG | *Moderate:* Increase from C, D or E to B score in any system<br>*Severe:* Increase to A score in any system |
| SLAM | Increase by ≥3 |
| LAI | Increase by >0.26 |

(BILAG: British Isles Lupus Assessment Group; CNS: central nervous system; NSAID: nonsteroidal anti-inflammatory drugs; LAI: Lupus Activity Index; PGA: Physician Global Assessment; SLEDAI: SLE Disease Activity Index; SFI: SELENA-SLEDAI Flare Index; SLAM: SLE activity measure)

Risk factors for disease flares in patients with SLE are given in **Box 1**.

**BOX 1:** Risk factors for disease flares in patients with SLE.

- African–American race
- Male gender
- Age of SLE onset ≤25 years
- Major organ disease (major cytopenias, neuropsychiatric lupus, nephritis, and vasculitis)
- Persistent clinical disease activity
- Immunological activity (low serum C3/C4 and high anti-dsDNA)
- Poor compliance to treatment
- No use or discontinuation of hydroxychloroquine
- Quick tapering or withdrawal of maintenance immunosuppressive treatment
- Serum BLyS levels ≥2 ng/mL

Flare mimics are listed in **Box 2**.

**BOX 2:** Flare mimics.

- Fibromyalgia
- Drug reaction
- Infection
- Metabolic (e.g., iron deficiency)
- Endocrine disorder
- Malignancy

## DIFFERENTIATION BETWEEN INFECTION AND SLE FLARE IN SLE PATIENT

| *Findings favoring infection* | *Findings favoring SLE* |
|---|---|
| • Fever with chills<br>• Fever persists despite treatment with prednisone >40 mg/day<br>• Leukocytosis and/or neutrophilia (especially in the absence of steroid therapy), increased numbers of band forms or metamyelocytes on peripheral blood smear, concomitant immunosuppressive treatment | Leukopenia (not explained by cytotoxic therapy), normal or only slightly increased C-reactive protein (CRP), coexisting serological activity (low complement factors C3/C4, elevated anti-DNA titers) |

## BIOMARKERS INTO DIFFERENTIATE INFECTION AND LUPUS FLARE

- *C-reactive protein:* Low diagnostic specificity
- Serum procalcitonin (PCT)
  - Low serum PCT levels (<0.17 ng/mL) had >90% negative predictive value for ruling out bacterial infection in SLE patients
  - A review of the literature published until 2014 indicated that raised PCT levels ≥0.5 µg/L should strongly suggest bacterial infection in the context of SLE.
- Delta neutrophil index (DNI) reflects the fraction of peripheral blood immature granulocytes, to differentiate infection from SLE flare.

DNI value >2.8% had 54% sensitivity and 88% specificity for diagnosing infection in febrile SLE patients

All the above-mentioned biomarkers require further standardization and validation

## SEROLOGICAL TESTS IN THE DIAGNOSIS OF LUPUS FLARE

- *Anti-ds DNA:* Patients with surges in anti-dsDNA titers should be monitored closely for the early recognition of objective features of active lupus. An increase in anti-dsDNA serum levels some weeks before an exacerbation followed by a moderate decrease at the time of the flare has also been described, especially in patients with lupus nephritis. However, not all lupus exacerbations are accompanied by changes in anti-dsDNA titres.
- *Antibodies to complement 1q (anti-C1q)* have also been described as indicators of disease activity, especially nephritis, in SLE. Additional benefit noted in assessing titers of anti-C1q in conjunction with anti-dsDNA for diagnosing renal flares. At present, the clinical use of anti-C1q is limited due to lack of standardization of the ELISA assay and its cut-off levels.
- *Serum C4 (but not C3) levels* tend to decrease approximately two months prior to clinical appearance of a renal flare, reflecting the early activation of the classical complement pathway. *Serum C3 levels have been reported to be abnormally low around the time of flare at a higher prevalence compared to serum C4.*
  - Together, serum C3 levels may be more sensitive and specific than C4 to diagnose an SLE flare, which has led to the suggestion of measuring only C3 - rather than both C3 and C4 - in monitoring disease activity.
- *Antibodies to the ribosomal P proteins* (anti-P) have been associated with specific organ activity in SLE, namely renal, liver and central nervous system (CNS) disease, particularly psychosis. However, the frequency in which they occur is rather low and ranges 6–20% in different ethnic groups.

## PREVENTION OF LUPUS FLARE

- *Hydroxychloroquine:* Patients with inactive disease who continued treatment with hydroxychloroquine had 74% lower risk for developing severe flares compared to those who discontinued the drug.

  A similar protective effect been demonstrated in patients with stable lupus nephritis on maintenance treatment.

  Apart from its immunomodulatory properties, hydroxychloroquine seem to exhibit also anti-thrombotic and anti-lipidemic effects. These effects, along with the long-term safety of the drug, have led to the suggestion of continuing it lifelong in patients with SLE, including during the period of pregnancy and lactation.
- *Belimumab* has emerged as a biologic agent capable of stabilizing SLE activity. When added to the conventional treatment in patients with active moderate-to-severe lupus, belimumab leads to significantly reduced (by 36%) risk of major flare-ups over a period of one year.
- *Mycophenolate mofetil* may be preferred as maintenance regimen in patients with more severe (clinically or histologically) lupus nephritis, black or Hispanic ethnicity, or when mycophenolate was used as induction regimen.

- Discontinuation or switching from mycophenolate to less potent agents such as azathioprine or calcineurin inhibitors, earlier than 18–24 months after attaining renal response, carries almost 2-fold increased risk for subsequent flare. Consequently, although the optimal duration of maintenance therapy in SLE has not been definitely established, we generally recommend a period of at least 2–3 years (5–7 years in lupus nephritis).

## SUGGESTED READING

1. Castrejón I, Tani C, Jolly M, Huang A, Mosca M. Indices to assess patients with systemic lupus erythematosus in clinical trials, long-term observational studies, and clinical care. Clin Exp Rheumatol. 2014;32(5 Suppl 85):S85-95.
2. Costedoat-Chalumeau N, Dunogué B, Morel N, Le Guern V, Guettrot-Imbert G. Hydroxychloroquine: A multifaceted treatment in lupus. Presse Med. 2014;43(6 Pt 2):e167-80.
3. Manzi S, Sanchez-Guerrero J, Merrill J T, Furie R, Gladman D, Navarra S V, et al. Effects of belimumab, a B lymphocyte stimulator-specific inhibitor, on disease activity across multiple organ domains in patients with systemic lupus erythematosus: combined results from two phase III trials. Ann Rheum Dis. 2012;71(11):1833-8.
4. McElhone K, Abbott J, Hurley M, Burnell J, Lanyon P, Rahman A, et al. Flares in patients with systemic lupus erythematosus. Rheumatology (Oxford). 2021;60(7):3262-7.
5. Tamirou F, D'Cruz D, Sangle S, Remy P, Vasconcelos C, Fiehn C, et al. Long-term follow-up of the MAINTAIN Nephritis Trial, comparing azathioprine and mycophenolate mofetil as maintenance therapy of lupus nephritis. Ann Rheum Dis. 2016;75(3):526-31.
6. Thanou A, Jupe E, Purushothaman M, Niewold TB, Munroe ME. Clinical disease activity and flare in SLE: Current concepts and novel biomarkers. J Autoimmun. 2021;119:102615.

CHAPTER 118

# Catastrophic Antiphospholipid Syndrome

## INTRODUCTION

Antiphospholipid syndrome (APS) is a systemic autoimmune disease characterized by thrombotic or obstetric events in patients who have persistent antiphospholipid antibodies (APLA), which include lupus anticoagulant (LA), anti-2-glycoprotein I (anti-2GPI), and/or anticardiolipin antibodies (aCL).

It can cause venous, arterial, or microvascular thrombosis in the deep veins of the lower limbs, as well as in cerebral arterial circulation. Although uncommon, thrombosis can occur in hepatic veins, visceral veins, or the cerebral venous circulation. Primary APS can develop alone or together with other autoimmune diseases, especially systemic lupus erythematosus (SLE).

Summary of the 2023 ACR/EULAR APS classification criteria is given in **Box 1**.

**BOX 1:** Summary of the 2023 ACR/EULAR APS classification criteria.

*Clinical criteria:*
- *Domain 1—macrovascular:* Venous thromboembolism
- *Domain 2—macrovascular:* Arterial thrombosis
- Domain 3—microvascular
  - *Suspected:* Livedo racemosa, livedoid vasculopathy lesions, antiphospholipid antibody (aPL) nephropathy, pulmonary hemorrhage
  - *Established:* Livedoid vasculopathy, aPL nephropathy, Pulmonary hemorrhage, Myocardial disease, Adrenal hemorrhage or microthrombosis
- *Domain 4—obstetric:* Prefetal death, fetal death, preeclampsia with severe features, central nervous system dysfunction, placental insufficiency with severe features
- *Domain 5—cardiac valve:* Valve thickening and valve vegetation
- *Domain 6—Hematology:* Thrombocytopenia

*Laboratory criteria:* Domain 7—aPL test by coagulation-based functional assay

*Clinical criteria:* Domain 8—aPL test by solid phase-based assay

Catastrophic APS (CAPS) is a life-threatening variant of APS characterized by the rapid onset of thrombotic events involving multiple organ systems, including large vessels and microvascular involvement. Approximately 1% of patients with APS develop the severe clinical picture of CAPS.

## CRITERIA FOR DIAGNOSIS OF CATASTROPHIC ANTIPHOSPHOLIPID SYNDROME

- Evidence of involvement of three or more organs, systems and/or tissues
- Development of manifestations simultaneously or in less than a week
- Confirmation by histopathology of small vessel occlusion in at least one organ or tissue
- Laboratory confirmation of the presence of antiphospholipid antibodies (lupus anticoagulant and/or anticardiolipin antibodies)

*Definite catastrophic APS*
- All four criteria

*Probable catastrophic APS*
- All four criteria, except for only two organs, systems and/or tissues involvement
- All four criteria, except for the absence of laboratory confirmation at least six weeks apart due to the early death of a patient never tested for aPL before the catastrophic APS
- 1, 2, and 4
- 1, 3, and 4 and the development of a third event in more than a week but less than a month, despite anticoagulation

## PATHOGENIC MECHANISMS

| | |
|---|---|
| *Cellular activation* | • Endothelial cell activation<br>• Immune cell activation<br>• Platelet activation |
| *Inhibition of anticoagulants* | • Inhibition of the protein C pathway<br>• Disruption of annexin A5 shield |

*Contd...*

*Contd...*

| | |
|---|---|
| *Inhibition of fibrinolysis* | • Inhibition of plasminogen activator inhibitor-1B<br>• Blocking of β2-glycoprotein I<br>• Blocking of annexin A2 |
| *Complement activation* | • Endothelial cell activation by C5a and MAC<br>• Immune cell activation by C5a<br>• Platelet activation by C3a<br>• MAC inhibition of fibrinolysis by C5a |

## PRECIPITATING FACTORS

| | |
|---|---|
| Infection | • Respiratory<br>• Urinary tract<br>• Skin<br>• Gastrointestinal tract |
| Surgery or trauma | |
| Malignancy | Hodgkin's and non-Hodgkin's lymphoma, acute lymphocytic leukemia, angiocentric lymphoma, and chronic myelocytic lymphoma<br>*Solid tumors:* Most often lung or colon adenocarcinoma |
| Anticoagulation withdrawal, or subtherapeutic anti-coagulation | |
| Pregnancy complications or initiation of oral contraception | • HELLP syndrome<br>• Placental infarction<br>• Pelvic thrombosis |
| Medications | |
| Flare of underlying autoimmune disease | |

## CLINICAL MANIFESTATIONS

| | |
|---|---|
| Renal involvement | • Acute kidney injury proteinuria hematuria occur<br>• *Histopathology:* Thrombotic microangiopathy and proliferative glomerulonephritis |
| Respiratory involvement | • ARDS due to pneumonia and diffuse alveolar hemorrhage<br>• Pulmonary embolism |
| Neurologic involvement | Encephalopathy, seizures, stroke, and cerebral venous occlusion |
| Cardiac involvement | • Myocardial infarction<br>• Myocarditis<br>• Takotsubo cardiomyopathy<br>• Libman–Sacks endocarditis |
| Skin manifestations | • Livedo reticularis<br>• Cutaneous necrosis with digital gangrene<br>• Purpura and splinter hemorrhages |
| Gastrointestinal | • Small and large bowel infarction<br>• Pancreatitis<br>• Budd–Chiari syndrome |
| Others | Infarction of adrenals, testes, ovary, and prostate |

## LABORATORY INVESTIGATION OF POSSIBLE CATASTROPHIC ANTIPHOSPHOLIPID SYNDROME

- Electrolytes
- Complete blood count, with blood smear examination for schistocytes
- Urinalysis and spot urine protein/creatinine ratio
- Coagulation studies (including INR, PTT, and D-dimer)
- Lactate dehydrogenase (LDH) and haptoglobin
- Evaluation for antiphospholipid syndrome (if not already diagnosed):
    - Anti-cardiolipin IgG and IgM
    - Anti-beta-2-glycoprotein type I IgG and IgM
    - *Evaluation for lupus anticoagulant:* Dilute Russell viper venom test
    - Antinuclear Antibody (ANA)

## DIFFERENTIAL DIAGNOSIS

- Microangiopathic hemolytic anemia:
    - Thrombotic thrombocytopenic purpura (TTP)
    - Hemolytic uremic syndrome (HUS) and atypical HUS
    - Heparin induced thrombocytopenia (HIT)
    - Purpura fulminans
    - Medication-related thrombotic microangiopathy
    - Malignant hypertension
    - Disseminated malignancy
- Sepsis
- Adrenal insufficiency (*Note:* CAPS may *cause* adrenal insufficiency)
- Endocarditis
- Vasculitis
- Cholesterol emboli

## TREATMENT

### General Measures

- Identify and treat any underlying cause, for example, treat any underlying infection.
- Aggressive antihypertensive therapy (uncontrolled hypertension may worsen intravascular hemolysis)
- Avoid intravascular catheters as they can undergo thrombosis

### Heparin Anticoagulation

- Heparin is probably the most important treatment (correlating most strongly with good outcomes in retrospective series). Heparin may exert some anti-inflammatory and complement-inhibitory effects).
- Heparin infusion is used initially, although low molecular weight heparin also seems to work.
    - Ideally, heparin infusions should be titrated against anti-Xa level (because many patients will have lupus anticoagulant, which artificially increases the PTT).
- Anticoagulant therapy (direct oral anticoagulants NOT recommended) vitamin K antagonist with INR target 2–3 Antiaggregation low-dose aspirin (100 mg/day)
- Glucocorticoids methylprednisolone, 0.5–1 g intravenously, once daily for three or more days, followed by oral or parenteral therapy with the equivalent of 1 mg/kg prednisone per day with tapering initiated once the patient improves clinically.
- Therapeutic plasmapheresis exchanges are typically performed once daily for five days (longer in patients with refractory disease).
- Intravenous immunoglobulin a typical dose is between 400 mg per kg per day for 5 days.
- Rituximab (a monoclonal antibody against the B-cell antigen CD20) 375 mg/$m^2$ once a week for four weeks, or 500–1,000 mg administered twice, at intervals of 7 or 14 days
- Studies suggest the use of eculizumab at a dose of 900 mg per week for 4 weeks, followed by 1,200 mg once every two weeks is effective.

## CATASTROPHIC ANTIPHOSPHOLIPID SYNDROME IN PREGNANCY

- Can occur in third trimester or in puerperium
- Clinical signs of pregnancy can include dyspnea, elevated blood pressure, abdominal discomfort, convulsions, chest pain, proteinuria, and pulmonary embolism. Fetal morbidities, such as premature birth, growth restriction, or mortality, are associated with placental insufficiency.
- DD-HELLP syndrome, acute fatty liver of pregnancy, TTP
- *Management:* Anticoagulants, plasmapheresis, corticosteroids, IVIG
- *Refractory cases:* Hydroxychloroquine and eculizumab

## ALGORITHM FOR CATASTROPHIC ANTIPHOSPHOLIPID SYNDROME

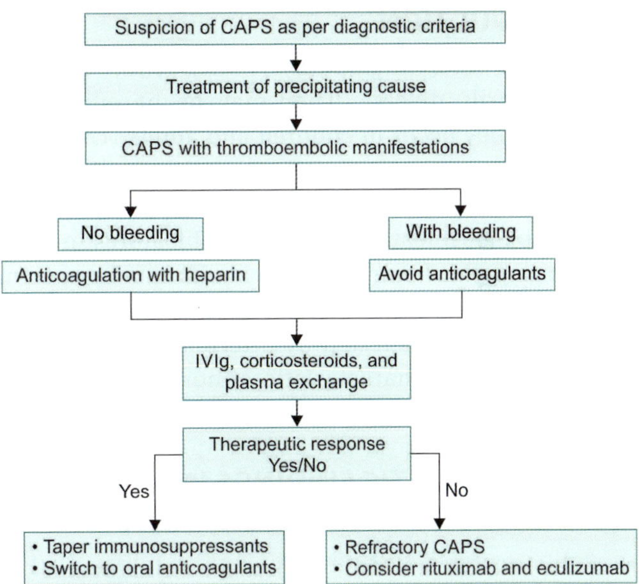


## SUGGESTED READING


1. Barbhaiya M, Zuily S, Naden R, Hendry A, Manneville F, Amigo MC, et al; ACR/EULAR APS Classification Criteria Collaborators. The 2023 ACR/EULAR Antiphospholipid Syndrome Classification Criteria. Arthritis Rheumatol. 2023;75(10):1687-702.
2. Cervera R, Rodríguez-Pintó I, Espinosa G. The diagnosis and clinical management of the catastrophic antiphospholipid syndrome: A comprehensive review. J Autoimmun. 2018; 92:1-11.
3. Kazzaz NM, McCune WJ, Knight JS. Treatment of catastrophic antiphospholipid syndrome. Curr Opin Rheumatol. 2016;28(3):218-27.
4. Legault K, Schunemann H, Hillis C, Yeung C, Akl EA, Carrier M, et al. McMaster RARE-Bestpractices clinical practice guideline on diagnosis and management of the catastrophic antiphospholipid syndrome. J Thromb Haemost. 2018;16(8):1656-64.
5. Siniscalchi C, Basaglia M, Riva M, Meschi M, Meschi T, Castaldo G, et al. Catastrophic antiphospholipid syndrome: A review. Immuno. 2024;4(1):1-13.

CHAPTER 119

# TTP/HUS/MAHA

## INTRODUCTION

Thrombotic microangiopathy (TMA) syndromes are extraordinarily diverse. They may be hereditary or acquired. They occur in children and adults. The onset can be sudden or gradual. Despite their diversity, TMA syndromes are united by common, defining clinical and pathological features. The clinical features include microangiopathic hemolytic anemia, thrombocytopenia, and organ injury. The pathological features are vascular damage that is manifested by arteriolar and capillary thrombosis with characteristic abnormalities in the endothelium and vessel wall.

## KEY DIAGNOSTIC FINDINGS IN ACUTE THROMBOTIC MICROANGIOPATHY

- Schistocytes within the peripheral blood at a pathological level
- Absence of an obvious alternative explanation for schistocytes
- Elevated serum LDH
- Thrombocytopenia
- Reduced serum haptoglobin
- Ischemic tissue damage due to microvascular occlusion; organs involved may include the kidney, brain, heart, lungs, gut, or skin. Different microangiopathies tend to involve different organs.
  - Acute kidney injury (AKI) may also result from plasma-free hemoglobin.

## PRIMARY THROMBOTIC MICROANGIOPATHY SYNDROMES

| *Hereditary disorders* | *Acquired disorders* |
|---|---|
| ADAMTS13 deficiency-mediated TMA (TTP) | ADAMTS13 deficiency-mediated TMA ( TTP) |
| Complement-mediated TMA | Shiga toxin–mediated TMA (ST-HUS) |
| Metabolism-mediated TMA | Drug-mediated TMA (immune reaction) |
| Coagulation-mediated TMA | Complement-mediated TMA |

**Likely causes of microangiopathic hemolytic anemia and thrombocytopenia according to presenting findings**

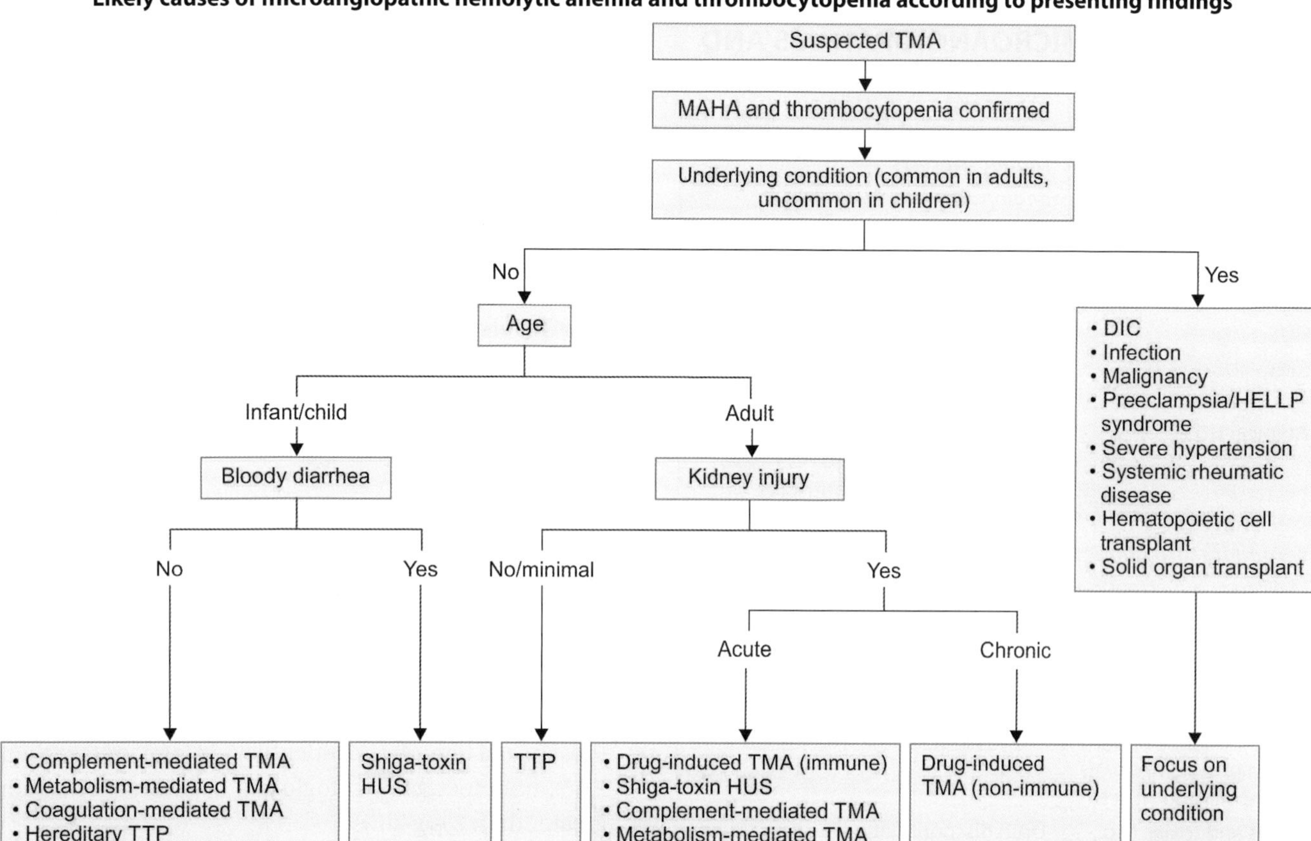


- CBC with differential
- Hemolysis labs:
  - Manual blood smear
  - Lactate dehydrogenase (LDH)
  - Haptoglobin
  - Direct antiglobulin test (direct Coombs)
- DIC labs:
  - INR
  - PTT
  - Fibrinogen
  - D-dimer
- Organ damage evaluation:
  - Liver function tests (including indirect bilirubin)
  - Troponin and ECG
  - Urinalysis and microscopic examination of the urine sediment
- Pregnancy testing as appropriate
- Infectious workup:
  - Blood cultures
  - Other relevant infectious evaluation (e.g., HIV testing and urine pneumococcus antigen)
- ADAMTS13 antigen level and anti-ADAMTS13 antibodies or inhibitor (depending on which tests are available)
- Antinuclear antibodies (ANA).
- Stool PCR analysis for Shiga-toxin genes, stool culture, and/or bioassay of stool for Shiga toxin (depending on the local availability of these tests)
- Other studies to consider:
  - Skin biopsy if there are worrisome skin lesions
  - Renal biopsy may help confirm the diagnosis of TMA and exclude other causes of renal failure
  - *B12 deficiency is suspected:* B12 level.
  - *CAPS is suspected:* Anticardiolipin antibody (IgG and IgM), anti-beta-2-glycoprotein type I (IgG and IgM), and dilute Russell viper venom time

## DIFFERENTIAL DIAGNOSES OF THROMBOTIC MICROANGIOPATHIES AND DIAGNOSTIC INVESTIGATIONS

| ***Differential diagnoses*** | ***Diagnostic tests*** |
|---|---|
| ***Primary thrombotic microangiopathy*** | |
| *TTP* | |
| Congenital TTP | Mutations of *ADAMTS13* gene |
| Acquired TTP | ADAMTS13 activity and inhibitor |
| HUS | |
| STEC-HUS | PCR for the Shiga toxin, or stool culture for STEC or *Shigella* |
| Atypical HUS | Genetic mutations in complement regulatory proteins (e.g., CFH, CFI, MCP, C3, CFB, THBD); anti-CFH autoantibodies |
| ***Secondary thrombotic microangiopathy*** | |
| Malignant hypertension | • Blood pressure and renal function<br>• Investigation for other causes of thrombotic microangiopathy associated with hypertension |
| Pregnancy-associated thrombotic microangiopathy, preeclampsia/eclampsia, and HELLP | • Pregnancy testing<br>• Elevated liver transaminase levels |
| Drugs and toxins (e.g., calcineurin inhibitors, quinine, and ticlopidine) | Drug discontinuation |
| Infections (e.g., influenza, HIV, Epstein–Barr virus, and parvovirus) | Infection-specific testing |
| Cancer | Imaging and other investigations including paraneoplastic syndromes |
| Autoimmune disease (e.g., systemic lupus erythematosus) | Autoimmune serologic markers, clinical symptoms or signs as per diagnostic criteria |
| Transplantation (e.g., solid organ and bone marrow) | Consider graft-versus-host disease, graft rejection, conditioning regimen, antirejection therapy |
| Disseminated intravascular coagulation | • Abnormal coagulation testing, reduced fibrinogen<br>• Assess for underlying causes (e.g., sepsis, malignancy) |
| Metabolic (e.g., cobalamin C deficiency) | Elevated serum homocysteine and serum or urine methylmalonic acid |

(C3: complement component 3; CFB: complement factor B; CFH: complement factor H; CFI: complement factor I; HELLP: hemolysis, elevated liver enzymes and low platelet count; HSCT: hematopoietic stem cell transplant; HUS: hemolytic uremic syndrome; MCP: membrane cofactor protein (CD46); PCR: polymerase chain reaction; STEC: Shiga toxin–producing *Escherichia coli*; THBD: thrombomodulin; TTP: thrombotic thrombocytopenic purpura)

## THROMBOTIC THROMBOCYTOPENIC PURPURA

Thrombotic thrombocytopenic purpura (TTP) is characterized by the pentad of fever, thrombocytopenia, hemolytic anemia, renal dysfunction, and neurologic dysfunction.

Thrombotic thrombocytopenic purpura results from either a congenital or acquired decrease/absence of the von Willebrand factor-cleaving protease ADAMTS13.

Low levels of ADAMTS13 result in microthrombi formation, which leads to end-organ ischemia and damage.

### PLASMIC SCORE

The PLASMIC score is calculated using findings on presentation and predicts the likelihood of ADAMTS13 activity being less than or equal to 10%.

The presence of peripheral schistocytes is required to apply this score. One point is given for each of the following features:

- Platelet count <30,000/μL
- Presence of hemolysis (reticulocyte count greater than 2.5%, undetectable haptoglobin, or indirect bilirubin greater than 2 mg/dL)
- Mean corpuscular volume (MCV) <90 fL
- International normalized ratio (INR) <1.5
- Creatinine <2.0 mg/dL
- Absence of cancer
- Absence of solid organ or stem cell transplant
  The score >5 suggests a high probability of TTP
  A score <5 suggests a low probability of TTP

Due to its high negative predictive value, it is recommended as a screening tool for patients who are unlikely to have TTP.

ADAMTS13 activity assays. An activity level of less than 10% confirms the diagnosis of TTP in patients with evidence of hemolysis and thrombocytopenia.

### TREATMENT

- Mainstay of treatment in TTP is plasma exchange (PEX) with high-dose corticosteroid therapy.
- The recommended volume of exchange volume (usually 40 mL/kg of body weight)/day
- Plasma repletes ADAMTS13. The treatment should be provided once daily.
- Recommended dose for corticosteroids is 1 mg/kg per day of prednisone in neurologically intact patients.

- In severely ill patients, intravenous methylprednisolone 1,000 mg as a single daily dose for three days or 125 mg two to four times daily may be more appropriate.
- Corticosteroids are continued as long as PEX is continued and subsequently tapered off based on clinical response.
- Other treatments used include splenectomy, cyclosporine, cyclophosphamide, vincristine, and rituximab.
- The addition of glucocorticoids and rituximab to PEX has been shown to decrease the required duration of therapeutic plasma exchange.
- Rituximab is an anti-CD20 monoclonal antibody with a good response rate in refractory and relapsed TTP.
- Vincristine, cyclophosphamide, and cyclosporine - used in refractory cases or when first-line therapy has failed.
- A newer agent, caplacizumab, has a high potential for the treatment of TTP. It is a humanized monoclonal antibody fragment (a bivalent, variable-domain-only fragment) that attacks the A1 section of VWF and prevents platelet adhesion.
- Caplacizumab is given as an initial intravenous dose followed by subcutaneous injections for 30 days after PEX has been stopped. This should coincide with an increase in ADAMTS13 activity to above 20%.
- Caplacizumab can increase the risk of bleeding, and clinically significant bleeding attributable to caplacizumab should warrant discontinuation of therapy and/or VWF concentrate infusion.

## BLOOD PRODUCTS TRANSFUSION

- Fresh frozen plasma if plasma exchange is going to be delayed (e.g., >6–8 hours) fluid overload to be prevented.
- *Platelets:* Giving platelets may *worsen* thrombosis and tissue ischemia., platelet administration should be avoided unless there is a clinically significant hemorrhage.
- *Red blood cell transfusion:*
  - Avoid overtransfusion, which may simply aggravate hemolysis.
  - Consider transfusion only if hemoglobin is <7 mg/dL and this is causing symptoms.
- *Folate* should be supplemented to promote endogenous hematopoiesis.

*2020 Treatment Guidelines by the International Society on Thrombosis and Hemostasis*

- For initial treatment of TTP a strong recommendation for the addition of corticosteroids to therapeutic plasma exchange (PEX) over PEX alone. No specific recommendation regarding a preferred dosage or type of corticosteroids.
- For patients with the first acute event, the panel suggested the addition of rituximab to corticosteroids and PEX.
- For patients with relapsing TTP, the panel recommended PEX, corticosteroids, and rituximab as recommended for initial treatment, with the addition of caplacizumab.
- For patients with TTP who are in remission but still have low plasma ADAMTS13 activity without any evidence of clinical signs/symptoms, they recommended using rituximab for prophylaxis.
- For patients who are pregnant and have decreased plasma ADAMTS13 activity but have no clinical signs/symptoms of TTP, the panel recommended prophylactic treatment with plasma infusion products.

## HEMOLYTIC UREMIC SYNDROME

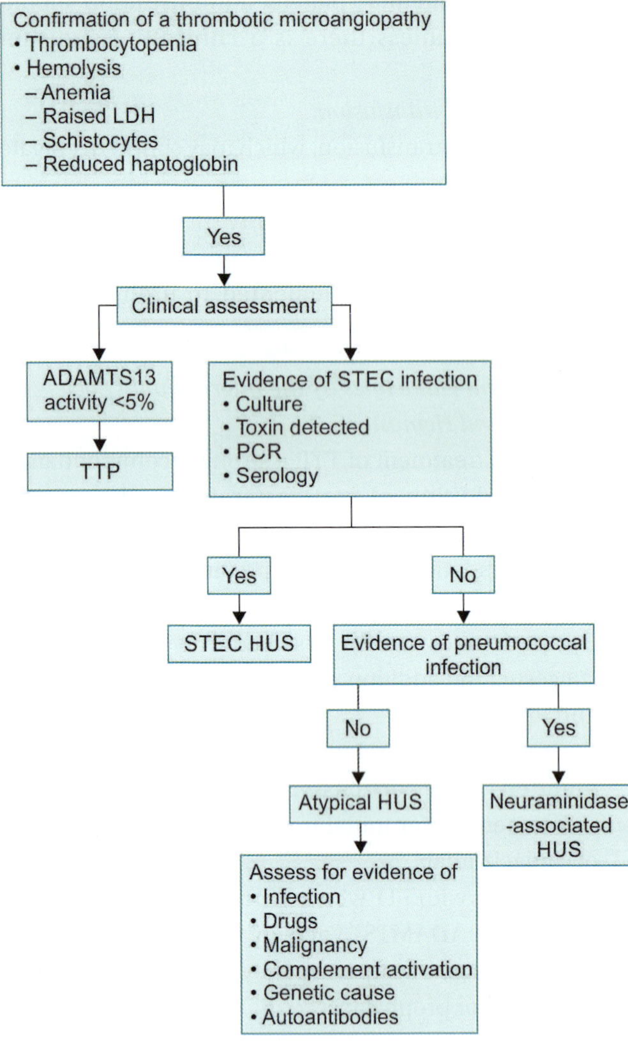


Other causes of secondary aHUS are as follows:

- Inherited vitamin $B_{12}$ (cobalamin) metabolism disorders
- DGKE mutation—Diacylglycerol kinase Epsilon
- HIV
- Influenza virus
- Autoimmune disease, for example, systemic lupus erythematosus and antiphospholipid antibody syndrome
- Drugs, for example, quinine, calcineurin inhibitors, chemotherapeutic agents, and malignant hypertension

## CLINICAL FEATURES OF STEC HUS

- Common in child younger than 5 years
- Painful diarrhea and abdominal pain
- Fever and vomiting may also be present.
- HUS symptoms include renal symptoms, such as anuria, oliguria, and fluid overload.
- Symptoms related to anemia, such as syncope, fatigue, and pallor
- Petechiae and easy bleeding may be notable due to thrombocytopenia
- Although less common in adults, an unfavorable prognosis. Notably, most HUS-related deaths occur in adults older than 60.
- In adult patients, neurological symptoms such as confusion, seizures, and coma are markedly more prevalent than in children. Older patients often also have neuropsychiatric symptoms.

## CLINICAL FEATURES OF ATYPICAL HEMOLYTIC UREMIC SYNDROME

- The initial clinical presentation as fatigue, pallor, or somnolence, which can progress to signs of AKI, such as oliguria, uremia, and fluid overload.
- If the inciting factor is *S. pneumoniae*, patients may have underlying pneumonia, empyema, or meningitis. Diarrhea, including bloody diarrhea, can also be prominent in atypical HUS.

## EVALUATION

- The diagnosis of HUS requires a high index of suspicion based on symptoms, travel history, laboratory data, and dietary history.
- A complete blood count with differential and comprehensive blood metabolic panel.
- Elevated LDH and indirect bilirubin, as well as low haptoglobin and elevated plasma hemoglobin, are diagnostic of hemolytic anemia, as are schistocytes on peripheral smear. A Coombs test should be negative, with the exception of HUS caused by *S. pneumoniae*.
- Up to 20% of patients have elevated amylase and lipase due to pancreatic damage, which may be accompanied by hyperglycemia.
- A stool sample should be collected to test for Shiga toxin whenever diarrhea is present. The results may not be positive for the Shiga toxin if it has been cleared or is avidly bound to the endothelium. If clinically indicated, testing for the presence of *S. dysenteriae* and *S. pneumoniae* should also be performed.
- Low complement levels are suggestive of, but not specific to aHUS, as typical HUS also causes immune system abnormalities.

- Patients may have hyponatremia, hyperkalemia, and other electrolyte abnormalities from acute kidney injury as the disease progresses. Genetic testing can also be sent to evaluate for genetic causes of aHUS.
- An ADAMTS13 level should be sent to rule out TTP. Abnormal coagulation studies, such as prolonged prothrombin time (PTT), activated partial thromboplastin time (aPTT), elevated D dimer, and elevated fibrin degradation products, are suggestive of DIC.

## TREATMENT/MANAGEMENT

- The management of typical HUS caused by STEC is generally supportive. Patients are often volume depleted, and less volume resuscitation has been linked to an increased need for renal replacement therapy. Blood transfusions are provided as clinically needed, and platelet transfusions should be given sparingly to avoid thrombotic complications.
- Antimotility agents and antibiotics are avoided in typical HUS caused by STEC, as they correlate with poorer outcomes, likely due to heightened Shiga toxin exposure.
- If *S. dysenteriae* or *S. pneumoniae* is present, early antibiotics are associated with improved outcomes.
- For aHUS, early treatment is crucial to avoid end-stage renal disease (ESRD) and mortality. The cornerstones of treatment for aHUS are first-line treatment with eculizumab and second-line with plasma exchange. Eculizumab is a recombinant monoclonal antibody that targets the C5 component of complement activation by preventing its cleavage; early eculizumab administration improves its effectiveness. The advent of eculizumab treatment has decreased progression to ESRD or death in children from 30 to 50% down to 9% and in adults from 60% down to 6 to 15%.
- Ravulizumab is a new C5 inhibitor approved for use in the USA in 2019 and the EU in 2020. Ravulizumab also binds to C5, preventing cleavage, and it has similar efficacy to eculizumab but with 4 times as long of a half-life. Prior to eculizumab, plasma exchange was the standard of care for HUS and is still used if eculizumab is not available or in addition if clinically indicated.

## SUGGESTED READING


1. Arnold DM, Patriquin CJ, Nazy I. Thrombotic microangiopathies: a general approach to diagnosis and management. CMAJ. 2017;189(4):E153-9.
2. Bhandari J, Rout P, Sedhai YR. Hemolytic Uremic Syndrome. In: StatPearls [Internet]. Treasure Island (FL): StatPearls Publishing; 2024. Available from: https://www.ncbi.nlm.nih.gov/books/NBK556038/ [Last accessed February, 2025].
3. George JN, Nester CM. Syndromes of thrombotic microangiopathy. N Engl J Med. 2014;371(7):654-66.
4. Kavanagh D, Raman S, Sheerin NS. Management of hemolytic uremic syndrome. F1000Prime Rep. 2014;6:119.
5. Stanley M, Killeen RB, Michalski JM. Thrombotic thrombocytopenic purpura. In: StatPearls [Internet]. Treasure Island (FL): StatPearls Publishing; 2024. Available from https://www.ncbi.nlm.nih.gov/books/NBK430721/ [Last accessed February, 2024].
6. Zheng XL, Vesely SK, Cataland SR, Coppo P, Geldziler B, Iorio A, et al. ISTH guidelines for treatment of thrombotic thrombocytopenic purpura. J Thromb Haemost. 2020; 18(10):2496-502.

CHAPTER 120

# Stevens–Johnson Syndrome: Toxic Epidermal Necrolysis

## INTRODUCTION

Stevens-Johnson syndrome (SJS) and toxic epidermal necrolysis (TEN) are rare, potentially life-threatening, severe mucocutaneous adverse reactions characterized by extensive epidermal detachment, erosion of mucosae, and severe constitutional symptoms.

## CLASSIFICATION

Classification of bullous erythema multiforme and epidermal necrolysis as proposed by Bastuji-Garin et al.

| ***Classification*** | ***Type of lesion*** | ***Distribution*** | ***Percentage of body surface area detached/ detachable*** |
|---|---|---|---|
| Bullous erythema multiforme | Typical targets | Acral | <10 |
| Overlap SJS–TEN | Spots with or without atypical targets | Generalized | >10–<30 |
| TEN with spots | Spots with or without atypical targets | Generalized | 30 and above |
| TEN without spots | Diffuse erythema, no spot or target | Generalized | >10 |

Most cases of SJS and TEN are drug-induced.

*Mycoplasma pneumoniae* and *Cytomegalovirus* infections are the next most common triggers of SJS/TEN, particularly in children.

## DRUGS ASSOCIATED WITH STEVENS-JOHNSON SYNDROME–TOXIC EPIDERMAL NECROLYSIS

| | |
|---|---|
| Sulfonamides | Cotrimoxazole, sulfadoxine, and sulfadiazine |
| Anticonvulsant | Carbamazepine, barbiturates, phenytoin, and lamotrigine |
| Antiviral | Nevirapine and abacavir |
| Antibiotics | Cephalosporins, fluoroquinolones, vancomycin, doxycycline, aminopenicillins, erythromycin, and ciprofloxacin |
| ATT | Thiacetazone, rifampicin, isoniazid, and ethambutol |
| NSAID | Piroxicam, diclofenac, ibuprofen, naproxen, celecoxib, and rofecoxib |
| Uric acid lowering agent | Allopurinol |

## DIFFERENTIAL DIAGNOSES

- Erythema multiforme major
- Staphylococcal scalded skin syndrome
- Pemphigus vulgaris, paraneoplastic pemphigus, bullous pemphigoid
- Bullous fixed drug eruption
- Drug induced linear IgA bullous dermatosis
- Acute GVHD
- Acute generalized exanthematous pustulosis
- Drug eruption with eosinophilia and systemic symptoms (DRESS)
- Acute lupus erythematosus

## FACTORS AFFECTING OUTCOME IN STEVENS–JOHNSON SYNDROME–TOXIC EPIDERMAL NECROLYSIS

| | |
|---|---|
| Age | Elderly age—increased complications |
| Sex | No difference in outcome |
| Coexisting diseases | DM poorly controlled, HIV SLE, cancer, heart disease-poor outcome |
| Metabolic parameters | Hypo and hyperglycemia, hypoand hyperkalemia, and hyponatremia can worsen condition |
| Sepsis | Onset of sepsis poor prognostic sign |
| Nosocomial infections | CAUTI, CLABSI, and CAP can occur |
| Extent of involvement | Risk of morbidity mortality directly proportional to percentage of skin involvement and type, severity and number of mucosae involved |
| Time of detection | Early detection improves prognosis |

## SEVERITY OF ILLNESS SCORE FOR TOXIC EPIDERMAL NECROLYSIS

A validated mathematical tool named "severity-of-illness score for toxic epidermal necrolysis (SCORTEN)" for the prognostication of SJS/TEN patients has been developed. It should be computed within 24 h after admission and again on the 3rd day.

Is widely used to evaluate and predict mortality due to SJS/TEN.

SCORTEN consists of seven independent risk factors, each given a point including

- Age > 40 years
- Malignancy
- Tachycardia > 120 beats/minute
- Skin detachment > 10%
- Serum urea > 10 mmol/L
- Glucose > 14 mmol/L,
- Serum bicarbonate < 20 mmol/L

| ***SCORTEN*** | ***Mortality rate (%)*** |
|---|---|
| 1 | 3.2 |
| 2 | 12.1 |
| 3 | 35.3 |
| 4 | 58.3 |
| 5 and above | 90 |

(SCORTEN: severity of illness score for toxic epidermal necrolysis)

Algorithm for management of SJS/TEN:

- Stop offending drug.
- Shift to intensive care unit under cover of multidisciplinary team and sterile precautions
- Assess airway, breathing, circulation. Assess the extent of body surface and mucosal involvement. Calculate SCORETEN.
- *Parameters to be monitored:* BP, pulse, urine output, body temperature, respiratory rate
- *Investigations:* Hemogram, renal and liver function tests, blood glucose, urine routine, blood culture, skin swab culture. FDP, D-Dimer, PCT, if needed
- *Supportive therapy:*
  - Barrier nursing
  - Strict temperature management-hypothermia common
  - Topical antiseptics and dressing of denuded skin
  - Start antibiotics if suspicion of sepsis—hypothermia, altered sensorium, increased bacterial count in skin swab or urine sample
  - Mouth care and eye care,
  - Nutrition—Oral nutrition preferred fluid or semi solid diet initially. 30–35 kcal/kg and 1.5 g/kg protein intake per day
  - Antacids, analgesics, and anxiolytics
  - Anticoagulation
- Fluid and electrolyte management
  - The early fluid requirement of TEN patients is two-third to three-fourth of that of a burn patient with the same extent of skin involvement Ringer lactate or saline solutions. The fluid requirements of burn patients is calculated by the Parkland formula, as follows:
    - Fluid requirement = 4 mL/kg body weight × percentage of body surface area involved.
    - For the first 24 hours, half the calculated fluid is administered in the first 8 hours and the other half in the next 16 hours. Fluid requirements beyond the first 24 hours should be managed according to the patient's condition.
    - Strict intake output chart to maintain urine output of 1500 mL/day
- Specific therapy
  - *Corticosteroids:* Prednisolone, dexamethasone or methylprednisolone should be given early (preferably within 72 hours) in high dosage (1–2 mg/kg/day prednisolone or 8–16 mg/day of dexamethasone intravenous or intramuscular).

    - A daily assessment of disease activity (such as the appearance of new lesions, perilesional erythema and skin tenderness) should be done and steroids should be maintained at the same dose till disease activity ceases.
    - Thereafter, dosage should be tapered quickly such that the total duration of steroid therapy is around 7–10 days.
    - Steroids can also be administered in pulse form employing slow intravenous infusion of methylprednisolone (500–1,000 mg/day) or dexamethasone (100 mg) for 3 days.
  - *Cyclosporine:* Cyclosporine can also be employed alone (3–5 mg/kg/day for 10–14 days), especially in patients with relative contraindications to corticosteroid use (e.g., patients with tuberculosis and severe hyperglycemia)
    - If both steroids and cyclosporine are used, steroids can be tapered even more quickly (2–3 days) and cyclosporine (3–5 mg/kg/day) can be continued for 7–10 days.
  - IVIG significant lack of consistency in the efficacy of intravenous immunoglobulin in different reports.
- Other therapies (low evidence)
  - Plasmapheresis, etanercept, infliximab, cyclophosphamide, pentoxifylline, n acetyl
  - Cysteine
- *Special situations*
  - *Pregnancy:* Avoid steroid in first trimester
  - IVIG
  - Cyclosporine second-line
  - *Children:* Early short course of iv steroids
  - *Low-dose IVIG:* 0.2–0.5 mg/kg
  - *HIV patients:* Low dose IVIG -0.2–0.5 mg/kg

## MARKERS OF STEVENS–JOHNSON SYNDROME–TOXIC EPIDERMAL NECROLYSIS

- *Granulysin:* Most useful of these markers. A rapid immunochromatographic assay capable of detecting high levels of serum granulysin (>10 ng/mL) has been developed with a sensitivity of 80% and a specificity of 95.8% in detecting SJS/TEN when compared to ordinary cutaneous drug reactions.
- Soluble Fas ligand
- Perforin/granzyme B,
- Soluble CD40 ligand

The other emerging markers for the early detection of SJS/TEN are serum lactate dehydrogenase, thymus and activation-regulated chemokine (TARC/CCL17), glutathione-S-transferase-pi (GSTpi) and high-mobility group protein B1 (HMGB1), alpha-defensins 1–3 in blister fluid and Bcl-2 expression in dermal infiltrate.

## SUGGESTED READING

1. Bastuji-Garin S, Rzany B, Stern RS, Shear NH, Naldi L, Roujeau JC. Clinical classification of cases of toxic epidermal necrolysis, Stevens-Johnson syndrome, and erythema multiforme. Arch Dermatol. 1993;129(1):92-6.
2. Chang HC, Wang TJ, Lin MH, Chen TJ. A Review of the systemic treatment of Stevens-Johnson Syndrome and Toxic epidermal necrolysis. Biomedicines. 2022;10(9):2105.
3. Dobry AS, Himed S, Waters M, Kaffenberger BH. Scoring assessments in Stevens-Johnson Syndrome and toxic epidermal necrolysis. Front Med (Lausanne). 2022;9: 883121.
4. Gupta LK, Martin AM, Agarwal N, D'Souza P, Das S, Kumar R, et al. Guidelines for the management of Stevens–Johnson syndrome/toxic epidermal necrolysis: An Indian perspective. Indian J Dermatol Venereol Leprol. 2016;82(6):603-25.
5. Kumar R, Das A, Das S. Management of Stevens-Johnson Syndrome-toxic epidermal necrolysis: Looking beyond guidelines! Indian J Dermatol. 2018;63(2):117-24.

CHAPTER 121

# Necrotizing Fasciitis

## INTRODUCTION

Necrotizing soft-tissue infections are rare infections of the skin and soft tissues with a high morbidity and mortality rate. They need prompt diagnosis and early surgical intervention. These represent a spectrum of disease resulting in tissue necrosis that is rapidly progressive; however, they remain a diagnostic challenge. Diagnosis is largely clinical and based on subtle physical examination findings, physiologic instability, and laboratory derangements.

## RISK FACTORS FOR NECROTIZING FASCIITIS

- Diabetes
- Chronic disease
- Immunosuppressive drugs
- Malnutrition
- Age >60 years
- Intravenous drug misuse
- Peripheral vascular disease
- Renal failure
- Underlying malignancy
- Obesity

## NECROTIZING FASCIITIS CLASSIFICATION

| *Type* | *Organism* | *Characteristics* |
|---|---|---|
| Type 1 | Polymicrobial<br>• Typically, 4–5 aerobic and anaerobic species cultured:<br>• Non-group A Streptococci<br>• Anaerobes including *Clostridia*<br>• Facultative anaerobes<br>• Enterobacteria<br>• Synergistic virulence between organisms | • Most common (80–90%)<br>• Seen in immunosuppressed (diabetics and cancer patients)<br>• Postop abdominal and perineal infections |
| Type 2 | • Monomicrobial<br>• Group A β-hemolytic streptococci is most common organism isolated | • 5% of cases<br>• Seen in healthy patients<br>• Extremities |
| Type 3 | Marine *Vibrio vulnificus* (gram-negative rods) | Marine exposure |
| Type 4 | Fungal | |

## ORGANISMS IDENTIFIED IN NECROTIZING FASCIITIS

| | |
|---|---|
| Gram-positive aerobic bacteria | • *Group A:* Hemolytic *Streptococcus*<br>• Group B *Streptococcus*<br>• Enterococci<br>• Coagulase-negative staphylococci *Staphylococcus aureus*<br>• *Bacillus spp.* |
| Gram-negative aerobic bacteria | *Escherichia coli, Pseudomonas aeruginosa Enterobacter cloacae, Klebsiella* spp., *Proteus, Serratia* spp., *Acinetobacter calcoaceticus, Citrobacter freundii,* and *Pasteurella multocida* |
| Anaerobic bacteria | *Bacteroides* spp., *Clostridium* spp, and *Peptostreptococcus* spp. |
| Marine *Vibrio* spp. | Vibrio vulnificus, *Vibrio parahaemolyticus*, Vibrio damsela, and *Vibrio alginolyticus* |
| Fungi | *Candida* spp., *Aspergillus* spp., and *Rhizopus* |

## SYMPTOMS AND SIGNS

| | |
|---|---|
| Early signs | • Localized abscess or cellulitis with rapid progression<br>• Minimal swelling<br>• No trauma or discoloration |
| Late signs | • Severe pain<br>• High fever, chills, and rigors<br>• Tachycardia<br>• Hypotension |
| Physical exam | • Skin bullae<br>• Discoloration<br>• Ischemic patches<br>• Cutaneous gangrene<br>• Swelling and edema<br>• Dermal induration and erythema<br>• Subcutaneous emphysema and crepitus (gas-producing organisms) |

## THE LABORATORY RISK INDICATOR FOR NECROTIZING FASCIITIS SCORE (LRINEC SCORE)

| *Variable* | *Value* | *Score* |
|---|---|---|
| C-reactive protein (mg/L) | ≤150 | 0 |
| | >150 | 4 |
| Total white blood cell count (1,000 cells/µL) | <15 | 0 |
| | 15–25 | 1 |
| | >25 | 2 |
| Hemoglobin (g/dL) | >13.5 | 0 |
| | 11–13.5 | 1 |
| | <11 | 2 |
| Sodium (mmol/L) | <135 | 0 |
| | >135 | 2 |
| Creatinine (mg/dL) | ≤1.6 | 0 |
| | >1.6 | 2 |
| Glucose (mg/dL) | ≤180 | 0 |
| | >180 | 1 |

## LRINEC RISK ASSESSMENT

| *Risk category* | *LRINEC points* | *Probability for presence of NF* |
|---|---|---|
| Low | ≤5 | <50% |
| Medium | 6–7 | 50–75% |
| High | ≥8 | >75% |

## RADIOLOGICAL FINDINGS IN NECROTIZING FASCIITIS (NOT SPECIFIC)

*X-ray:*

- Soft-tissue swelling
- Gas in soft tissues

*CT scan:*

- Soft-tissue edema
- Thrombosis of superficial vessels
- Gas tracking along fascial planes*
- Lack of soft-tissue enhancement
- Fluid collections within muscle or fascial planes

**Absence of gas tracking does not rule out necrotizing fasciitis*

## TREATMENT ALGORITHM FOR NECROTIZING FASCIITIS

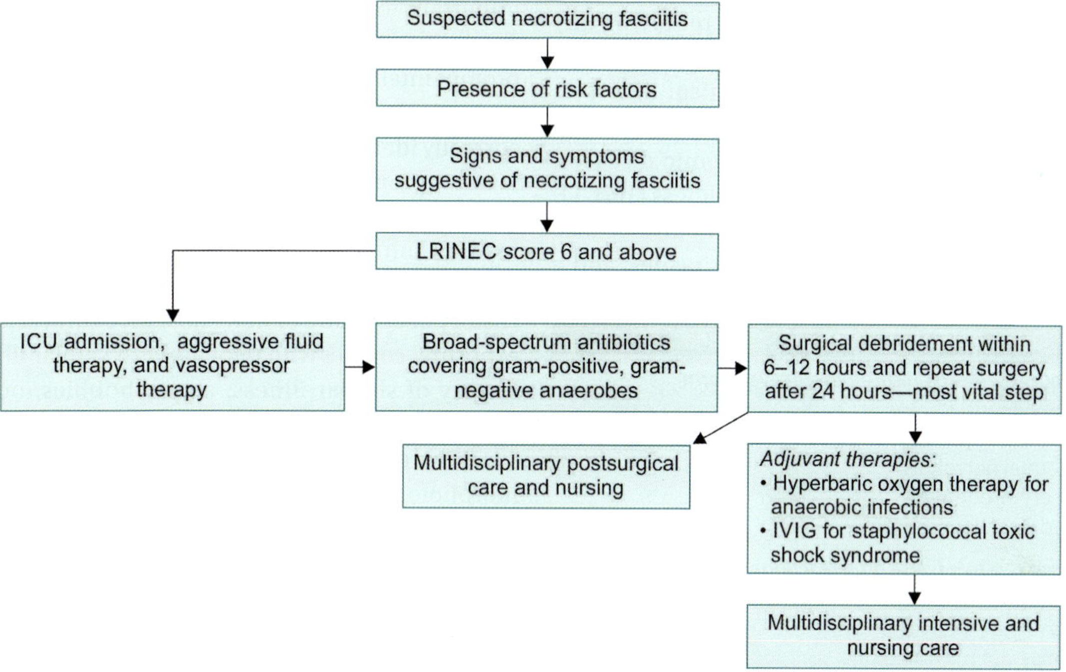


## SUGGESTED READING

1. Bisgaard EK, Bulger EM. Current diagnosis and management of necrotizing soft tissue infections: What you need to know. J Trauma Acute Care Surg. 2024;97(5):678-86.
2. Green RJ, Dafoe DC, Raffin TA. Necrotizing fasciitis. Chest. 1996;110(1):219-29.
3. Hoesl V, Kempa S, Prantl L, Ochsenbauer K, Hoesl J, Kehrer A, et al. The LRINEC Score-An Indicator for the Course and Prognosis of Necrotizing Fasciitis? J Clin Med. 2022;11(13):3583.
4. Misiakos EP, Bagias G, Patapis P, Sotiropoulos D, Kanavidis P, Machairas A. Current concepts in the management of necrotizing fasciitis. Front Surg. 2014;1:36.
5. Puvanendran R, Huey JC, Pasupathy S. Necrotizing fasciitis. Can Fam Physician. 2009;55(10):981-7.
6. Wallace HA, Perera TB. Necrotizing Fasciitis. In: StatPearls. Treasure Island (FL): StatPearls Publishing; 2025. Available from https://www.ncbi.nlm.nih.gov/books/NBK430756/ [Last accessed February, 2025].

CHAPTER 122

# Generalized Rash and Purpura in Intensive Care Unit

## INTRODUCTION

Differentiating among different rash is important for early initiation of life saving therapy as well as removing any offending agent. Rashes in intensive care unit are classified into four groups: (1) Primary dermatological illness in severe form, (2) rashes associated with adverse drug reactions, (3) rashes associated with systemic diseases, and (4) rashes as a consequence of critical illness **(Box 1)**.

Differentiating different rashes are difficult because many different conditions produce similar rashes, and a single condition can result in different rashes with varied appearances. A rapid and accurate diagnosis is critically important to make treatment decisions, especially when mortality or significant morbidity can occur without prompt intervention.

In evaluating a patient with rash initial step is to correctly identify the rash correctly so that with associated features proper differential diagnosis can be formulated to arrive at a diagnosis **(Table 1)**. History of onset of the rash, its duration, areas affected, associated itching or pain, fever, bleeding or discharge from the rash is important. History of exposure to new substances, travel history, drug exposure, contact with persons with similar illness, family history of similar illness, atopy, hobbies, occupational exposure, sexual history are important.

During examination site and distribution of rash, morphological features of the rash like color, size, shape,

**BOX 1:** Classification of rashes in intensive care unit.

*Group 1: Primary dermatological illness in severe form*
- Pemphigus vulgaris
- Stevens–Johnson syndrome
- Toxic epidermal necrolysis
- Exfoliative erythroderma
- Generalized pustular psoriasis

*Group 2: Rashes due to adverse drug reactions*
- Nonsteroidal anti-inflammatory drugs
- Antibiotics
- Antiepileptics
- Contrast
- Angiotensin converting enzyme Inhibitors

*Group 3: Rash due to systemic illness*
- Erythema multiforme
- Vitiligo
- Erythema nodosum
- Sweet syndrome
- Cutaneous leukocytoclastic vasculitis
- Pyoderma gangrenosum

*Group 4: Critical illness related*
- Skin infections
- Pressure sores
- Rashes due to vasopressors
- Disseminated intravascular coagulation
- Contact dermatitis

*Source:* Al Bshabshe et al. (2023).

**TABLE 1:** Glossary of dermatological terms.

| | |
|---|---|
| Macule | Non palpable are of altered color |
| Papule | Palpable elevated small area of skin <0.5 cm |
| Plaque | Palpable flat topped discoid lesion >2 cm |
| Nodule | Solid palpable lesion within the skin >0.5 cm |
| Vesicle | Small fluid filled blister <0.5 cm |
| Bulla | Large fluid filled blister >0.5 cm |
| Pustule | Blister containing pus |
| Wheal | Elevated lesion, often white with red margin due to dermal edema |
| Petechiae | Pinhead-sized macules of blood <2 mm |
| Purpura | Large petechiae that do not blanch on pressure more than 3 mm |
| Ecchymosis | Large extravasation of blood in skin |
| Erythema | Redness of skin |

*Source:* Glynn M, et al. (2017).

and scale are important. Characteristics of individual lesions, such as; areas of involvement and sparing, with particular attention to palms, soles, face, nails, sun-exposed areas, and extensor and flexor surfaces of extremities; pruritic or painful lesions; systemic symptoms, specially fever; and dermatologic signs, such as blanching, and the Koebner phenomenon.

## ALGORITHMIC APPROACH TO DIAGNOSE SKIN RASH

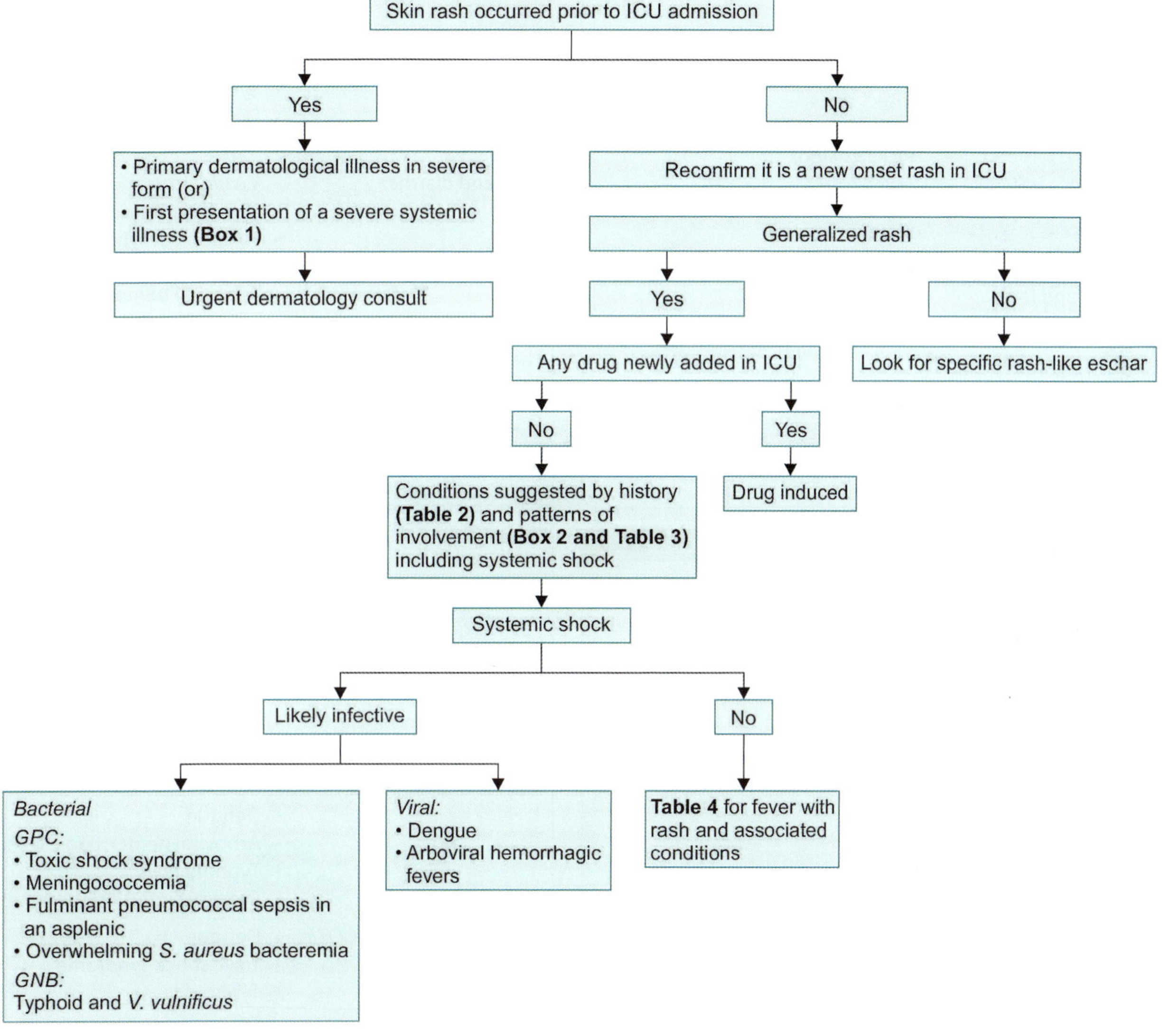

**TABLE 2:** Generalized rash: Conditions suggested by patient history.

| *Historical finding* | *Conditions* |
|---|---|
| Chemicals | Contact dermatitis |
| Contact with ill persons | • Meningococcemia<br>• Varicella<br>• Viral exanthem, nonspecific |
| Drug exposure | • Drug eruption<br>• Urticaria (i.e., hives) |
| Hobbies | Contact dermatitis |
| Insect and arthropod exposure | • Insect bites<br>• Lyme disease<br>• Rickettsialpox |
| Occupational exposure | Contact dermatitis |
| Plant exposure | Contact dermatitis |
| Recent systemic symptoms and fever | • HIV acute exanthem<br>• Meningococcemia<br>• Varicella<br>• Viral exanthem, nonspecific |
| Sexual history | HIV acute exanthem |
| Travel | • Insect bites<br>• Rickettsialpox |

*Source:* Ely JW et al. (2010).

**BOX 2:** Generalized rash: Involvement of palms and soles.

- Staphylococcal scalded skin syndrome
- Stevens–Johnson syndrome
- Toxic epidermal necrolysis
- Toxic shock syndrome
- Erythema multiforme
- Drug eruption
- HIV acute exanthem
- Meningococcemia
- Psoriasis (plaque psoriasis)
- Insect bites
- Varicella
- Viral exanthem, nonspecific

*Source:* Ely JW et al. (2010)

**TABLE 3:** Generalized rash: Conditions associated with pruritus.

| *Common* | *Rare* |
|---|---|
| • Contact dermatitis<br>• Insect bites<br>• Varicella<br>• Drug eruption<br>• Erythema multiforme<br>• Toxic epidermal necrolysis<br>• Toxic shock syndrome (late)<br>• Viral exanthem, nonspecific | • Meningococcemia<br>• Staphylococcal scalded skin syndrome<br>• Stevens–Johnson syndrome |

*Source:* Ely JW et al. (2010).

**TABLE 4:** DD for ICU patients with fever and rash.

| | |
|---|---|
| Rash and shock | • Toxic shock syndrome<br>• MC meningococcemia<br>• Fulminant pneumococcal sepsis in an asplenic<br>• Overwhelming *S. aureus* bacteremia<br>• Dengue<br>• Arboviral hemorrhagic fevers |
| Rash and abdominal pain | • Typhoid fever<br>• Cholesterol emboli syndrome<br>• Systemic lupus erythematosus<br>• Dengue<br>• Arboviral hemorrhagic fevers |
| Rash and diarrhea | • *V. vulnificus*<br>• Gas gangrene<br>• Toxic shock syndrome<br>• Dengue<br>• Arboviral hemorrhagic fevers |
| Rash and mental status changes | • Systemic lupus erythematosus (if cerebritis)<br>• Meningococcemia<br>• Typhoid fever<br>• *Staphylococcus aureus* bacteremia |
| Rash and relative bradycardia | • Typhus<br>• Typhoid fever<br>• Arboviral hemorrhagic fevers<br>• Drug fever |
| Rash and splenomegaly | • Typhoid fever<br>• Rubella<br>• Systemic lupus erythematosus |
| Rash and eosinophilia | • Dengue<br>• Cholesterol emboli syndrome |
| Rash and leukopenia | • Measles<br>• Dengue<br>• Arboviral hemorrhagic fever<br>• Typhoid fever<br>• Systemic lupus erythematosus |
| Rash and elevated SGOT/SGPT | • Dengue<br>• Toxic shock syndrome<br>• Typhoid fever |
| Rash and thrombocytopenia | • Meningococcemia<br>• Dengue<br>• Toxic shock syndrome<br>• Measles<br>• Systemic Lupus Erythematous |

*Source:* Burke A et al. (1998).

## PURPURA AND PETECHIAE

Purpura are due to red blood cells extravasation, and they do not blanch on pressure. Erythema is due to vasodilation, and it blanches with pressure.

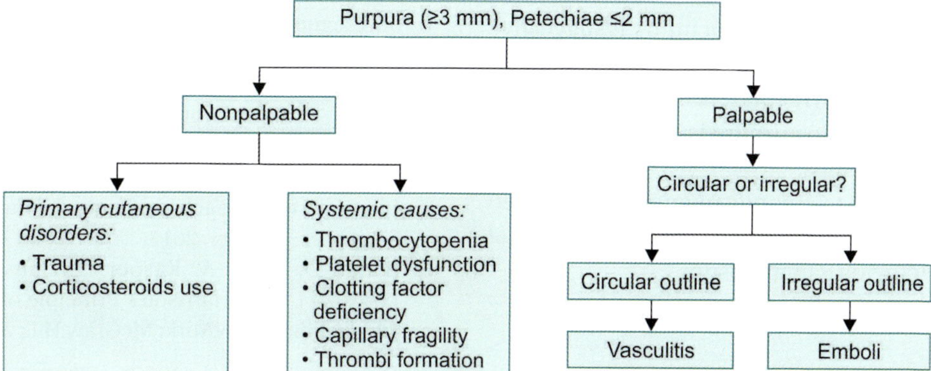


## ALGORITHMIC APPROACH FOR PURPURA

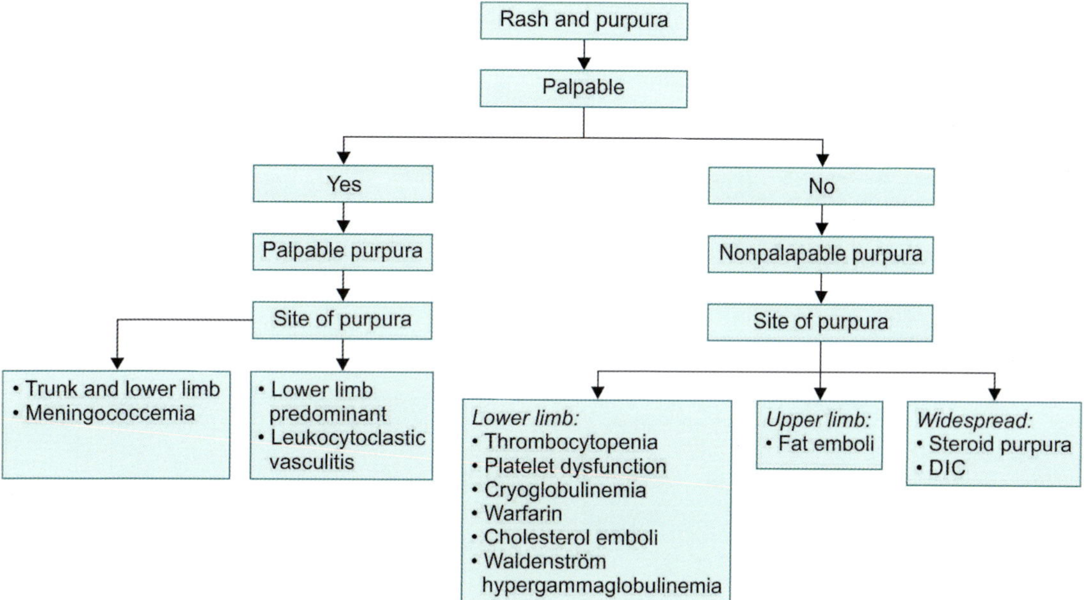


## SPECIFIC FEATURES

- Initial site of purpura in thrombocytopenia induced purpura is the distal lower extremity.
- In monoclonal cryoglobulinemia-related purpura, lower limb will be involved and hemorrhagic infarct of fingers, toes and ears will be present. Lesion will be increased by cold exposure.
- Purpura with jaundice and neurological manifestation could be due to thrombotic thrombocytopenic purpura.
- Warfarin induced rash is seen between third to tenth days of therapy in areas of abundant subcutaneous fat.
- Cholesterol emboli related purpura predominantly involves lower limb.
- Thrombi formation is seen in: (a) Disseminated intravascular coagulation, purpura fulminans; (b) warfarin (Coumadin)-induced necrosis; (c) heparin-induced thrombocytopenia and thrombosis; (d) anti phospholipid antibody syndrome; (e) monoclonal cryoglobulinemia; (f) vasculopathy induced by

levamisole-adulterated cocaine; (g) SARS-CoV-2 infection; (h) thrombotic thrombocytopenic purpura; (i) thrombocytosis; (j) Homozygous protein C or protein S deficiency.

- Petechiae in upper body after major injury is suggestive of fat emboli.
- If palpable purpura is irregular, it is due to embolic phenomenon. If palpable purpura is circular its due to leukocytoclastic vasculitis.
- Palpable purpura due to embolic phenomenon is seen in acute meningococcemia, disseminated gonococcal infection and Ecthyma gangrenosum.

## SUGGESTED READING

1. Al Bshabshe A, Mousa WF, Nor El-Dein N. An Overview of Clinical Manifestations of Dermatological Disorders in Intensive Care Units: What Should Intensivists Be Aware of? Diagnostics (Basel). 2023;13(7):1290
2. Cunha BA. Rash and fever in the critical care unit. Crit Care Clin. 1998;14(1):35-53.
3. Ely JW, Seabury Stone M. The generalized rash: Part II. Diagnostic approach. Am Fam Physician. 2010;81(6):735-9.
4. Glynn M, Drake WM. Hutchisons's Clinical Methods: An Integrated Approach to Clinical Practice, 24th edition. Singapore: Elsevier; 2017.
5. Longo D, Fauci A, Kasper D, Hauser S, Jameson JL, Loscalzo J, et al. Harrison's Principle of Internal Medicine, 22nd edition. New York: McGraw Hill; 2025.

# PART 12

# HEMATOLOGY

***Editor:*** Raymond Dominic Savio

***Associate Editors:*** Suresh Kumar Sundaramurthy, Naveen Chandra Chinni

CHAPTER **123**

# Pancytopenia

## OVERVIEW

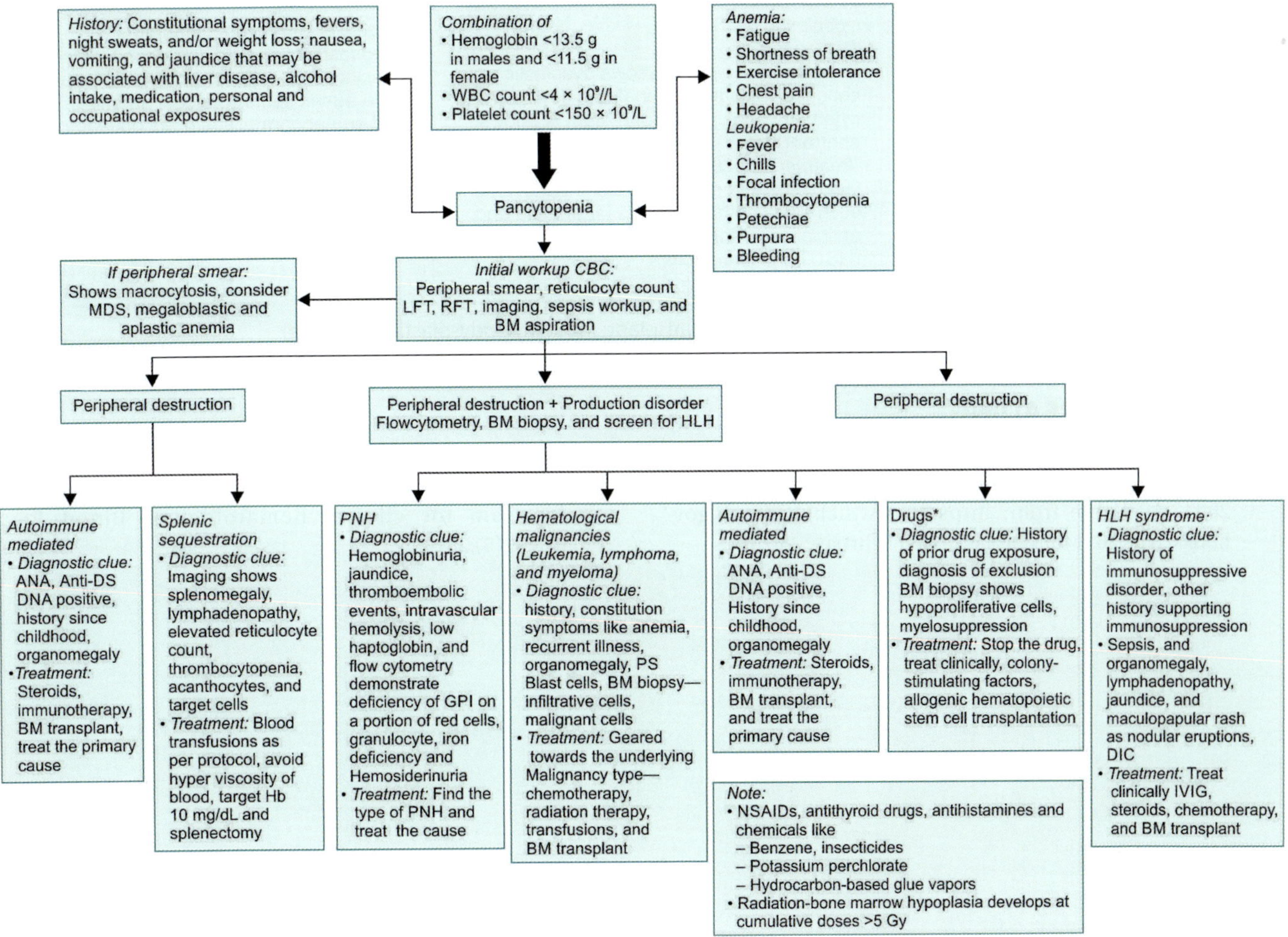


(ANA: antinuclear antibody; anti-DS DNA: antidouble-stranded DNA antibody; CBC: complete blood count; HLH: hemophagocytic lymphohistiocytosis; LFT: liver function test; MDS: myelodysplastic syndrome; RFT: renal function test)

## PRODUCTION DISORDER

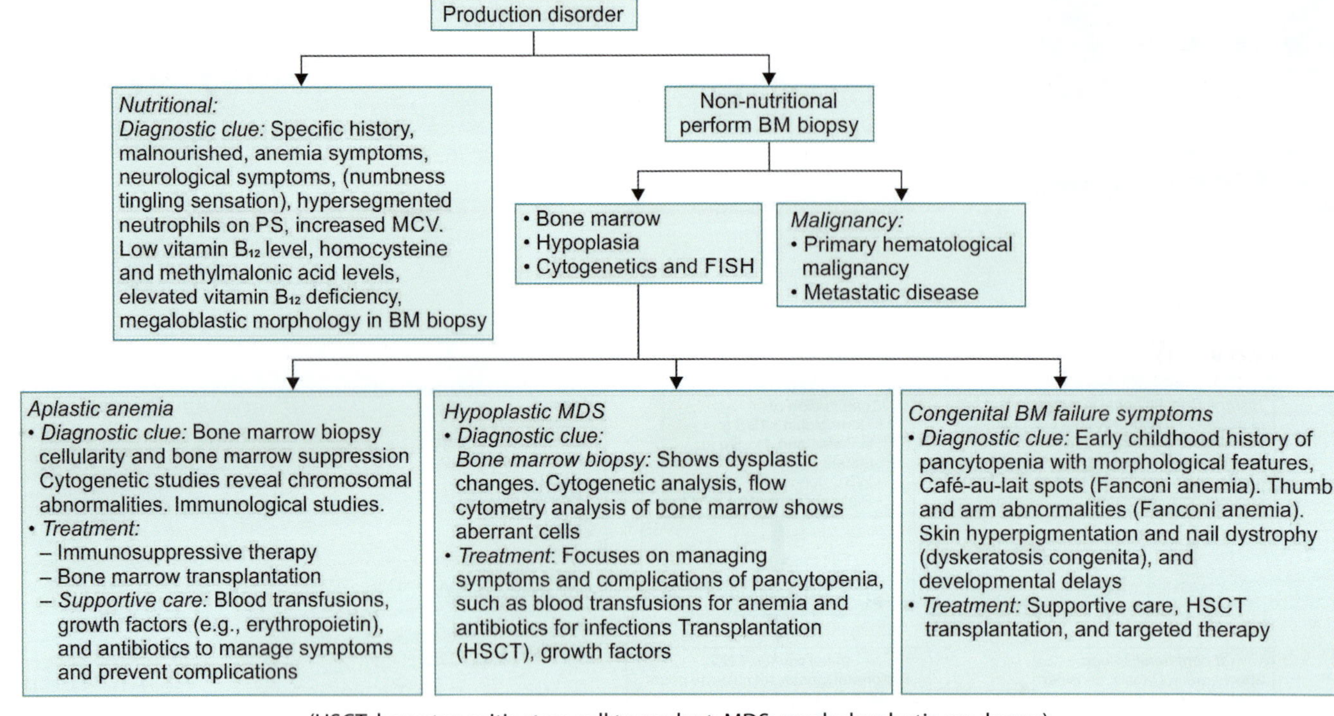


(HSCT: hematopoeitic stem cell transplant; MDS: myelodysplastic syndrome)

## SUGGESTED READING


1. Chiravuri S, De Jesus O. Pancytopenia. In: StatPearls [Internet]. Treasure Island (FL): StatPearls Publishing; 2024. Available from: https://www.ncbi.nlm.nih.gov/books/NBK563146/ [Last accessed February, 2025].
2. Gnanaraj J, Parnes A, Francis CW, Go RS, Takemoto CM, Hashmi SK. Approach to pancytopenia: Diagnostic algorithm for clinical hematologists. Blood Rev. 2018;32(5):361-7.

CHAPTER

# 124 Hemophagocytic Lymphohistiocytosis

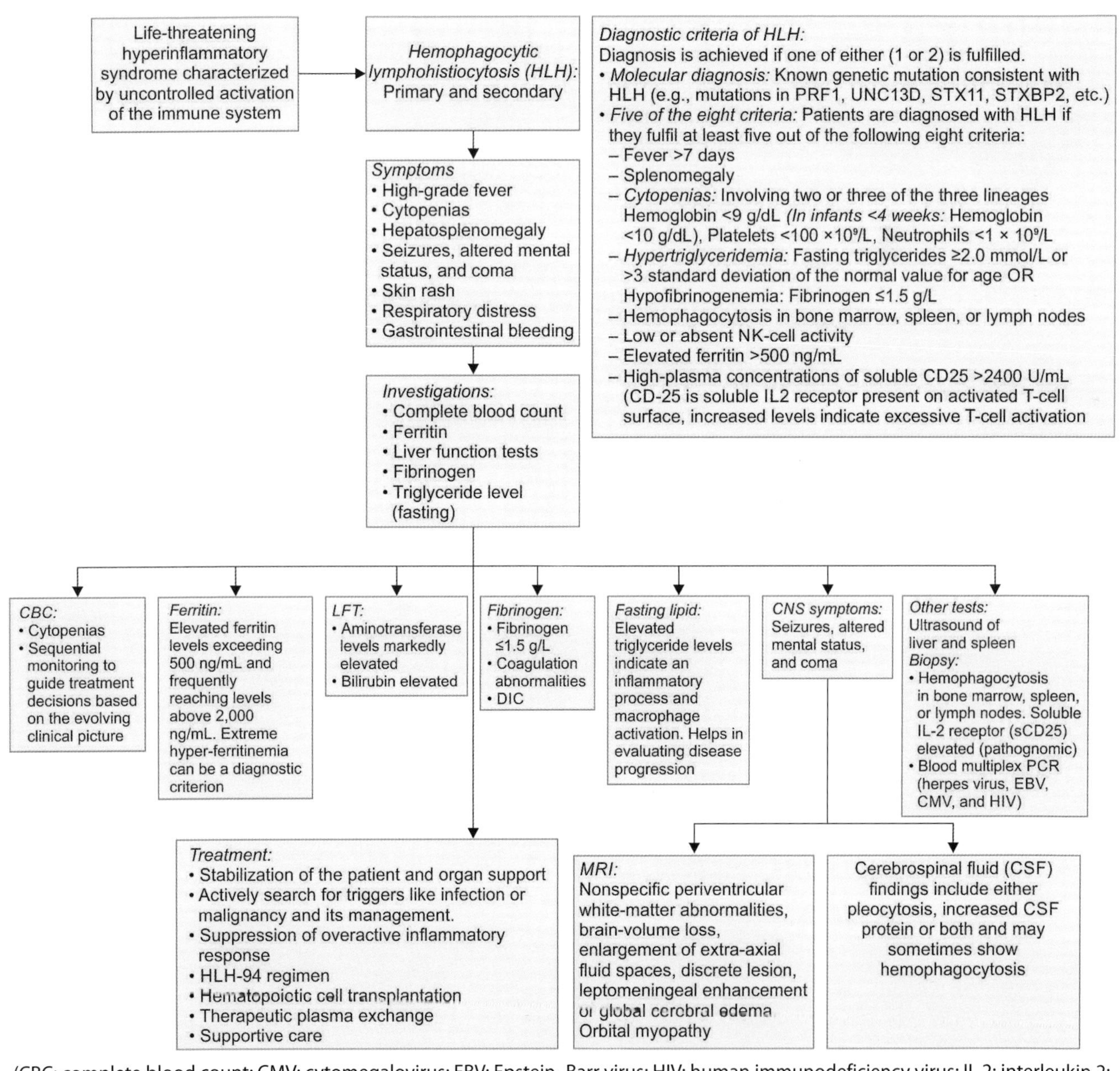


(CBC: complete blood count; CMV: cytomegalovirus; EBV: Epstein–Barr virus; HIV: human immunodeficiency virus; IL 2: interleukin 2; LFT: liver function test; MCV: mean corpuscular volume; NK cell: natural killer cell; RFT: renal function test)

## SUGGESTED READING

1. Barba T, Maucort-Boulch D, Iwaz J, Bohé J, Ninet J, Hot A, et al. Hemophagocytic lymphohistiocytosis in intensive care unit: A 71-Case strobe-compliant retrospective study. Medicine (Baltimore). 2015;94(51):e2318.
2. Bauchmuller K, Manson JJ, Tattersall R, Brown M, McNamara C, Singer M, et al. Haemophagocytic lymphohistiocytosis in adult critical care. J Intensive Care Soc. 2020;21(3):256-68.
3. Bichon A, Bourenne J, Allardet-Servent J, Papazian L, Hraiech S, Guervilly C, et al. High mortality of HLH in ICU regardless etiology or treatment. Front Med (Lausanne). 2021;8:735796.

CHAPTER

# 125 Thrombocytopenia

## EVALUATION AND DIAGNOSIS

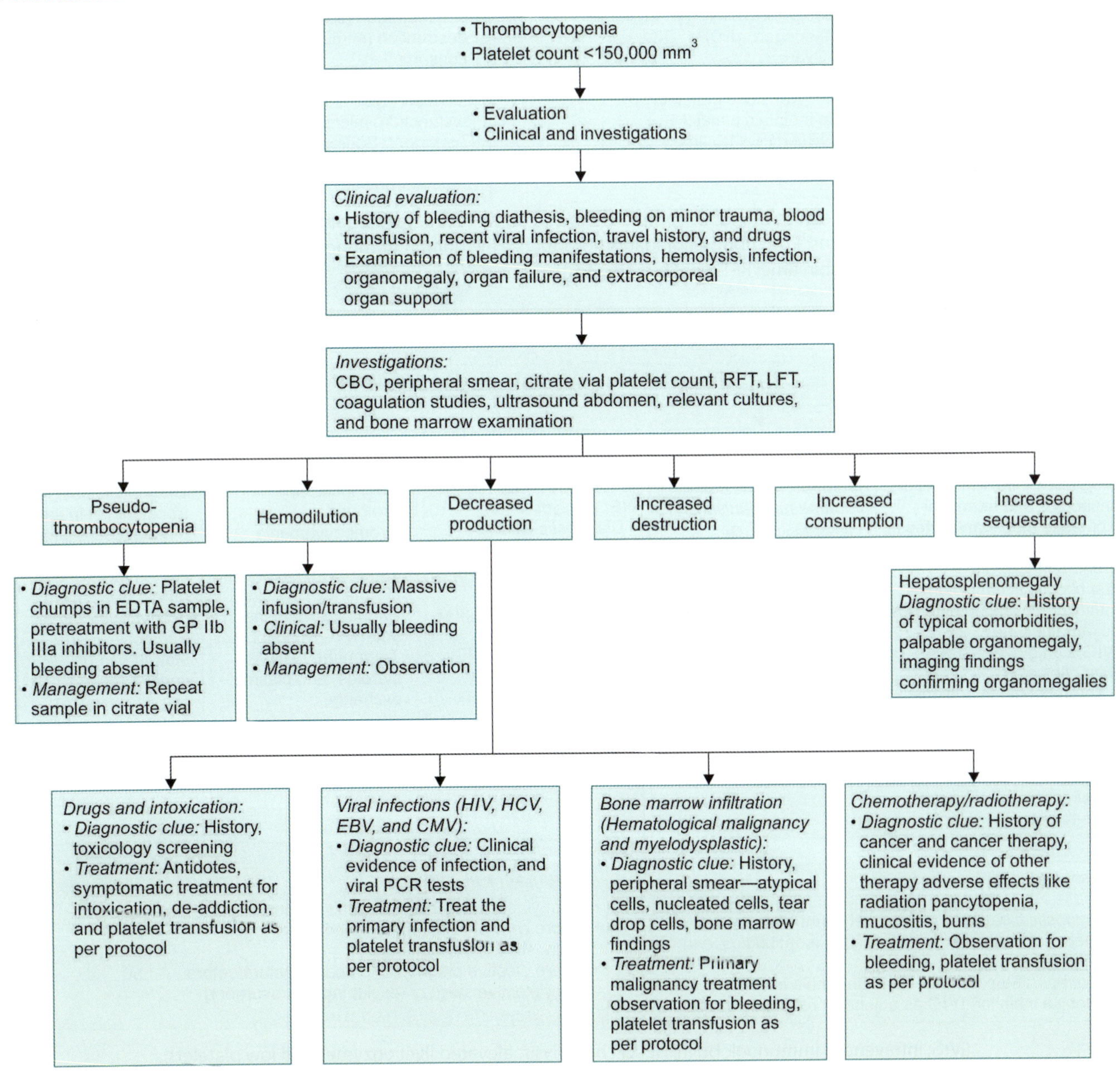

## THROMBOCYTOPENIA DUE TO PLATELET CONSUMPTION

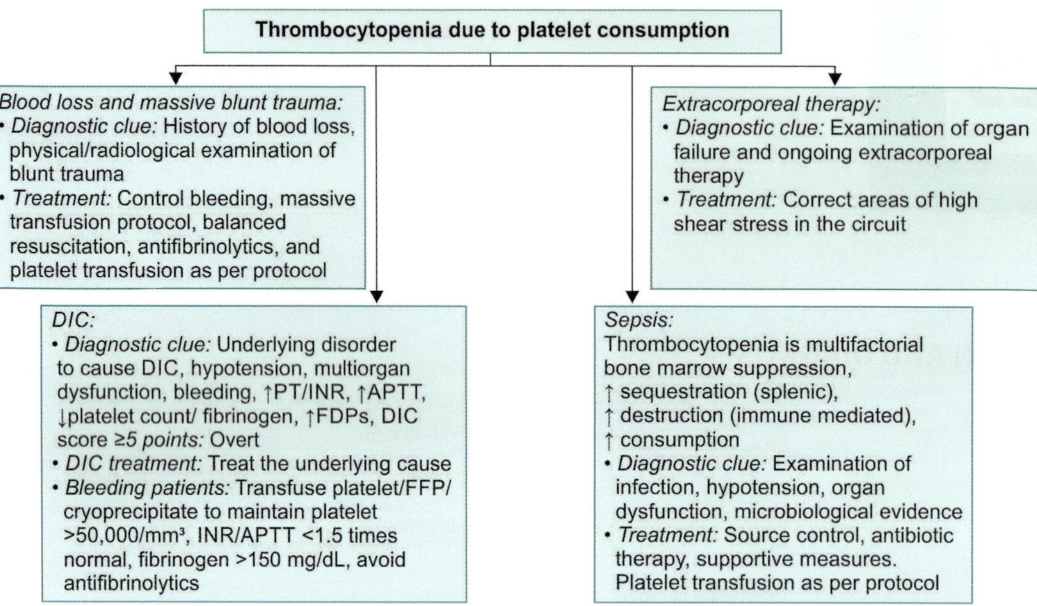


(APTT: activated partial thromboplastin time; CBC: complete blood count; CMV: cytomegalovirus; DIC: disseminated intravascular coagulopathy; EBV: Epstein–Barr virus; FDP: fibrin degradation products; HIV: human immunodeficiency virus; HCV: hepatitis C virus; LFT: liver function test; PT: prothrombin time; RFT renal function test)

## THROMBOCYTOPENIA DUE TO PLATELET DESTRUCTION

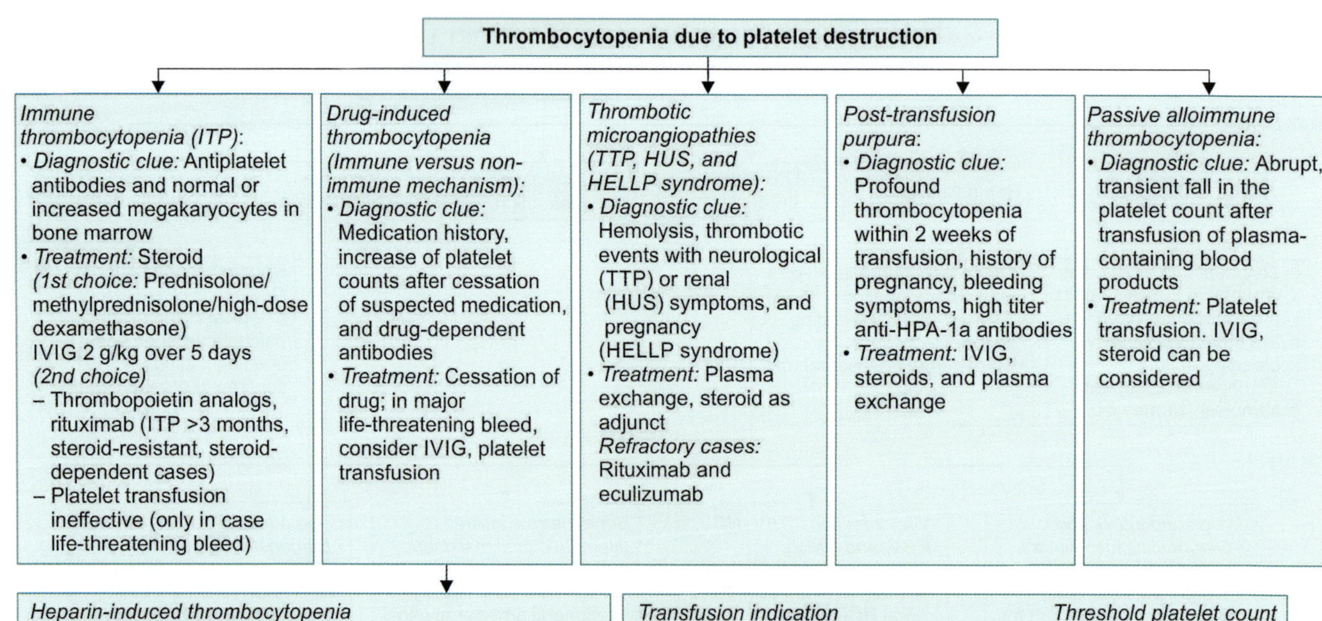


| Transfusion indication | Threshold platelet count |
|---|---|
| • Prophylactic transfusion of adult patients | 10 |
| • Before central vein catheter placement/urgent diagnostic lumbar puncture | 20 |
| • Before elective diagnostic lumbar puncture/before major elective surgery (excluding neurosurgery) | 50 |

(IVIG: intravenous immunoglobulin; HELLP: hemolysis, elevated liver enzymes and low platelets; HUS: hemolytic uremic syndrome; TTP thrombotic thrombocytopenic purpura)

## SUGGESTED READING

1. Aluru N, Samavedam S. Thrombocytopenia in Intensive Care Unit. Indian J Crit Care Med. 2019;23(Suppl 3): S185-8.
2. Greinacher A, Selleng S. How I evaluate and treat thrombocytopenia in the intensive care unit patient. Blood. 2016;128(26):3032-42.
3. Ostadi Z, Shadvar K, Sanaie S, Mahmoodpoor A, Saghaleini SH. Thrombocytopenia in the intensive care unit. Pak J Med Sci. 2019;35(1):282-7.
4. Zarychanski R, Houston DS. Assessing thrombocytopenia in the intensive care unit: The past, present, and future. Hematology Am Soc Hematol Educ Program. 2017;(1): 660-6.

# CHAPTER 126

# Anemia

## EVALUATION AND INVESTIGATIONS

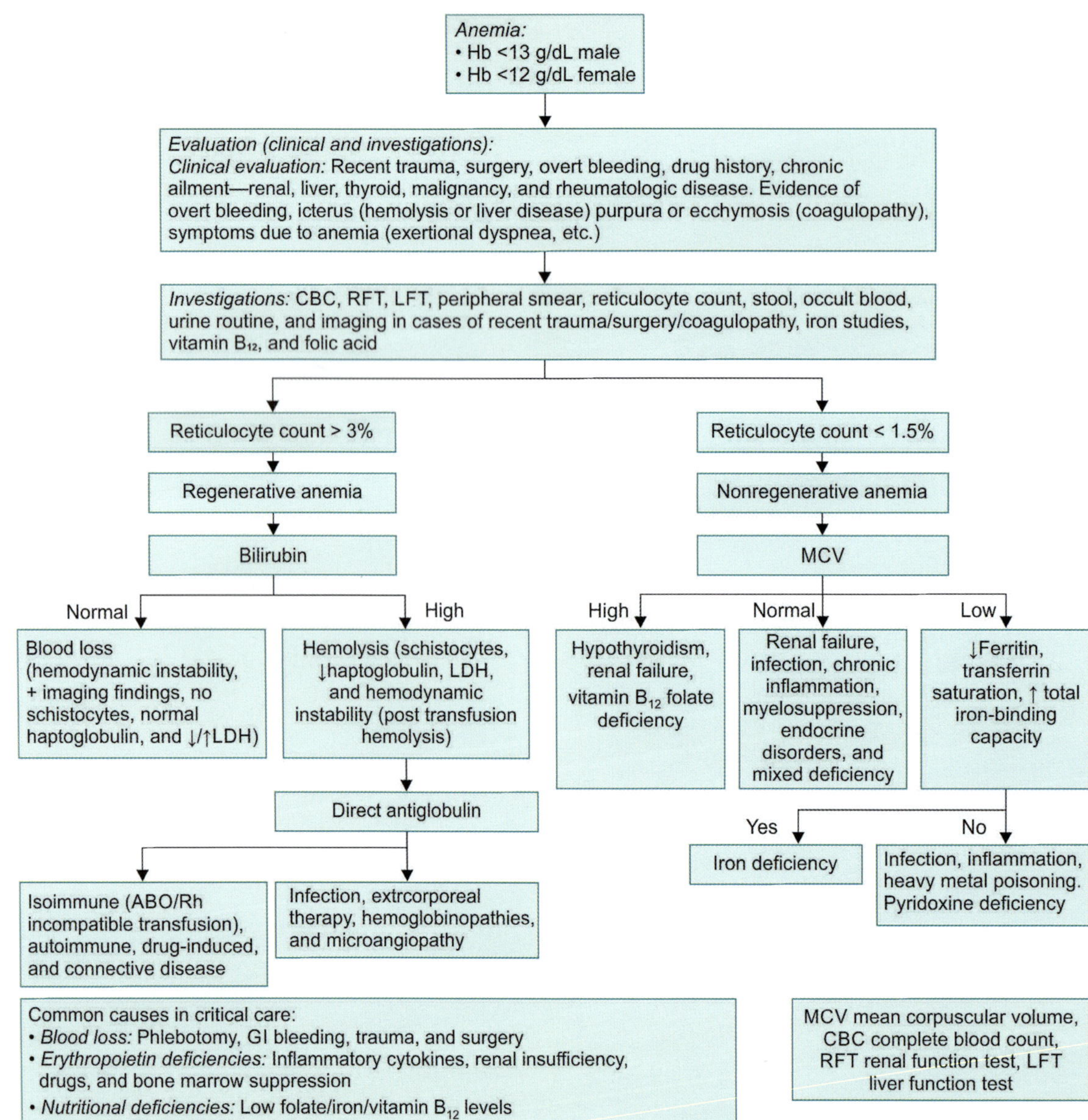

## IMPACT OF ANEMIA ON CRITICAL ILLNESS

- *Anemia and cardiac disease:* ↑mortality, recurrent ischemia in ACS patients, and ↑ adverse postoperative neurologic and renal outcomes in patients undergoing CABG and patients with preoperative anemia
- *Anemia and respiratory failure:* ↑rate of extubation failure and reintubation in patients with anemia, poor outcomes in COPD patients on invasive mechanical ventilation
- *Anemia and sepsis:*
  - ↑frequency in sepsis patients
  - TRICC trial-no difference in 30-day mortality between restrictive and liberal transfusion strategies in older or more severally ill patients. Better outcomes with a more restrictive transfusion approach in younger and less ill patients

## ANEMIA TREATMENT

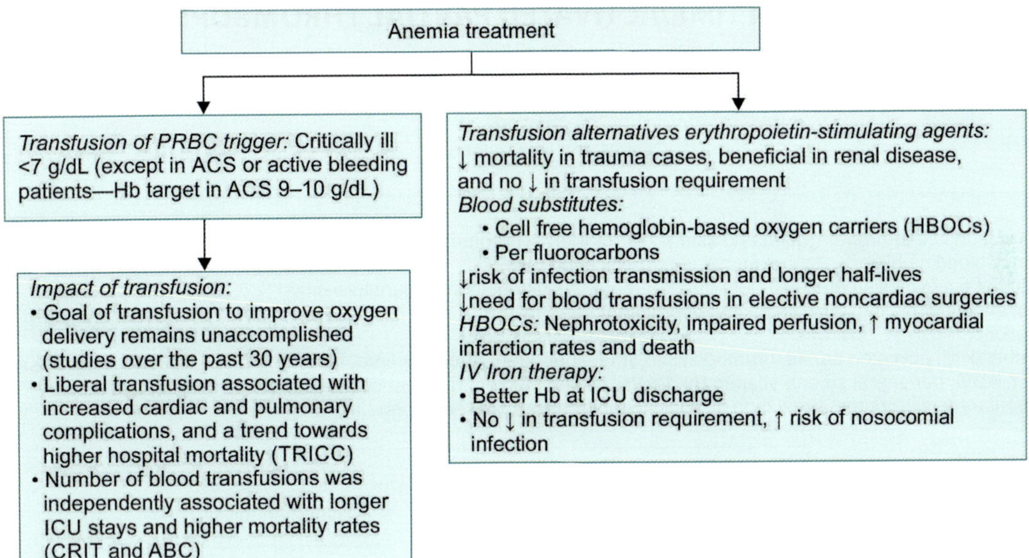


## SUGGESTED READING

1. Hegde A. Approach to an anemic critically ill patient. Indian J Crit Care Med. 2019;23(Suppl 3):S178-80.
2. Lasocki S, Pène F, Ait-Oufella H, Aubron C, Ausset S, Buffet P, et al. Management and prevention of anemia (acute bleeding excluded) in adult critical care patients. Ann Intensive Care. 2020;10(1):97.

CHAPTER **127**

# Deranged Prothrombin Time/ Activated Partial Thromboplastin Time

## ABNORMAL PROTHROMBIN TIME/ACTIVATED PARTIAL THROMBOPLASTIN TIME

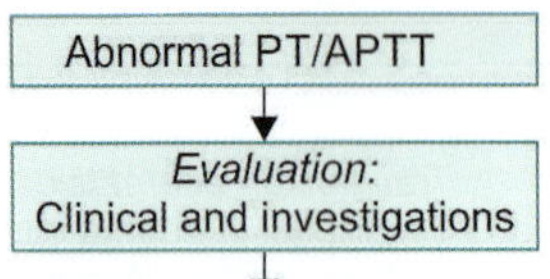


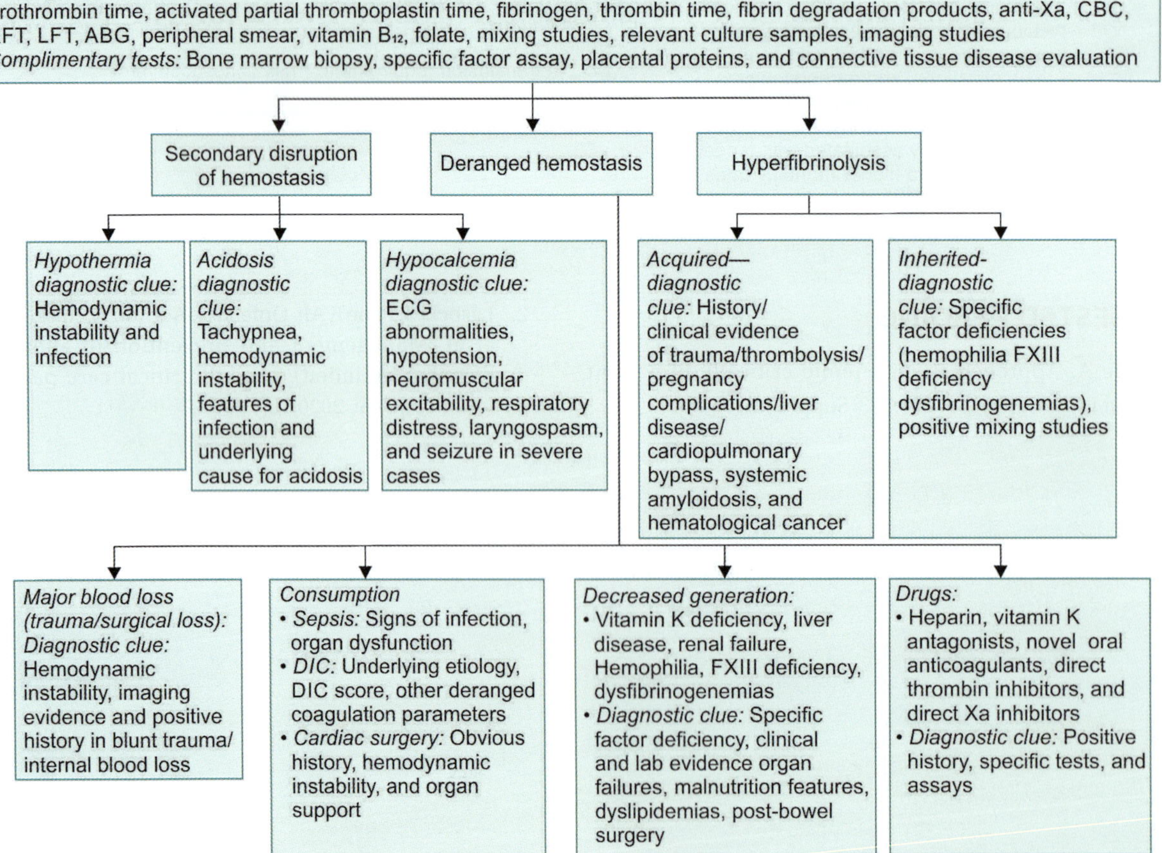


(ABG: arterial blood gas; APTT: activated partial thromboplastin time; CBC: complete blood count; LFT: liver function test; PT: prothrombin time; RFT: renal function test)

## TREATMENT

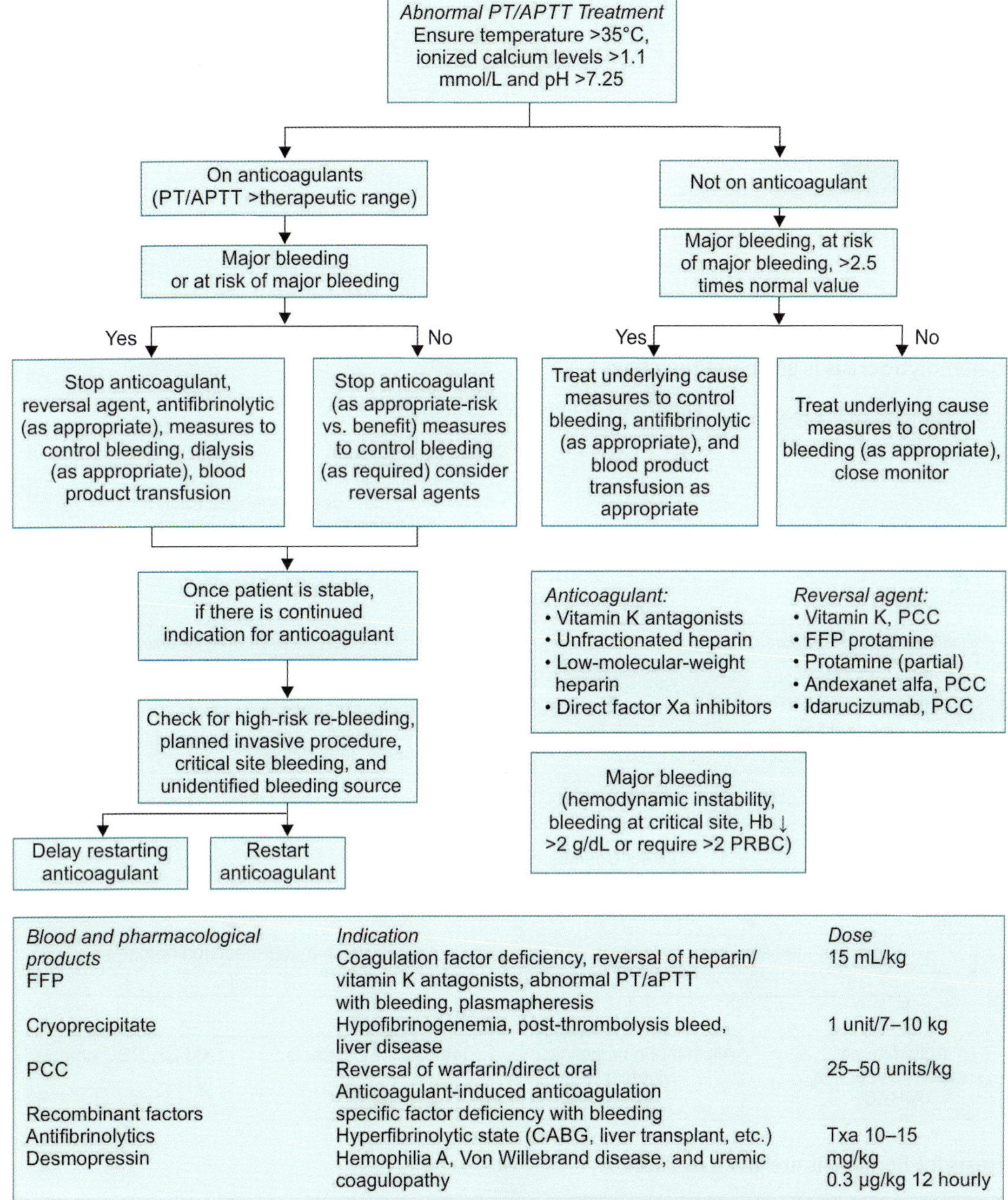


| *Blood and pharmacological products* | *Indication* | *Dose* |
|---|---|---|
| FFP | Coagulation factor deficiency, reversal of heparin/ vitamin K antagonists, abnormal PT/aPTT with bleeding, plasmapheresis | 15 mL/kg |
| Cryoprecipitate | Hypofibrinogenemia, post-thrombolysis bleed, liver disease | 1 unit/7–10 kg |
| PCC | Reversal of warfarin/direct oral Anticoagulant-induced anticoagulation | 25–50 units/kg |
| Recombinant factors | specific factor deficiency with bleeding | |
| Antifibrinolytics | Hyperfibrinolytic state (CABG, liver transplant, etc.) | Txa 10–15 mg/kg |
| Desmopressin | Hemophilia A, Von Willebrand disease, and uremic coagulopathy | 0.3 µg/kg 12 hourly |

(APTT: activated partial thromboplastin time; CABG: coronary artery bypass grafting; FFP: fresh frozen plasma; PCC: prothrombin complex concentrate; PT: prothrombin time; Txa: tranexamic acid)

## SUGGESTED READING

1. Chornenki NLJ, Fralick M, Sholzberg M. International normalized ratio and activated partial thromboplastin time testing. CMAJ. 2022;194(33):E1135.
2. Neuenfeldt FS, Weigand MA, Fischer D. Coagulopathies in intensive care medicine: Balancing act between thrombosis and bleeding. J Clin Med. 2021;10(22):5369.
3. Singh MY. Approach to the coagulopathic patient in the intensive care unit. Indian J Crit Care Med. 2019;23(Suppl 3):S215-20.

CHAPTER 128

# Hemolytic Crisis

## HEMOLYTIC CRISIS

Approach to hemolytic crisis is given in **Flowchart 1**.

**Flowchart 1:** Approach to hemolytic crisis.

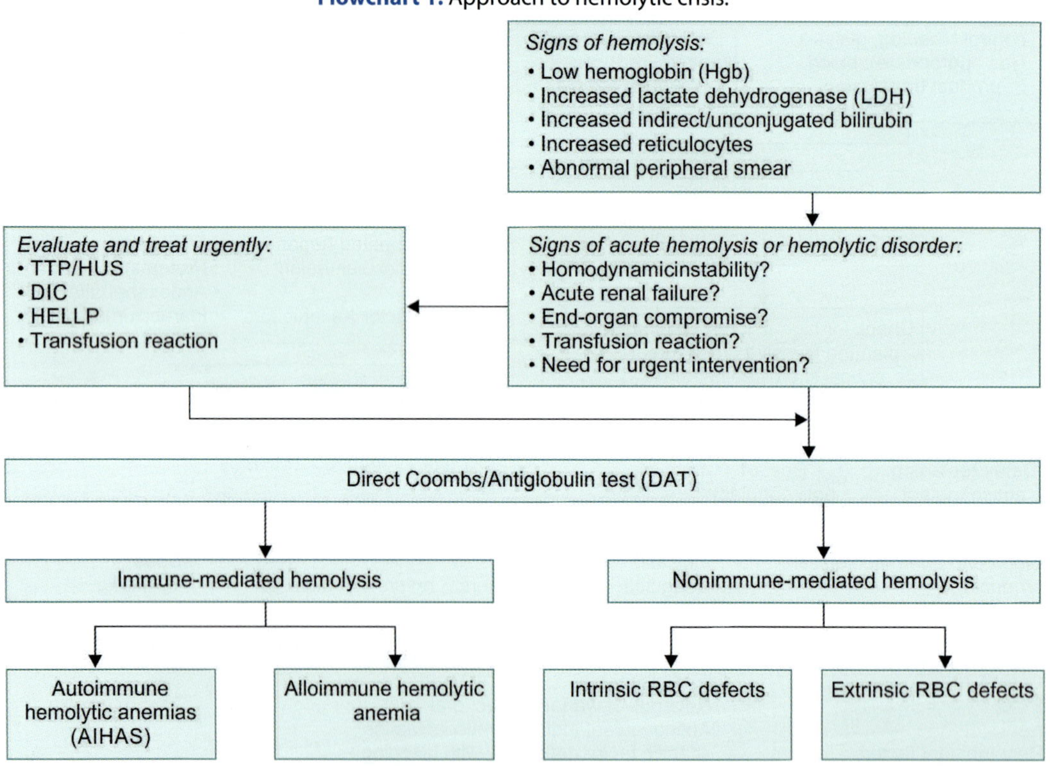


Laboratory tests for hemolysis are given in **Table 1**.

**TABLE 1:** Laboratory tests for hemolysis.

| *Tests* | *Findings in hemolysis* | *Cause* |
|---|---|---|
| Haptoglobin | Decreased | Binds free hemoglobin released from lysed red blood cells |
| Lactate dehydrogenase (LDH) | Elevated | Released from lysed RBC |
| Peripheral blood smear | Abnormal red blood cells | Depends on the underlying cause of anemia |
| Reticulocyte count | Increased | Marrow response to anemia |
| Unconjugated bilirubin | Increased | Hemoglobin breakdown |
| Urinalysis | Urobilinogen, positive for blood | Free Hb and its metabolites |

Approach to immune hemolytic anemia is given in **Flowchart 2**.

**Flowchart 2:** Immune hemolytic anemia.

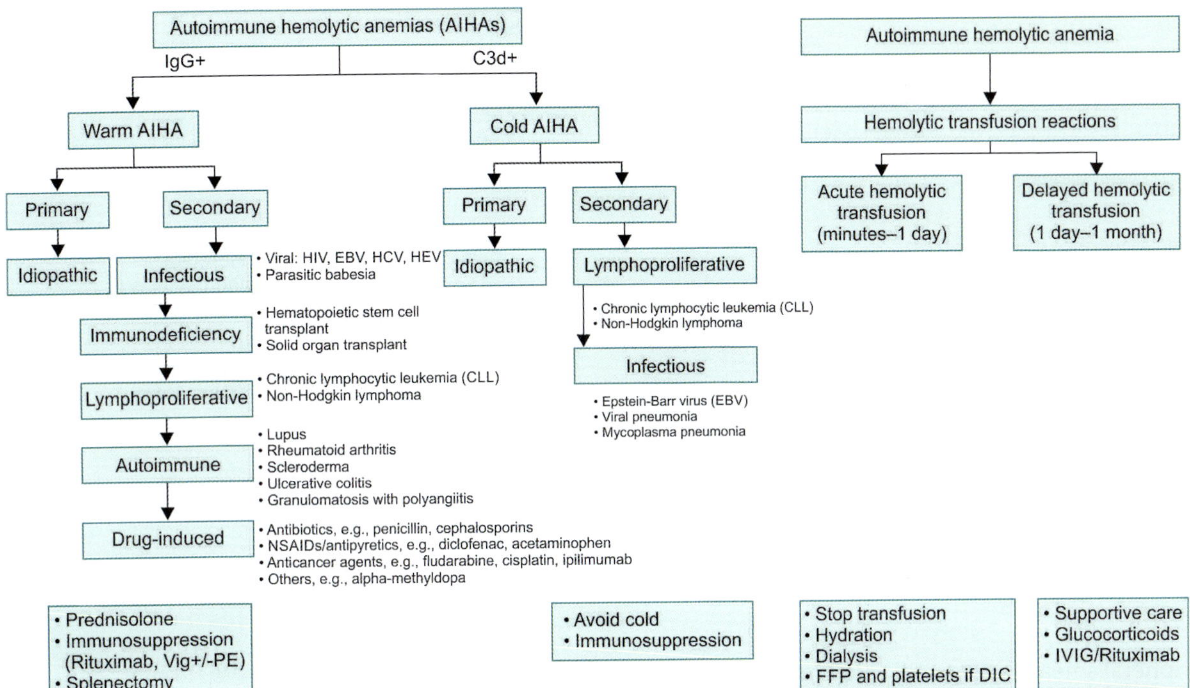


The comparison between intravascular hemolysis and extravascular hemolysis is given in **Table 2**.

**TABLE 2:** Intravascular hemolysis versus extravascular hemolysis.

| | *Intravascular hemolysis* | *Extravascular hemolysis* |
|---|---|---|
| Site of hemolysis | Within the circulation (vasculature) | Mononuclear phagocytes of RES—spleen and liver macrophages |
| Free hemoglobin | Released in blood | Engulfed by macrophages |
| Serum haptoglobin | Decreased or absent | Normal or slightly decreased |
| In blood | • Hemoglobinemia<br>• Methemoglobinemia<br>• Mild unconjugated hyperbilirubinemia | Unconjugated hyperbilirubinemia |
| In urine | • Hemoglobinuria (brown)<br>• Hemosiderinuria | Increased urobilinogen and urobilin (yellow) |
| Spleen and liver | Normal | Enlarged |

Approach to nonimmune hemolytic anemia (intrinsic RBC defects) is given in **Flowchart 3**.

**Flowchart 3:** Nonimmune hemolytic anemia (intrinsic RBC defects).

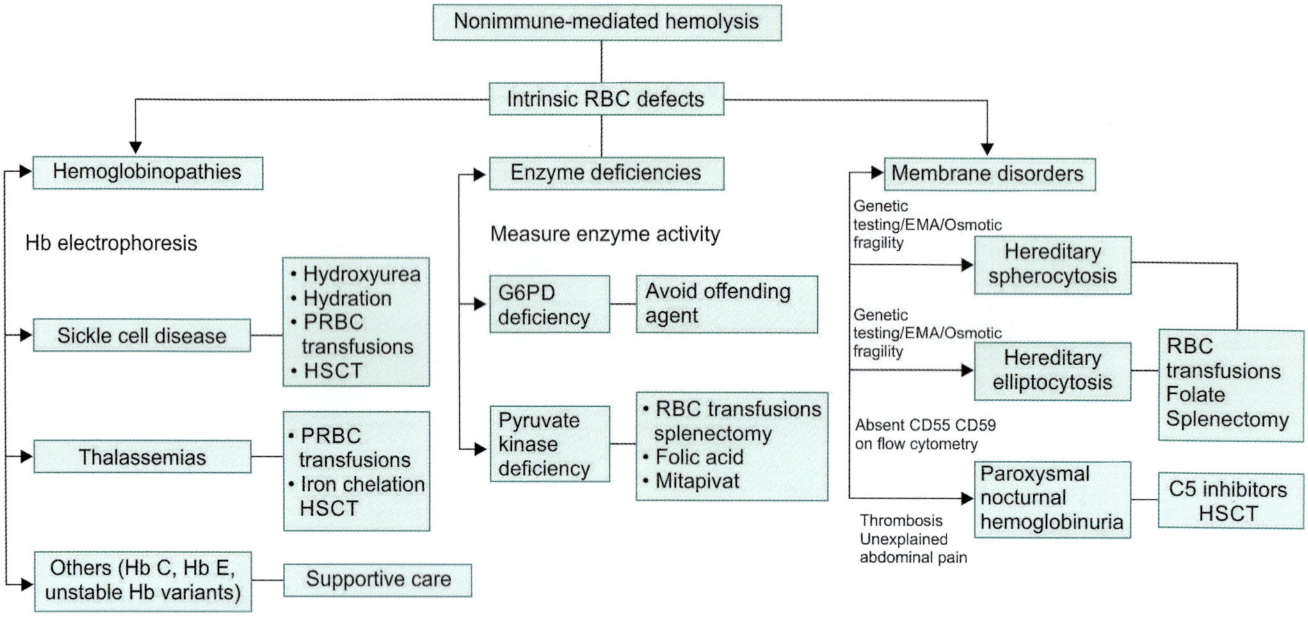

- Nonimmune-mediated hemolysis
  - Intrinsic RBC defects
    - Hemoglobinopathies
      - Hb electrophoresis
      - Sickle cell disease — • Hydroxyurea • Hydration • PRBC transfusions • HSCT
      - Thalassemias — • PRBC transfusions • Iron chelation HSCT
      - Others (Hb C, Hb E, unstable Hb variants) — Supportive care
    - Enzyme deficiencies
      - Measure enzyme activity
      - G6PD deficiency — Avoid offending agent
      - Pyruvate kinase deficiency — • RBC transfusions splenectomy • Folic acid • Mitapivat
    - Membrane disorders
      - Genetic testing/EMA/Osmotic fragility → Hereditary spherocytosis — RBC transfusions Folate Splenectomy
      - Genetic testing/EMA/Osmotic fragility → Hereditary elliptocytosis — RBC transfusions Folate Splenectomy
      - Absent CD55 CD59 on flow cytometry; Thrombosis Unexplained abdominal pain → Paroxysmal nocturnal hemoglobinuria — C5 inhibitors HSCT

Peripheral smear as diagnostic aid is detailed in **Table 3**.

**TABLE 3:** Peripheral smear as diagnostic aid.

| *Morphological observation* | *Significance* | *Further tests indicated* |
|---|---|---|
| Oval macrocytes and basophilic stippling | Megaloblastic anemia | Serum vitamin $B_{12}$ and folate levels |
| Microcytosis | Chronic disorder; thalassemia trait | Hb electrophoresis/HPLC |
| Hypochromia | Iron deficiency anemia | Serum ferritin, transferrin, and iron levels |
| Sickle cells | Sickle cell disease | Hb electrophoresis to confirm presence of HbS |
| Spherocytes | Hereditary spherocytosis | Red cell membrane analysis |
| Elliptocytes/ovalocytes | Hereditary elliptocytosis/ovalocytosis | Red cell membrane analysis |
| Red-cell fragmentation | • *If platelets decreased:* Microangiopathic hemolysis<br>• *If platelets normal:* Macroangiopathic hemolysis | • *Microangiopathic hemolysis:* DIC screen → consumptive coagulopathy<br>• *U&E:* Marked renal dysfunction in HUS<br>• *Altered neurological status:* Suspect TTP |

Approach to nonimmune hemolytic anemia (extrinsic RBC defects) is given in **Flowchart 4**.

**Flowchart 4:** Nonimmune hemolytic anemia (extrinsic RBC defects).

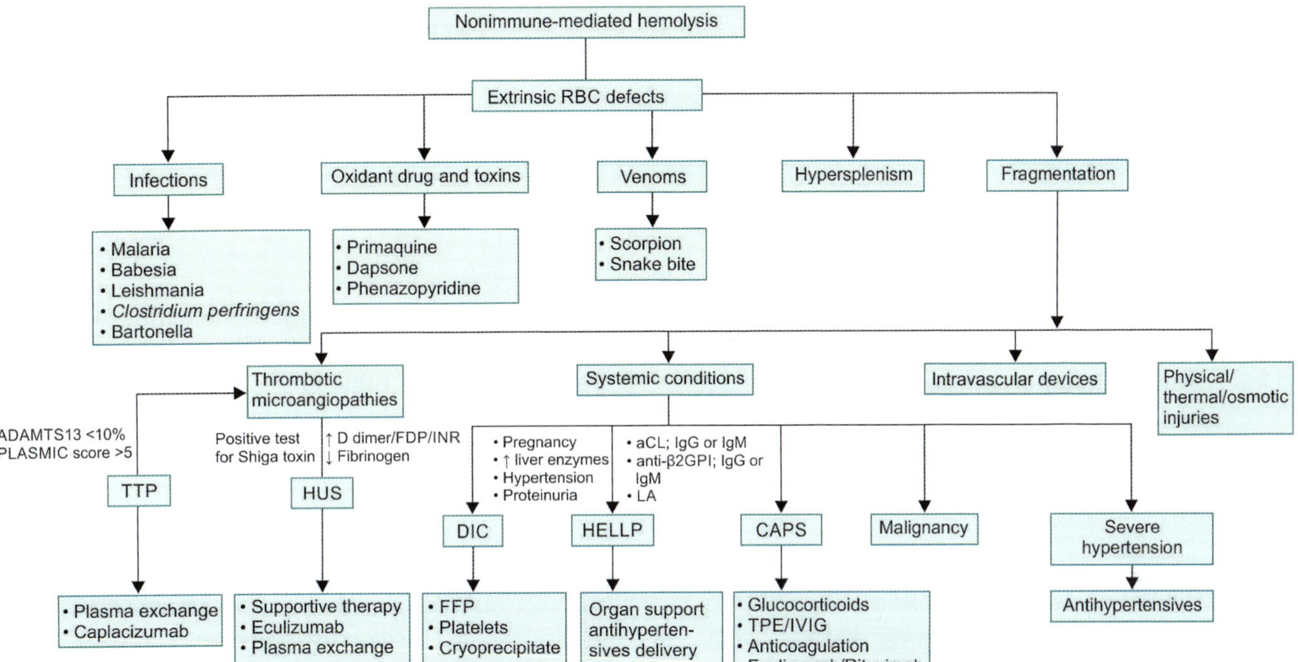


**TABLE 4:** PLASMIC score for predicting ADAMTS13 activity.

| *Variable* | *Score* |
|---|---|
| Platelet count <30 × $10^9$/L | 1 |
| Hemolysis | 1 |
| No cancer history | 1 |
| No transplantation history | 1 |
| MCV <90 fL | 1 |
| Creatinine <2 mg/dL | 1 |
| INR <1.5 | 1 |

*(Note: 0–4 (low risk)*: 4.3%; *5–6 (intermediate risk)*: 56.8%; and *7 (high risk)*: 96.2%)

PLASMIC score for predicting ADAMTS13 activity is given in **Table 4**.

## SUGGESTED READING

1. Berentsen S, Barcellini W. Autoimmune Hemolytic Anemias. N Engl J Med. 2021;385:1407-19.
2. Jamwal M, Sharma P, Das R. Laboratory approach to hemolytic anemia. Indian J Pediatr. 2020;87(1):66-74.

CHAPTER

# 129 Tumor Lysis Syndrome

## CRITERIA FOR LABORATORY AND CLINICAL TUMOR LYSIS SYNDROME AS DEFINED BY CAIRO–BISHOP

Laboratory tumor lysis syndrome (TLS) is defined by any 2 or more of the listed values within 3 days before or 7 days after initiation of chemotherapy, in the setting of adequate hydration (with or without alkalinization) and use of a hypouricemic agent **(Table 1)**.

Clinical TLS **(Table 2)** is defined by the presence of laboratory TLS plus 1 of the listed features in the absence of some other cause.

**TABLE 1:** Laboratory tumor lysis syndrome.

| *Variable* | *Value* | *Change from baseline* |
|---|---|---|
| Uric acid | >8 mg/dL | >25% increase |
| Potassium | >6 mEq/L | >25% increase |
| Phosphorus | >4.5 mg/dL | >25% increase |
| Calcium | <7 mg/dL | >25% decrease |

**TABLE 2:** Clinical tumor lysis syndrome.

| *Variable* | *Grade 0* | *Grade 1* | *Grade 2* | *Grade 3* | *Grade 4* | *Grade 5* |
|---|---|---|---|---|---|---|
| Creatinine | <1.5 × ULN | 1.5 ULN | >1.5–3 × ULN | >3–6 × ULN | >6 × ULN | Death |
| Cardiac arrythmia | None | Nil intervention | Medical intervention | Controlled with device (defib) | Life-threatening arrythmia | Death |
| Seizures | None | | Generalized seizure (controlled by drugs) | Poorly controlled with drugs | Status epilepticus and intractable epilepsy | Death |

## APPROACH TO MANAGEMENT OF TUMOR LYSIS SYNDROME

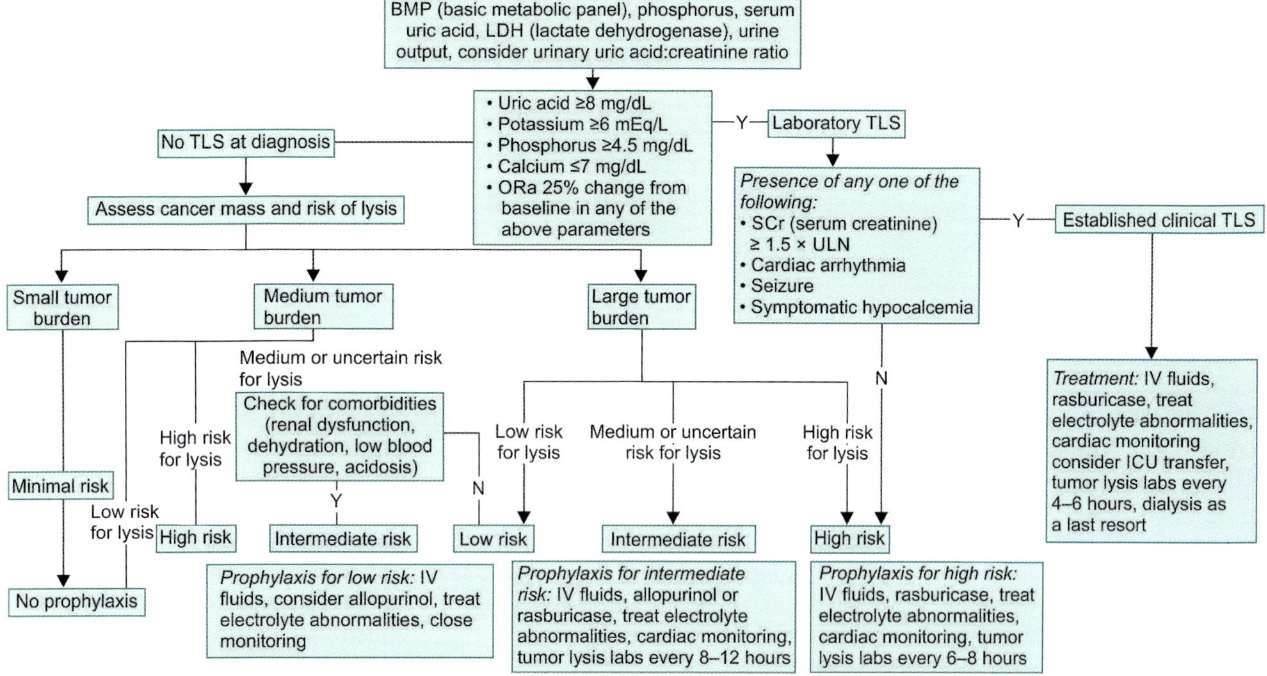


Low-, intermediate- and high-risk groups are given in **Table 3**.

**TABLE 3:** Low-, intermediate- and high-risk groups.

| ***Low-risk group (<5% risk of TLS)*** | ***Intermediate-risk group (1–5% risk of TLS)*** | ***High-risk group (>5% risk of TLS)*** |
|---|---|---|
| • *Acute myeloid leukemia* with WBC <25,000/µL and serum LDH <2 times ULN<br>• *Chronic lymphocytic leukemia* with WBC ≤50,000/µL and not treated with fludarabine/rituximab or venetoclax<br>• *Multiple myeloma and chronic myeloid leukemia*<br>• *Non-Hodgkin lymphoma* with normal serum LDH and not meeting high- or intermediate-risk criteria<br>• Other solid tumors | • Adult T-cell lymphoma/leukemia, DLBCL, peripheral T-cell lymphoma, transformed lymphoma, mantle-cell lymphoma with serum LDH above ULN but without bulky disease<br>• *Childhood anaplastic large cell lymphoma* (stage III/IV) with serum LDH <2 times ULN<br>• *Burkitt lymphoma* (early stage) with serum LDH <2 times ULN<br>• *Acute lymphoblastic leukemia* with WBC <100,000/µL and serum LDH <2 times ULN<br>• *Acute myeloid leukemia* with WBC 25,000–100,000/µL or WBC <25,000 and serum LDH = 2 times ULN<br>• Lymphoblastic lymphoma (early stage) with serum LDH <2 times ULN<br>• *Chronic lymphocytic* leukemia treated with fludarabine/rituximab, or lenalidomide, or venetoclax with lymph nodes ≥5 cm or absolute lymphocyte count ≥25 × $10^9$/L, and/or WBC ≥50,000/µL<br>• *Solid tumors (bulky and highly thermosensitive):* Neuroblastoma, germ cell cancer, small cell lung cancer | • *Burkitt lymphoma* with serum LDH ≥2 times ULN<br>• *Acute lymphoblastic leukemia* with WBC ≥100,000/µL and/or serum LDH ≥2 times ULN<br>Acute myeloid leukemia with WBC ≥100,000/µL<br>• *Lymphoblastic lymphoma* with serum LDH ≥2 times ULN or stage III/IV lymphoblastic lymphoma<br>• *Chronic lymphocytic leukemia* treated with venetoclax + hyperuricemia + lymph node ≥10 cm or lymph nodes ≥5 cm + absolute lymphocyte count ≥25 × $10^9$/L<br>• *Childhood DLBC* (stage III/IV) with serum LDH ≥2 times ULN<br>• Intermediate-risk disease with renal dysfunction and/or uric acid, potassium, or phosphate levels above ULN |

## SUGGESTED READING

1. Ho M, Zanwar S, Duggan P, Carr R, Habermann T, Navin PJ, et al. Hiding in (not so) plain sight: Spontaneous tumor Lysis syndrome due to intravascular large B cell lymphoma. Am J Hematol. 2022;97(1):151-9.
2. Howard SC, Jones DP, Pui CH. The tumor lysis syndrome. N Engl J Med. 2011;364(19):1844-54.

CHAPTER 130

# Mismatched Blood Transfusion

## BLOOD TRANSFUSION REACTIONS

| *Type of reaction* | *Important features* | *Management* |
|---|---|---|
| Acute hemolytic transfusion reaction (AHTR) | Caused by ABO or non-ABO incompatibility. Leads to intravascular hemolysis of donor red blood cells (RBCs) | Supportive therapy. Ensure adequate renal perfusion. Manage DIC |
| Delayed hemolytic transfusion reaction (DHTR) | Caused by antibodies against non-ABO RBC antigens, usually Duffy or Kidd antigens. Antibodies are often acquired through previous transfusions or pregnancy | Withhold further transfusions until the antibody is determined. Intravenous immunoglobulin (IVIG) as a treatment option |
| Febrile nonhemolytic transfusion reaction (FNHTR) | Second most common transfusion reaction. Cytokines from Leukocytes | Antipyretic medications. Incidence decreased with leukoreduction |
| Allergic reactions—Urticarial | IgE-mediated reaction leading to histamine release. Mostly associated with fresh frozen plasma (FFP) and platelets transfusion | Mild reactions usually respond to antihistamines |
| Allergic reactions—Anaphylactic | Severe, but very rare. Higher risk in IgA-deficient patients | Fluids, vasopressors, corticosteroids, antihistamines, epinephrine, and bronchodilators |
| Transfusion-related acute lung injury (TRALI) | Presents as noncardiogenic pulmonary edema. Highest risk with plasma-containing products | Supportive therapy. Usually does not respond to diuretics |
| Transfusion-associated circulatory overload (TACO) | Most common cause of transfusion-related mortality. Pulmonary edema due to excessive volume or rapid transfusion | Diuretics. Slow down the rate of transfusion |
| Transfusion-associated graft-versus-host disease (TA-GVHD) | Extremely rare late reaction. Donor leukocytes attack recipient cells | Prevented by irradiation of units for at-risk patients. Steroids and immunosuppressive drugs. High mortality rate despite treatment |
| Post-transfusion purpura (PTP) | Rare, delayed reaction. Recipient's alloantibodies attack donor platelet antigens | Hematology consultation. Intravenous Immunoglobulin (IVIG) is the favored treatment |

## PATHOPHYSIOLOGY OF MISMATCHED TRANSFUSION

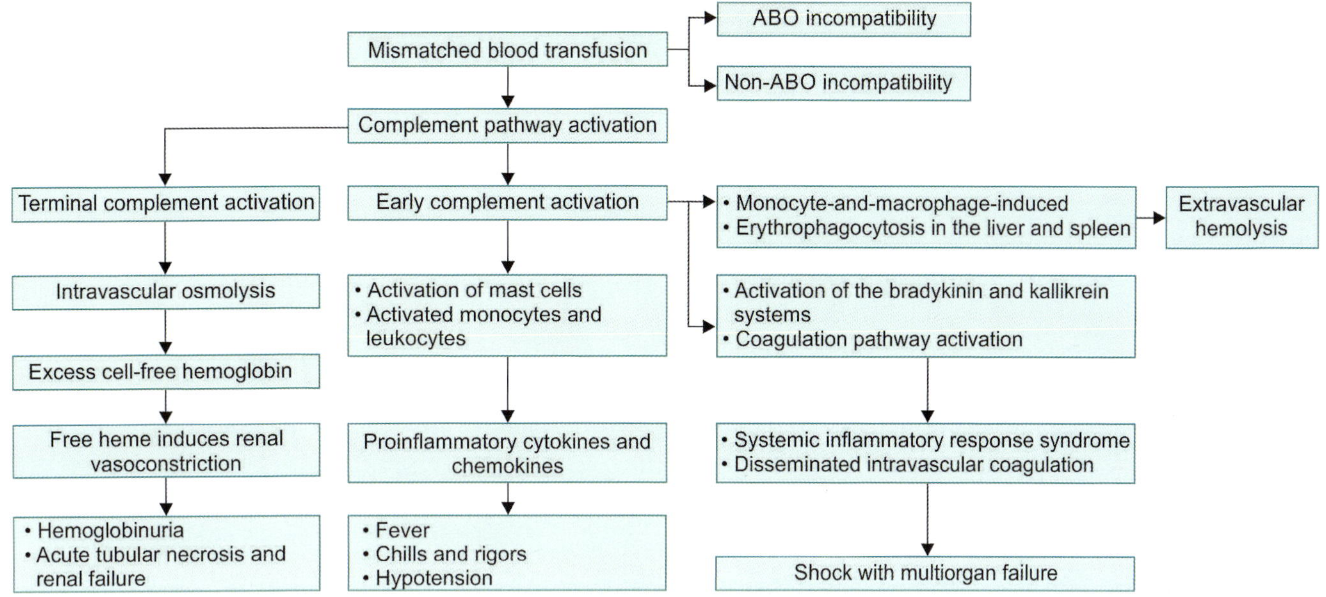


## MANAGEMENT OF MISMATCHED TRANSFUSION

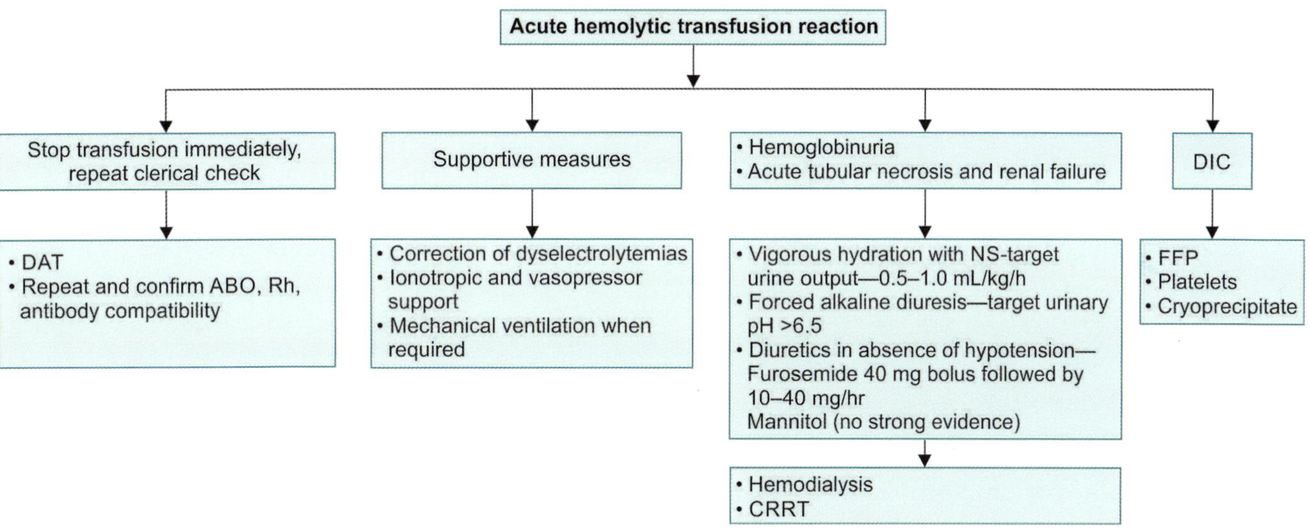


## SUGGESTED READING


1. Ackfeld T, Schmutz T, Guechi Y, Le Terrier C. Blood Transfusion Reactions-A Comprehensive Review of the Literature including a Swiss Perspective. J Clin Med. 2022;11(10):2859.
2. Panch SR, Montemayor-Garcia C, Klein HG. Hemolytic transfusion reactions. N Engl J Med. 2019;381(2):150-62.

# PART 13

# INFECTIONS

***Editors:*** Saswati Sinha, Vaishali Solao
***Associate Editor:*** Mohit Kharbanda

CHAPTER

# 131 Approach to a Patient with Fever and Thrombocytopenia

## INTRODUCTION

Fever and thrombocytopenia may occur due to a wide variety of clinical conditions and can often be multifactorial especially in a critically ill or hospitalized patient. Prompt recognition of the cause and timely management can be lifesaving in conditions such as thrombotic microangiopathies, disseminated intravascular coagulation (DIC) and Acute promyelocytic leukemia and Heparin induced thrombocytopenia (HIT). Identification of "red flag" signs in history, clinical examination, associated organ involvement and certain basic investigations can help in appropriate diagnosis and management.

## HISTORY

- Clinical context—outpatient/critically ill/pregnancy
- Past history—autoimmune disorders, infections, malignancy, and previous history of thrombocytopenia
- Recent history—medications (including chemotherapy and alternative medications) and vaccination
- Travel history/endemic—tropical infections
- Risk factors—retroviral infections/viral hepatitis
- History of alcohol consumption

## PHYSICAL EXAMINATION

- Overt bleeding—petechiae, purpura, mucocutaneous bleeding
- Hepatosplenomegaly—infections, hematological disorders
- Altered mental status—TMA/ fulminant hepatic failure
- Thrombotic manifestations—TMA/DIC/HIT
- Lymphadenopathy—Infections, lymphoma
- Jaundice—Infections, hepatitis
- Joint/soft tissue bleed—additional coagulopathy

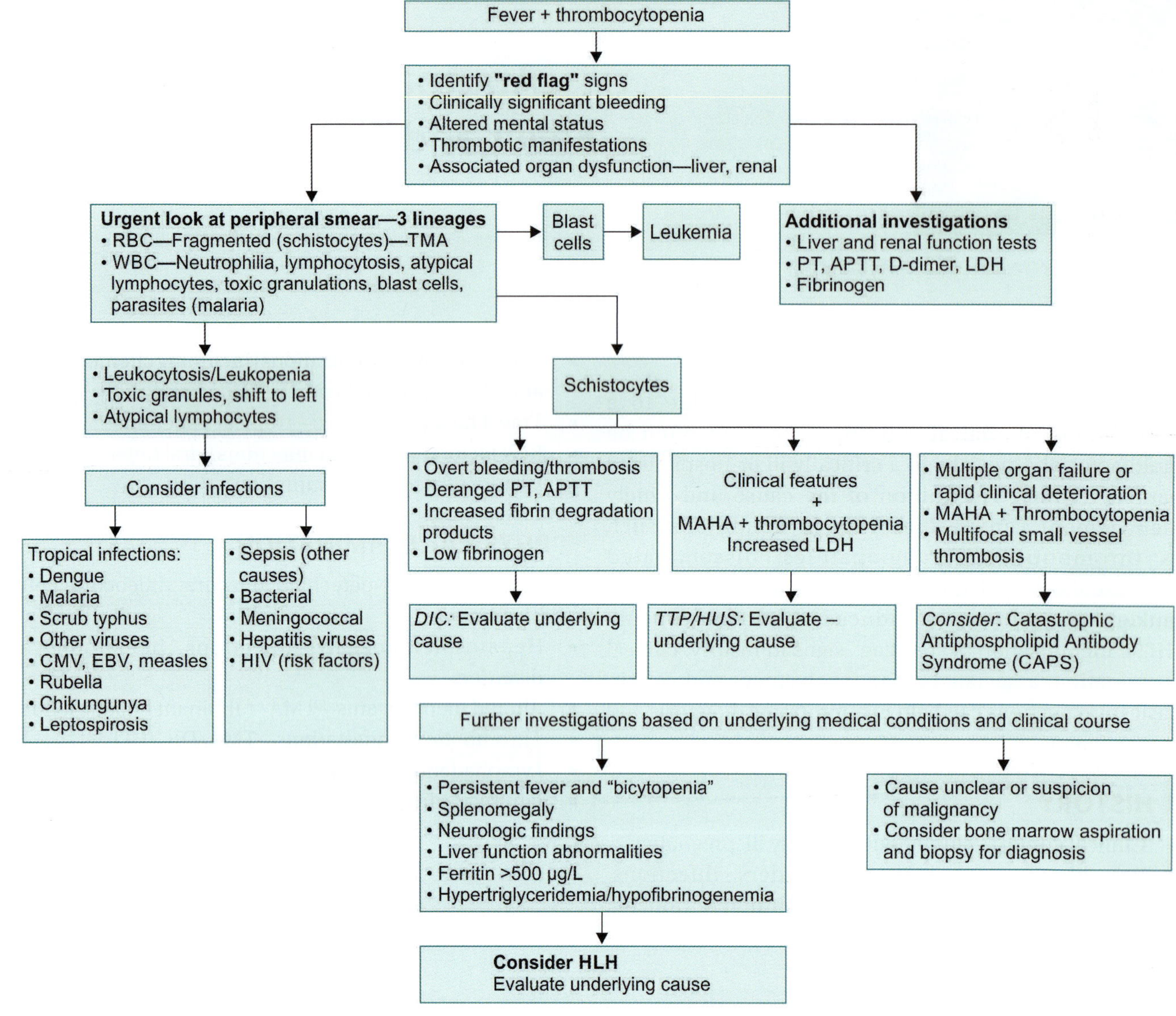
Fever + thrombocytopenia
• Identify "red flag" signs
• Clinically significant bleeding
• Altered mental status
• Thrombotic manifestations
• Associated organ dysfunction—liver, renal
Urgent look at peripheral smear—3 lineages
• RBC—Fragmented (schistocytes)—TMA
• WBC—Neutrophilia, lymphocytosis, atypical lymphocytes, toxic granulations, blast cells, parasites (malaria)
Blast cells
Leukemia
Additional investigations
• Liver and renal function tests
• PT, APTT, D-dimer, LDH
• Fibrinogen
• Leukocytosis/Leukopenia
• Toxic granules, shift to left
• Atypical lymphocytes
Consider infections
Tropical infections:
• Dengue
• Malaria
• Scrub typhus
• Other viruses
• CMV, EBV, measles
• Rubella
• Chikungunya
• Leptospirosis
• Sepsis (other causes)
• Bacterial
• Meningococcal
• Hepatitis viruses
• HIV (risk factors)
Schistocytes
• Overt bleeding/thrombosis
• Deranged PT, APTT
• Increased fibrin degradation products
• Low fibrinogen
Clinical features + MAHA + thrombocytopenia Increased LDH
• Multiple organ failure or rapid clinical deterioration
• MAHA + Thrombocytopenia
• Multifocal small vessel thrombosis
DIC: Evaluate underlying cause
TTP/HUS: Evaluate – underlying cause
Consider: Catastrophic Antiphospholipid Antibody Syndrome (CAPS)
Further investigations based on underlying medical conditions and clinical course
• Persistent fever and "bicytopenia"
• Splenomegaly
• Neurologic findings
• Liver function abnormalities
• Ferritin >500 µg/L
• Hypertriglyceridemia/hypofibrinogenemia
• Cause unclear or suspicion of malignancy
• Consider bone marrow aspiration and biopsy for diagnosis
Consider HLH
Evaluate underlying cause

CHAPTER 132

# Fever with Jaundice

## INTRODUCTION

Fever with jaundice is quite common in the ICU and can present as a diagnostic dilemma as there can be multiple causes and can often be multifactorial. Meticulous history taking, clinical examination and analysis of the abnormalities in biochemical as well as synthetic functions of the liver can help narrow down the differential diagnosis and guide the proper choice of imaging if necessary to find out the cause.

## HISTORY

### Clues to Likely Diagnosis

- Fever, chills, abdominal pain, or influenza-like symptoms—acute infection
- Typical prodromal symptoms with jaundice and right upper abdominal pain—viral hepatitis
- Acute right upper quadrant pain, fever, chills, nausea, and vomiting—choledocholithiasis/cholangitis
- Associated symptoms—rash, altered sensorium, bleeding, joint pains, and myalgias
- History of travel—exposure to ticks
- History of trauma
- Careful history of alcohol, drugs (including alternative medicines, herbal medications, over the counter medications, illicit drugs)
- History of blood transfusion, surgery or other procedures (hepatitis B and C), exposure to patient with jaundice—hepatitis A
- Occupational or recreational exposure to industrial toxins—vinyl chloride, mushrooms (Amanita phalloides)
- Other associated medical conditions

## PHYSICAL EXAMINATION

- *Stigmata of chronic liver disease*—palmar erythema, spider nevi, caput medusae, gynecomastia
- Rash, eschar, joint swelling, altered consciousness, prostration, seizures, respiratory distress—*tropical infections*
- *Tenderness and respiratory arrest on deep palpation of right hypochondrium (Murphy's sign)*—acute cholecystitis
- Consistency of the liver on palpation, splenomegaly, and ascites
- Supraclavicular (Virchow node) or peri umbilical nodule (Sister Mary Joseph nodule)—abdominal malignancy

## BASIS OF DIAGNOSTIC EVALUATION

*Goal of laboratory testing*—pattern of the disease process (prehepatic, hepatocellular, or obstructive)

- *CBC*—relative erythrocyte numbers/hemoglobin mass, Schistocytes in peripheral smear (intravascular hemolysis)
- *Aminotransferases (ALT/AST)*—ALT is more specific for liver parenchymal damage, AST/ALT ratios and magnitude of elevation may indicate the underlying pathology (limited utility in chronic liver disease).
- *Gamma glutamyl transferase (GGT)*—similar to AST/ALT, may be elevated in alcohol related liver disease, less specific
- *Alkaline phosphatase (ALP)*—marker of cholestatic disease
- *Albumin, prothrombin time (INR)*—synthetic function of liver, need to be assessed as per clinical context.

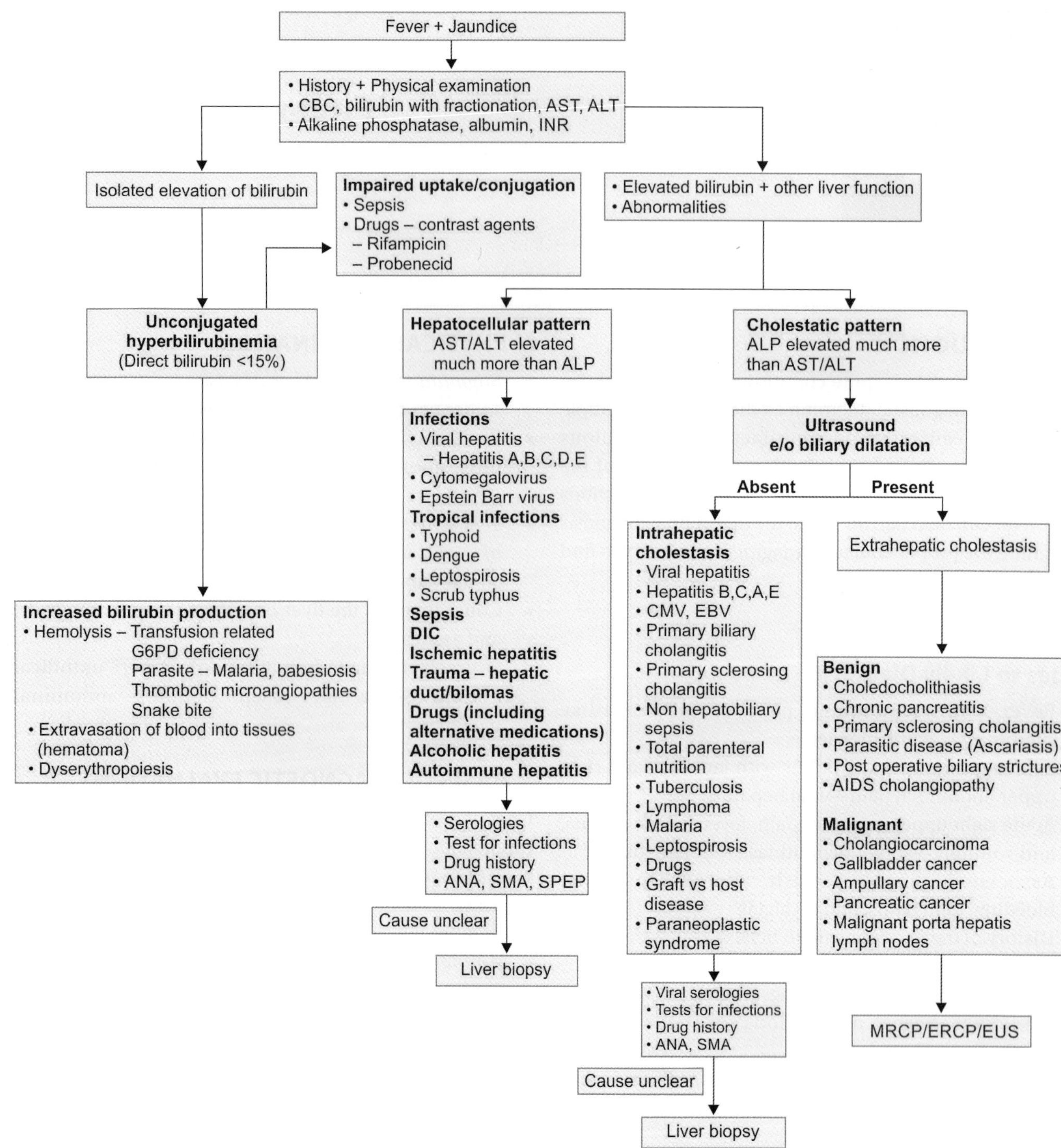
Fever + Jaundice
• History + Physical examination
• CBC, bilirubin with fractionation, AST, ALT
• Alkaline phosphatase, albumin, INR
Isolated elevation of bilirubin
Impaired uptake/conjugation
• Sepsis
• Drugs – contrast agents
– Rifampicin
– Probenecid
• Elevated bilirubin + other liver function
• Abnormalities
Unconjugated hyperbilirubinemia
(Direct bilirubin <15%)
Hepatocellular pattern
AST/ALT elevated much more than ALP
Cholestatic pattern
ALP elevated much more than AST/ALT
Infections
• Viral hepatitis
– Hepatitis A,B,C,D,E
• Cytomegalovirus
• Epstein Barr virus
Tropical infections
• Typhoid
• Dengue
• Leptospirosis
• Scrub typhus
Sepsis
DIC
Ischemic hepatitis
Trauma – hepatic duct/bilomas
Drugs (including alternative medications)
Alcoholic hepatitis
Autoimmune hepatitis
Ultrasound
e/o biliary dilatation
Absent
Present
Intrahepatic cholestasis
• Viral hepatitis
• Hepatitis B,C,A,E
• CMV, EBV
• Primary biliary cholangitis
• Primary sclerosing cholangitis
• Non hepatobiliary sepsis
• Total parenteral nutrition
• Tuberculosis
• Lymphoma
• Malaria
• Leptospirosis
• Drugs
• Graft vs host disease
• Paraneoplastic syndrome
Extrahepatic cholestasis
Increased bilirubin production
• Hemolysis – Transfusion related
G6PD deficiency
Parasite – Malaria, babesiosis
Thrombotic microangiopathies
Snake bite
• Extravasation of blood into tissues (hematoma)
• Dyserythropoiesis
Benign
• Choledocholithiasis
• Chronic pancreatitis
• Primary sclerosing cholangitis
• Parasitic disease (Ascariasis)
• Post operative biliary strictures
• AIDS cholangiopathy
Malignant
• Cholangiocarcinoma
• Gallbladder cancer
• Ampullary cancer
• Pancreatic cancer
• Malignant porta hepatis lymph nodes
• Serologies
• Test for infections
• Drug history
• ANA, SMA, SPEP
Cause unclear
Liver biopsy
• Viral serologies
• Tests for infections
• Drug history
• ANA, SMA
Cause unclear
Liver biopsy
MRCP/ERCP/EUS

CHAPTER

# 133 Fever in an Immunocompromised Host

The proportion of critically ill immunocompromised patients have increased over the past several years. Immunocompromised patients include patients receiving long-term (>3 months) or high-dose (>0.5 mg/kg/day) steroids or other immunosuppressant drugs, solid-organ transplant recipients, patients with solid tumor requiring chemotherapy in the last 5 years or with hematological malignancy. Increased aggressiveness and duration of cancer treatments, greater use of organ and hematopoietic cell transplantation, and introduction for the treatment of autoimmune and autoinflammatory diseases of steroid sparing agents that induce specific immune defects. The type of immune deficit (T-cell, B-cell, complement, phagocyte) is likely to predict the kind of infection (bacterial, viral, fungal, parasitic).

## CHALLENGES

Both common and uncommon pathogens can cause infection in these patients—high index of suspicion is necessary.

Non-infectious syndromes can mimic infections - can make diagnosis challenging.

Clinical presentation may be altered due to the immune deficit—thorough history and physical examination is mandatory to identify the nature and severity of immunosuppression and the exposure to specific pathogens.

Invasive diagnostic procedures may be required to establish a confirmed diagnosis.

Molecular diagnostic testing and biomarkers need to be appropriately utilized to diagnose and guide therapy.

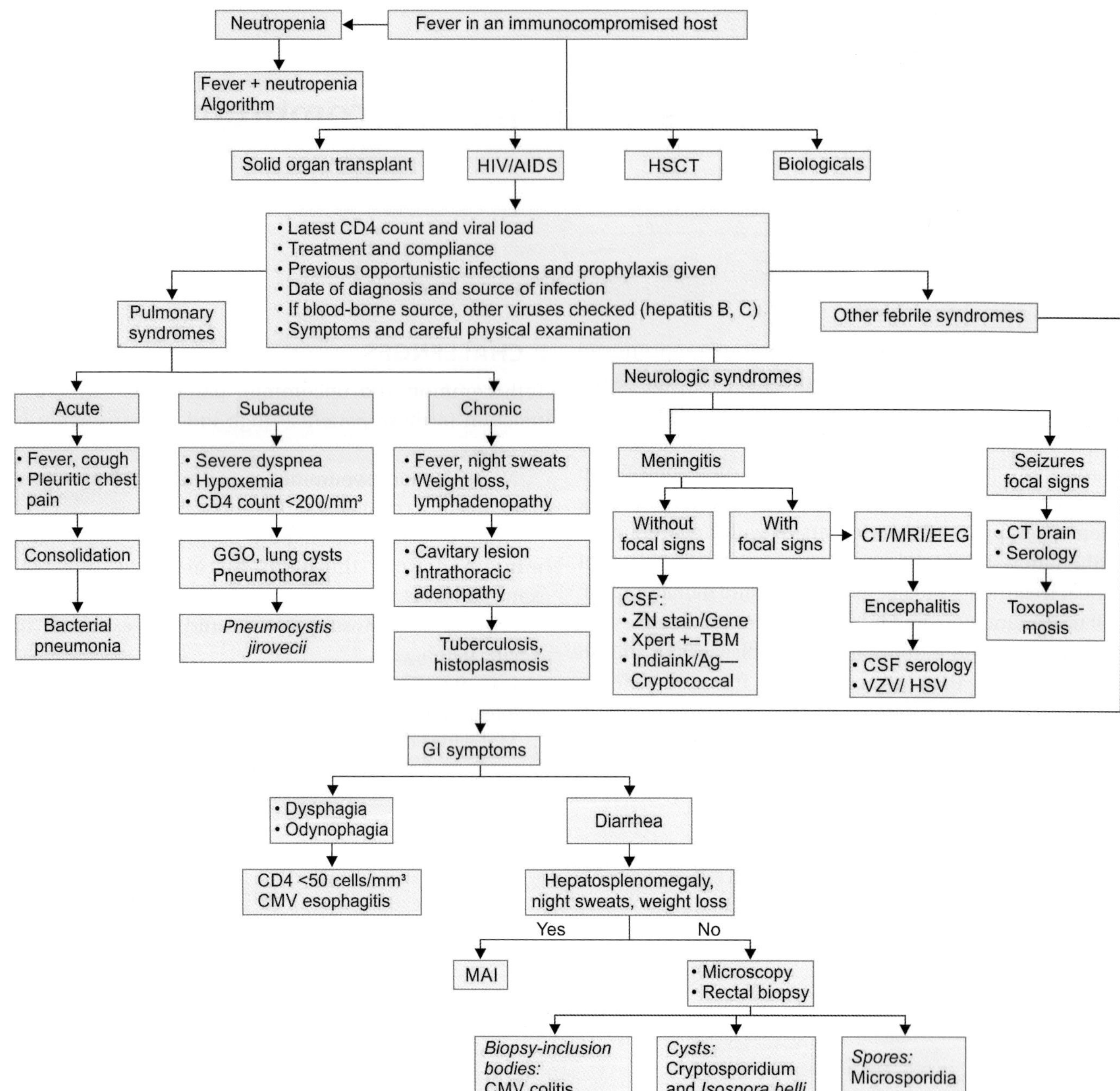
Fever in an immunocompromised host
Neutropenia
Fever + neutropenia Algorithm
Solid organ transplant
HIV/AIDS
HSCT
Biologicals
• Latest CD4 count and viral load
• Treatment and compliance
• Previous opportunistic infections and prophylaxis given
• Date of diagnosis and source of infection
• If blood-borne source, other viruses checked (hepatitis B, C)
• Symptoms and careful physical examination
Pulmonary syndromes
Other febrile syndromes
Neurologic syndromes
Acute
Subacute
Chronic
• Fever, cough
• Pleuritic chest pain
• Severe dyspnea
• Hypoxemia
• CD4 count <200/mm³
• Fever, night sweats
• Weight loss, lymphadenopathy
Consolidation
Bacterial pneumonia
GGO, lung cysts Pneumothorax
Pneumocystis jirovecii
• Cavitary lesion
• Intrathoracic adenopathy
Tuberculosis, histoplasmosis
Meningitis
Seizures focal signs
Without focal signs
With focal signs
CT/MRI/EEG
• CT brain
• Serology
CSF:
• ZN stain/Gene
• Xpert +–TBM
• Indiaink/Ag—Cryptococcal
Encephalitis
• CSF serology
• VZV/ HSV
Toxoplas-mosis
GI symptoms
• Dysphagia
• Odynophagia
Diarrhea
CD4 <50 cells/mm³ CMV esophagitis
Hepatosplenomegaly, night sweats, weight loss
Yes
No
MAI
• Microscopy
• Rectal biopsy
Biopsy-inclusion bodies: CMV colitis
Cysts: Cryptosporidium and Isospora belli
Spores: Microsporidia

**Fever in solid organ transplant recipient**

↓

**History**:
- Time since transplant
- Epidemiological exposures + pretransplant serologies (donor + recipient)
- Antimicrobial prophylaxis
- Immunosuppressive regimen
- Prior cultures (colonization with MDR pathogens)

↓

**Physical examination (may be altered due to immunosuppression):**
- *Surgical site:* Wound infection, dehiscence, hematoma
- *Hardware:* Indwelling catheters, drains, signs of inflammation
- *Systemic examination:* Neurological, lungs, abdomen, skin, axilla, groin, perianal region, spine, calves

**Investigations:**
- Urinalysis and urine culture
- 2 sets of blood culture
- Radiography, CT/ MRI—directed as per clinical presentation
- Invasive diagnostic procedures maybe needed:
  – Bronchoscopy—pulmonary infiltrates
  – Lumbar puncture—altered sensorium

**Time since transplantation**

| 0–30 days | 30–180 days | >180 days |
|---|---|---|
| • *Procedure related:* Wound infection, Anastomotic leaks, Organ ischemia, Line related<br>• Donor derived<br>• Recipient colonizers<br>• Nosocomial infections | • Period of most intense immunosuppression<br>• Residual infection<br>• Relapsed infection<br>• Opportunistic infections<br>• Re-activation of latent infection | • Community acquired<br>• Depends on net state of immune suppression |
| *OrganismsL*<br>• Drug-resistant pathogens<br>• MRSA, VRE<br>• *Candida*<br>• *Clostridium difficile* | *Organisms:*<br>• *Bacteria:* CRE, MRSA, VRE, *C. difficile, Mycobacterium tuberculosis, Nocardia*<br>• *Virus:* HSV, CMV, EBV, VZV, influenza, adenovirus Hepatitis B,C, BK polyoma virus<br>• *Fungal: Candida, Cryptococcus neoformans, Pneumocystis jirovecii*<br>• *Parasitic: Leishmania, Strongyloides, Trypanosoma cruzi, Toxoplasma* | *Organisms:*<br>• *Bacteria: M. tuberculosis Nocardia* sp<br>• *Virus:* HSV, CMV, EBV, VZV Influenza, hepatitis BK polyoma<br>• *Fungal:* Aspergillus (GVHD)<br>– Mucor<br>– Atypical molds |

Graft rejection should also be considered

## HEMATOPOIETIC CELL TRANSPLANT

### Definition

Transplantation of hematopoietic cells from any source (bone marrow, peripheral blood, umbilical cord blood).

### Risk Factors for Infection

- *Source*: Depending on *source* they are classified as
  - *Autologous*—patient's own cells
  - *Syngeneic*—identical twin (HLA identical)
  - *Allogeneic*—sibling, related or unrelated donor (HLA identical, haploidentical or mismatched)
  - *Umbilical cord blood*—HLA identical, haploidentical or mismatched
- *Time since transplant*: *Timelines*—type of infections can be divided based on the time elapsed since transplantation *(Day 0 - stem cells infused)*
  - Pre-engraftment—from transplantation to neutrophil recovery, approximately day 20 to 30
  - Early postengraftment—from engraftment to day 100
  - Late postengraftment—after day 100
- *Pretransplant patient factors:* Indication for transplant with infectious burden, infections prior to transplant (bacterial, viral, fungal) age, obesity (immobility/skin breakdown), psychological issues (compliance), surgical history geography (endemicity of infections), malnutrition, and indwelling devices
- *Post-transplant patient factors:* Graft versus host disease (GVHD)—skin, gut, indwelling devices—increased immunosuppression. Relapse of underlying disease, veno-occlusive disease, graft failure

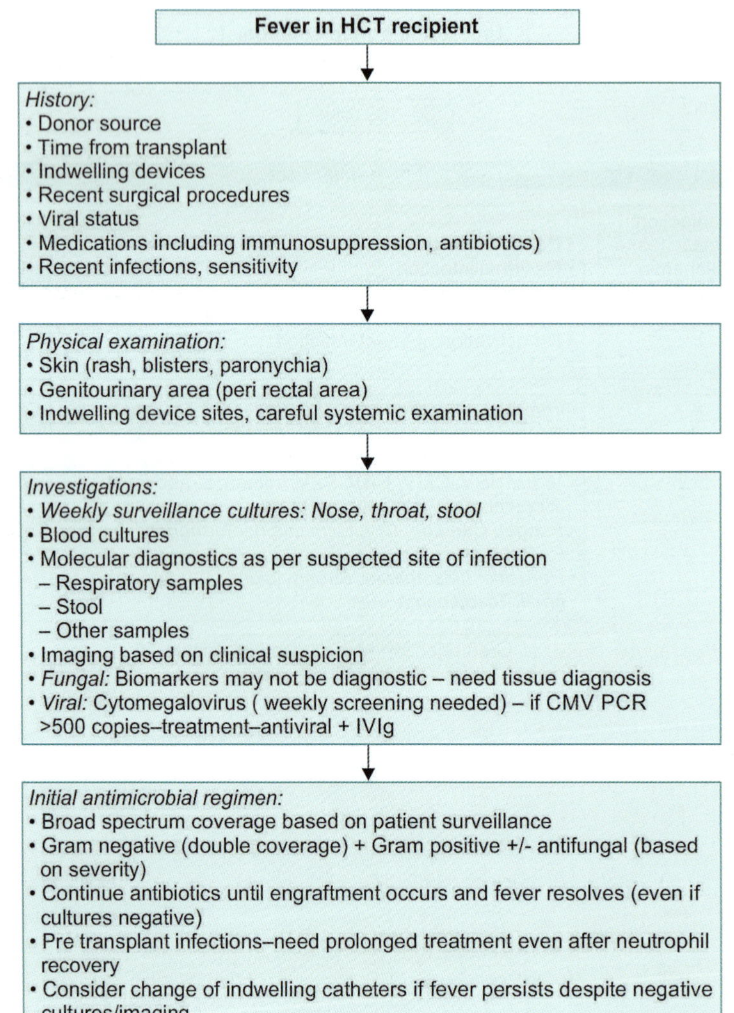

## COMMON INFECTIONS AFTER HCT AS PER TIMELINE

| *Site of infection* | *Early (<1 month)* | *Intermediate (1–4 months)* | *Late (>6 months)* |
|---|---|---|---|
| Disseminated | Gram negative/Gram positive | *Candida*, *Aspergillus*, EBV | Encapsulated bacteria (*S. pneumoniae*, *N. meningitis*, *H. influenzae*) |
| Skin and mucous membranes | HSV | HHV6 | VZV, HPV (warts) |
| Gastrointestinal tract | *Clostridium difficile* | CMV, Adenovirus, *Bradyrhizobium enterica* (cord blood cells) | EBV, CMV, *B. enterica* (cord blood cells) |
| Lungs | Aerobic bacteria (gram positive, gram negative), *Aspergillus*, *Candida*, other molds, HSV | *Pneumocystis*, seasonal respiratory viruses, *Toxoplasma* | *Pneumocystis*, *Nocardia*, *S. Pneumoniae* |
| Kidney | | BK virus, Adenovirus | |
| Brain | | HHV6, *Toxoplasma* | |
| Bone marrow | | CMV, HHV6 | CMV, HHV6 |

| *Clinical syndrome* | *Infectious differential diagnosis* | *Noninfectious differential diagnosis* |
|---|---|---|
| CLABSI | Gram positive, Gram negative bacteria, *Candida* | Infusion or Transfusion-related event |
| Diarrhea | Bacteria, virus, parasite, *Clostridium difficile*, CMV colitis | Graft vs Host disease |
| Enterocolitis | Infectious causes of diarrhea/dysentery, CMV | Conditioning related (Chemotherapy or TBI) |
| Encephalitis | HSV, VZV, CMV | Septic or metabolic encephalopathy |
| Hepatitis | CMV, HBV reactivation | GVHD of liver, Veno-occlusive disease of liver |
| Sepsis/septic shock | Bacterial, fungal | Cytokine release syndrome |
| Pneumonia | Respiratory viruses, CMV, Adenovirus, Gram positive, Gram negative bacteria, *Aspergillus*, Mucor, PCP, *Legionella* | Transfusion related acute lung injury, Aspiration, Pulmonary edema, Peri-engraftment respiratory distress syndrome (PERDS) |
| Pancytopenia | CMV, Bacterial sepsis | Nonengraftment or delayed engraftment, HLH |
| Skin and soft tissue infection/rash | Bacterial, viral, fungal | GVHD, disease infiltration, drug rash |
| Oral mucositis | HSV | Conditioning related |

# CHAPTER 134 Patient with Fever and Rash in the ICU

## INTRODUCTION

The diagnostic approach to the patient with rash and fever depends on the proper association of clinical findings using the syndromic approach. The appearance of the rash, epidemiologic information, and acuteness/severity of illness should be assessed diagnostically and combined with the pattern of organ involvement, which is the essence of the diagnostic process.

## HISTORY

Duration, onset site, history of exposure to any other patient, injury, surgery, drugs, insect bites, endemicity, spread, and systemic symptoms.

## EXAMINATION

Type of rash, spread, mucosal involvement, involvement of palms and feet, and systemic examination to look at other involved organs.

## INVESTIGATIONS

- CBC and CRP
- Renal function tests and liver function test
- ECG, echocardiography, X-ray chest
- Coagulation profile
- Blood and other appropriate cultures
- Dengue serology
- HIV, IgM *Leptospira*, IgM rubeola, HSV PCR, etc. depending on the type of rash

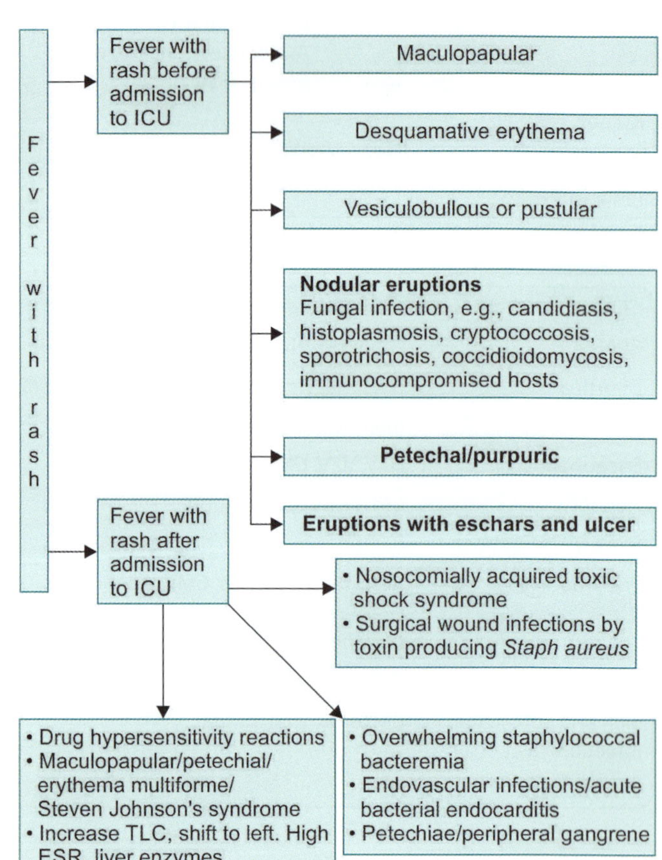

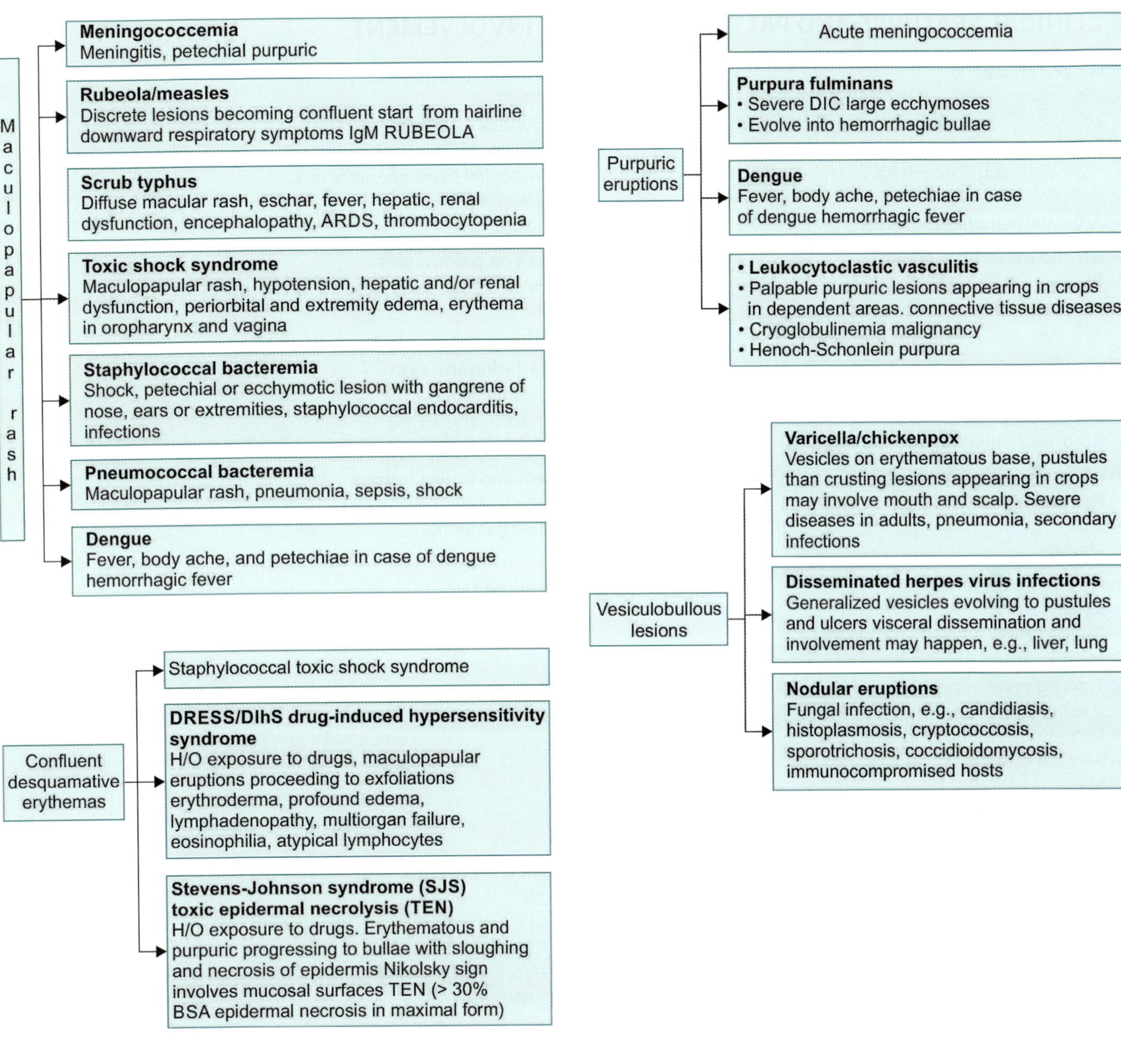
Maculopapular rash
Meningococcemia
Meningitis, petechial purpuric
Rubeola/measles
Discrete lesions becoming confluent start from hairline downward respiratory symptoms IgM RUBEOLA
Scrub typhus
Diffuse macular rash, eschar, fever, hepatic, renal dysfunction, encephalopathy, ARDS, thrombocytopenia
Toxic shock syndrome
Maculopapular rash, hypotension, hepatic and/or renal dysfunction, periorbital and extremity edema, erythema in oropharynx and vagina
Staphylococcal bacteremia
Shock, petechial or ecchymotic lesion with gangrene of nose, ears or extremities, staphylococcal endocarditis, infections
Pneumococcal bacteremia
Maculopapular rash, pneumonia, sepsis, shock
Dengue
Fever, body ache, and petechiae in case of dengue hemorrhagic fever
Purpuric eruptions
Acute meningococcemia
Purpura fulminans
• Severe DIC large ecchymoses
• Evolve into hemorrhagic bullae
Dengue
Fever, body ache, petechiae in case of dengue hemorrhagic fever
• Leukocytoclastic vasculitis
• Palpable purpuric lesions appearing in crops in dependent areas. connective tissue diseases
• Cryoglobulinemia malignancy
• Henoch-Schonlein purpura
Vesiculobullous lesions
Varicella/chickenpox
Vesicles on erythematous base, pustules than crusting lesions appearing in crops may involve mouth and scalp. Severe diseases in adults, pneumonia, secondary infections
Disseminated herpes virus infections
Generalized vesicles evolving to pustules and ulcers visceral dissemination and involvement may happen, e.g., liver, lung
Nodular eruptions
Fungal infection, e.g., candidiasis, histoplasmosis, cryptococcosis, sporotrichosis, coccidioidomycosis, immunocompromised hosts
Confluent desquamative erythemas
Staphylococcal toxic shock syndrome
DRESS/DIhS drug-induced hypersensitivity syndrome
H/O exposure to drugs, maculopapular eruptions proceeding to exfoliations erythroderma, profound edema, lymphadenopathy, multiorgan failure, eosinophilia, atypical lymphocytes
Stevens-Johnson syndrome (SJS) toxic epidermal necrolysis (TEN)
H/O exposure to drugs. Erythematous and purpuric progressing to bullae with sloughing and necrosis of epidermis Nikolsky sign involves mucosal surfaces TEN (> 30% BSA epidermal necrosis in maximal form)

## CLINICAL FEATURES AND PATTERN OF ORGAN INVOLVEMENT

| | |
|---|---|
| **Rash and shock**<br>• TSS<br>• MC<br>• Fulminant pneumococcal sepsis in an asplenic<br>• Overwhelming *S. aureus* bacteremia<br>• DHF/DSS<br>• Arboviral hemorrhagic fevers | **Rash and relative bradycardia**<br>• RMSF<br>• Typhus<br>• Typhoid fever<br>• Arboviral hemorrhagic fevers<br>• Drug fever |
| **Rash and periorbital edema**<br>• RMSF | **Rash on palms/soles**<br>• RMSF<br>• DF<br>• TSS |
| **Rash and conjunctival suffusion**<br>• RMSF<br>• DHF/DSS<br>• Arboviral hemorrhagic fevers | **Scarlatiniform rash**<br>• Scarlet fever<br>• Kawasaki's disease<br>• Arboviral hemorrhagic fevers |
| **Rash and conjunctivitis**<br>• Kawasaki's disease<br>• TSS<br>• Measles | **Rash and bullae lesions**<br>• *V. vulnificus*<br>• Gas gangrene |
| **Rash and abdominal pain**<br>• RMSF<br>• Scarlet Fever<br>• Measles<br>• Typhoid Fever<br>• *V. vulnificus*<br>• Cholesterol emboli syndrome<br>• Atypical measles<br>• SLE<br>• DHF/DSS<br>• Arboviral hemorrhagic fevers | **Livedoid rash**<br>• SLE<br>• Cholesterol emboli syndrome |
| **Rash and diarrhea**<br>• *V. vulnificus*<br>• Gas gangrene<br>• TSS<br>• DHF/DSS<br>• Arboviral hemorrhagic fevers | **Rash and purpura**<br>• MC<br>• RMSF<br>• Cholesterol emboli syndrome<br>• Hypersensitivity vasculitis<br>• DHF/DSS<br>• Arboviral hemorrhagic fevers |
| **Rash and CVA**<br>• SLE<br>• Cholesterol emboli syndrome<br>• *S. aureus* ABE | **Rash and edema of hands/feet**<br>• Kawasaki's disease<br>• TSS<br>• RMSF |
| **Rash and mental status changes**<br>• SLE (if cerebritis)<br>• RMSF<br>• MC<br>• Typhoid fever<br>• *S. aureus* ABE | **Rash and adenopathy**<br>• SLE<br>• Rubella<br>• Scarlet fever<br>• Kawasaki's disease |
| **Rash and pulmonary infiltrates**<br>• RMSF<br>• Atypical measles<br>• SLE | **Rash and splenomegaly**<br>• Typhoid fever<br>• Rubella<br>• SLE<br>• RMSF |

## Laboratory Features

| **Rash and eosinophilia** | **Rash and thrombocytopenia** |
|---|---|
| • Scarlet fever RMSF<br>• DHF/DSS DHF/DSS<br>• Cholesterol emboli syndrome | • MC<br>• RMSF<br>• DHF/DSS<br>• TSS<br>• MEASLES<br>• SLE |
| **Rash and leukopenia**<br>• RMSF SLE<br>• Measles Rash and Thrombocytosis<br>• DH F/DSS<br>• Arboviral hemorrhagic fever<br>• Typhoid fever<br>• SLE | **Rash and thrombocytosis**<br>• Kawasaki's disease |
| **Rash and leukocytosis**<br>• *V. vulnificus*<br>• MC<br>• Gas gangrene<br>• Scarlet fever<br>• Cholesterol emboli syndrome | **Rash and elevated SGOT/SGPT**<br>• RMSF<br>• DHF/DSS<br>• TSS<br>• Typhoid fever |
| (DHF/DSS: dengue hemorrhagic fever/dengue shock syndrome; MC: meningococcemia; RMSF: Rocky Mountain spotted fever; SLE: systemic lupus erythematosus; TSS: toxic shock syndrome) | |

CHAPTER

# 135 Fever with Altered Sensorium

## INTRODUCTION

Airway management, history, and clinical examination are of paramount importance in fever with altered sensorium.

## HISTORY

- Onset of fever grade/type
- Onset of altered sensorium
- Temporal relation between fever and altered sensorium
- Headache
- Nausea/vomiting
- Seizures
- Focal deficits
- Comorbidities
- *Geographical area*: Viral encephalitis or tropical infection prevalent in the area
- Drug addictions/antipsychotics, prescription drugs, and alcohol
- Travel history
- Rashes, jaundice, cough, and burning micturition

## EXAMINATION

- Vital parameters
- Look specifically for rash, bite marks, jaundice, lymph nodes, abdominal organomegaly, murmurs, lung findings, urinary retention, etc.

## INVESTIGATIONS

Investigations including ruling out tropical fevers:

- CBC, CRP, urea, creatinine, sodium, potassium, LFT, TSH, and RBS
- Blood culture aerobic x 2. ABG
- X-ray chest, ECG, ECHO, X-ray chest ± USG whole abdomen
- Malaria card test (RDT) (kit must use HRP/LDH antigen)/malarial smearsx 3
- Dengue card tests for NS1antigen, IgM, and IgG
- Typhidot, IgM Scrub Typhus, IgM Leptospira

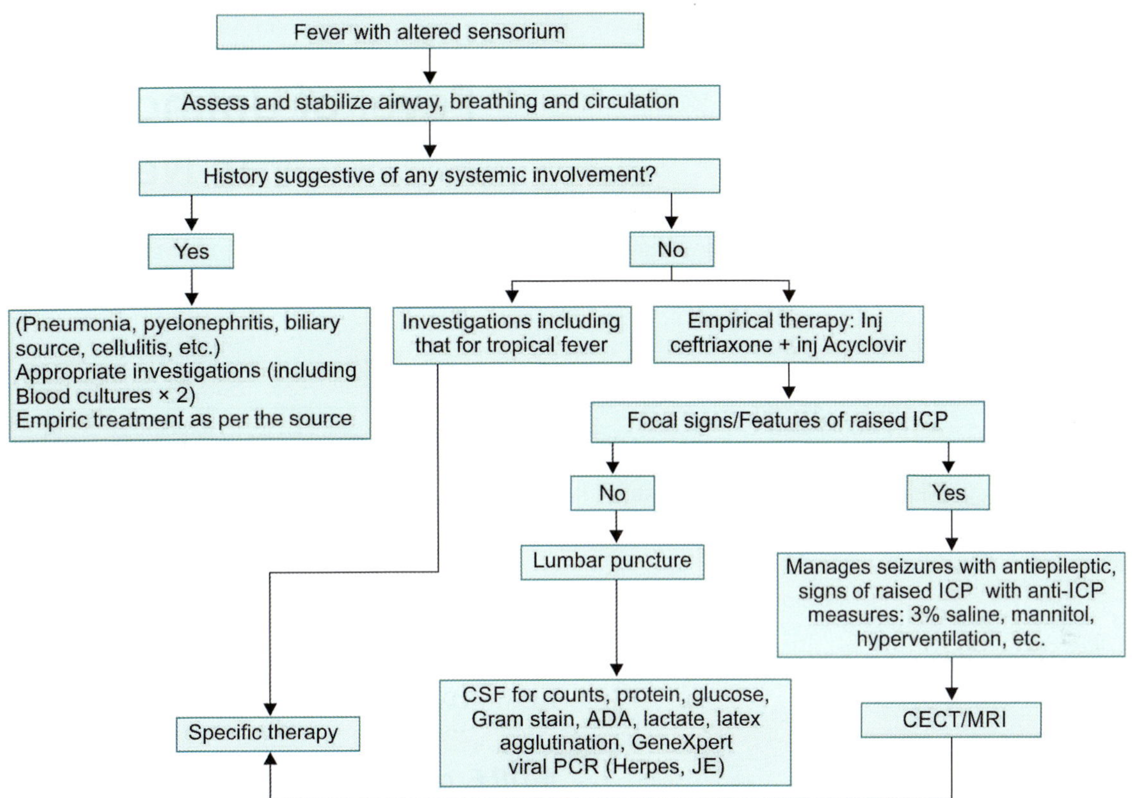


| | ***Gross*** | ***Protein mg/dL*** | ***Glucose mg/dL*** | ***Cells/cmm*** |
|---|---|---|---|---|
| Normal | Clear | 15–40 | 50–80 | 0–5 Lymphocytes |
| Bacterial | Cloudy | >250 | <45 | > 1,000 mostly neutrophils |
| (Viral) Aseptic | Clear | ↑ but < 150 | N or LOW | ↑ but less than 250 |
| Tubercular | Clear/clot | Moderate ↑ (100–500) | <45 | 100–500 |
| Fungal | Clear | Moderate to highly increased | Normal or slightly decreased | Variably increased |

CHAPTER 136

# Fever of Unknown Origin in Neutropenia

| *IDSA* | *ESMO 2011* | *ECIL 4* | *NCCN* |
|---|---|---|---|
| • Until ANC >500 and recovering<br>• And Afebrile for >48 hours | • If ANC <500<br>• Afebrile for 5–7 days consider discontinuation | • Afebrile >48 hours<br>• Stable 72–96 hours<br>• Discontinue regardless of ANC | • ANC >500 and recovering discontinue antibiotics<br>• If ANC <500 consider any of below discontinue de-escalate to prophylaxis until neutropenia resolves |

## MICROBIOLOGICALLY DOCUMENTED INFECTION

7–14 days based on site and organism

### MDR/XDR Infections

MDR is defined as acquired nonsusceptibility to at least one agent in three or more antimicrobial categories

Extensively drug resistant (XDR) is defined as nonsusceptibility to at least one agent in all but two or fewer antimicrobial categories

### MDR *Klebsiella pneumoniae*

NDM +

OXA 48 +

NDM + OXA 48 +

### *MDR E. coli*

- NDM
- MDR *Pseudomonas aeruginosa* (Carbapenem resistant)/DTR difficult to treat *Pseudomonas*
- *Acinetobacter baumannii* CRAB (Carbapenem resistant)
- Vancomycin-resistant *Enterococcus* VRE
- MRSA

## DRUG OF CHOICE FOR ABOVE ORGANISMS

| *MDR Kleb* | *MDR E. coli* | *DTR Pseudomonas (Metallo-beta-lactamase +)* |
|---|---|---|
| • NDM<br>• Aztreonam + Avibactam<br>• OXA 48 only<br>• Ceftazidime + Avibactam | • NDM<br>• Polymyxin B + fosfomycin<br>Or<br>• Polymyxin B + Tigecycline | • Carbapenem resistant<br>• Ceftazidime avibactam + Aztreonam<br>• Cefiderocol<br>• Ceftolozane + Tazobactam<br>• Colistin + Meropenem + Amikacin |

| *CRAB* | *VRE* | *MRSA* |
|---|---|---|
| • Polymyxin B + Minocycline<br>or<br>• Polymyxin B + high dose sulbactam 96–9 g)<br>or<br>• Eravacycline | • Linezolid<br>• Daptomycin<br>• Tigecycline<br>• Fosfomycin | • Vancomycin<br>or<br>• Teicoplanin |

## ANTIBIOTIC OF CHOICE

While choosing appropriate antibiotic for MDRO things to keep in mind:

- Site of infection and antibiotic penetration at the site. For example, tigecycline has poor concentration in lungs so should not be preferred to treat VAP especially never as a single agent. Tigecycline on the other hand has excellent biliary concentration so can be agent of choice for cholangitis if MDRO is susceptible.
- PK/PD of the drug chosen especially if renal or liver dysfunction present.
- Always better to know the enzyme responsible for resistance in case of *Klebsiella* and *E coli*.
- Pseudomonas has multiple mechanism of carbapenem resistance so only enzyme detection does not help, like PBP proteins.
- Correct dosing is most crucial and therapeutic drug monitoring ideal if available
- Colistin and polymyxin B have different PK/PD and penetration, for example polymyxin b does not concentrate in urine so colistin preferred in pyelonephritis. Polymyxin B dosing is easier especially in presence of AKI. Only colistin can be given intrathecally for ventriculitis.
- For NDM *Klebsiella*, essential to do synergy testing for aztreonam + Avibactam. Both should be given simultaneously over 3 hours infusion. Aztreonam Avibactam therapy has better bacteremia clearance and mortality advantage over colistin based therapy.
- When awaiting cultures are always better to give polymyxin combined with other agents like fosfomycin, tigecycline or ceftazidime Avibactam as Acinetobacter cover is essential till organism is identified.

# CHAPTER 137 Pyrexia of Unknown Origin

Fever >101°F or more for >3 weeks despite 1 week of baseline evaluation.

| *Infections* | *Malignancies* | *Inflammation* | *Miscellaneous* |
|---|---|---|---|
| *Bacterial*<br>• SABE<br>• Abdominal or pelvic abscess (prostatic abscess in male)<br>• Septic phlebitis<br>• Infected<br>• Prosthesis (joints)<br>• TB<br>• Atypical mycobacterial infections<br>*Others*<br>• Endemic mycoses<br>• Bartonella<br>• Brucellosis<br>• Toxoplasmosis<br>• *VIRAL*<br>• CMV<br>• EBV<br>• Parvovirus | *Hematological*<br>• Lymphoma<br>• AML<br>• Hairy cell leukemia<br>• Myeloproliferative disease<br>*Solid organ*<br>• Atrial myxoma<br>• Hepatic carcinoma<br>• Metastatic disease<br>• Glioblastoma multiforme<br>• Renal cell carcinoma | *CTD*<br>• SLE<br>• Stills disease<br>• Takayasu arteritis<br>• Giant cell arteritis<br>• Wegner's disease<br>*Others*<br>• Crohn's disease<br>• Macrophage activation syndrome<br>• sarcoidosis | • Drug fever<br>• Factitious fever<br>• Addison's disease<br>• Thyroiditis<br>• Hypothalamic dysfunction (central fever)<br>• Thromboembolism |

## INVESTIGATIONS

### Infection

- Cultures, appropriate site specific and blood cultures
- PET CT
- TEE
- Bone marrow biopsy plus culture
- CMV/EBV PCR
- Syphilis serology
- Urine TB culture
- MRI abdomen pelvis (abscess deep seated)

### Malignancies

- Tumor markers
- CEA
- CA 19.9
- Alpha fetoprotein
- Biopsy of index organ involvement lymph node or liver or peritoneum or pleura
- Serum electrophoresis
- Bone marrow biopsy
- TEE

### Inflammation

- ANA
- ANA blot
- ANCA
- APLA
- Cryoglobulins
- Joint aspirations to detect crystals
- PET CT ( Takayasu arteritis )
- Temporal artery biopsy
- Serum ferritin
- Triglyceride levels
- SACE levels

## MISCELLANEOUS

- Thyroid function test
- TPO antibodies
- TSH receptor antibodies
- ESR
- Serum cortisol levels
- Synacthen stimulation test
- Doppler for DVT

CHAPTER 138

# MDR/XDR Infections

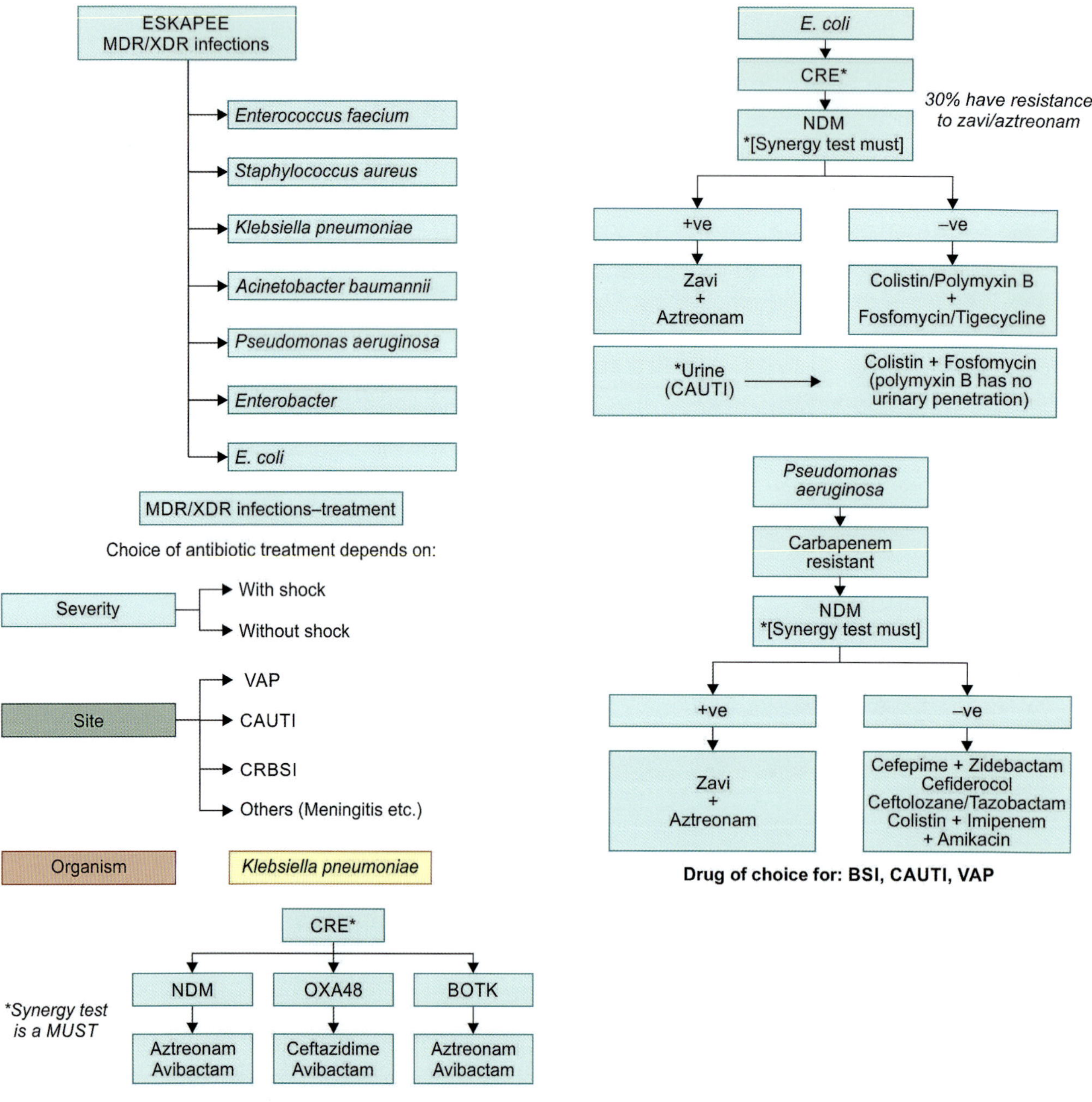

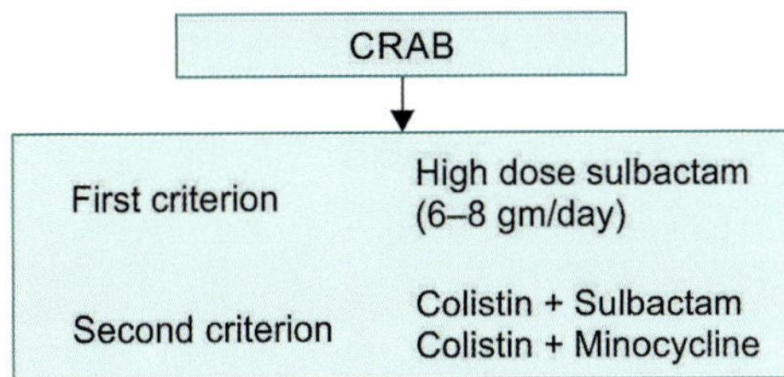


**Drug of choice for: BSI, CAUTI, VAP**

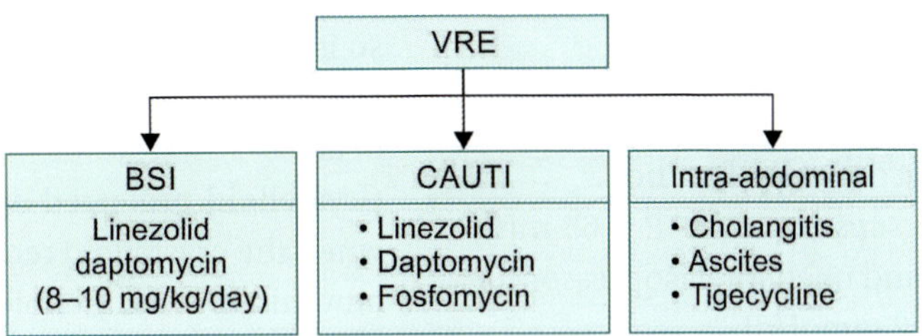


**Drug of choice for: BSI, CAUTI, VAP**

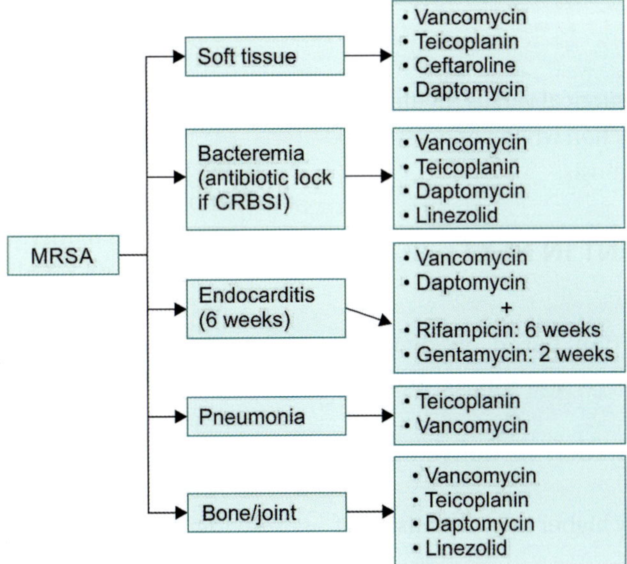

CHAPTER

# 139 Septic Shock

## INTRODUCTION

Sepsis is defined as dysregulated host response to infective agent leading to life threatening organ dysfunction.

Septic shock is defined as sepsis and MAP < 65 mm Hg despite fluid resuscitation and need for vasopressor to maintain MAP and Sr lactate > 2 mmol/dL

## FIRST 1-HOUR BUNDLE

- Blood culture preferable two sets (four bottles)
- Appropriate broad-spectrum antibiotic intravenously after cultures taken
- Fluid resuscitation
- Search for source of sepsis (surgical versus medical)
- Use PCR techniques for detection wherever possible ex lungs or blood for rapid diagnosis.

## ADVANCE MANAGEMENT IN NEXT 24 HOURS IN ICU

- Continued fluid resuscitation based on dynamic parameters like PPV/SVV if patient is sedated ventilated
- ECHO-based fluid resuscitation in nonventilated patients (LVOT VTI guided)
- Target MAP > 65 occasionally higher in hypertensives if situation demands
- Capillary refill time is a good marker of coherence between microcirculation and microcirculation
- Measure serum lactate at 4–6 hours, lactate clearance of more than 2 mmol/h is a marker of good resuscitation. Lactate clearance can lag clinical improvement so is not best endpoint of resuscitation, CRT and MAP UOP better markers. It is ideal to use combination of all.
- Crystalloid preferred over colloids. In extreme cases when the crystalloid requirement is extremely high 5% albumin may be a choice to avoid massive crystalloid loading and interstitial oedema which will harm the microcirculation.
- Balanced crystalloid preferred over normal saline
- *Vasopressors:*
    - Noradrenaline first drug of choice 0.1–1 μm/kg/min
    - Vasopressin is added if Noradrenaline requirement goes above 0.3 μg/kg/min
    - Adrenaline is the third drug of choice
- Renal replacement therapy in AKI sepsis:
    - No advantage of early versus conventional indication of RRT
    - Continuous renal replacement therapy is better tolerated if patient on dual or triple vasopressors, can also be combined with blood purification therapies. Trials have not shown mortality advantage of CRRT over SLEDD in septic shock.
- *Steroids in septic shock:* The pendulum keeps swinging for and against low-dose hydrocortisone (200 mg/24 h) in septic shock. SSG currently do recommend low dose hydrocortisone in septic shock.
- *Controlling hyperglycemia:* Insulin infusions are indicated if persistent hyperglycemia with a target blood sugar of 150–180 mg/dL

- *Source control:* In case of surgical source, it is essential to consider curative surgery or temporizing drains (percutaneous cholecystostomy for empyema GB) if possible.
- *Elective ventilation:* Worsening septic shock in terms of rising vasopressors and lactates must consider elective ventilation to take away the work of breathing. Use low tidal volume ventilation strictly.
- *Immunomodulation by blood purification:* No evidence to support such therapies as yet. Oxiris and toramyxin filters remain the most studied with considerable promise in various studies. We need large RCT to support the use of these filters in all septic shocks, yet in right situation (young patient with good source control) in more than two-thirds organ failures blood purification is a step to consider as salvage therapy (albeit despite lack of robust evidence).

CHAPTER

# 140 New-onset Fever in Intensive Care Unit

## INTRODUCTION

Fever of > 38.3°Celsius or 101° Fahrenheit after 48 hours of ICU stay.

## CAUSES

| *Infections:* | *Noninfectious:* |
|---|---|
| • CLABSI<br>• VAP<br>• CAUTI<br>• SSI<br>• Aspiration pneumonia<br>• Clostridium difficile diarrhea<br>• Meningitis (postneurosurgery)<br>• Endocarditis<br>• Sinusitis<br>• DEEP SSI postabdominal surgery collections or leaks<br>• Acalculous cholecystitis<br>• Superficial SSI skin and soft tissue infections | • Pancreatitis<br>• Central fever<br>• Drug fever<br>• DVT ? PE<br>• Neuroleptic malignant syndrome<br>• Serotonin syndrome<br>• Drug withdrawal<br>• Transfusion reactions<br>• Adrenal/thyroid disorders |

## DIAGNOSTIC APPROACH

Clinical suspicion for site of infection:

- *VAP:*
  - After 48 hours of intubation
  - Change in quantity and quality of secretions
  - Increase in $FiO_2$ requirements by 0.2 or PEEP > 3
  - Chest X-ray/HRCT showing new onset consolidation
  - ET secretion culture > $10^6$ colony count or BAL culture (>25 neutrophil/HPF) >$10^4$ colony count
- *CAUTI:*
  - Patient has urinary catheters for >48 hours
  - Fever, suprapubic pain
  - Culture positive of single organism >100,000 CFU/mL
- *CLABSI:*
  - Bacteremia in a patient who has CVC >48 hours with no other possible source
  - Differential time to positivity should be >2 hours
- *Clostridium difficile:*
  - Stool GDH
  - Stool toxin A and B
  - Stool PCR in case GDH (positive but toxin negative)
- *Superficial and deep SSI*:
  - Postsurgical local site related infections
  - Appropriate CT scans with or without contrast
  - CT-guided aspirations of collections and culture
  - Swab or pus from infected suture site for culture
  - TEE for endocarditis
- *Biomarkers*:
  - Procalcitonin
  - BDG
  - Galactomannan

## MANAGEMENT

### Empiric Antibiotic for VAP/CAUTI/CLABSI

- Treat underlying cause with knowledge of local antibiogram
- Duration of antibiotics 7–14 days if GNB CLABSI
- 14 days if *Staph aureus* CLABSI
- 7 Days if CONS CLABSI
- 14 days after culture negative for fungal CLABSI
- 6–8 weeks if endocarditis or osteomyelitis
- VAP 10–14 days appropriate antibiotic
- CAUTI 7 days if prompt response to antibiotic or 10–14 days for delayed response
- Removal of CVC/urinary catheter as the case maybe
- Titrating antibiotics after positive culture is very crucial
- In case proven to be noninfectious revisiting the need for antibiotics

# PART 14

# AIRWAY

***Editors:*** Vikrant Shamrao Pawar, Ketan Kargirwar

***Associate Editor:*** Dnyanesh Kashikar

CHAPTER 141

# Postextubation Stridor

## DEFINITION AND IDENTIFICATION

Postextubation stridor is defined as a high-pitched sound produced by turbulent airflow through a narrowed airway occurring after the removal of an endotracheal tube. Incidence is 1.5–26%.

Identification is done by history taking and clinical examination.

## CLASSIFICATION

| *Types* | *Site of obstruction* | *Causes* | |
|---|---|---|---|
| | | ***Acute*** | ***Subacute/chronic*** |
| Inspiratory | At or above the level of the vocal cords | • Croup<br>• Epiglottitis<br>• Foreign body aspiration<br>• Anaphylaxis | • Laryngomalacia (in infants)<br>• Vocal cord paralysis<br>• Subglottic stenosis<br>• Tumors (e.g., laryngeal cancer) |
| Expiratory | Obstruction below the level of vocal cords | • Asthma<br>• Bronchial obstruction (e.g., foreign body, tumor) | |
| Biphasic | Involvement of both upper and lower airways | • Laryngeal edema<br>• Tracheal or laryngeal tumors | |

## RISK FACTORS FOR POSTEXTUBATION STRIDOR

| | | |
|---|---|---|
| Intubation related | • Excessive airway manipulation<br>• Traumatic intubation<br>• Prolonged intubation attempt (>10 min) | • Larger tubes<br>• Recurrent intubations |
| Post-intubation related | • Prolonged intubation >36 hours<br>• Agitation while intubated<br>• High cuff pressure | |
| Patient factors | • Female<br>• Short neck<br>• Known airway pathology (tracheal stenosis, tracheomalacia) | • Small height to internal endotracheal tube diameter ratio<br>• Children<br>• Trauma |

## PREVENTIVE APPROACH TO POSTEXTUBATION STRIDOR

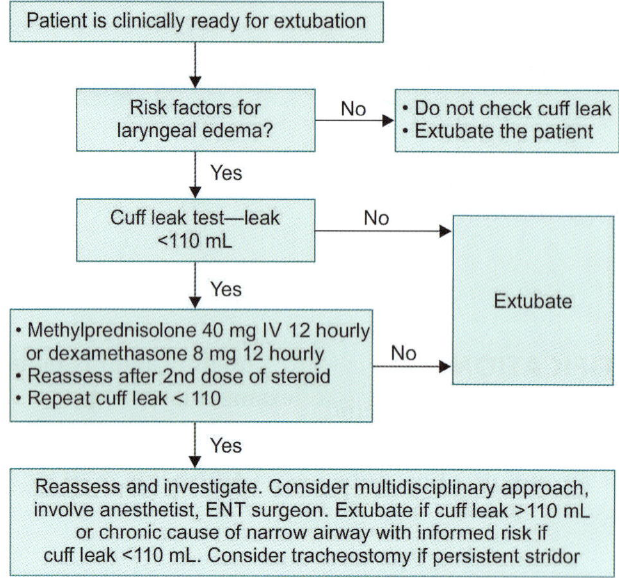


## TREATMENT ALGORITHM FOR POSTEXTUBATION STRIDOR

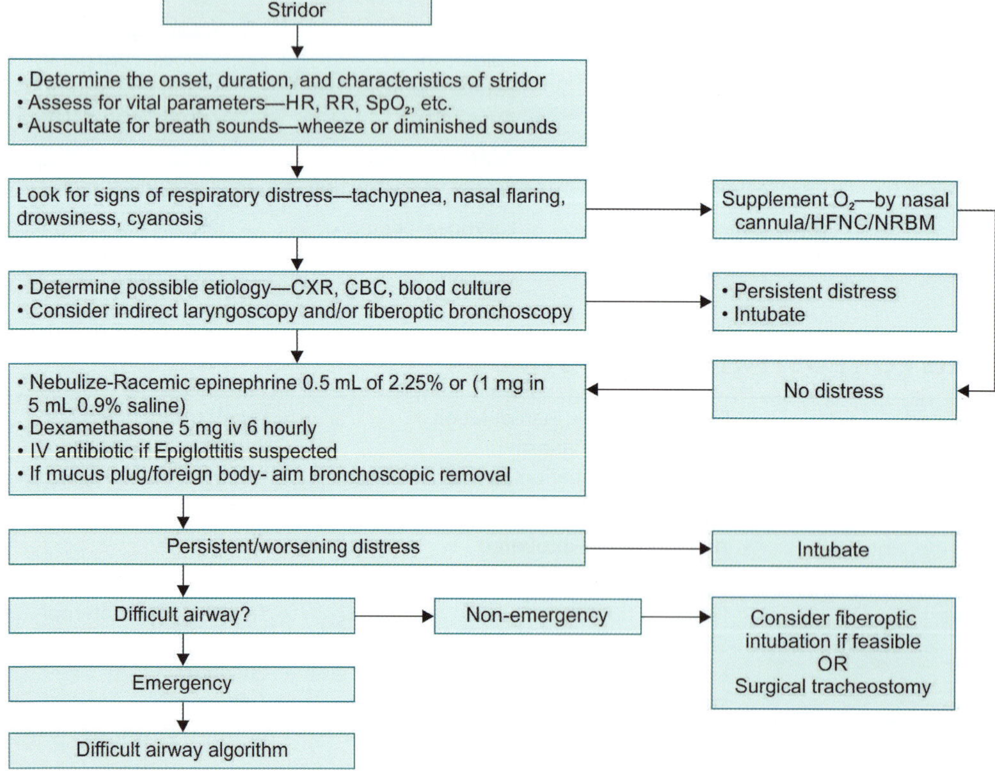


## SUGGESTED READING

1. AK AK, Cascella M. Post-Intubation Laryngeal Edema. In: StatPearls [Internet]. Treasure Island (FL): StatPearls Publishing; 2024.
2. Epstein SK. Corticosteroids to prevent postextubation upper airway obstruction: the evidence mounts. Crit Care. 2007;11(4):156.
3. Pluijms WA, van Mook WN, Wittekamp BH, Bergmans DC. Postextubation laryngeal edema and stridor resulting in respiratory failure in critically ill adult patients: updated review. Crit Care. 2015;19(1):295.

CHAPTER 142

# Difficult Airway Management

## DEFINITION OF DIFFICULT AIRWAY

A difficult airway is defined as a clinical situation in which a trained anesthesiologist has difficulty with:

- Bag-mask ventilation
- Endotracheal intubation
- The combination of both

## ASSESSMENT OF AIRWAY (TABLE 1)

**TABLE 1:** Points to consider in assessment of airway.

| | |
|---|---|
| History | • Previous intubation difficulties<br>• Head and neck surgery, trauma, or anatomical abnormalities |
| Physical examination | Assess airway predictors, including:<br>• Mallampati classification (I-IV)<br>• Thyromental distance<br>• Neck circumference and flexibility<br>• Interincisor gap<br>• Ability to protrude the mandible |
| Imaging | • X-ray neck AP/lateral. Chest X-ray<br>• CT head, neck, thorax wherever needed |

## PREPARATIONS

- Develop a comprehensive airway management plan based on the assessment.
- Identify and prepare for potentially difficult airway scenarios.
- Each ICU, OR and emergency room must have difficult airway trolley. Contents mentioned in **Table 2**.

**TABLE 2:** Contents of difficult airway trolley.

| | | |
|---|---|---|
| • Laryngoscope 2 with at least one alternative blade (e.g. straight, McCoy)<br>• Miller blades<br>• Flexible fiberoptic laryngoscope (with portable/ battery light source)<br>• Aintree Intubation Catheter<br>• Bougie<br>• Stylet | Cricothyroid cannulas with high pressure jet ventilation system (Manujet)<br>OR<br>Large bore cricothyroid cannulas (e.g. cuffed Melker)<br>OR<br>Surgical cricothyroidotomy kit; Tracheostomy kit | • Intubating LMA (Size 3,4,5 with dedicated tubes and pushers)<br>• Proseal LMA<br>• Supreme LMA |

## DIFFICULT AIRWAY ALGORITHM

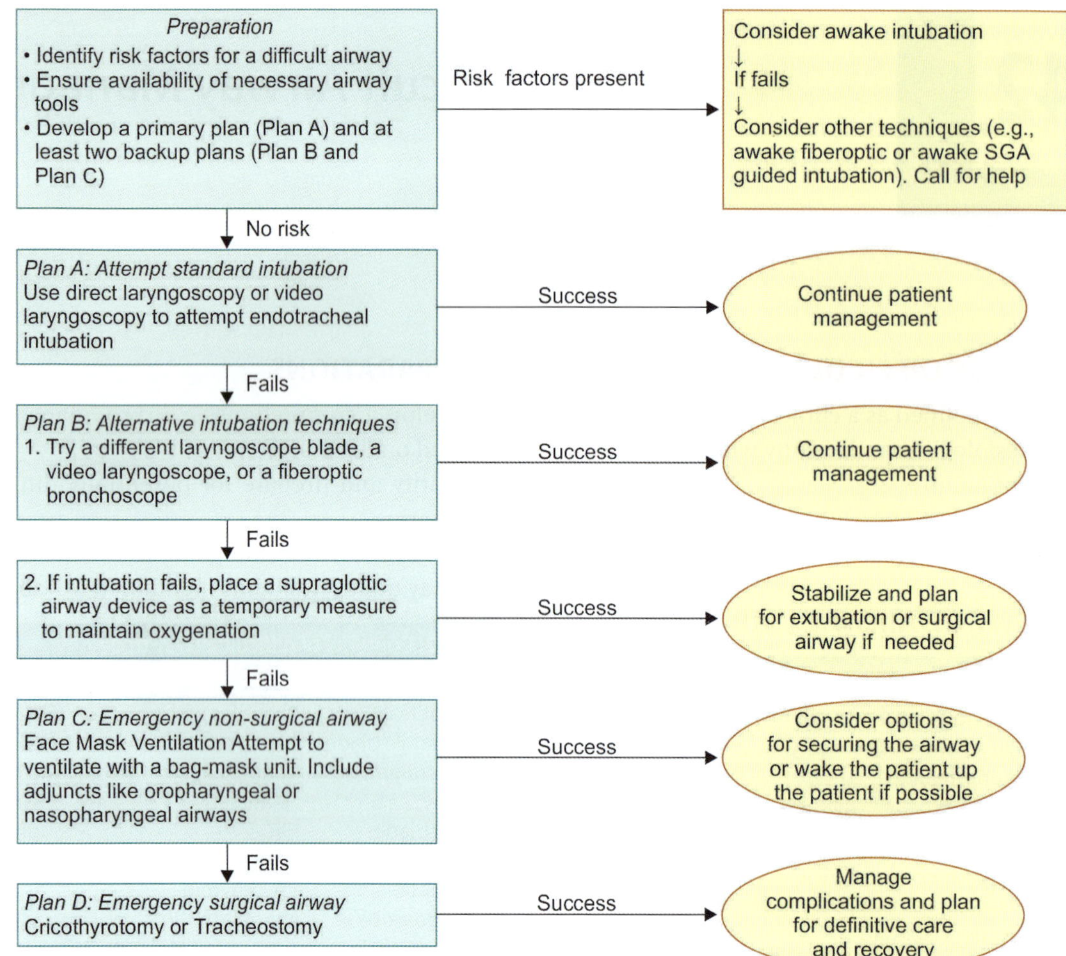


## SUGGESTED READING

1. Apfelbaum JL, Hagberg CA, Connis RT, Abdelmalak BB, Agarkar M, Dutton RP, et al. 2022 American Society of Anesthesiologists Practice Guidelines for Management of the Difficult Airway. Anesthesiology. 2022;136(1):31-81.
2. Bjurström MF, Bodelsson M, Sturesson LW. The Difficult Airway Trolley: A Narrative Review and Practical Guide. Anesthesiol Res Pract. 2019;2019:6780254.
3. Fuchs A, Haller M, Riva T, Sabine N, Robert G, Joana BE, et al. Translation and application of guidelines into clinical practice: A colour-coded difficult airway trolley. Trends Anaesth Crit Care. 2021;40:46-54.

CHAPTER 143

# Emergency Airway Access

## INTRODUCTION

Emergency airway access is a critical intervention when conventional methods of securing the airway (e.g., intubation) fail or are not feasible. This procedure is often necessary in cases of severe airway obstruction, facial trauma, or when a patient cannot be ventilated or intubated through standard means. Below is a structured approach to emergency airway access, focusing on the techniques and considerations.

## INDICATIONS FOR EMERGENCY AIRWAY ACCESS

- Inability to ventilate or intubate after multiple attempts
- Severe airway obstruction (e.g., due to foreign body, swelling)
- Facial or neck trauma compromising airway anatomy
- Rapid deterioration of respiratory status

## TECHNIQUES FOR EMERGENCY AIRWAY ACCESS

### Cricothyrotomy

#### *Indications*

Preferred in pediatric patients when other methods are not successful or feasible.

#### *Procedure*

- Identify the cricoid membrane located between the thyroid and cricoid cartilages.
- Clean the area with antiseptic.
- Use a scalpel to make a vertical incision through the skin over the cricoid membrane.
- Insert a large bore cannula (e.g., 14-gauge) through the membrane into the trachea.
- Confirm placement by observing for airflow and/or auscultation.

### Surgical Cricothyrotomy

#### *Indications*

When immediate airway access is required, especially in adults.

#### *Procedure*

- Position the patient supine with the neck extended.
- Identify the cricoid membrane and clean the area.
- Make a vertical incision through the skin over the cricoid membrane, followed by a
- horizontal incision through the membrane.
- Insert a tracheostomy tube or endotracheal tube through the incision into the trachea.
- Secure the tube and confirm correct placement through ventilation.

### Tracheostomy

#### *Indications*

For prolonged airway access in patients requiring long-term ventilation or airway support.

#### *Procedure*

- Assess the anatomy and position the patient appropriately.
- Make a surgical incision at the second or third tracheal ring.
- Dissect through the tissue to expose the trachea carefully.
- Insert the tracheostomy tube into the trachea and secure it.
- Confirm placement by auscultation and capnography.

## POSTPROCEDURE MANAGEMENT

### Monitoring

- Monitor oxygen saturation and vital signs. Get chest X-ray done.
- Assess for complications such as pneumothorax, subcutaneous emphysema, or accidental extubation.

## Ventilation Support

- Provide appropriate ventilatory support through the newly established airway.
- Ensure the airway is secured and free from obstruction.

## Documentation

Document the indication for the procedure, the technique used and the patient's response.

# COMPLICATIONS

## Short Term

Bleeding, infection, and injury to surrounding structures.

## Long Term

Tracheal stenosis, tracheoesophageal fistula, or difficulty weaning from mechanical ventilation **(Fig. 1)**.

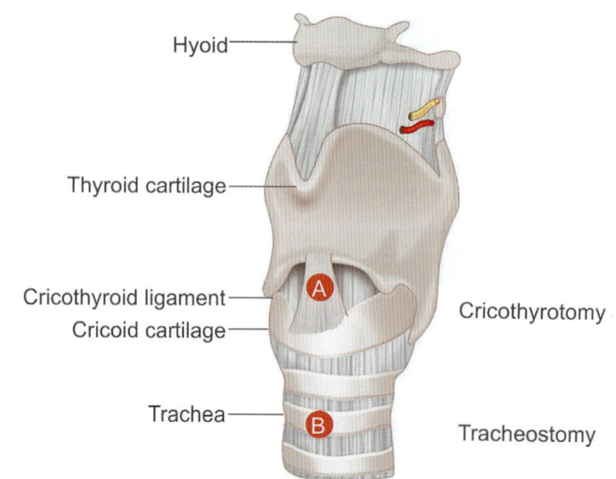


**Fig. 1:** Point A: Site of access for cricothyrotomy. Point B: Site of access for tracheostomy.

# EMERGENCY AIRWAY ACCESS ALGORITHM

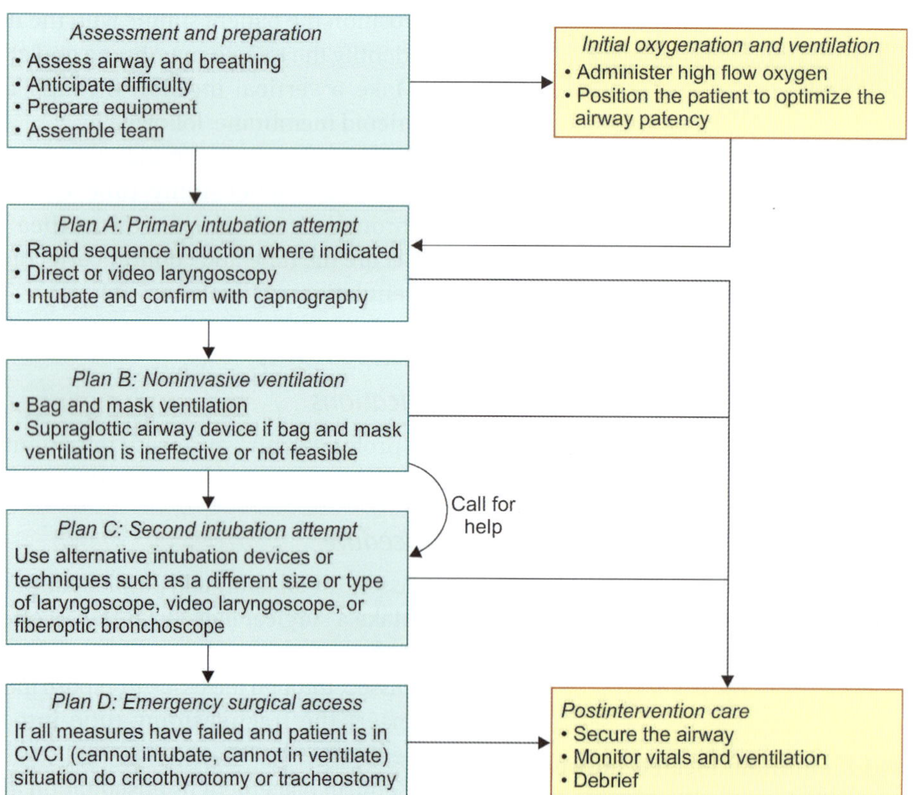


# SUGGESTED READING

1. Frerk C, Mitchell VS, McNarry AF, Mendonca C, Bhagrath R, Patel A, et al. Difficult Airway Society 2015 guidelines for management of unanticipated difficult intubation in adults. Br J Anaesth. 2015;115:827-48.
2. Kristensen MS, Teoh WH, Baker PA. Percutaneous emergency airway access; prevention, preparation, technique and training. Br J Anaesth. 2015;114(3):357-61.
3. Ramkumar V, Dinesh E, Shetty SR, Shah A, Kundra P, Das S, et al. All India difficult airway association 2016 guidelines for the management of unanticipated difficult tracheal intubation in obstetrics. Indian Journal of Anaesthesia 2016;60:899-905.

# PART 15

# OBSTETRICS

***Editors:*** Gunchan Paul, Leena Patil
***Associate Editor:*** Basjinder Kaur

CHAPTER 144

# Jaundice in Pregnancy

**TABLE 1:** Normal ranges for liver function tests to evaluate pregnant women with liver disorders.

| | ***Nonpregnant*** | ***Pregnant*** | | |
|---|---|---|---|---|
| | | ***1st trimester*** | ***2nd trimester*** | ***3rd trimester*** |
| *Liver tests* | | | | |
| Bilirubin (umol/L) | 0–17 | 4–16 | 3–13 | 3–14 |
| Albumin (g/L) | 35–46 | 28–37 | | |
| AST (IU/L) | 7–40 | 10–28 | 11–29 | 11–30 |
| ALT (IU/L) | 0–40 | 6–32 | | |
| GGT (IU/L) | 11–50 | 5–37 | 5–43 | 3–41 |
| ALP (IU/L) | 30–130 | 32–100 | 43–135 | 133–418 |
| Bile acids (umol/L) | 0–6 (fasting)<br>0–10 (nonfasting) | | | 19 (nonfasting) |

**TABLE 2:** Data regarding the safety of radiological investigations used to assess pregnant women with liver disorders.

| ***Ultrasound*** | ***Safe at any gestation in pregnancy*** |
|---|---|
| Liver elastography | • Safe at any gestation in pregnancy<br>• It should be noted that there may be a small increase in liver stiffness and controlled attenuation parameter in the third trimester, which reflects the normal physiology of pregnancy |
| MRCP | • Safe at any gestation in pregnancy |
| ERCP | • Fetal radiation estimated between <0.1–0.5 mGy (threshold for malformation = 50 mGy) can be performed in pregnancy, ideally in the 2nd/3rd trimester |
| OGD (esophagogastric duodenoscopy) | • Safe in pregnancy, ideally performed in the 2nd trimester in the left lateral position<br>• Midazolam may be used judicially |
| Liver biopsy | • It can be performed where clinical need/diagnostics uncertainty dictates, and delay in diagnostic would be more dangerous for the pregnant women<br>• Ensure coagulopathy corrected |

**Flowchart 1:** Initial workup for pregnant woman with abnormal liver function tests (LFTs).

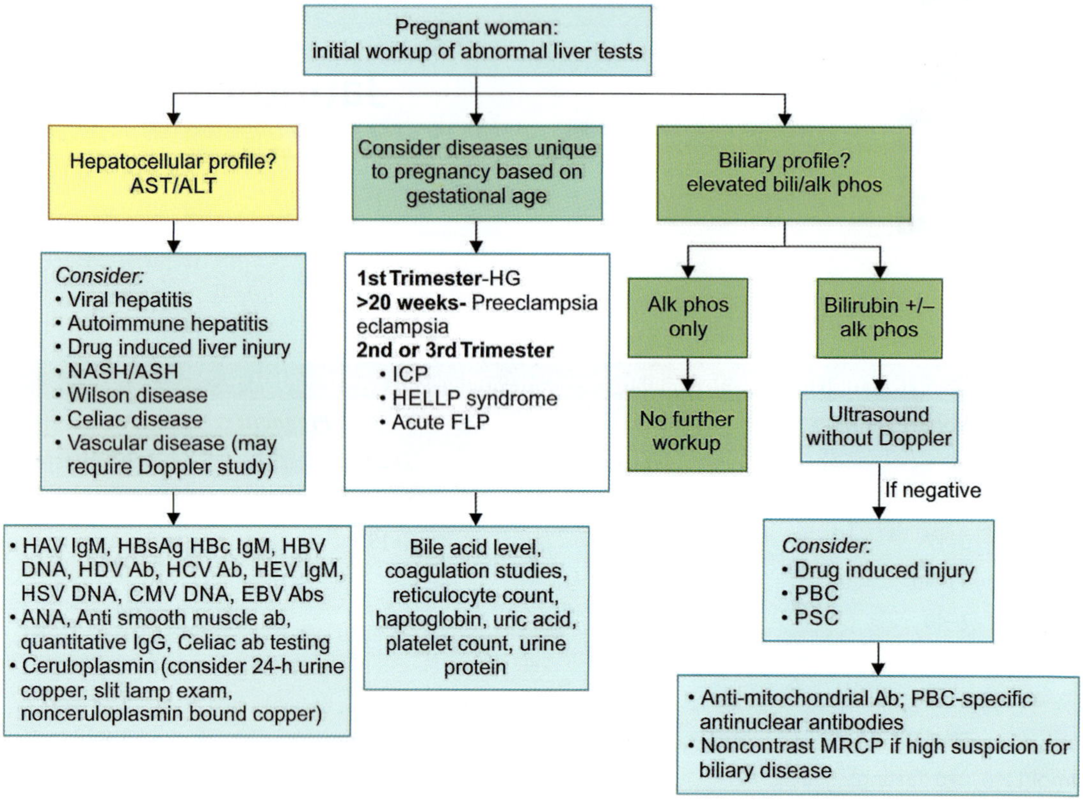

Pregnant woman:
initial workup of abnormal liver tests

Hepatocellular profile?
AST/ALT

*Consider:*
- Viral hepatitis
- Autoimmune hepatitis
- Drug induced liver injury
- NASH/ASH
- Wilson disease
- Celiac disease
- Vascular disease (may require Doppler study)

- HAV IgM, HBsAg HBc IgM, HBV DNA, HDV Ab, HCV Ab, HEV IgM, HSV DNA, CMV DNA, EBV Abs
- ANA, Anti smooth muscle ab, quantitative IgG, Celiac ab testing
- Ceruloplasmin (consider 24-h urine copper, slit lamp exam, nonceruloplasmin bound copper)

Consider diseases unique to pregnancy based on gestational age

**1st Trimester**-HG
**>20 weeks-** Preeclampsia eclampsia
**2nd or 3rd Trimester**
- ICP
- HELLP syndrome
- Acute FLP

Bile acid level, coagulation studies, reticulocyte count, haptoglobin, uric acid, platelet count, urine protein

Biliary profile?
elevated bili/alk phos

Alk phos only → No further workup

Bilirubin +/– alk phos → Ultrasound without Doppler → If negative →

*Consider:*
- Drug induced injury
- PBC
- PSC

- Anti-mitochondrial Ab; PBC-specific antinuclear antibodies
- Noncontrast MRCP if high suspicion for biliary disease

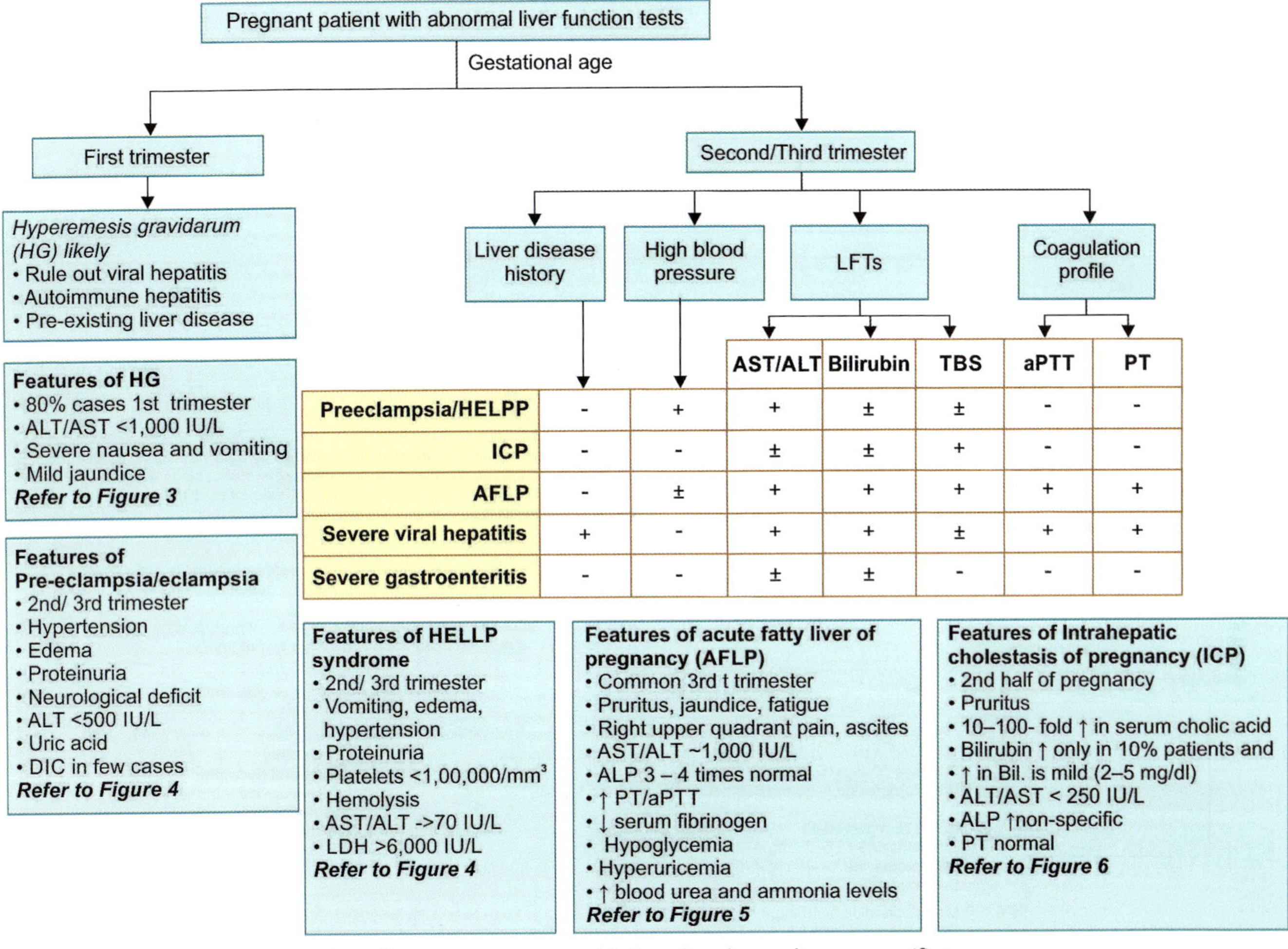


| | Liver disease history | High blood pressure | AST/ALT | Bilirubin | TBS | aPTT | PT |
|---|---|---|---|---|---|---|---|
| **Preeclampsia/HELPP** | - | + | + | ± | ± | - | - |
| **ICP** | - | - | ± | ± | + | - | - |
| **AFLP** | - | ± | + | + | + | + | + |
| **Severe viral hepatitis** | + | - | + | + | ± | + | + |
| **Severe gastroenteritis** | - | - | ± | ± | - | - | - |

**Fig. 2:** Work-up for pregnant woman with Jaundice due to diseases specific to pregnancy.

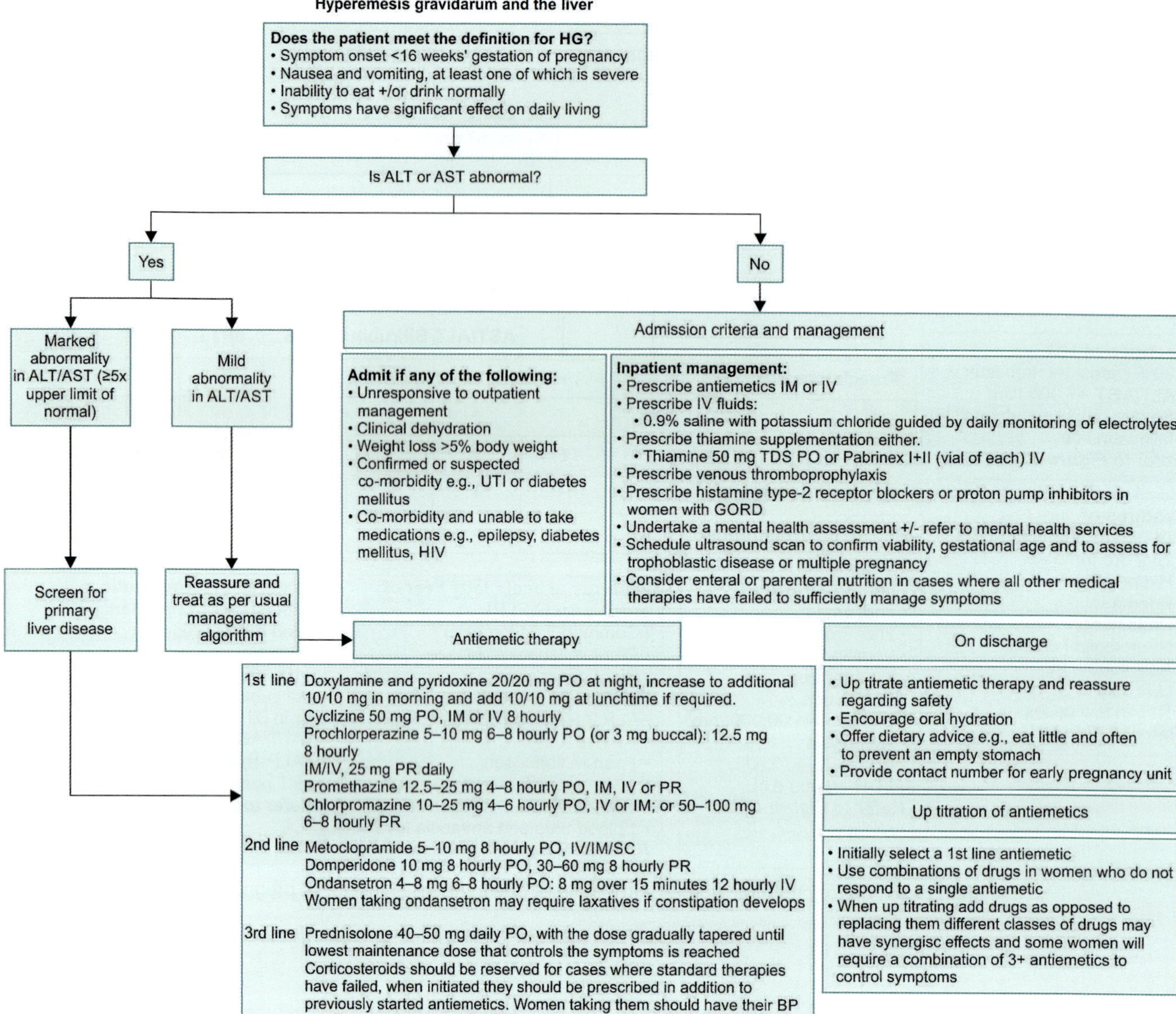


**Fig. 3:** Management of hyperemesis gravidarum.

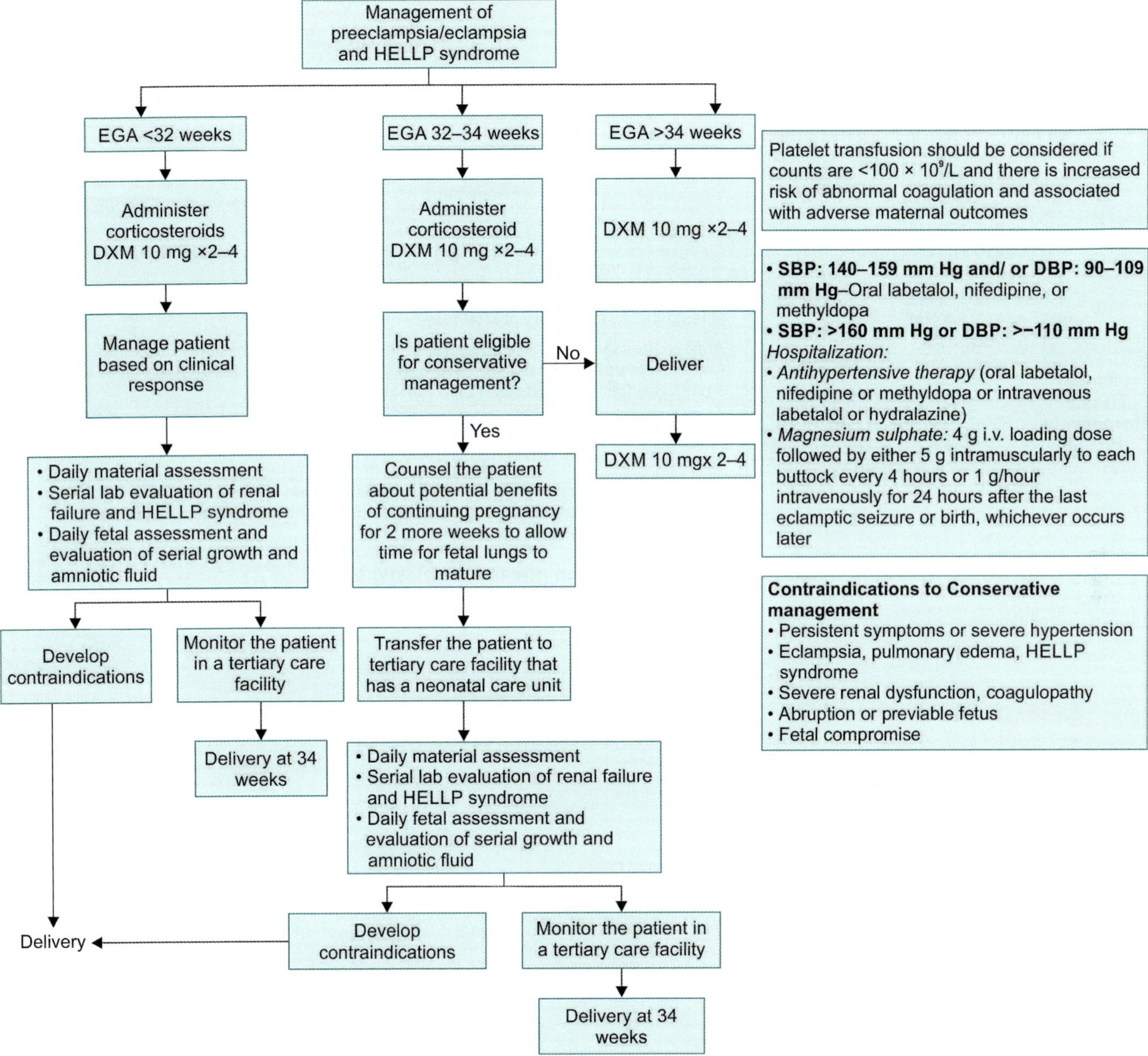
Management of preeclampsia/eclampsia and HELLP syndrome
EGA <32 weeks
EGA 32–34 weeks
EGA >34 weeks
Administer corticosteroids DXM 10 mg ×2–4
Administer corticosteroid DXM 10 mg ×2–4
DXM 10 mg ×2–4
Manage patient based on clinical response
Is patient eligible for conservative management?
No
Deliver
Yes
DXM 10 mgx 2–4
• Daily material assessment
• Serial lab evaluation of renal failure and HELLP syndrome
• Daily fetal assessment and evaluation of serial growth and amniotic fluid
Counsel the patient about potential benefits of continuing pregnancy for 2 more weeks to allow time for fetal lungs to mature
Develop contraindications
Monitor the patient in a tertiary care facility
Delivery at 34 weeks
Transfer the patient to tertiary care facility that has a neonatal care unit
• Daily material assessment
• Serial lab evaluation of renal failure and HELLP syndrome
• Daily fetal assessment and evaluation of serial growth and amniotic fluid
Delivery
Develop contraindications
Monitor the patient in a tertiary care facility
Delivery at 34 weeks
Platelet transfusion should be considered if counts are <100 × 10⁹/L and there is increased risk of abnormal coagulation and associated with adverse maternal outcomes
• SBP: 140–159 mm Hg and/ or DBP: 90–109 mm Hg–Oral labetalol, nifedipine, or methyldopa
• SBP: >160 mm Hg or DBP: >–110 mm Hg
Hospitalization:
• Antihypertensive therapy (oral labetalol, nifedipine or methyldopa or intravenous labetalol or hydralazine)
• Magnesium sulphate: 4 g i.v. loading dose followed by either 5 g intramuscularly to each buttock every 4 hours or 1 g/hour intravenously for 24 hours after the last eclamptic seizure or birth, whichever occurs later
Contraindications to Conservative management
• Persistent symptoms or severe hypertension
• Eclampsia, pulmonary edema, HELLP syndrome
• Severe renal dysfunction, coagulopathy
• Abruption or previable fetus
• Fetal compromise

*Contd…*

*Contd…*

| HELLP class | Mississippi classification | Tennessee classification |
|---|---|---|
| 1 | Platelet count ≤50,000/uL<br>AST or ALT ≥70 IU/L<br>LDH ≥600 IU/L | Platelet count ≤100,000/uL<br>AST ≥70IU/L<br>LDH ≥600 IU/L |
| 2 | 50,000/uL <Platelet Count ≤100,000/uL<br>AST or ALT ≥70IU/L<br>LDH ≥600 IU/L | NA |
| 3 | 100,000/uL<Platelet Count ≤150,000/uL<br>AST or ALT ≥40IU/L<br>LDH ≥600 IU/L | NA |
| Partial HELLP/ Incomplete HELLP | N/A | (Severe preeclampsia + one of the following ELLP, EL, LP) |

**Indications**

**All patients with class 1 or 2 HELLP syndrome**

Or

Patients with class 3 HELLP syndrome complicated by eclampsia, severe epigastric pain, end organ damage (i.e. Brain, kidney, heart, liver, lungs) and/or placental abruption-disseminated intravascular coagulation

↓

**Implementation**

- *Magnesium sulphate IV:* Loading dose and continuous infusion during antepartum and at least the first 24 hours postpartum
- *Antihypertensives:* (Labetalol, hydralazine, nifedipine) aggressively utilized to minimum or prevent sustained severe systolic hypertension (≥160 mm Hg) or sustained severe diastolic hypertension (≥110 mm Hg)
- *IV dexamethasone:* 10 mg every 12 hours until delivery and recovery postpartum is assured by normalizing of HELLP lab indices at which time IV dexamethasone is decreased to 5 mg every 12 hours × 2 and stopped
- *Management in intense care or hospital labor and delivery setting:* Where OBGYN/ MFM professional expertise and around the clock medical staff and blood bank are immediately available

**Fig. 4:** Management of preeclampsia and HELLP syndrome.

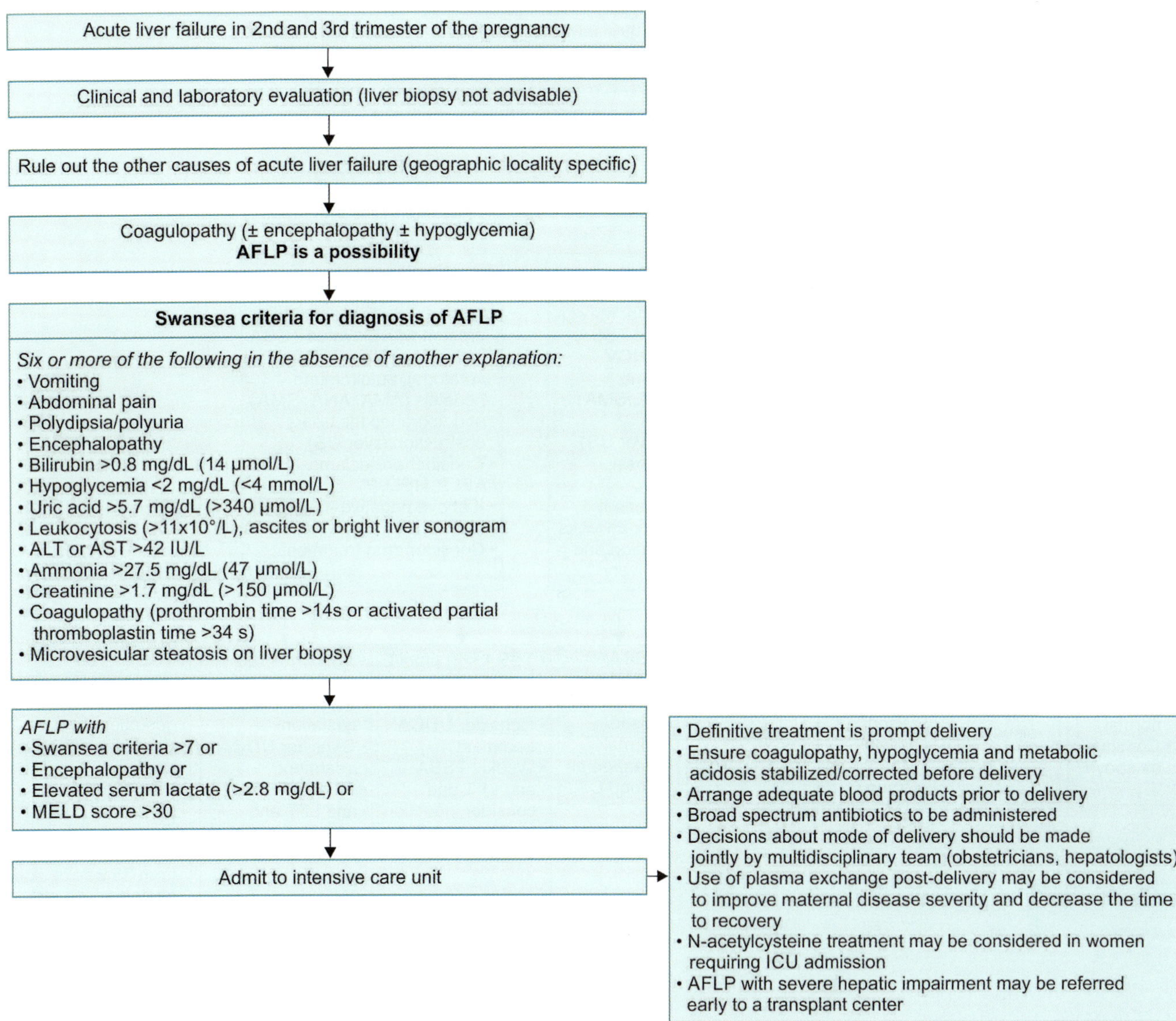


**Fig. 5:** Management of Acute Fatty Liver of Pregnancy (AFLP).

Woman presents with pruritus, with or without a rash or if ICP suspected
**Initial assessment**
Total serum bile acids (TSBA), liver transaminases (AST/ALT), bilirubin

**Group A**
TSBA normal
ALT/AST normal

If pruritus persists, repeat TSBA, ALT/AST every 2–3 weeks <32/40 weeks' gestation and then at least weekly until delivery

- TSBA normal
- ALT/AST normal
- Continue as above

- TSBA normal
- ALT/AST raised
- Manage as Group B

- TSBA raised
- ALT/AST raised/ normal
- Manage as Group C

**Group B**
TSBA normal
ALT/AST raised

*Exclude other causes of hepatic impairment:*
- Maternal diseases that may present with elevated TSBA include hepatitis C (HCV serology), autoimmune hepatitis (AMA, ANA, SMA) and extrahepatic biliary obstruction (liver US)
- Consider pre-eclampsia, AFLP, HELLP
- If pruritus persists, repeat TSBA and LFT every 2 weeks <32/40 weeks' gestation and then weekly until delivery

- TSBA normal
- ALT/AST raised
- Continue as above

- TSBA raised
- ALT/AST raised/ normal
- Manage as Group C

**Group C**
TSBA raised
ALT/AST raised/normal

*Exclude other causes of hepatic impairment:*
- Maternal diseases that may present with elevated TSBA include hepatitis C (HCV serology), autoimmune hepatitis (AMA, ANA, SMA) and extrahepatic biliary obstruction (liver US)
- Consider pre-eclampsia, AFLP, HELLP
- If above negative–diagnose ICP
- Consider drug treatment

- TSBA <40 μmol/L and <34/40 weeks' gestation
- Consider UDCA treatment
- Weekly TSBA and LFT and consider induction by 39 completed weeks' gestation

- TSBA 40–100 μmol/L and <37/40 weeks' gestation
- Consider UDCA treatment
- Weekly TSBA and LFT and consider induction by 39/40 weeks' gestation

Stop treatment with UDCA at time of delivery

- TSBA >100 μmol/L and/or >34/40 weeks gestation
- Consider UDCA treatment
- Weekly BA and LFT
- Recommend delivery from 35 weeks' gestation‡

Reduce UDCA gradually 2–4 weeks post-delivery if ongoing symptoms

Ensure TSBA, ALT/AST and bilirubin return to normal within 3 months of delivery, and if not investigate for underlying liver disease. Consider genetic screening if family history of hepatobiliary disease, early onset or severe disease

**Fig. 6:** Management of Intra-hepatic Cholestasis of Pregnancy (ICP).

## CLINICAL GUIDELINE: LIVER DISEASE AND PREGNANCY (STRONG RECOMMENDATIONS WITH LOW/ VERY LOW LEVEL OF RECOMMENDATION)

### Primary Biliary Cholangitis and Primary Sclerosing Cholangitis

- Ursodeoxycholic acid should be continued during pregnancy in primary biliary cholangitis (and primary sclerosing cholangitis when treated) as it is safe in pregnancy and breastfeeding (strong recommendation, strong consensus).
- For women with de novo or worsening pruritus, suggested treatments include rifampicin (300–600 mg daily) and anion exchange resins (cholestyramine, 4–8 g/day or colestipol, 5–10 g/day), the latter given at least 4 hours after ursodeoxycholic acid (weak recommendation, consensus)

### Autoimmune Hepatitis

Pregnant women with AIH should be continued on their treatment. For de novo AIH (as in non-pregnant women), induction with corticosteroids (prednisolone-0.5-1 mg/kg/day or budesonide-6-9 mg/day) and maintenance therapy with thiopurines (azathioprine) should be given 2 weeks later or when serum bilirubin <100 µmol/L. Treatment is associated with better maternal and fetal outcomes (strong recommendation, strong consensus)

### Viral Hepatitis

- Pregnant women presenting with acute hepatitis should be tested for common etiologies of acute liver injury, including viral hepatitis, hepatitis A virus (HAV), hepatitis B virus (HBV), hepatitis E virus (HEV), and herpes simplex virus (HSV)
- Pregnant women with acute hepatitis suspected from HSV should be initiated on acyclovir
- Active-passive immunoprophylaxis with hepatitis B immune globulin and the HBV vaccination series should be administered to all infants born to HBV-infected mothers to prevent perinatal transmission.
- Women chronically infected with HBV and high viral load (>200,000 U/mL or >10 6 log copies/ml and higher) should be offered antiviral medication with tenofovir or telbivudine in the third trimester to reduce perinatal transmission of HBV
- C-section should not be performed electively in HAV, HBV, or HCV-positive mothers to prevent fetal infection.
- Caesarean section may be performed only in Asian HBeAg-positive women with high HBV DNA titer (>7 log10 copies/mL; 6.14 log10 IU/mL) who have not received antiviral therapy during pregnancy (open recommendation).
- All pregnant women with risk factors for HCV should be screened with anti-HCV antibody. Screening should not be performed in women without risk factors for HCV acquisition
- Invasive procedures (e.g., amniocentesis, invasive fetal monitoring) should be minimized in infected mothers and their fetus to prevent vertical transmission of hepatitis C
- Hepatitis C therapy should not be offered to pregnant women to either treat HCV or decrease the risk for vertical transmission
- Women chronically infected with HBV or HCV should be allowed to breastfeed as indicated for infant health

### Wilson's Disease

Pregnant women with Wilson's disease (WD) should be continued on their treatment with penicillamine, trientine, or zinc with a dose reduction of chelators in the second and third trimesters.

## SUGGESTED READING

1. European Association for the Study of the Liver. EASL Clinical Practice Guidelines on the management of liver diseases in pregnancy. J Hepatol. 2023;79(3):768-828.
2. Tran TT, Ahn J, Reau NS. ACG Clinical Guideline: Liver Disease and Pregnancy. Am J Gastroenterol. 2016;111(2): 176-94; quiz 196.

CHAPTER 145

# Thrombocytopenia in Pregnancy

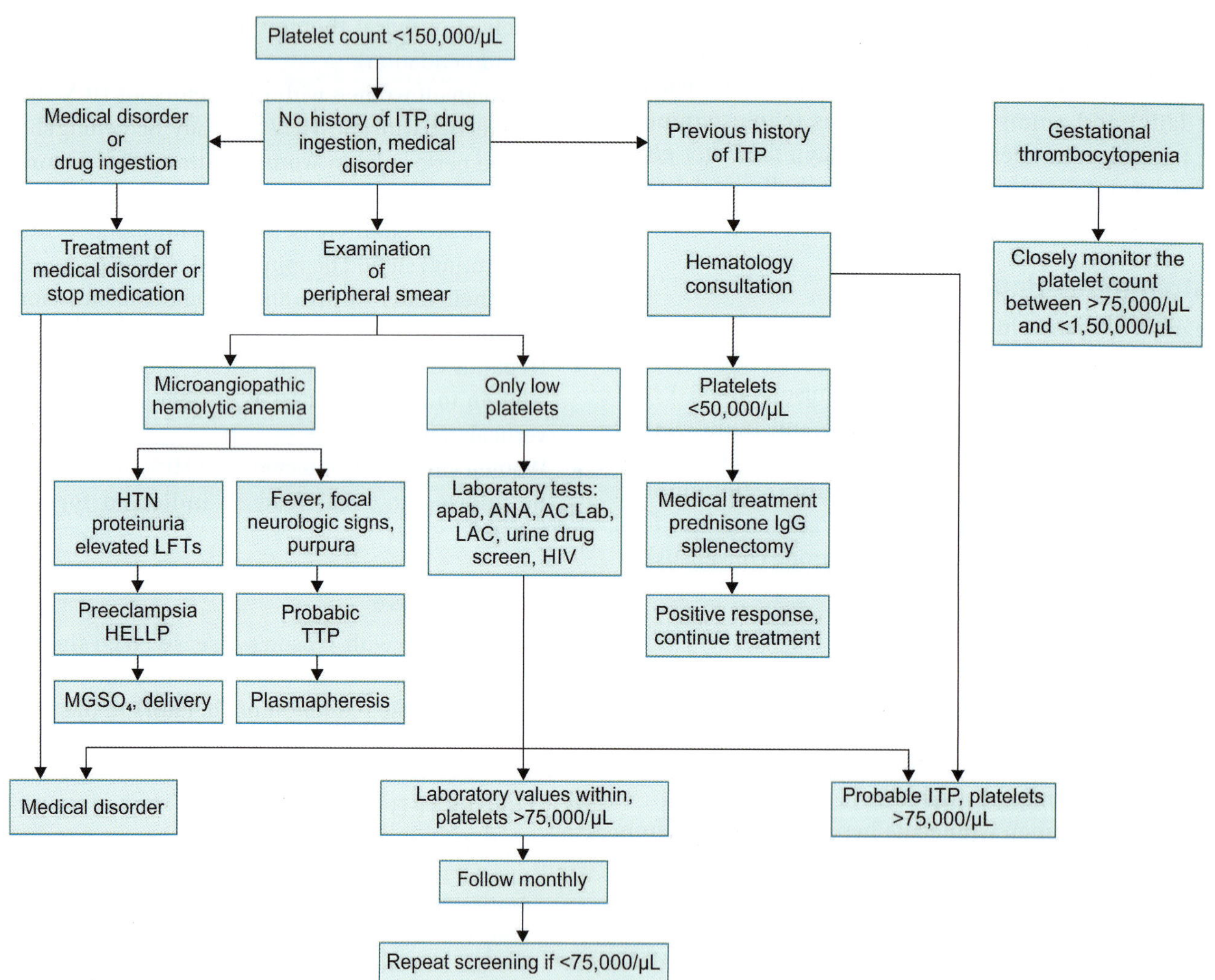


## SUGGESTED READING


1. Cines DB, Levine LD. Thrombocytopenia in pregnancy. Blood. 2017;130(21):2271-7.
2. Provan D, Arnold DM, Bussel JB, Chong BH, Cooper N, Gernsheimer T, et al. Updated international consensus report on the investigation and management of primary immune thrombocytopenia. Blood Adv. 2019;3(22): 3780-817.
3. Reese JA, Peck JD, Deschamps DR, McIntosh JJ, Knudtson EJ, Terrell DR, et al. Platelet counts during pregnancy. N Engl J Med. 2018;379(1):32-43.
4. Valera MC, Parant O, Vayssiere C, Arnal JF, Payrastre B. Physiologic and pathologic changes of platelets in pregnancy. Platelets. 2010;21(8):587-95.
5. Zainal A, Salama A, Alweis R. Immune thrombocytopenic purpura. J Community Hosp Intern Med Perspect. 2019; 9(1):59-61.

CHAPTER 146

# Hypertension in Pregnancy

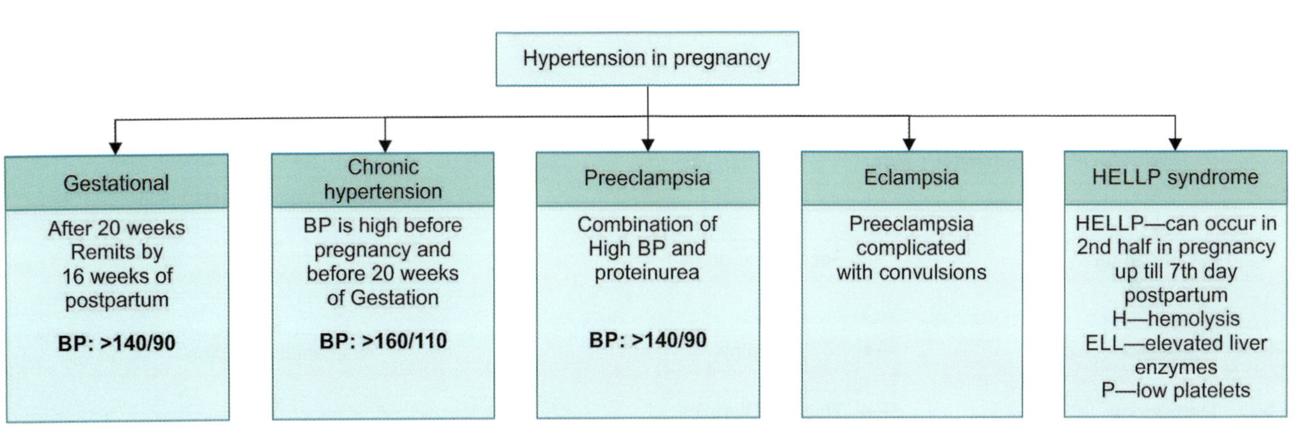


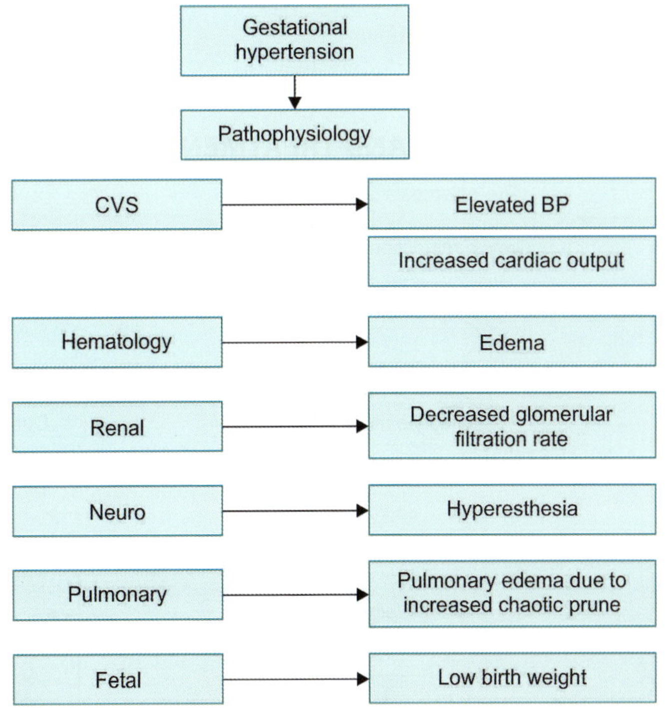

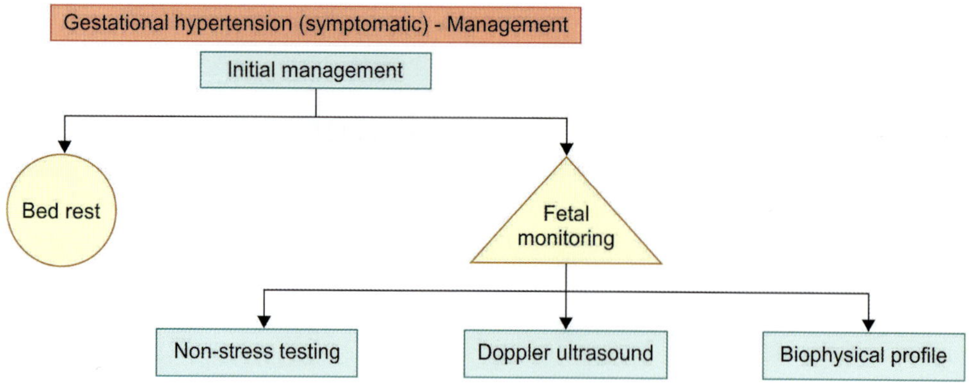

Gestational hypertension (symptomatic) - Management
Initial management
Bed rest
Fetal monitoring
Non-stress testing
Doppler ultrasound
Biophysical profile

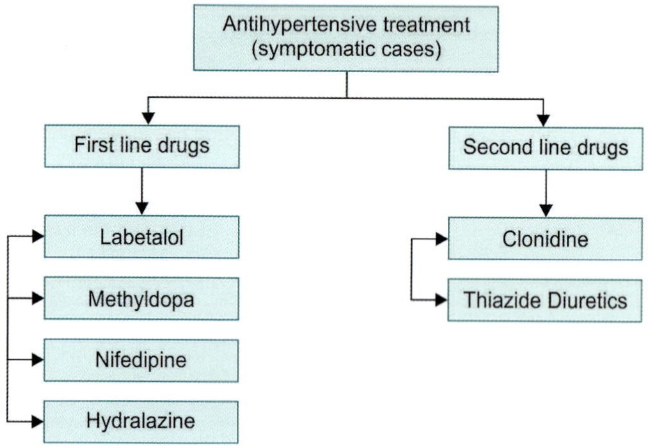

Antihypertensive treatment (symptomatic cases)
First line drugs
Second line drugs
Labetalol
Methyldopa
Nifedipine
Hydralazine
Clonidine
Thiazide Diuretics

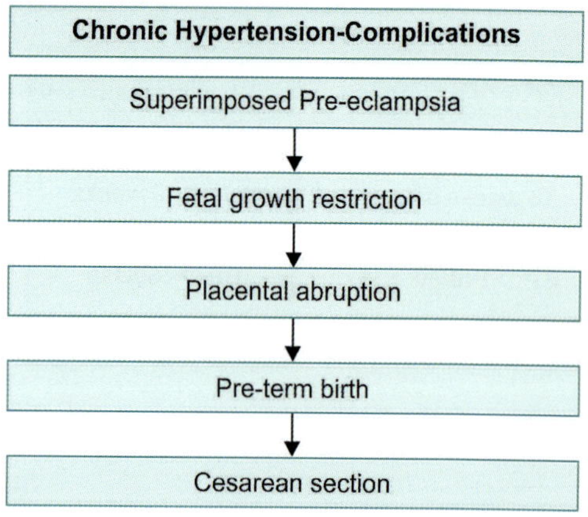

Chronic Hypertension-Complications
Superimposed Pre-eclampsia
Fetal growth restriction
Placental abruption
Pre-term birth
Cesarean section

## CHRONIC HYPERTENSION: DIAGNOSIS AND TREATMENT

Diagnosis
Pre-eclampsia
Growth restriction
Treatment plan
Pre-pregnancy care
Lifestyle modifications
During pregnancy
Optimize Anti-hypertensive therapy
Prevent end-organ damage
Sodium restriction
Weight reduction
DASH diet (Dietary approaches to Stop Hypertension)
Adjust blood pressure targets higher than outside pregnancy
Lower antihypertensive dose during the second trimester
Initiate antihypertensives if: BP >160 systolic BP >70 diastolic

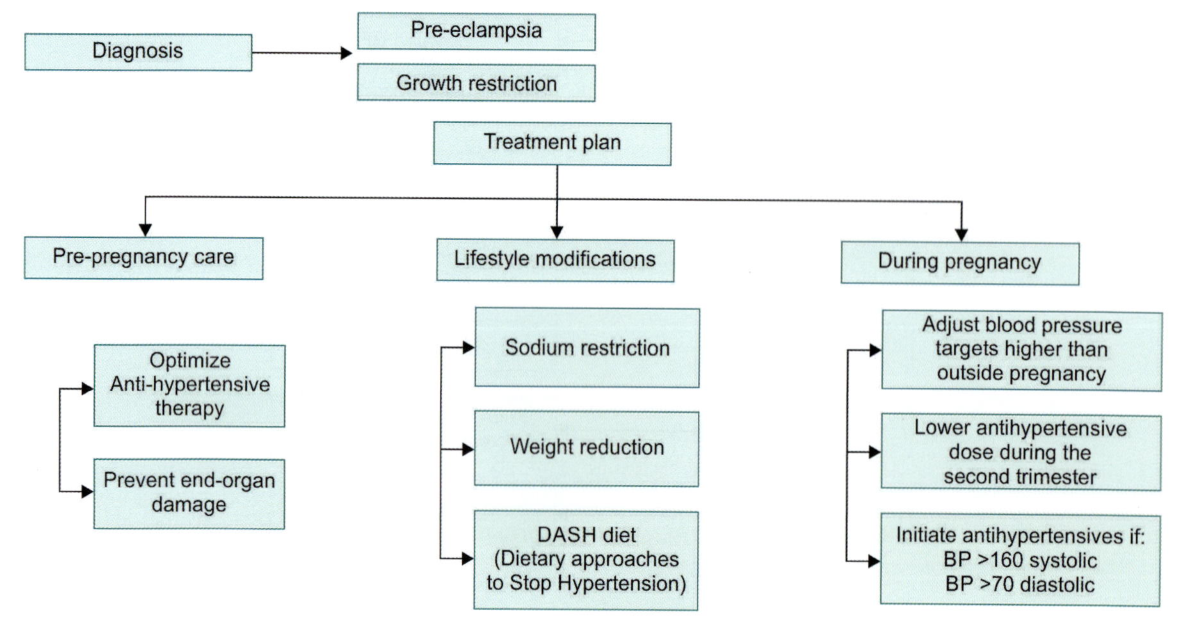

## Treatment of Severe Preeclampsia

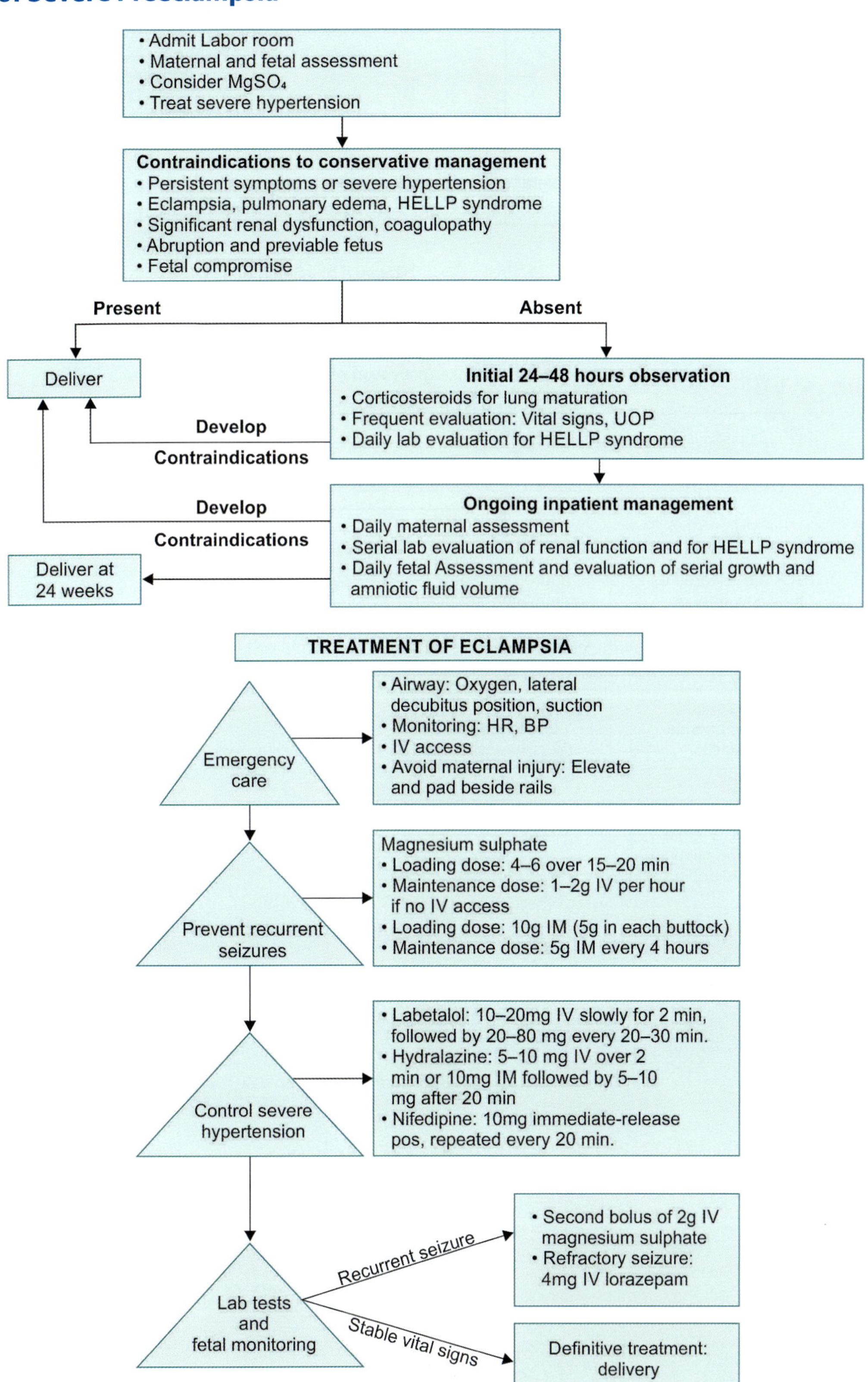

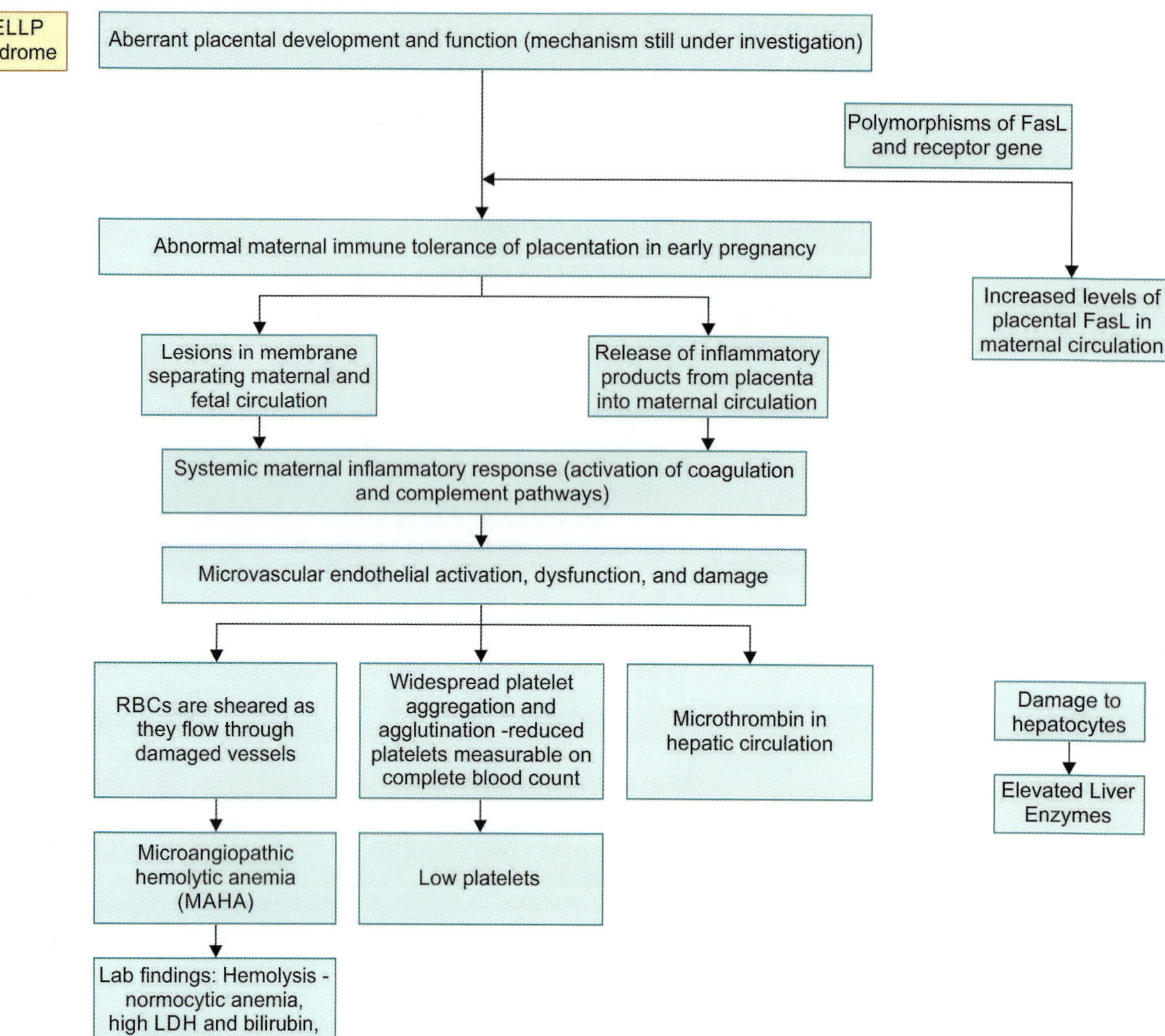
HELLP Syndrome
Aberrant placental development and function (mechanism still under investigation)
Polymorphisms of FasL and receptor gene
Abnormal maternal immune tolerance of placentation in early pregnancy
Increased levels of placental FasL in maternal circulation
Lesions in membrane separating maternal and fetal circulation
Release of inflammatory products from placenta into maternal circulation
Systemic maternal inflammatory response (activation of coagulation and complement pathways)
Microvascular endothelial activation, dysfunction, and damage
RBCs are sheared as they flow through damaged vessels
Widespread platelet aggregation and agglutination -reduced platelets measurable on complete blood count
Microthrombin in hepatic circulation
Damage to hepatocytes
Elevated Liver Enzymes
Microangiopathic hemolytic anemia (MAHA)
Low platelets
Lab findings: Hemolysis - normocytic anemia, high LDH and bilirubin, low haptoglobin

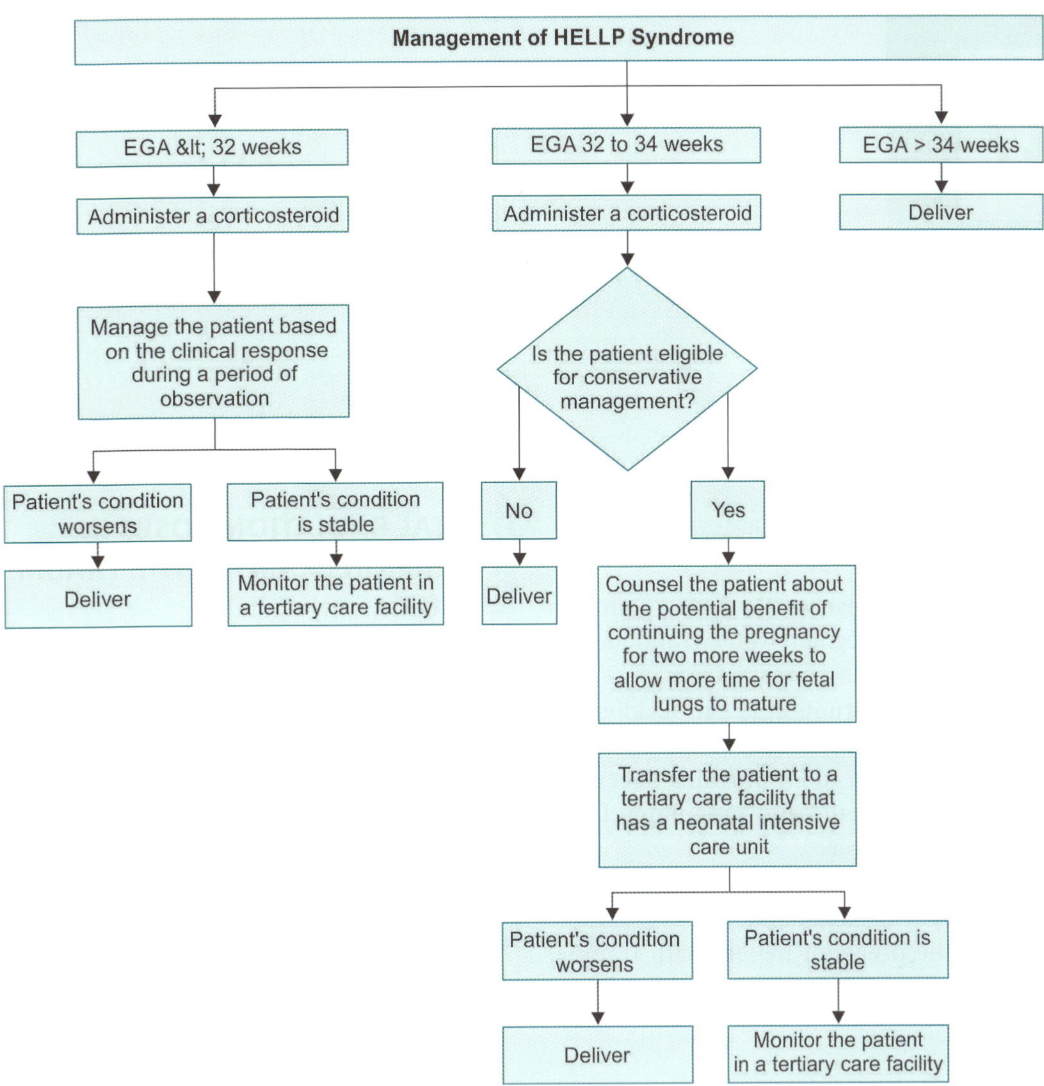


## SUGGESTED READING


1. ACOG Practice Bulletin No. 222: gestational hypertension and preeclampsia: ACOG Practice Bulletin, Number 222. Obstet Gynecol. 2020;135(6):1492-5.
2. American College of Obstetricians and Gynecologists. Preeclampsia and High Blood Pressure During Pregnancy. [online] Available from https://www.acog.org/womens-health/faqs/preeclampsia-and-high-blood-pressure-during-pregnancy [Last accessed February, 2025].
3. American Heart Association. Understanding blood pressure readings. [online] Available from https://www.heart.org/en/hea/thtopics/high-blood-pressure/understandingblood-pressure-readings [Last accessed February, 2025].
4. Moser M, Brown CM, Rose CH, Garovic VD. Hypertension in pregnancy: is it time for a new approach to treatment? J Hypertens. 2012;30(6):1092-100.

CHAPTER 147

# Trauma Management of Pregnant Patient

## KEY POINTS

- Incidence of trauma during pregnancy is 6–8% (severe trauma: 3–6%).
- Of pregnant women hospitalized due to trauma, 60% progress to delivery.
- Domestic violence represents the most common trauma mechanism for pregnant women, and ideally, it should be identified during antenatal care.
- Diagnosis of placental abruption in car accidents is important.
- Ultrasound in the trauma room provides necessary information about the fetus and pregnancy (fetal FAST), enabling quick action
- Most imaging exams required for good trauma care do not represent harm to the pregnancy
- Management of the pregnant patient with trauma, especially in severe cases over 20–24 weeks, is essentially a multidisciplinary approach of the trauma surgeon and the obstetrician

## FETAL RADIATION DOSES IN COMMON EXAMS IN THE TRAUMA ROOM

| *Exam* | *Fetal dose (mGy)* |
|---|---|
| Head or neck CT scan | 0.001–0.01 |
| Extremity X-ray | <0.001 |
| 2-view chest X-ray | 0.0005–0.01 |
| Abdominal or pelvic X-ray | 0.1–3.0 |
| Chest tomography | 0.1–0.66 |
| Lumbosacral spine X-ray | 1–10 |
| Abdominal tomography | 1.3–35 |
| Pelvic tomography | 10–50 |

| | *Physiological changes* | *Clinical implications* |
|---|---|---|
| **Cardiovascular** | • Blood volume ↑↑ × erythrocyte mass↑<br>• ↑Heart rate (15–20 bpm)<br>• ↓ Blood pressure (2nd trimester)<br>• ↑ Plasma volume (30–40%)<br>• ↓↓ Peripheral resistance (20%)→<br>• ↓ Diastolic blood pressure<br>• ↑ Uterine volume (3rd trimester) → cava compression | • Physiological "anemia" (normal Hb ≥ 11 g/dL)<br>• Physiological changes may obscure the diagnosis of hypovolemia or hemorrhagic shock<br>• Hypotension in pregnant trauma patient usually indicates profound hemorrhagic shock with substantial loss of circulating volume, necessitating initiation of a massive transfusion protocol<br>• ↓ Venous return when a patient is in the supine position (↓ preload)—Supine hypotension may occur as early as 20 weeks GA<br>• It can be alleviated by left lateral tilt of 30°. Lesser degrees tilt is not effective, while larger degrees are not beneficial<br>• Avoid placing the patient in the supine position during the initial survey and while imaging<br>• If CPR is deemed necessary, place the patient supine on a firm backboard and 2-handed manual left uterine displacement (LUD) |

*Contd...*

*Contd…*

| | *Physiological changes* | *Clinical implications* |
|---|---|---|
| **Pulmonary** | • ↑ Tidal volume<br>• Respiratory rate unchanged<br>• ↑ Minute ventilation<br>• Elevation of the diaphragmatic dome by 4 cm → Functional residual capacity ↓ 20% ↓Inspiratory capacity<br>• ↑Oxygen consumption<br>• ↑ Rib cage circumference and cephalad displacement of the diaphragm | • *Respiratory alkalosis:*<br>– $pO_2$ ↑ to 105 mm Hg from 75 to 100 mm Hg<br>– $pCO_2$ ↓ to 32 mm Hg from 37 to 40 mm Hg<br>– pH ↑ to 7.40 to 7.45 from 7.35 to 7.40<br>– Bicarbonate ↓ to 18 to 21 mmol/L from 22 to 26 mmol/L<br>• Lower apnea time tolerance → induction and tracheal intubation should occur with precision and hastened<br>• Thoracostomy tubes need to be placed more cephalad by 1 or 2 intercostal spaces |
| **Airway** | • ↑ Airway edema<br>• ↑ Vascular engorgement<br>• ↑ Tissue fragility | • Even favorable-appearing airways may prove to be difficult to intubate<br>• Smaller tracheal tubes (6–6.5 mm internal diameter) should be chosen due to edema<br>• Tissue friability may lead to increased risk of bleeding, obscuring laryngoscope views<br>• Avoid nasopharyngeal airway<br>• Practitioner and technique with the highest chance of first-pass intubation is warranted |
| **Renal** | • ↑ Glomerular filtration<br>• ↑ Plasma volume<br>• ↓ Creatinine, urea, and plasma uric acid | • Reduced creatinine and blood urea nitrogen values may obscure the diagnosis of AKI<br>• Renal compensation of respiratory alkalosis ↓ serum bicarbonate to 18–21 mmol/L<br>• Normal base deficit is around 2–3 mEq/L |
| **Coagulation** | • Increased anemia<br>• ↑ Factors I, VII, VIII and X, and XII<br>• ↑ Fibrinogen ↑ Von WF<br>• Resistance to activated C protein | • Physiological changes help mitigate acute blood loss and may actually prove protective during trauma<br>• Normalization of fibrinogen values may be a warning sign of severe hemorrhage and impending DIC<br>• Viscoelastic testing (TEG and ROTEM) may be used to diagnose and manage trauma-induced coagulopathy<br>• ↑ Risk of thromboembolism |
| **Gastrointestinal** | • ↑ Gastrin<br>• ↓ Esophageal sphincter activity<br>• ↓ Gastrointestinal motility<br>• ↑ Production of gastric secretion<br>• ↑ Risk of bronchoaspiration | • ↑Risk for aspiration begins as early as 18–20 weeks gestation<br>• Use rapid sequence induction during intubation with succinylcholine or high-dose rocuronium (1.2 mg/kg)<br>• Both succinylcholine and rocuronium are unlikely to cross the placenta and are low risk for the fetus<br>• Avoid sugammadex due to unknown safety profile and potential for precipitating preterm labor |

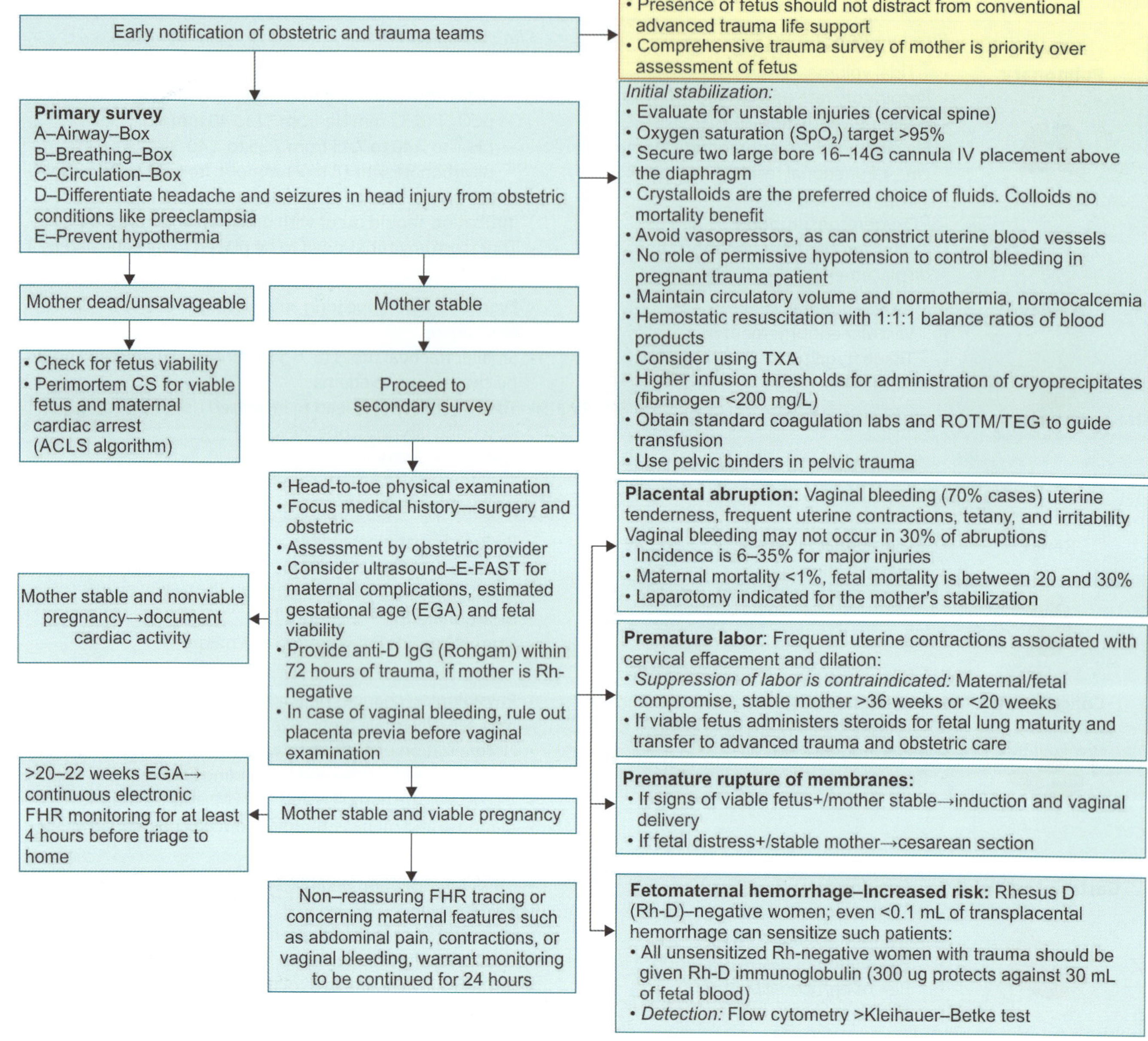


## SUGGESTED READING

1. Febrasgo position statement trauma and pregnancy DOI: https://doi.org/10.1055/s-0043-1777339. Number 10 - October 2023. The National Specialized Commission on High-Risk Pregnancy of the Brazilian Federation of Gynecology and Obstetrics Associations (Febrasgo) and the Brazilian Society of Integrated Trauma Care (SBAIT) endorse this document. Content production is based on scientific evidence on the proposed theme and the results presented contribute to clinical practice.
2. Lopez CE, Salloum J, Varon AJ, Toledo P, Dudaryk R. The Management of Pregnant Trauma Patients: A Narrative Review. Anesth Analg. 2023;136(5):830-40.

CHAPTER 148

# Shock during Pregnancy

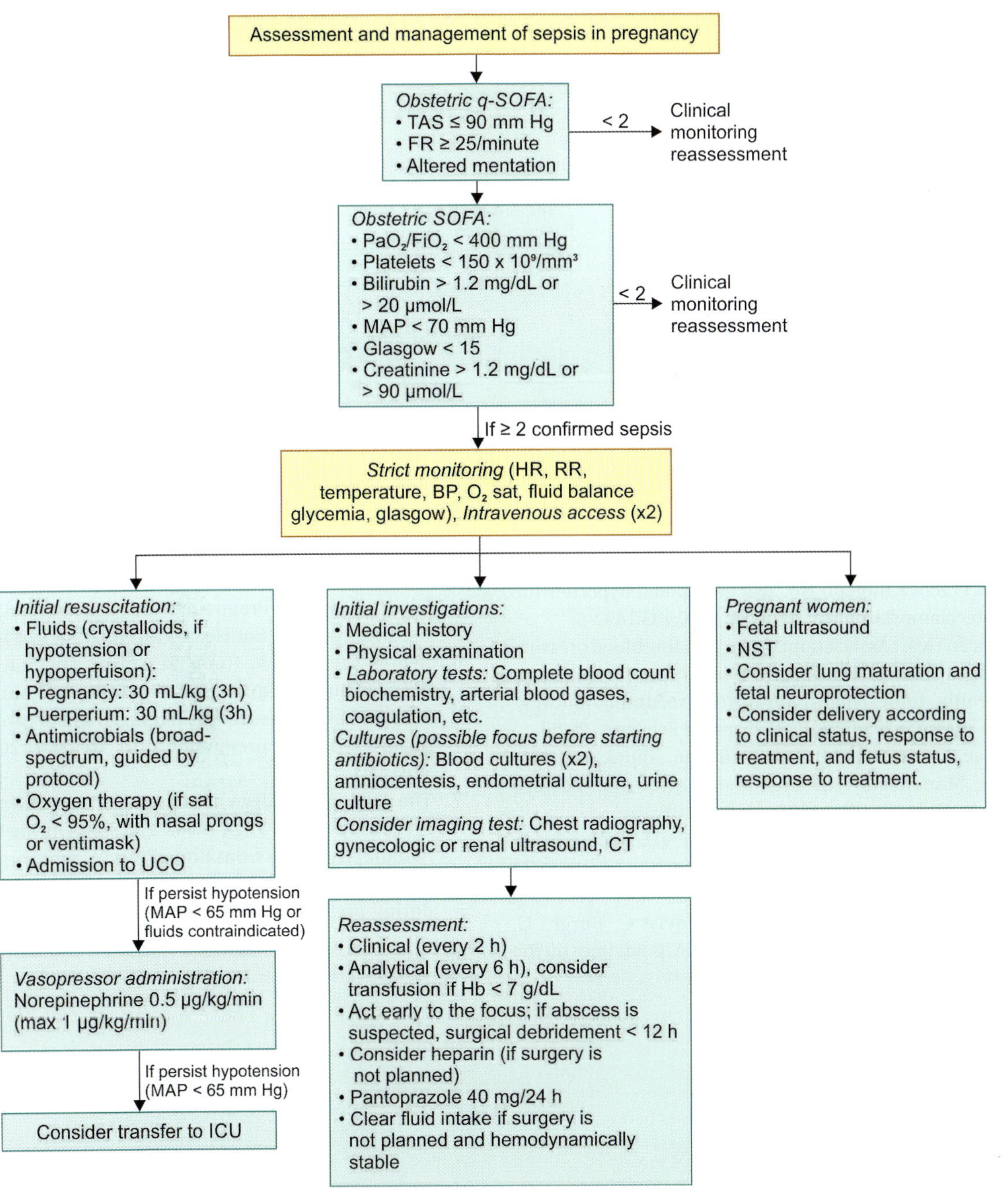

**Cardiogenic Shock during Pregnancy**

Peripartum cardiomyopathy patient in cardiogenic shock

**Medications**

*Targeted therapies:*
- Bromocriptine

*Vasodilators/inodilators:*
- Nitroglycerine > nitroprusside
- Milrinone or levosimendan > dobutamine

*Anticoagulation*:
- Low molecular weight heparin or unfractionated Heparin

*Diuretics:*
- Loop or thiazide diuretics
- Avoid aldosterone antagonists

*Neurohormonal blockade:*
- Beta blocker when stable
- Avoid ACEi/ARB and aldosterone antagonists

**Mechanical circulation support**

Consider early!

*IABP:*
- *Pros:* Anticoagulation not mandatory
- *Cons:* Limited hemodynamic support

*Impella:*
- *Pros:* Increased hemodynamic support
- *Cons:* Strict anticoagulation requirements

*ECMO:*
- *Pros:* Increased hemodynamic support, supports oxygenation
- *Cons:* Strict anticoagulation requirements, may increase prolactin

**Cardiac transplantation**

Last resort in the acute setting given high rate of ejection fraction recovery and poorer outcomes in PPCM

**Delivery**

*Obstetrics:*
- Avoid prostaglandin E analogues if possible
- Left lateral decubitus position
- Minimize maternal pushing

*Anesthesia:*
- Epidural analgesia preferred

**Arrhythmia management**

**Medications**
- Avoid amiodarone and dronedarone

**Electrical cardioversion**
- Generally safe

**Ablation**
- Last resort

## SUGGESTED READING


1. ACOG Practice Bulletin No. 222: gestational hypertension and preeclampsia. Obstet Gynecol. 2020;135:1492-5.
2. American Heart Association. Understanding blood pressure readings. [Online] Available from https://www. heart.org/en/health- topics/high-blood-pressure/understanding-blood-pressure-readings [Last accessed February, 2025].
3. Cardiac disease in pregnancy guideline - quick reference guide. Manchester: Greater Manchester and Eastern Cheshire Strategic Clinical Networks; 2018.
4. Moser M, Brown CM, Rose CH, Garovic VD. Hypertension in pregnancy: is it time for a new approach to treatment? J Hypertens. 2012;30(6):1092-100.
5. Regitz-Zagrosek V, Blomstrom Lundqvist C, Borghi C, Cifkova R, Ferreira R, Foidart JM, et al. ESC guidelines on the management of cardiovascular diseases during pregnancy: the Task Force on the Management of Cardiovascular Diseases during Pregnancy of the European Society of Cardiology (ESC). Eur Heart J. 2011;32(24):3147-97.
6. Regitz-Zagrosek V, Roos-Hesselink JW, Bauersachs J, Blomström-Lundqvist C, Cífková R, De Bonis M, et al. 2018 ESC guidelines for the management of cardiovascular diseases during pregnancy. Eur Heart J. 2018;39(34):3165-241.
7. The American College of Obstetricians and Gynecologists. Preeclampsia and High Blood Pressure During Pregnancy. [Online] Available from https://www. acog. org/womens-hea/th/faqs/preeclampsia-and-high-blood- pressure-during-pregnancy [Last accessed February, 2025].

CHAPTER 149

# Cardiac Arrest in Pregnancy

## MATERNAL CARDIAC ARREST

Complete cessation of cardiac activity of a woman during pregnancy and up to 6 weeks postdelivery

## BASIC LIFE SUPPORT IN PREGNANCY

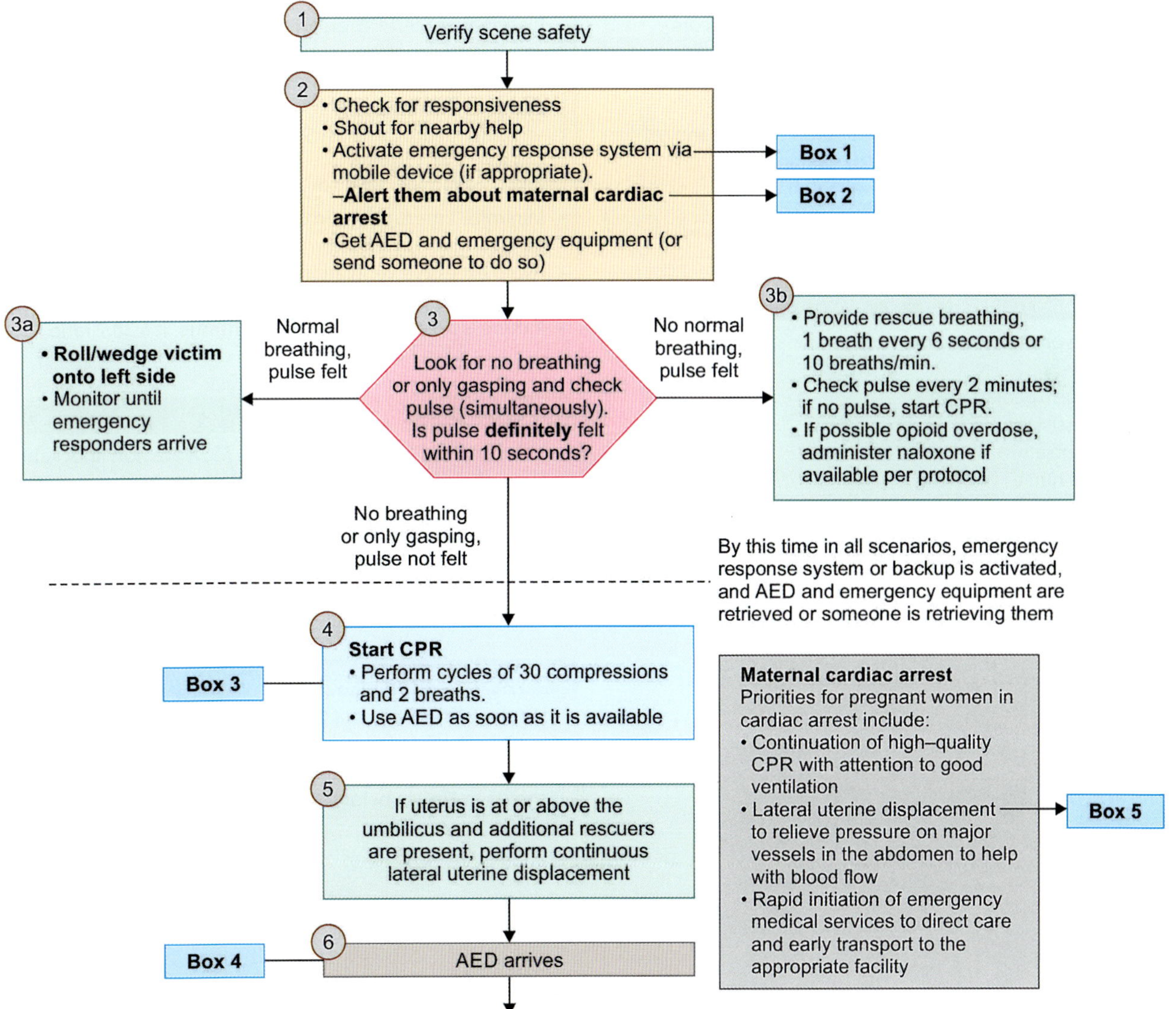


Contd...

*Contd...*

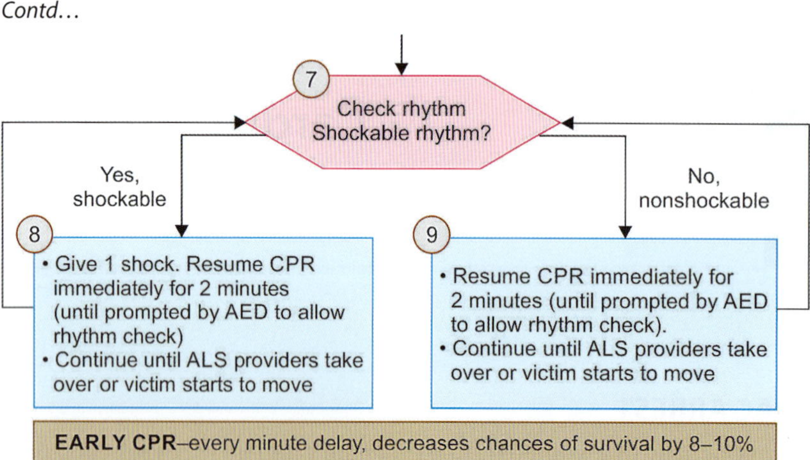


**EARLY CPR**–every minute delay, decreases chances of survival by 8–10%

**BOX 1:** How to activate the emergency response system.

- Call on a designated number from the nearest intercom number/your mobile number
- Introduce yourself to the call receiver
- Describe the location of the victim
- Describe the condition/expected duration of pregnancy of the patient (fundal height/history by bystander)
- Hang on the phone until the call receiver has fully understood your message

**BOX 2:** Personnel required.

- Critical care physician/anesthesiologist
- Obstetrician
- Neonatologist/pediatrician
- Technical assistant
- Obstetric nurse
- Critical care nurse
- Most experienced anesthesiologist to take care of airway challenges related to pregnancy
- One team member dedicated to LUD

**BOX 3:** High-quality CPR.

- Place patient SUPINE on firm backboard for chest compressions
- Locate the lower half of the sternum
- Compress-HARD and FAST
  - *HARD (depth):* At least 5 cm
  - *FAST:* 100-120/min
- Allow adequate chest recoil
- Minimize interruptions in compressions (<10 secs)
- CCF (cardiac compression fraction): Ideally > 80%
- Avoid excessive ventilation
- Change compressor every 2 mins, or sooner if fatigued
- If there is no advanced airway- continue at a 30:2 ratio

**BOX 4:** Defibrillation/AED.

- Most (90%) of the rhythms during MCA are non-shockable
- Nevertheless, defibrillation should be attempted by AED in shockable rhythms
- Same energy of defibrillation (biphasic 120-200 J)
- No harm to the fetus, so do not waste time in removing fetal monitors

**BOX 5:** Lateral Uterine Displacement (LUD).

- Displaces the weight of the gravid uterus from the major vessels- the inferior vena cava and aorta
- May be performed by one-hand or two-hand technique, as shown in **Figure** below

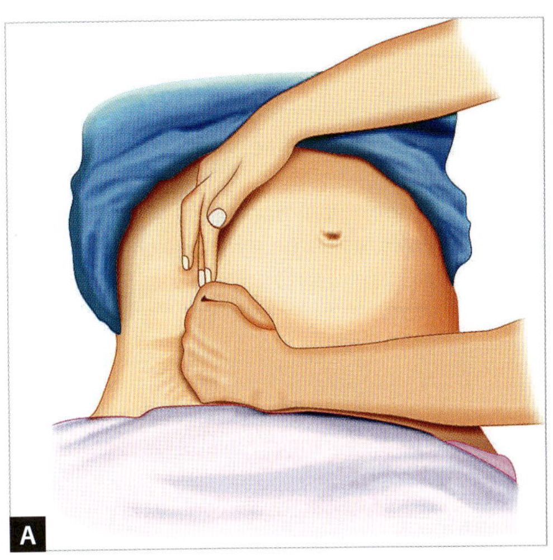


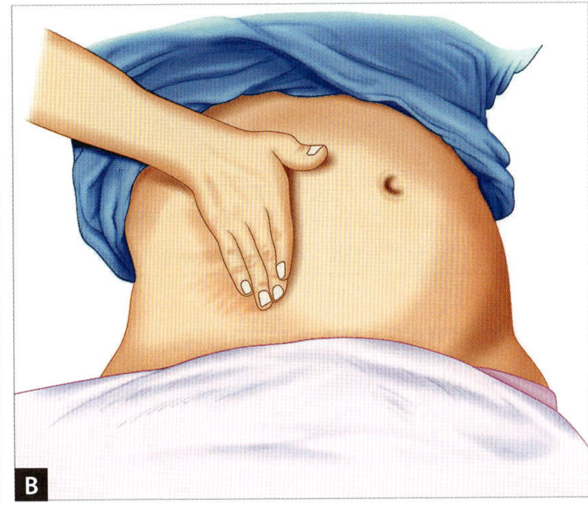


(A) Manual left lateral uterine displacement, performed with 2-handed technique; (B) 1-handed technique during resuscitation.

## PHYSIOLOGICAL CHANGES IN PREGNANT FEMALE-RELEVANT TO CARDIAC ARREST

| | |
|---|---|
| 1. Increased stroke volume and cardiac output (30%-50%) | → the ejection fraction produced by cardiac compressions is negligible to match this high C.O state |
| 2. Physiological anemia | → decreased oxygen delivery to the tissues during Maternal CPR |
| 3. Aortocaval compression | → decreased venous return, hypotension, decreased uteroplacental blood flow. Hence, must do LUD and early PMCD |

## CAUSES OF CARDIAC ARREST IN PREGNANCY (ABCDEFGH)

| | | |
|---|---|---|
| A | Anesthetic issues | • Hypoxia/anoxia (difficult airway, loss of airway, aspiration<br>• Hypotension |
| B | Bleeding | • Uterine (atony, rupture)<br>• Placental (abruption, previa, accrete<br>• Retained products of conception leading to DIC<br>• Comorbidities like liver failure |
| C | CVS | • Acute MI<br>• Congenital heart disease<br>• Valvular heart disease<br>• Aortic dissection,<br>• Peripartum cardiomyopathy<br>• Arrhythmias |
| D | Drug-related | • Magnesium sulphate<br>• Oxytocin overdose<br>• Anaphylaxis<br>• Medication error (overdose, drug interaction) |
| E | Embolic | • Amniotic fluid embolism<br>• Pulmonary thromboembolism |
| F | Fever | • Sepsis<br>• Blood transfusion reactions |

*Contd...*

*Contd...*

| G | General issues | 5Hs<br>• Hypovolemia<br>• Hypoxia<br>• Hydrogen ion (acidosis)<br>• Hypokalemia<br>• Hyperkalemia | 5Ts<br>• Tension pneumothorax<br>• Tamponade-cardiac<br>• Toxins<br>• Thrombosis-pulmonary<br>• Thrombosis-coronary |
|---|---|---|---|
| H | Hypertension | PIH, severe eclampsia | |

## ADVANCED CARDIAC LIFE SUPPORT

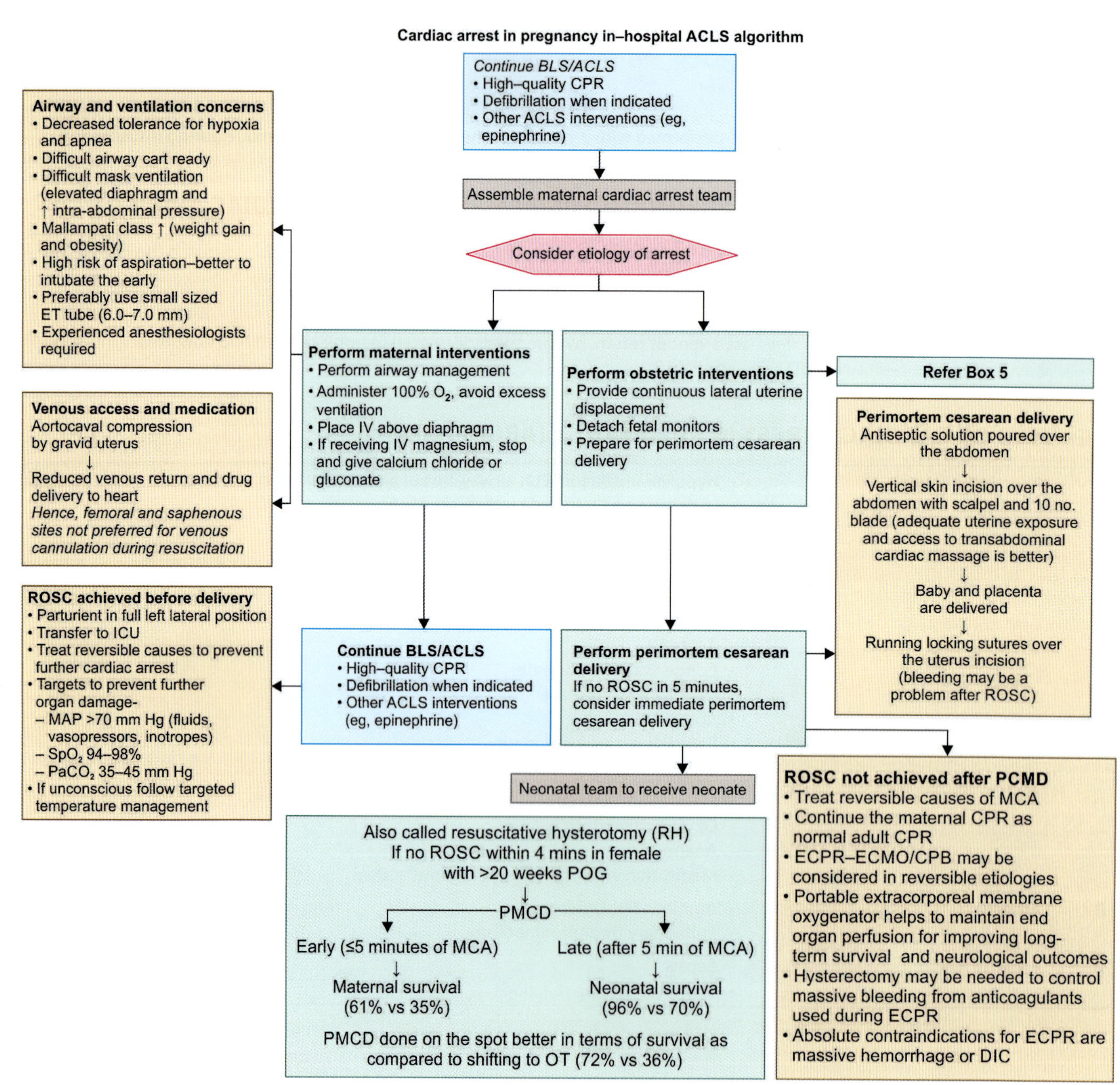

## DIFFERENCES BETWEEN PREGNANT AND NONPREGNANT CPR

| *Characteristics* | *Nonpregnant* | *Pregnant* |
|---|---|---|
| 1. Lives affected | One | Two-Mother and fetus |
| 2. Call for help | Trained personnel<br>+<br>AED | MCA team-<br>• Trained Anesthetist<br>• Obstetrician<br>• Neonatologist/Pediatrician<br>• OT/critical care assistant |
| 3. Chest compressions | Lower half of the sternum | Lower half of the sternum<br>+<br>Left uterine displacement/30° left tilt |
| 4. Airway management | Nasopharyngeal, oropharyngeal airway, ETT, and LMA can be used | • Difficult airway cart should be ready<br>• Airway resistance is high<br>• Avoid nasopharyngeal airway<br>• ETT 1mm smaller than the usual size<br>• Mallampati class ↑ due to weight gain and obesity<br>• Prefer early intubation by expert |
| 5. Breathing | • Single person can do bag and mask ventilation<br>• Hyperventilation is avoided →decreases C.O →decreases cerebral perfusion | • 2 persons required for bag-mask ventilation<br>• High risk of aspiration, so, intubate early<br>• Oxygenation is more important than aspiration as tolerance is decreased for hypoxia and apnea<br>• Hyperventilation is avoided →decreased C.O. →decreases cerebral perfusion and causes fetal acidosis |
| 6. Defibrillation | 120-200 J biphasic<br>Common rhythm encountered – shockable rhythms | • 120–200 J biphasic<br>• Common rhythm encountered – non-shockable rhythm<br>• Same energy is not harmful to the fetus |
| 7. Intravenous access | Preferably upper limb | Above the level of the diaphragm is a must |
| 8. Drugs | Adrenaline<br>Amiodarone | Specific drugs-<br>1. Calcium gluconate – magnesium sulfate toxicity<br>2. Intralipid emulsion-local anesthetic (LA) toxicity |
| 9. Advanced cardiac life support | ECHO/$EtCO_2$<br>USG<br>ECMO | ECMO-for reversible causes-amniotic fluid embolism, LA toxicity<br>PMCD should be done if there is no ROSC in 4 mins of CPR, if uterine height is >20 weeks |

## DRUGS USED DURING MATERNAL CARDIAC ARREST

| *Drug* | *Indication* | *Dose* |
|---|---|---|
| Adrenaline /epinephrine | MCA during ACLS to maintain ROSC and cardiac activity | 1 mg IV Every 3–5 minutes |
| Amiodarone | Ventricular fibrillation or pulseless ventricular tachycardia that is unresponsive to CPR, defibrillation, and epinephrine | 300 mg rapid IV infusion and repeat dose of 150 mg |
| Calcium gluconate | Antidote for magnesium toxicity | 10 mL of 10% calcium gluconate/chloride IV |
| Atropine | Symptomatic bradycardia | 1 mg IV push, may repeat every 3–5 minutes |
| Lipid emulsion 20% | Suspected local anesthetic toxicity | 1.5 mL/kg IV over 1 minute |
| Naloxone | Narcotic-induced respiratory depression | 0.4 mg IV bolus followed by 0.2–0.4 mg/h if the patient continues to be unresponsive |

*Contd…*

*Contd...*

| *Drug* | *Indication* | *Dose* |
|---|---|---|
| Tranexamic acid | Within 3 hours of postmortem hemorrhage | 1g IV at 1 mL/min,<br>repeat the same dose if bleeding continues after 30 minutes or if bleeding reoccurs after 24 hours of the first dose every 3–5 minutes |
| High-concentration dextrose solution | For hypoglycemic detected in the periarrest period | 0.5–1 g/kg IV 25% D solution contains 25 gm dextrose in 100 mL |
| *Oxytocin should be used cautiously as it can trigger MCA due to its vasodilatory properties. Lower doses should be used* | | |

## SUGGESTED READING


1. AHA 2020 CPR Guidelines
2. Beckett VA, Knight M, Sharpe P. The CAPS Study: incidence, management, and outcomes of cardiac arrest in pregnancy in the UK: a prospective, descriptive study. BJOG. 2017; 124(9):1374-81.
3. Fischer C, Bonnet MP, Girault A, Le Ray C. Update: Focus in-hospital maternal cardiac arrest. J Gynecol Obstet Hum Reprod. 2019;48(5):309-14.

CHAPTER 150

# Ovarian Hyperstimulation Syndrome

## INTRODUCTION

- Ovarian hyperstimulation syndrome (OHSS) is rare but an iatrogenic complication
- OHSS is due to an exaggerated response to ovulation therapy, typically, exogenous gonadotropin stimulation hormone, and rarely observed with other agents
- OHSS that is characterized by ovarian enlargement due to multiple ovarian cysts and an acute fluid shift into the extravascular space.
- Pregnancy complicated by OHSS may be at increased risk of pre-eclampsia and preterm delivery
- *Risk factors for OHSS*
  - A. *Primary risk factors (patient-related):*
    1. High basal AMH (>3.36 ng/mL (independent predictor).
    2. Young age (<33 years)
    3. Previous OHSS (Moderate and severe cases/ hospitalization)
    4. PCO-like ovaries (>24 antral follicles in both ovaries combined).
  - B. *Secondary risk factors (ovarian response related); On day of hCG trigger:*
    1. High number of medium/large follicles (≥13 follicles ≥11 mm in diameter or ≥11 follicles ≥10 mm in diameter)
    2. High or rapidly rising E2 levels and high number of follicles (E2 5,000 pg/mL and/or ≥18 follicles predictive of severe OHSS)
    3. Number of oocyte retrieved (≥11 predicts OHSS)
    4. Elevated inhibin—B levels (Elevated levels on day 5 of gonadotropin stimulation, at oocyte retrieval and 3 days before)
    5. hCG administration for luteal phase supp.

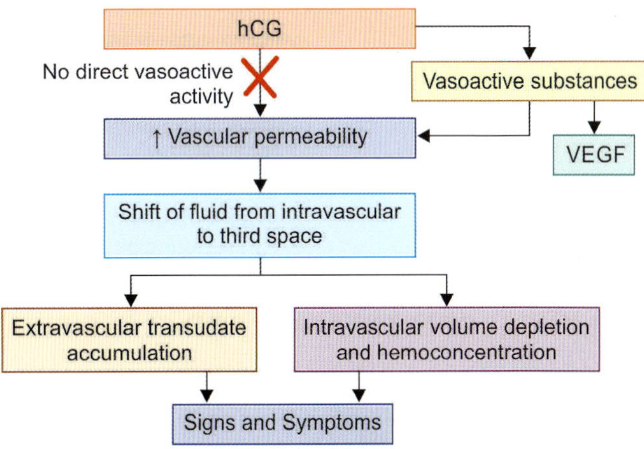


| | | |
|---|---|---|
| *Mild OHSS* | • Abdominal bloating<br>• Mild abdominal pain | • No major abnormality<br>• Ovarian size usually <8 cm[a] |
| *Moderate OHSS*<br>(symptoms due to acute fluid shift into extra-vascular space) | • Moderate abdominal pain<br>• Nausea ± vomiting | • Ultrasound evidence of ascites<br>• Ovarian size is usually 8–12 cm[a] |
| *Severe OHSS*<br>(symptoms of moderate OHSS with extreme thirst and dehydration) | • Clinical ascites (± hydrothorax)<br>• *Gastro-intestinal system*—Vomiting, rapid weight gain/increasing abdominal girth (due to ascites), paralytic ileus | • Oliguria <300 mL/day or < 30 mL/h)<br>• Hematocrit >0.45<br>• Hyponatremia (sodium <135 mmol/L)<br>• Hypoproteinemia (serum albumin <35 g/L)<br>• Ovarian size usually >12 cm[a] |

*Contd...*

*Contd...*

| | | |
|---|---|---|
| | • *Pulmonary system*—Respiratory distress (due to ascites, pleural and pericardial effusion, pulmonary thromboembolism, rarely pulmonary edema)<br>• *Cardiovascular system*—Hypotension and tachycardia (due to hypovolemia), pericardial effusion<br>• *Renal system*—Renal failure, oliguria (due to hypovolemia)<br>• *Hepatobiliary system*—liver edema<br>• *Constitutional symptoms*—pyrexia (non-infectious origin—due to release of prostaglandins) leg/vulval swelling<br>• *Cystic enlargement of ovaries*—ovarian torsion and hemorrhage | |
| Critical OHSS | • Tense ascites<br>• Large hydrothorax<br>• Thromboembolism/hypercoagulability (due to high serum E2 estrogen levels)<br>• Acute respiratory distress syndrome<br>• Sepsis | • Worsening of previous findings<br>• Hematocrit > 0.55<br>• White cell count > 25 000/mL<br>• Oliguria/anuria |

(RCOG: Royal College of Obstetricians and Gynecologists; OHSS: Ovarian Hyperstimulation Syndrome)
[a]Ovarian size may not correlate with severity of OHSS in cases of assisted reproduction because of the effect of follicular aspiration. Women demonstrating any feature of severe or critical OHSS should be classified in that category.

**Clinical mimics.**

- Ovarian torsion or cyst rupture
- Pelvic infection/abscess
- Appendicitis
- Bowel perforation
- Ectopic pregnancy
- FSH secreting pituitary adenoma

## CLINICAL PRESENTATION AND CLASSIFICATION

According to the time of presentation, there are two main types of OHSS.

| ***Early OHSS*** | ***Late OHSS*** |
|---|---|
| 3–7 days after hCG administration | 10–12 days after hCG administration |
| Correlates to ovarian response to exogenous hCG administration | Correlates to endogenous hCG release by implanting embryo or to hCG administration for luteal phase support |
| Predicted by a higher number of growing follicles and elevated E2 levels | Predicted by a higher number of gestational sacs |
| Higher risk of preclinical miscarriage | More likely to be severe |

Mild to moderate OHSS—excellent prognosis

Severe OHSS—Morbidity is clinically significant, fatality occurs mainly due to hypovolemic shock, electrolyte imbalance, hemorrhage, and thromboembolism. However, the prognosis is optimistic with adequate treatment.

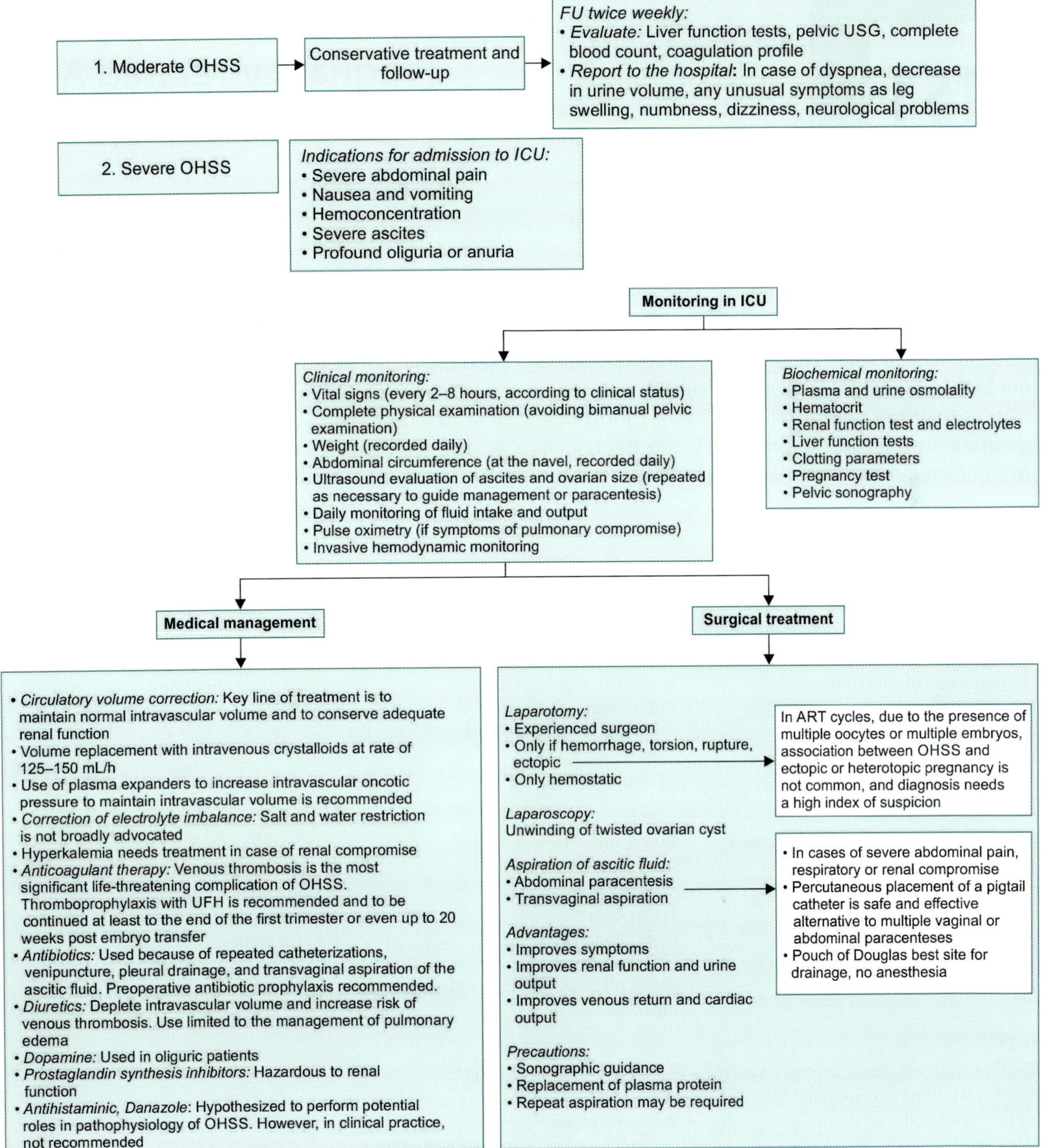


## SUGGESTED READING

1. Jahromi NB, Parsanezhad ME, Shomali Z, Bakhshai P, Alborzi M, Vaziri MN, et al. Ovarian Hyperstimulation Syndrome: A Narrative Review of Its Pathophysiology, Risk Factors, Prevention, Classification, and Management. Iran J Med Sci May. 2018;43(3):248-60.

CHAPTER

# 151

# Pregnancy-related Acute Kidney Injury

## INTRODUCTION

Pregnancy-related acute kidney injury (PRAKI) refers to acute kidney injury (AKI) occurring during pregnancy or the postpartum period. The causes of PRAKI vary depending on the stage of pregnancy and the region, with common factors including postpartum hemorrhage, puerperal sepsis, pre-eclampsia, eclampsia, and placental previa. Diagnostic criteria for PRAKI include a serum creatinine (SCr) level exceeding 1 mg/dL, an increase in SCr by 0.3 mg/dL within 48 hours, a 50% rise in SCr from baseline within 7 days, or a urine output of less than 0.5 mL/kg/h for at least 6 hours.

## CAUSES

| ***Prerenal*** | ***Intrinsic renal*** | ***Postrenal*** |
|---|---|---|
| *Early pregnancy* | | |
| • Bleeding—miscarriage<br>• Hyperemesis gravidarum<br>• Ovarian hyperstimulation syndrome<br>• Ectopic pregnancy | • Anticardiolipin antibody syndrome<br>• Sepsis (i.e., septic abortion)<br>• Autoimmune disease<br>• Glomerulonephritis, interstitial nephritis, lupus nephritis<br>• CKD progression | • Renal Stones<br>• Ureteral obstruction |
| *Late pregnancy* | | |
| Bleeding—second-trimester miscarriage, placenta previa, placental abruption | • Severe pre-eclampsia, HELLP<br>• Acute fatty liver of pregnancy<br>• HUS/TTP<br>• Pyelonephritis<br>• Chorioamnionitis<br>• CKD Progression<br>• Glomerulonephritis, interstitial nephritis, lupus nephritis | • Polyhydramnios<br>• Multifetal gestation<br>• Large uterine fibroids<br>• Ureteral obstruction<br>• Renal stones |
| *Postpartum* | | |
| Bleeding—uterine atonia, uterine rupture, obstetrical trauma (vulvovaginal and perineal tears and lacerations) | • Severe pre-eclampsia, HELLP<br>• HUS<br>• Puerperal sepsis<br>• Glomerulonephritis, interstitial nephritis, lupus nephritis Nephrotoxic drugs (NSAIDS, antibiotics, proton-pump inhibitors, H2 antagonists)<br>• CKD Progression | Renal Stones |

| First trimester | Second trimester | Third trimester | D | Postpartum |
|---|---|---|---|---|
| ***Septic abortion***<br>*Clinical features:*<br>• Prerenal azotemia or ATN<br>*Treatment:*<br>> Volume resuscitation, antibiotics | ***Preeclampsia/HELLP***<br>*Clinical features:*<br>~ Hypertension and proteinuria after 20 weeks of gestation Headache, visual disturbance, seizures, abdominal pain<br>• Hemolytic anemia, transaminitis, thrombocytopenia, high LDH<br>*Treatment:*<br>> Delivery, IV magnesium for seizure prevention | | | |
| ***Hyperemesis gravidarum***<br>*Clinical features:*<br>• Prerenal azotemia or ATN<br>• Evaluate for molar pregnancy<br>*Treatment:*<br>• Volume resuscitation | ***TTP/aHUS***<br>*Clinical features:*<br>• TTP is more common in the 20 d/3 m trimester, and aHUS is more common in the postpartum period<br>• Neurological involvement is more common in TTP than in aHUS<br>• Hemolytic anemia, thrombocytopenia, elevated LDH and bilirubin<br>*Laboratory testing*<br>• *TTP:* ADAMTS-13 activity <10%<br>• *PaHUS:* Genetic testing for complement cascade gene mutations<br>*Treatment:*<br>• *TTP:* Plasma exchange<br>• *PaHUS:* Plasma exchange + eculizumab | | | |
| | ***Acute Fatty Liver of Pregnancy***<br>*Clinical features:*<br>• Nausea, vomiting, abdominal pain, jaundice, ascites<br>• Transaminitis, low platelets, hypoglycemia, lactic acidosis<br>*Laboratory testing:*<br>• Maternal and fetal testing for *LCHAD* gene mutation<br>*Treatment:*<br>• Delivery, plasmapheresis, and/or liver transplant in severe cases | | | |
| ***Lupus nephritis and/or antiphospholipid antibody syndrome***<br>*Clinical features:*<br>• Dysmorphic red blood cells on urine sediment, extra-renal lupus manifestations<br>• Low complements, positive anti-dsDNA, anti-cardiolipin antibodies, and/or anti-p2 glycoprotein antibodies<br>• Kidney biopsy is only recommended if pathology will change management<br>*Treatment:*<br>• Lupus nephritis: steroids + hydroxychloroquine + azathioprine/tacrolimus<br>• Antiphospholipid antibody syndrome: aspirin +/- low molecular weight heparin | | | | |

## SUGGESTED READING


1. Bellomo R, Ronco C, Kellum JA, Mehta RL, Palevsky P; Acute Dialysis Quality Initiative workgroup. Acute renal failure - definition, outcome measures, animal models, fluid therapy and information technology needs: the Second International Consensus Conference of the Acute Dialysis Quality Initiative (ADQI) Group. Crit Care. 2004;8(4):R204-12.
2. Mehta RL, Kellum JA, Shah SV, Molitoris BA, Ronco C, Warnock DG, et al. Acute Kidney Injury Network: report of an initiative to improve outcomes in acute kidney injury. Crit Care. 2007;11(2):R31.
3. Tran TT, Ahn J, Reau NS. ACG Clinical Guideline: Liver Disease and Pregnancy. Am J Gastroenterol. 2016;111(2):176-194; quiz 196.
4. Vigil-De Gracia P Acute fatty liver and HELLP syndrome: two distinct pregnancy disorders. Int J Gynaecol Obstet. 2001;73(3):215-20.
5. Ye W, Shu H, Yu Y, Li H, Chen L, Liu J, et al. Acute kidney injury in patients with HELLP syndrome. Int Urol Nephrol. 2019;51(7):1199-206.

CHAPTER 152

# Peripartum Cardiomyopathy

## ALGORITHM FOR THE DIAGNOSIS OF PERIPARTUM CARDIOMYOPATHY

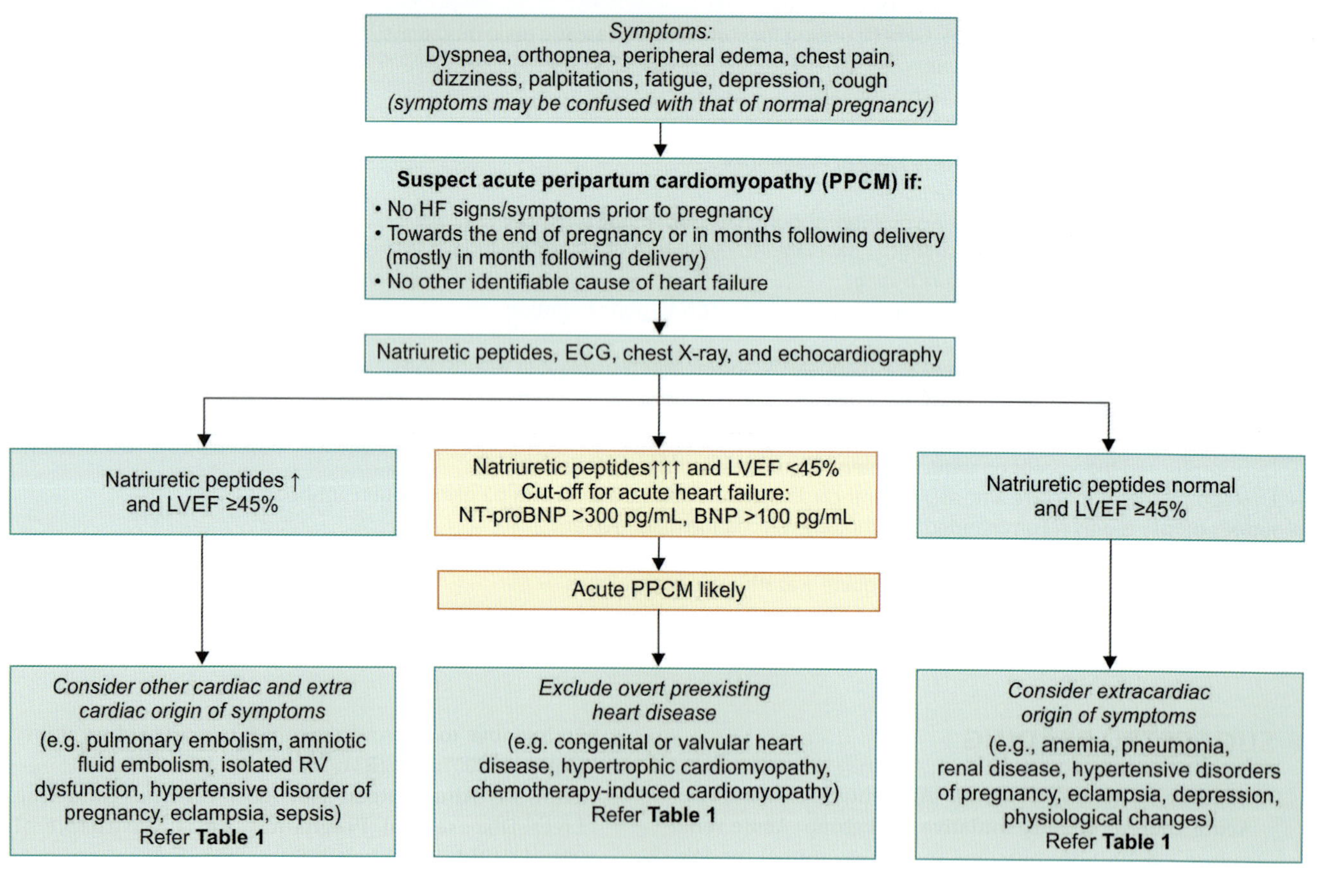

**TABLE 1:** Differentials for heart failure during pregnancy.

| ***Differential diagnosis*** | ***Considerations*** |
|---|---|
| *Acute onset, during stressful delivery or immediate postpartum* | |
| Takotsubo cardiomyopathy | Echocardiogram may show classic apical ballooning symptoms of HF during a prior pregnancy |
| Recurrent peripartum cardiomyopathy | |
| Myocarditis | Consider if viral prodrome, fulminant presentation, normal to reduced LV function |
| Pregnancy-related myocardial infarction | ECG changes, regional wall abnormality on ECHO |
| Pulmonary embolism | Dyspnea, tachycardia with preserved LVEF |
| Preeclampsia | Preserved systolic function on echocardiogram |
| *During the second trimester, commonly* | |
| Pre-existing cardiomyopathy | History of HF prior to pregnancy; prior echo studies with low LVEF before pregnancy |
| Hypertrophic cardiomyopathy | Left ventricular hypertrophy, LVOT obstruction, preserved systolic function; familial predisposition |
| Valvular heart disease | • HF signs/symptoms prior to pregnancy<br>• Echocardiographic findings; congenital aortic stenosis; mitral stenosis from rheumatic heart disease in endemic country. Patients with PPCM may also have valve disease, i.e., mitral regurgitation |
| Congenital heart disease | • HF signs/symptoms prior to pregnancy<br>• May be diagnosed for the first time during pregnancy by echocardiography |
| Hypertensive heart disease | • During the second trimester, commonly<br>• Left ventricular hypertrophy; diastolic dysfunction; less common in young people unless there is a very longstanding history of hypertension |
| Ischemic heart disease | Cardiovascular risk factors; angina; prior CAD |
| Chemotherapy-related cardiomyopathy | History of chemotherapy, particularly doxorubicin |
| Cardiomyopathy due to other systemic diseases | SLE, antiphospholipid syndrome, hemochromatosis |

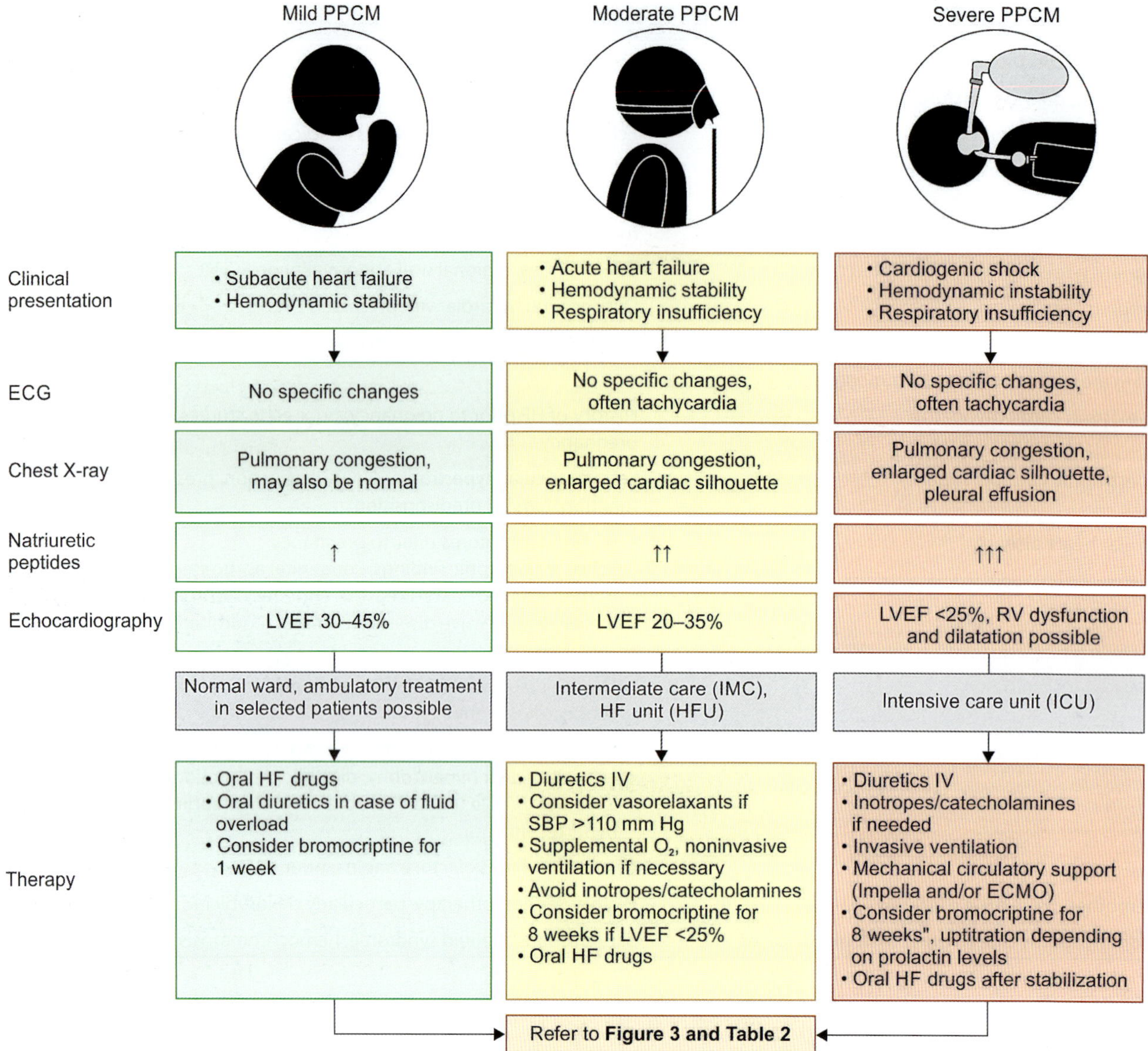


**Fig. 1:** Clinical scenarios of varying severity of PPCM with results of diagnostic tests and monitoring and treatment plans.

## LABOR AND DELIVERY

- Plan with cardio obstetric team
- An attempt to stabilize the mother to avoid potential fetal complications of prematurity is reasonable.
- Hemodynamic instability despite medical therapy should prompt early delivery (or termination if prior to fetal viability).
- Stable patients are delivered vaginally unless there are obstetric reasons for cesarean section
- Caution for fluid overload especially after delivery

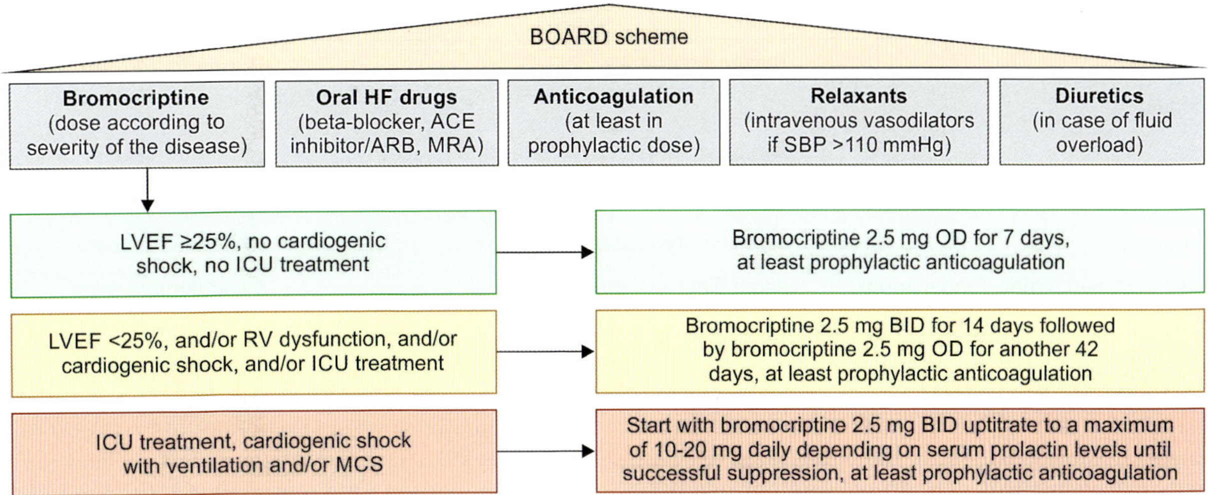


**Fig. 2:** BOARD scheme for management of clinical scenarios of varying severity of PPCM.

**TABLE 2:** Heart failure and anticoagulant drugs: Safety in pregnancy and lactation.

| ***Medications*** | ***During pregnancy*** | ***During lactation*** |
|---|---|---|
| *Heart failure medications* | | |
| Beta-blockers—standard treatment of HF (metoprolol tartrate is used most commonly) | • Yes, Use with caution<br>• IUGR<br>• If used near delivery, monitor for hypoglycemia and bradycardia in newborns for 24-48 hours, regardless of breastfeeding | • Yes (limited data)<br>• Metoprolol is present in small amounts in breast milk |
| Loop diuretics and Thiazide diuretics | • Use with caution<br>• Potential reduction in blood flow, but use is often unavoidable | Yes, use with caution as over-diuresis decreases milk production |
| Relaxants (Vasodilators) (hydralazine/nitrates) | Yes, caution for hypotension | Yes, Use with caution |
| Cardiac glycoside | • Yes, no congenital defects<br>• ESC guidelines suggest allowing use in atrial fibrillation if needed | Yes |
| ACE-I/ARB—as standard guideline-directed therapy for afterload reduction and LV remodeling | No, teratogenic | Enalapril and Captopril can be used |
| Aldosterone receptor antagonists—as guideline-directed therapy for HF | No | Spironolactone may be used |
| Ivabradine | No, scant human data but teratogenic in animals | Avoid |
| *Anticoagulants* | | |
| LMWH—for prevention and treatment of thromboembolic complications and as a bridge to VKA postpartum | Yes, caution at the time of delivery and neuroaxial block | Yes |

*Contd...*

*Contd...*

| ***Medications*** | ***During pregnancy*** | ***During lactation*** |
|---|---|---|
| *Anticoagulants* | | |
| VKA | Avoid, warfarin embryopathy and fetopathy | Yes |
| UFH | Use with caution | Use with caution |
| NOACS | Avoid (limited data) | Avoid (limited data) |
| Synthetic pentasaccharide (fondaparinux) | Avoid (limited data) | Avoid (limited data) |

## SUGGESTED READING

1. Bauersachs J, König T, van der Meer P, Petrie MC, Hilfiker-Kleiner D, Mbakwem A, et al. Pathophysiology, diagnosis and management of peripartum cardiomyopathy: a position statement from the Heart Failure Association of the European Society of Cardiology Study Group on peripartum cardiomyopathy. Eur J Heart Fail. 2019;21(7):827-43.
2. Davis MB, Arany Z, McNamara DM, Goland S, Elkayam U. Peripartum Cardiomyopathy: JACC State-of-the-Art Review. J Am Coll Cardiol. 2020;75(2):207-21.

CHAPTER 153

# Postpartum Hemorrhage

## POSTPARTUM HEMORRHAGE DURING PREGNANCY

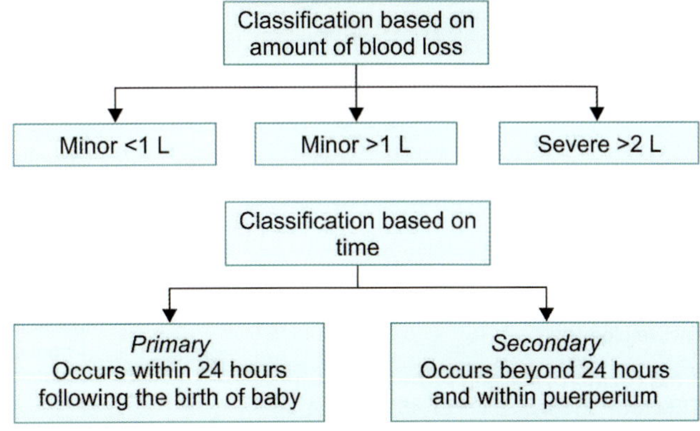


| ***3rd Stage Hemorrhage*** | ***True PPH*** |
|---|---|
| Bleeding occurs *before expulsion* of placenta | Bleeding occurs *subsequent to expulsion* of placenta |

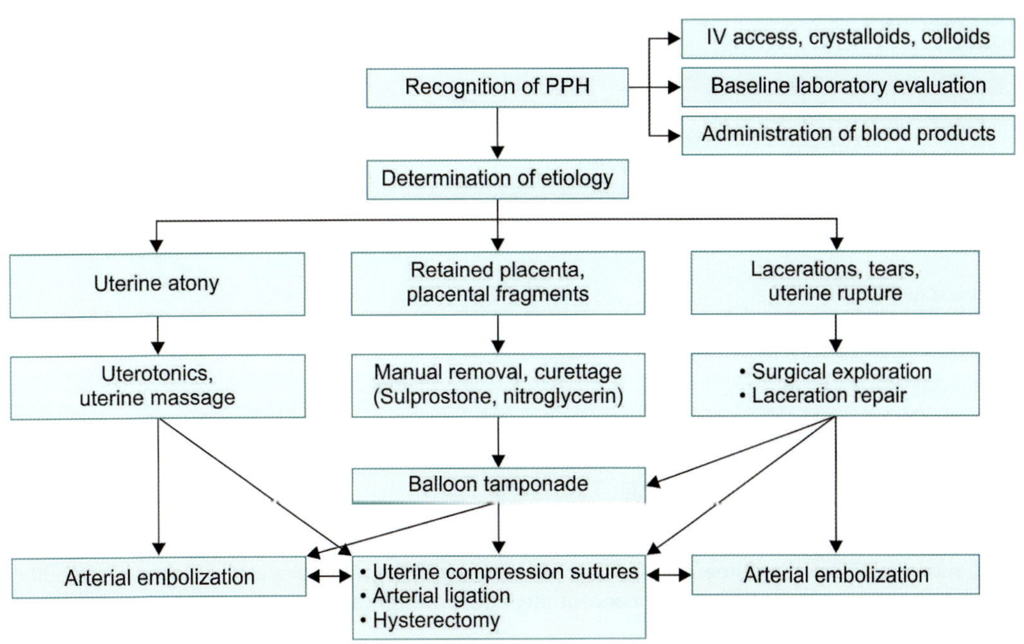

Surgical/mechanical control (uterine massage) and uterotonics administration
Hemogram, including platelets and coagulation (PT, aPTT and fibrinogen)
Basic preconditions adjustment: Targets—Ph > 7.2 Ca > 1 mmol/L Hb > 7 gram /dL

## Bleeding Persists, Despite Control of the Above Conditions?

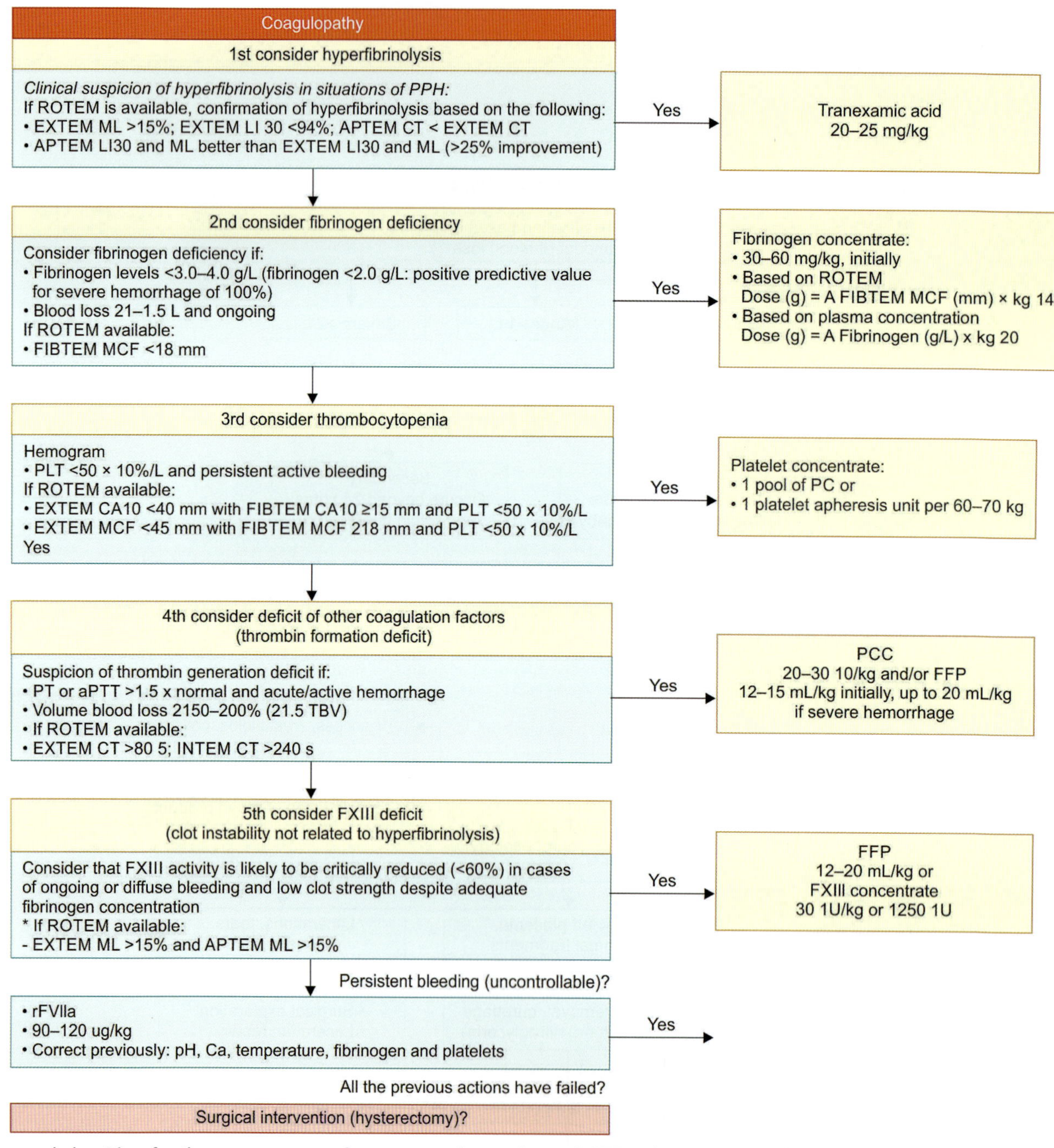


Proposed algorithm for the management of postpartum hemorrhage. A PTT indicates activated partial thromboplastin time; CA10, clot amplitude after 10 minutes. (CT: clotting time; FFP: fresh frozen plasma; Hb: hemoglobin; LI30: lysis index after 30 minutes; MCF: maximum clot firmness; ML: maximum lysis; PC: platelet concentrate; PCC: prothrombin complex concentrate; PLT: platelet count; PT: prothrombin time; TBV: total blood volume)

# PART 16

# CHECKLISTS

***Editors:*** Sachin Gupta, Deeksha Singh Tomar

CHAPTER 154

# Intrahospital Transport of Critically Ill

| ***Pretransport*** | ***Yes/No*** |
|---|---|
| Indication of transfer | |
| Communication to the receiving unit | |
| Information to the attendants | |
| Vitals checked and documented | |
| Resuscitation bag ready | |
| Oxygen cylinders | |
| If intubated, then endotracheal tube fixation checked | |
| All tubes and drainage tubes fixation checked | |
| ***During transport*** | |
| Multiparameter monitor is connected | |
| ECG, BP, $SpO_2$ is monitored | |
| Ongoing infusions are continued | |
| Sedatives and analgesics available | |
| Pressure transducers (if present) attached to the relevant landmarks | |
| ***Post-transport*** | |
| Monitor is attached back to the patient | |
| Vitals checked and documented | |
| Consciousness assessment done (if sedation given) | |
| Ventilator or other organ support connected to the machine (if present) | |

CHAPTER 155

# Intubation

| | *Yes/No* |
|---|---|
| Indication evaluated and re-evaluated | |
| Consent taken | |
| ***Equipment*** | |
| Adult artificial manual breathing unit (AMBU) bag with mask present | |
| Oral and nasal airway present | |
| Three size endotracheal tubes present (at least 7.5, 8, 8.5 mm ID) | |
| Intubating bougie present | |
| Laryngoscope checked with all sizes laryngoscope blades | |
| Yankauer suction present and connected | |
| Laryngeal mask airway present | |
| Cricothyroidotomy kit available | |
| Fiberoptic bronchoscopy facility available | |
| ***Patient variables*** | |
| Preoxygenation with 100% oxygen done for at least 3 minutes | |
| Positioning of patient done | |
| In-line stabilization if required | |
| ***Drugs*** | |
| Sedatives present (propofol, etomidate or midazolam) | |
| Analgesics present (opioids) | |
| Muscle relaxant present (rocuronium, atracurium, and cisatracurium) | |
| ***Monitoring*** | |
| $SpO_2$ monitored during the procedure | |
| Hemodynamics monitored during the procedure | |
| ***Postintubation*** | |
| Confirmation of tracheal intubation by 5-point auscultation done | |
| USG confirmation of intubation (if available) | |
| $ETCO_2$ confirmation of tracheal intubation | |
| Waveform confirmation on ventilator screen | |

CHAPTER

# 156 Extubation

| *Pre-extubation* | *Yes/No* |
|---|---|
| Indication for intubation resolved | |
| Sedation stopped >6 hours | |
| Conscious, obeying commands | |
| Hemodynamically stable or noradrenaline <5 mcg/min | |
| Respiratory rate < 35 breaths/min | |
| $SpO_2$ >90% with $FiO_2$ <0.4 and/or PEPP <5 cm $H_2O$ | |
| Tolerated spontaneous breathing trial (SBT) >30 minutes | |
| No respiratory or metabolic acidosis in arterial blood gas | |
| Minimal airway secretions | |
| ***Post-extubation*** | |
| Nebulization with bronchodilator done | |
| Oxygen therapy/BIPAP/HFNC (if required) | |
| Arterial blood gas after 1 hour of extubation | |
| No deterioration in consciousness | |
| No immediate new onset arrhythmia or hemodynamic instability | |

CHAPTER 157

# Bedside Percutaneous Tracheostomy

| ***Preprocedure*** | ***Yes/No*** |
|---|---|
| Elective or emergency tracheostomy | |
| Written consent taken | |
| Coagulation parameters checked | |
| Coagulation correction done if requested | |
| Oral hygiene with chlorhexidine mouthwash | |
| Endotracheal tube withdrawal done till vocal cords | |
| ***Periprocedure*** | |
| Positioning of patient with neck extension done | |
| Adequate sedation and muscle relaxant administered if prescribed | |
| $FiO_2$ on ventilator increased to 100% | |
| Controlled mode of ventilation switched on | |
| Anterior neck scanned with ultrasound, if available | |
| Tracheostomy kit checked before opening | |
| Proper suctioning done immediately after tracheostomy | |
| End-tidal carbon dioxide ($ETCO_2$) confirmation immediately after tracheostomy, if available | |
| Ventilation waveform confirmation done for ventilation | |
| ***Postprocedure*** | |
| Shoulder roll removed and patient position optimized | |
| Tracheostomy tube fixed as per institute protocol | |
| Sedation and muscle paralysis stopped if indicated | |
| Chest radiograph ordered and checked | |
| Ventilator weaning planned | |
| Tracheostomy care initiated by nurses | |

CHAPTER 158

# Intercostal Drainage

| Preprocedure | Yes/No |
|---|---|
| Is the clinical setting an emergency? | |
| Indication discussed | |
| Consent taken | |
| Site marked | |
| Radiological confirmation of insertion site done | |
| ***Intraprocedure*** | |
| Scrub and sterile gown worn by the operator | |
| Insertion site cleansed with 2% chlorhexidine | |
| Local anesthesia given at the incision site | |
| Intercostal drain inserted and connected to water seal | |
| Air column present | |
| ICD tube secured and taped | |
| ***Postprocedure*** | |
| Chest X-ray for confirmation | |
| Documentation in patient file | |

CHAPTER 159

# Proning

| | ***Preproning*** | ***Yes/No*** |
|---|---|---|
| General | *Rule out absolute contraindications:*<br>• Raised ICP<br>• Unstable pelvic fracture<br>• Spinal instability<br>• Open abdomen<br>• Anterior surface wounds/burns | |
| Airway management | Endotracheal tube/ tracheostomy tube secured and tied | |
| | Closed suction applied | |
| | Oral and ET/TT suctioning done | |
| | Adequate sedation and muscle paralysis given | |
| Face care | Eyes lubricated with eye drops | |
| | Eyes padded and covered properly | |
| | Forehead and chin padded | |
| | Orogastric/nasogastric tube secured tightly | |
| Lines/tubings care | Central venous catheters/hemodialysis catheters checked for sutures | |
| | Disconnect all non-essential IV lines | |
| | All essential IV lines should be long to allow easy maneuvering | |
| | Chest drains should be clamped and place at the foot end of the patient | |
| | Arterial line disconnected from transducer and syringe inserted at the end of pressure line | |
| Pressure areas | Pad the chest, nipples, elbows and knees | |
| Manpower | At least 4 people present with one at the head end | |
| | ***Postproning*** | |
| Airway assessment | Note the fixation of endotracheal tube | |
| | Check suction catheter passes freely | |
| | Check the ventilator parameters | |
| | Patient is connected to the monitor | |
| Body positioning | Head is placed in the ring and is kept in neutral position | |
| | Hands are placed facing head end | |
| | Abdomen is free between the two bolsters | |
| | All bony prominences are padded | |
| Lines/tubings | Feeding tube and urinary catheter are secured | |
| | Central line/arterial line if any are secured and connected to transducer | |

CHAPTER

# 160 Central Venous Line Cannulation

| | Yes/No |
|---|---|
| Indication for central line insertion | |
| Consent taken | |
| Vein identified with the help of ultrasound (when available) | |
| After hand washing, aseptic painting with 2% chlorhexidine solution for at least 30 seconds | |
| Local anesthesia given | |
| Central line insertion done and backflow ascertained | |
| All ports flushed and capped or connected to infusion lines | |
| Insertion site covered with a transparent dressing | |
| Insertion documentation complete | |

CHAPTER 161

# Arterial Cannulation

| | *Yes/No* |
|---|---|
| Indication for arterial cannulation | |
| Consent taken | |
| Site identified (if possible use ultrasound) | |
| Allen's test performed for radial cannulation | |
| Aseptic painting and draping of the site done | |
| Local anesthesia given | |
| Arterial cannulation done and arterial flow noted | |
| Arterial line fixed and secured | |
| Transducer connected and zeroing done | |
| Pressure bag with 300 mm Hg pressure | |

CHAPTER 162

# Brain Death Declaration

| ***Preapnea test*** | ***Yes/No*** |
|---|---|
| Patient suffering from irreversible brain damage | |
| Pupillary reflexes present | |
| Corneal reflexes present | |
| Gag or cough reflex present | |
| Pupils dilated, not responding to light | |
| Effect of sedation and/or muscle paralysis absent | |
| Triggering breath on ventilator | |
| ***During apnea test*** | |
| Pre-oxygenation performed for at least 3 minutes | |
| Arterial blood gas sample taken for baselines $CO_2$ before starting apnea test | |
| 6–8 liters of oxygen by cannula inside the endotracheal (ET)/Tracheostomy (TT) tube after disconnecting the ventilator | |
| Saturation and hemodynamics maintained for 10 minutes | |
| Arterial blood gas repeated for $CO_2$ level rise more 20 mm Hg from baseline | |
| Ventilator reconnected | |
| ***Postapnea test*** | |
| Time of first apnea test noted | |
| Family informed the result | |
| Second apnea test performed after 6 hours | |
| If positive, inform the concerned authorities | |
| Time of death reported as first apnea test time | |

CHAPTER 163

# Ends-of-Life

| | Yes/No |
|---|---|
| Life expectancy expected to be in days to weeks | |
| All potentially reversible causes of patient's condition excluded | |
| Clinician's consensus presents in the treatment | |
| Patient is able to take part in the decision making | |
| Any advanced directive available | |
| All decision makers within the family are able to make a decision | |
| Family is aware about the irreversible condition of the patient | |
| Family meeting is documented | |
| Family explained about further course of comfort care plan | |
| Guidance and care plan explained to the patient and the family | |
| Pain assessment and pain relief given | |
| Medication given for nausea (if any) | |
| Dyspnea assessment and management given | |
| Delirium assessment and medication given (if required) | |
| Airway secretions suctioning done | |
| Fever management done | |
| Spiritual needs of the patient/family met | |
| Visitation policy relaxed | |

CHAPTER 164

# Venovenous Extracorporeal Membrane Oxygenation

| ***Preinitiation*** | ***Yes/No*** |
|---|---|
| Indication confirmed as per Extracorporeal Life Support Organization (ELSO) criteria | |
| Consent taken | |
| Insertion venous site evaluated by ultrasound | |
| Circuit and cannula checked | |
| Circuit priming done | |
| Flow meter and pressure transducer zeroed | |
| Hand crank available | |
| Check battery life in minutes | |
| ***Initiation*** | |
| Insertion site cleansed with chlorhexidine solution and draped | |
| Femoral access secured first followed by internal jugular vein | |
| Priming bag disconnected | |
| Venous and arterial connections secured with air-free technique after heparin administration | |
| $FiO_2$ and sweep gas flow set | |
| Extracorporeal membrane oxygenation (ECMO) initiated with required settings | |
| Arterial and venous cannulas sutured and covered with sterile dressing | |
| Ventilator settings reduced as desired | |
| ***Postinitiation*** | |
| Documentation done in patient's records | |
| Set flow and pressure alarm | |
| Target ACT 160–180 sec | |

CHAPTER 165

# High Peak Pressure on Ventilator

| *Ventilator-related issues* | *Yes/No* |
|---|---|
| High pressure alarm setting too low | |
| Expiratory valve checked | |
| Heated moisture exchanger blocked with secretions | |
| ***Patient-related issues*** | |
| Is chest moving bilaterally? | |
| Patient coughing or biting the tube | |
| Is the endotracheal (ET) tube too deep in trachea | |
| Tracheal suctioning done to rule out mucus plugging | |
| Patient ventilator asynchrony present | |
| Artificial manual breathing unit (AMBU) Bag ventilation is possible | |
| Ultrasound sonography (USG) assessment or clinical assessment of pneumothorax | |
| Bronchospasm present | |
| Open chest binders if any | |

CHAPTER

# 166 Low Minute Ventilation

| | Yes/No |
|---|---|
| Endotracheal tube or tracheostomy tube cuff leak | |
| Leak in ventilator circuit | |
| Port open in heat moisture exchanger | |
| Tidal volume set is too low | |
| Intercostal drainage tubes allowing air to leak | |
| Pressure alarm settings too low | |
| Endotracheal tube partially dislodged | |
| Decreased tidal volume delivered due to poor lung compliance | |
| Decreased tidal volume delivered due to increased airway resistance | |

CHAPTER 167

# High Membrane Pressure on RRT

| ***High positive pressure alarm*** | ***Yes/No*** |
|---|---|
| Blue tubing (return line) connected to patient is kinked | |
| Blue tubing (return line) is clamped | |
| Hemodialysis catheter port is clamped where blue tubing (return line) is attached | |
| ***High negative pressure alarm*** | |
| Red tubing (access line) connected to patient is kinked | |
| Red tubing (access line) is clamped | |
| Hemodialysis catheter port is clamped where red tubing (access line) is attached | |
| Blood flow not coming from vein | |
| ***High transmembrane pressure*** | |
| Is the dialysis line kinked | |
| Dialyzer is clotted | |
| Dialysate line is kinked | |
| Vascular access flow is poor | |
| High ultrafiltrate rate | |

# Index

Page numbers followed by *b* refer to box, *f* refer to figure, *fc* refer to flowchart, and *t* refer to table.

## A

## D

## E



## F

## I



## J

## K



## L



## M

## T